Derrick Taylor MD

AF796792

Operative Strategy in General Surgery

An Expositive Atlas

Volume I

Operative Strategy in General Surgery

An Expositive Atlas

Volume I

Jameson L. Chassin
Professor of Clinical Surgery
New York University School of Medicine
Director of Surgery
Booth Memorial Medical Center

Illustrated by Caspar Henselmann
With 528 Illustrations

Springer-Verlag
New York Heidelberg Berlin

Jameson L. Chassin, M.D.
Professor of Clinical Surgery
New York University School of Medicine

Director of Surgery
Booth Memorial Medical Center
Flushing, New York 11355 U.S.A.
(*Use this address for correspondence.*)

Consultant Surgeon
University Hospital, New York University Medical Center
and
New York Veterans Administration Hospital

Attending Surgeon
Bellevue Hospital
and
Long Island Jewish-Hillside Medical Center

Library of Congress Cataloging in Publication Data

Chassin, Jameson L
Operative strategy in general surgery (v. 1)
Includes index.
1. Surgery, Operative—Atlases. I. Title.
[DNLM: 1. Surgery, Operative—Atlases. W0517 C488a]
RD32.C42 617'.91'00222 79-29758

All rights reserved.
No part of this book may be translated or reproduced in any form without written permission from Springer-Verlag.
The use of general descriptive names, trade names, trademarks, etc., in this publication, even if the former are not especially identified, is not to be taken as a sign that such names, as understood by the Trade Marks and Merchandise Marks Act, may accordingly be used freely by anyone.

© 1980 by Springer-Verlag New York Inc.
Printed in the United States of America.

9 8 7 6 5 4 3 2 1

ISBN 0-387-**90452**-2 Springer-Verlag New York Heidelberg Berlin
ISBN 3-540-**90452**-2 Springer-Verlag Berlin Heidelberg New York

To Charlotte

Contents

Foreword

This surgical atlas should be of great value to all clinical surgeons, both those in training and those in surgical practice, and Dr. Chassin is superbly qualified to author this work. During more than three decades as a member of the faculty of the New York University School of Medicine, he has taught countless residents many aspects of the art of surgical technique. One measure of Dr. Chassin's unusual teaching ability is that he is both Professor of Clinical Surgery at New York University and Director of Surgery at Booth Memorial Hospital, where our fourth-year surgical residents have rotated regularly for the past 12 years. Booth Memorial is the only hospital outside the New York University Medical Center to which New York University residents rotate. This simple fact well underlines Dr. Chassin's remarkable capability for teaching.

When a surgical complication develops after an operation, two or three possibilities should be considered. First, of course, was the diagnosis correct? If it was, then the cause of the complication is usually either an inadequate operative technique or a flawed concept underlying the selection of the operative procedure. When the surgical technique seems faultless, a postoperative complication would strongly indicate that the concept was erroneous, albeit cherished perhaps for decades.

Unlike any other atlas on operative technique, this book specifically discusses the conceptual basis of the operation as well as the strategy that will help the surgeon avoid common pitfalls. The operative technique is then described step by step.

I am confident that in the years ahead this atlas will be regarded as one of the major contributions to our literature of surgical technique.

Frank C. Spencer, M.D.
George David Stewart Professor and Chairman
Department of Surgery
New York University School of Medicine

Preface

Spectacular developments in applied physiology during the past two decades have markedly reduced the number of deaths from respiratory, cardiac, or renal complications following surgery. Currently the major cause of preventable postoperative fatality is sepsis. The mortality rate of such operations as esophagectomy, low anterior resection, and total gastrectomy will be no greater than 1%–2% if leakage from the anastomosis and contamination of the peritoneum are prevented. With proper technique and good surgical judgment, these complications are avoidable.

If we are to achieve this low mortality rate, scholarly attention must be focused on surgical technique and on methods of teaching surgical technique. This pedagogical problem first came to my attention in 1967 when, in addition to training my own residents, I accepted the assignment of teaching fourth-year residents from the New York University Medical School who began rotating to Booth Memorial Hospital for a period of 2 or 3 months each. In the past 20 years I have guided residents through more than 4000 major operations. It is obvious that we surgeons perform many intricate surgical maneuvers intuitively or automatically. Good teaching in the operating room, however, requires that the preceptor analyze and demonstrate the best way to perform each maneuver. He must also determine the pitfalls and danger points of each step of the operation and then articulate a strategy that will make the operation safe and efficient for the resident. This task stimulated my writing this book.

Each operation described in this atlas is preceded by a brief review of the indications for and the concept underlying the choice of the procedure among possible alternatives. Following this is a checklist of the main points of preoperative care, then a list of pitfalls and danger points that require the surgeon's advance planning if success is to be consistently achieved. Immediately preceding the description of each surgical technique, I have written a section on operative strategy that analyzes the danger points and the errors surgeons are prone to make; this analysis is accompanied by a detailed account of the maneuvers to be employed in avoiding these pitfalls.

This text is not a compendium of every operation of the gastrointestinal tract. For each disease state, I have described one operative technique, one that I have found to be valuable and safe when performed either by expert surgeons or by residents. Alternate techniques are included only when indicated by variations in the anatomy or pathology. This policy has provided the space required to describe in meticulous detail each operation that is included. Discussions of the postoperative care and complications are limited to those points that are pertinent to the operation described. Methods of preventing such complications as thromboembolism or atelectasis, which may occur after any operation, are not discussed since whole texts on this subject alone are available.

The descriptions of operative technique have been immensely aided by the excellent illustrations of Mr. Caspar Henselmann, whose drawings are based on actual observation of the operations. The illustrations are neither stylized nor idealized, but show the surgical field as the surgeon sees it. The drawings take the reader through the operation step by step. To further the teaching effectiveness, I have not separated the written description of operations into text and legends, but rather have provided a single narrative that follows the illustrations and explains those points an illustration cannot show. Citations of figures are set in bold type so that the reader can easily correlate the illustration with the corresponding text. The elements of the book are arranged so that related elements—text and illustrations—are placed together on the same or facing pages.

This volume describes the more common operations of the gastrointestinal tract. [Volume II will cover such areas as the biliary tract, pancreas, spleen, hernia (abdominal, inguinal, femoral, and hiatal), breast, and the thyroid and adrenal glands.] Considerable space is devoted to complicated operations, such as esophagogastrectomy and low anterior resection, to enable both the surgeon in training and the more experienced practitioner to study in detail those operations that he or she will not perform every day and that are fraught with many technical pitfalls. For the surgeon beginning training, I have emphasized in Appendixes A, B, and C the basic principles of foot, hand, and body stance; the use and abuse of various instruments; and the fundamentals of dissecting, sewing, and achieving hemostasis. Since brand names of surgical products and names of instruments vary with geography, an illustrated glossary (Appendix D) is included to explain these items.

Unique to this atlas is the detailed discussion of *stapled* gastrointestinal tract operations: indications, contraindications, precautions, complications, and selected techniques. After studying 472 such anastomoses my colleagues and I concluded that they are just as safe as sutured anatomoses provided they are performed with equal sophistication; otherwise, complications can be serious. Although surgical stapling has been widely adopted throughout the United States and elsewhere, this technology has attracted scant critical analysis in surgical texts or in the surgical literature, and coverage for the most part has been rather spotty. I have described the technical details of those stapling procedures whose safety and efficacy we have demonstrated by personal experience, including a number of new techniques and modifications.

Not for two decades has a completely new American atlas of general surgery by a single author been published. It was not a lack of humility which led me to undertake this awesome task. Rather, it was my observation that when many operative techniques by multiple authors are included in one text, the reader is confused as to which technique to use under which circumstances. Also, often the master surgeon will inadvertently fail to record some important details of technique that make a procedure safe in his hands. I hope that my description of operative techniques and strategies that I have found valuable both in my practice and in teaching will prove helpful to the reader. In writing about surgical concepts and techniques I have tried to indicate which statements are supported by data and which are still not thoroughly validated. The references at the end of each chapter were selected primarily to elucidate areas of controversy; a more exhaustive bibliography would be beyond the scope of this book.

In compiling this volume I received considerable advice and criticism from Drs. Kenneth M. Rifkind and James W. Turner, both Assistant Directors of Surgery at Booth Memorial Hospital, and from Dr. Simon D. Fink, for which I am grateful. I would like to record my debt to Dr. Frank C. Spencer, Chairman, Department of Surgery at New York University School of Medicine, for continually stimulating all of us in his department to analyze and improve our performance both as surgeons and as teachers. I would also like to thank Ms. Velinda Badaluco for efficiently overseeing the administration of my office and the Booth surgical department as well as the preparation of this manuscript. Mr. Walter Green and the staff of Springer-Verlag New York were also of great help in completing this project.

Words cannot express my gratitude to my wife Charlotte, without whose support and understanding this work could not have been accomplished.

Introduction

1 Concept and Strategy in Surgery

Developing a Concept

Successful surgery requires study, advance planning, clear thinking, and technical skill. Brilliant execution of the wrong operation at the wrong time can only lead to disaster. To achieve consistently good results for each surgical condition the surgeon has to develop a concept that combines analysis of the literature, study of the disordered physiology, and comprehension of the hypothesis underlying the contemplated operation.

To develop a concept properly a surgeon must:

Know the normal and pathological physiology and anatomy.

Explore the relative merits of alternative operations.

Analyze the operation selected for the problem at hand. Are there *valid data* to demonstrate that it will accomplish the desired goal? Is the mortality rate for the procedure such that the benefit outweighs the risk?

Reflect on his or her *own experience* of complications and deaths following the operation selected. This information is more relevant than are the results that may be reported from some renowned medical center, where one surgeon may have developed great expertise in a particular operation. Superior results under such circumstances obviously do not indicate that less-experienced surgeons will be as successful.

Review postoperative complications and poor results. When a complication or a death occurs, the surgeon must analyze the case carefully and attempt to make an objective appraisal of what went wrong. Was there poor judgment in the choice of operation? Was the diagnosis inaccurate? Was the assessment of the risk incorrect? Was there an error of technique? Did the surgeon lack the technical expertise to undertake the procedure?

Keep records of mortality and morbidity for each operation. Frequent analysis of results increases the data base of the surgeon's own experience. The knowledge the surgeon gains leads to self-renewal and improved performance; without it the surgeon learns nothing from experience.

Establishing Strategy

Establishing an *operative strategy*—the surgeon's advance planning of the technical steps in the operation—is vital to the safety and efficiency of complex surgical procedures. The operative strategy is what the surgeon ponders the night before the operation: Where are the pitfalls? How should they be avoided? The thesis of this book is that by studying strategy the surgeon can reduce the incidence of operative misadventures and postoperative complications.

Anticipating and analyzing potential problems and danger points before an operation will more likely lead to a successful result than will frenzied activity in the operating room after the surgeon and patient are already in deep trouble. Anticipation enhances the surgeon's capacity for prompt decision-making in the operating room.

Strategy also includes planning the sequence of an operation to clearly expose vital structures early in the dissection so as to avoid damaging them. Planning to *complete the simple steps first* improves the efficiency of an operation. Continuing in this manner will simplify the more difficult steps.

The reputation for being a rapid operator is highly prized by some surgeons. More important than speed, however, are accuracy and delicacy of technique, especially when good anesthesia and patient-support technology are available. Nevertheless, *time should not be wasted.* A reduction in operating time is not achieved merely by performing rapid hand motions. An operation can be expedited without sacrificing safety only when thoughtful advance planning, anticipation, and an alert recognition of anatomical landmarks are combined with efficiency of execution. Together, they will eliminate wasted motion and wasted time.

A discussion of the concept underlying an operation and of operative strategy will be found in the text preceding the description of each operative technique.

2 Management of the Contaminated Operation

The incidence of postoperative wound sepsis varies with the magnitude of contamination. The generally accepted classification of operative wounds according to contamination, as listed by Altemeier et al., is:

1) Clean

Nontraumatic

No inflammation encountered

No break in technique

Respiratory, alimentary, genitourinary tracts not entered

2) Clean–Contaminated

Gastrointestinal or respiratory tracts entered without significant spillage

Appendectomy—not perforated—no cloudy peritoneal exudate

Prepared oropharynx entered

Genitourinary or biliary tract entered in absence of infected urine or bile

Minor break in technique

3) Contaminated

Major break in technique, or gross spillage from gastrointestinal tract

Traumatic wound, fresh

Entrance of genitourinary or biliary tracts in presence of infected urine or bile

4) Dirty and Infected

Acute bacterial inflammation encountered, without pus

Transection of "clean" tissue for the purpose of surgical access to a collection of pus

Perforated viscus encountered

Dirty traumatic wound

Table 2–1 demonstrates the high incidence of postoperative wound infection in good hospitals, in which accurate observations were made and records kept. If proper surgical technique and sound strategy are employed, figures such as these can be substantially reduced. The methods that prevent wound infection generally are effective also in preventing deep abdominal and pelvic sepsis following operative contamination.

TABLE 2–1. Incidence of Infection in Relation to Wound Classification

	No. of Cases		Incidence of Wound Infection	
	Foothills Hospital[a]	Five Hospitals[b]	Foothills Hospital (%)[a]	Five Hospitals (%)[b]
Total	23,649	15,613	4.8	7.4
% Clean	76.4	74.8	1.8	5.0
% Clean–contaminated	17.5	16.5	8.9	10.8
% Contaminated	3.2	4.3	21.5	16.3
% Dirty	2.9	3.7	38.0	28.5

[a] Cruse JP, Foord R (1973) Arch Surg 107:206.
[b] Howard JM et al. (1964) Ann Surg 160 (Suppl.): 1.

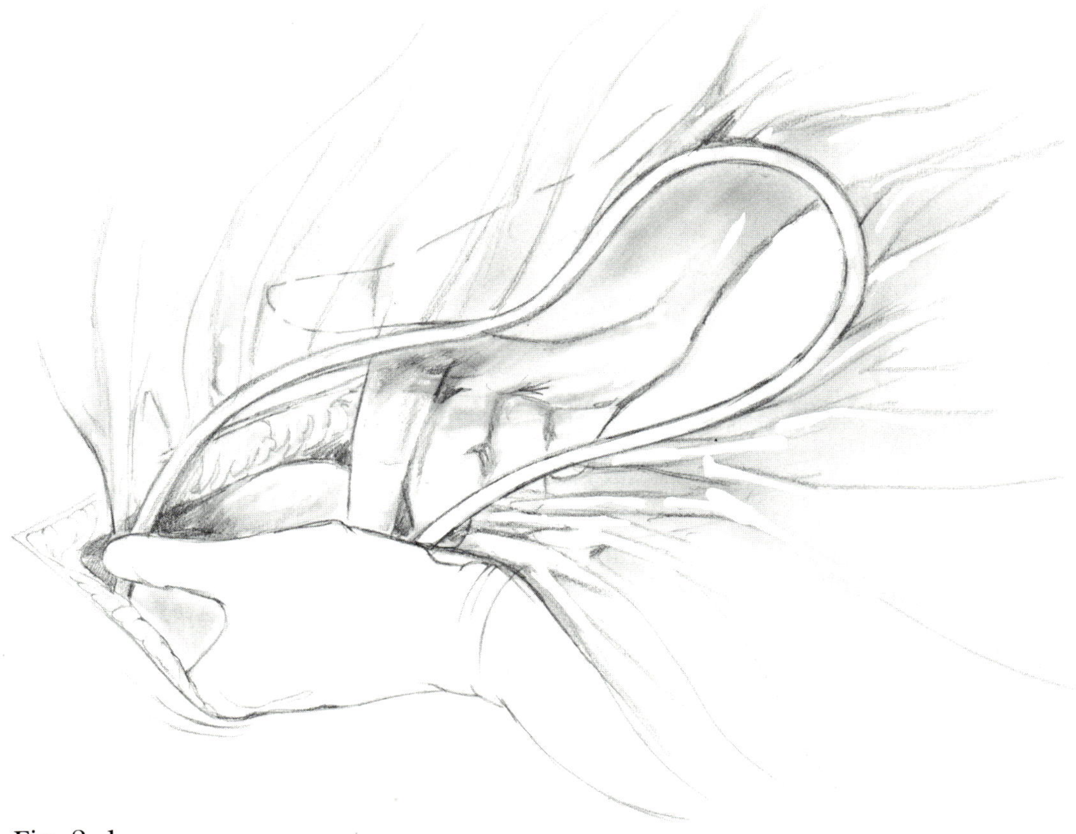

Fig. 2–1

Management should be aimed at (1) minimizing the bacterial inoculum and (2) enhancing host tissue defenses.

Minimizing Bacterial Inoculum

As it is not possible to eliminate local peritoneal contamination in operations upon the biliary or gastrointestinal tracts, the surgeon should concentrate on localizing the spill and minimizing the bacterial insult to the abdominal wound and especially to the subcutaneous fat. Applying wet gauze pads to the wound does not accomplish this as contaminated fluid can penetrate the gauze. Before initiating the contaminated portion of the operation, the surgeon should insert an impermeable plastic sheath to protect the wound and the subcutaneous fat from contamination. A device that may help accomplish this is the *Wound Protector*, a ring drape (**Figs. 2–1 and 2–2**). At the conclusion of the contaminated segment of the operation, the gauze pads, wound protector drape, gloves, and instruments all should be discarded.

While it has long been customary to pour several liters of saline into the peritoneal cavity just before closing the incision, the surgeon can achieve greater efficiency in washing bacteria out of the operative field with the method employed by chemists in preparing a chemically clean glass beaker: five or six rinsings with small quantities of liquid. During the contaminated portion of the operation, fre-

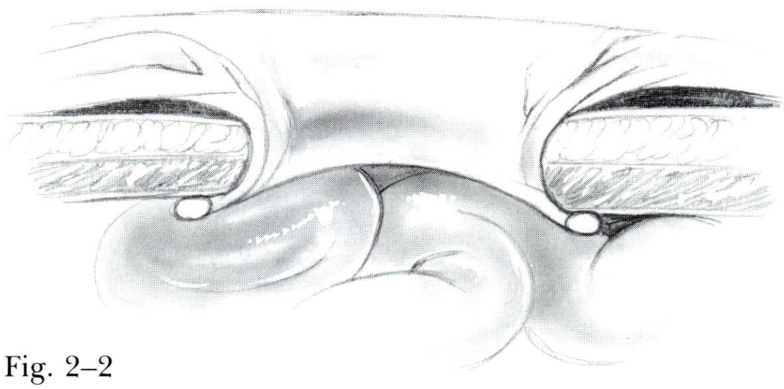

Fig. 2–2

quent *irrigations* with 100–200 ml saline, followed by aspiration, are effective in washing out bacteria as they are being spilled into the field. At the same time, be careful that this irrigation fluid does not spill over into the subcutaneous tissues. Replace the gauze pads after aspiration of the saline is *complete*.

Adding an appropriate *antibiotic* to the irrigating solution further enhances its efficacy. When antibiotic sensitivity studies are not available, a solution of 0.1% kanamycin is satisfactory in the abdomen, it has been found. In advanced sepsis, a dilute solution of an aminoglycoside and clindamycin may be preferred. In patients with renal failure use these drugs with caution as some absorption from the peritoneum is possible. Noon et al. reported that antibiotic irrigation of the abdominal cavity and the incision reduces the incidence of wound infection. For situations in which gram-positive organisms are a threat—such as in operations that use Marlex mesh to repair a hernia—50,000 units of bacitracin may be added to 500 ml of a 0.2% kanamycin solution. Lavage of the subcutaneous tissues with 10% povidone-iodine solution for a period of 60 seconds before closing the skin also has produced a significant reduction in wound infections, according to a study by Sindelar and Mason.

Mechanical and antibiotic *bowel preparation* (see p. 277) has been demonstrated, in random studies conducted by Clarke et al., to lower the incidence of wound infection after colon anastomoses. Similar preparation in patients who have cancer of the stomach is appropriate because the necrotic interstices of the tumor often harbor virulent bacteria.

When latex drains are brought from a contaminated area in the abdomen through the incision, bacteria enter the subcutaneous tissues. The contamination is lessened, Cruse and Foord found, if the drain is brought out through a separate stab wound, reducing the incidence of wound infection. Cruse and Foord also found that the adhesive plastic skin drape failed to reduce the incidence of wound infection.

Enhancing Host Tissue Defenses

The defenses of host tissues are tremendously impaired by such *poor surgical techniques* as traumatic dissection, clamping large bites of tissue in hemostats, and leaving too many ligatures of too heavy a material. All these make the tissues less able to conquer bacterial invasion. In Cruse's study the use of the electrosurgical knife almost doubled the wound infection rate. Other factors that were correlated with marked increases in the incidence of wound infection in clean wounds were malnutrition, obesity, and diabetes.

Nutritional rehabilitation, including the use of total parenteral nutrition when necessary, helps restore the impaired immunological defenses of the depleted patient.

Perioperative antibiotics (see p. 10) assure a therapeutic level in the serum and tissues before the incision. Even if minor hematomas should form, presumably they too will contain a therapeutic level of antibiotic. Polk and Lopez-Mayor proved that this reduces the incidence of wound infection.

Effective evacuation, by *suction catheters,* of blood, fibrin, and serum from the operative site restores the efficiency of phagocytosis, which these substances impair. Alexander et al. have noted that infections are prevented by this means. This is extremely important in the splenic bed following splenectomy and in the presacral space following low colorectal anastomosis. In both locations a relatively small inoculum of bacteria combined with blood and serum may produce an abscess, whereas bacteria without blood or blood without bacteria may prove harmless. In the low colorectal anastomosis, infected hematoma and the resultant abscess formation probably are common causes of anastomotic failure. In Cruse and Foord's study, the use of closed-suction drainage following cholecystectomy reduced the incidence of postoperative infection to 0% as compared to 9.9% following the use of Penrose latex drains.

Intermittent instillation of an antibiotic solution into closed-suction or sump catheters postoperatively is another method of enhancing the defenses of host tissues. The antibiotic selected depends on the nature of the contamination as well as on the pattern of bacterial resistance to antibiotics in each hospital. We have experienced favorable results with 0.1% kanamycin solution in the presacral space following low colorectal anastomosis and following total proctectomy when the perineum has been closed. In clean-contaminated and contaminated abdominal incisions, McIlrath et al. obtained excellent results postoperatively by injecting 10 ml Dab's solution into the closed-suction subcutaneous catheter every 8 hours for 4 days. Instilling an antibiotic solution has the additional advantage of preventing clotted serum from obstructing the suction catheters.

Schwab and Kelly prefer to administer continuous irrigation with a saline solution (50 ml per hour) in the presacral space after total proctectomy has been performed.

Leaving the skin and subcutaneous tissues completely unsutured, to close by granulation and contraction is an excellent method of preventing wound sepsis. To accomplish healing of the abdominal wall in the absence of skin sutures, the abdomen should be closed with a suture material that will not produce chronic draining sinuses. Sutures of monofilament wire, using a modified Smead-Jones technique, will achieve this end nicely.

Keep the skin edges separated postoperatively by inserting a light packing over fine mesh gauze for 5–10 days. Change the packing daily, using a sterile technique. If the wound is clean, secondary closure may be performed with sterile micropore adhesive strips. Interrupted nylon vertical mattress skin sutures may also be inserted in the operating room, about 2–3 cm apart. The sutures should be left untied beneath the gauze pack until the appropriate time.

This type of management is particularly suitable for the gross contamination that occurs in operations for advanced peritonitis, gangrenous appendicitis, or subphrenic abscess.

Management of Contaminated Operative Wound

The following is our method of managing a clean-contaminated incision. The example is of an abdomen that has been exposed to intestinal bacteria during an open colon anastomosis.

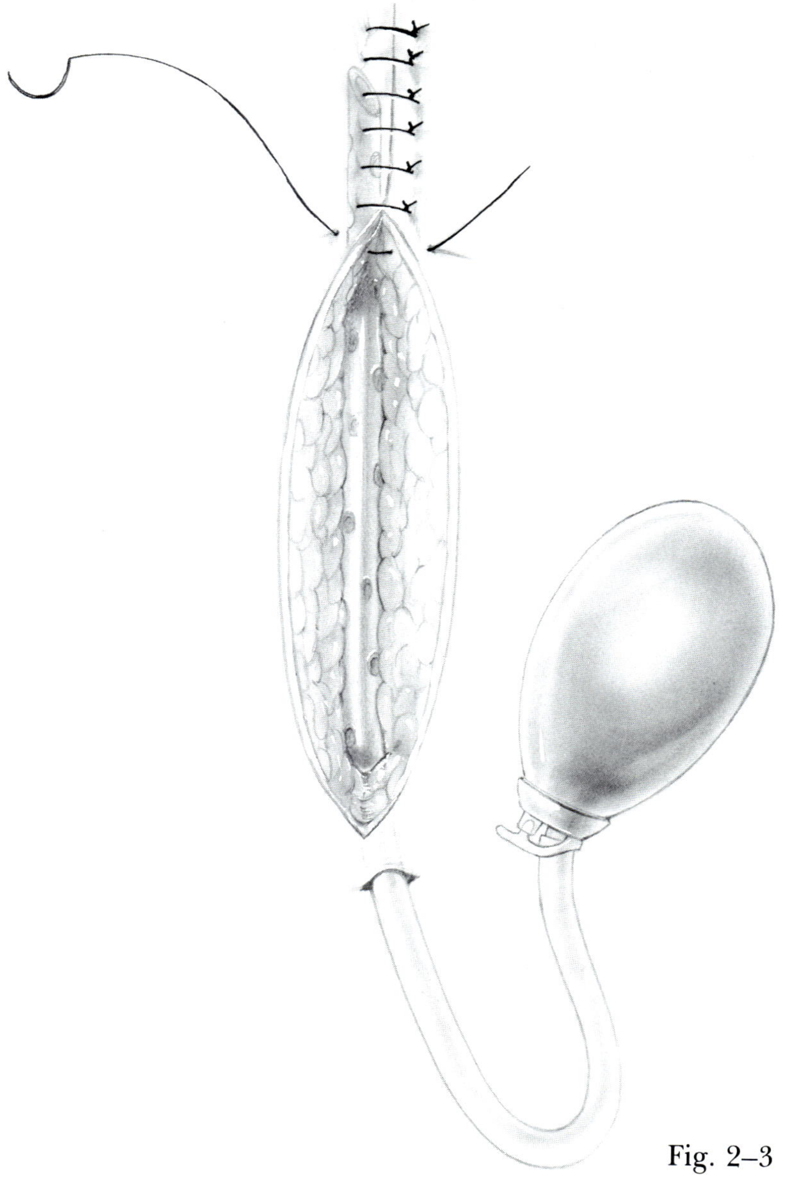

Fig. 2–3

Before the incision is closed, it is thoroughly irrigated with aliquots of 0.1% kanamycin solution. The incision is then closed with interrupted sutures of 2–0 monofilament stainless steel wire or No. 1 polyglycolic (PG) absorbable suture (see Chap. 5). The subcutaneous tissue is again irrigated with antibiotic solution. A section of Silastic Jackson-Pratt tubing is selected, 3–5 mm in external diameter, with multiple perforations, equal in length to the abdominal incision. The tube is brought out through a puncture wound near one pole of the incision, attached to a closed-suction drainage device (**Fig. 2–3**), and fixed to the skin by a suture. The skin incision is closed with a continuous 4–0 PG subcuticular stitch. Every 8 hours, following the method of McIlrath et al., 10 ml

Dab's solution is instilled into the subcutaneous catheter and the continuous suction omitted for 20 minutes. This is continued for 4 days after the operation, after which the catheter is removed. The gauze dressing on the wound is removed 2 days after the operation, leaving the incision uncovered. The exit puncture wound of the suction catheter is redressed daily with the application of a bit of povidone-iodine ointment.

Dab's solution contains 500 mg neomycin, 100 mg polymyxin, and 80 mg gentamycin in 1,000 ml normal saline; other formulas may prove equally successful.

If the wound has been exposed to particularly heavy or virulent contamination during the course of the operation, we prefer to leave the skin open rather than use the suction-catheter technique.

Management of Infected Operative Wound

Infection of the operative wound may be revealed by such signs as local erythema, tenderness, fever, or tachycardia. If local pain and systemic toxicity are out of proportion to the degree of local findings in the wound, one should suspect infection by anaerobic organisms, especially Clostridia.

If there is the slightest suspicion of infection, the incision should be explored by opening the skin down to the fascia. Obtain samples for bacteriological identification. If infection is found, the skin should be opened over the entire length of the infected part of the wound, which should then be irrigated. Necrotic tissue should be debrided. The skin edges should be kept open with gauze packing, which should be changed once or twice daily. This gives the surgeon the opportunity to observe the area closely. Serious infections, such as necrotizing fasciitis or myositis, must be diagnosed early and treated with appropriate systemic antibiotics and debridement.

Perioperative Antibiotics

Studies by Polk and Lopez-Mayor and by Altemeier et al. have demonstrated that when significant contamination may be anticipated because of the nature of the operation, the incidence of wound infection is reduced if an adequate blood level of the proper antibiotic is provided before the incision is made. This type of management is appropriate for patients who undergo open colon anastomosis, exploration of an infected common bile duct, cholecystectomy for acute cholecystitis, or gastrectomy for carcinoma. Some institutions use prophylactic antibiotics for elective cholecystectomy in the elderly because patients over age 60 who suffer gallstones have a high incidence of gram negative and anaerobic bacteria in their bile.

Antibiotics should be initiated intravenously 2 hours before surgery and repeated after 4 hours and then every 6 hours for 3 doses. As a rule, continuing the prophylactic antibiotic beyond 3–4 doses is of no value and raises the risk of encouraging the development of antibiotic resistance. Exceptions to this rule usually are made for patients who have drainage tubes in the pleural cavity or the common bile duct. Whether these exceptions are valid is not entirely clear from the data currently available.

Which antibiotic to employ for prophylaxis varies with the proposed operation and with the bacterial sensitivity pattern in each hospital. Polk used cephaloridine. We use cefazolin now because we prefer intravenous administration. Cephalothin should not be used for this purpose because of its extremely rapid excretion after intravenous administration.

Throughout this book, reference to the use of prophylactic antibiotics immediately before, during, and for 24 hours following surgery will be indicated by the term "perioperative antibiotics."

References

Alexander JW et al. (1976) Prevention of wound infections: a case for closed suction drainage to remove wound fluids deficient in opsonic properties. Am J Surg 132:59

Amer Coll of Surg Subcommittee, Altemeier WA et al. (1976) Manual on control of infection in surgical patients. Lippincott, Philadelphia

Clarke JS et al. (1977) Preoperative oral antibiotics reduce septic complications of colon operations. Ann Surg 186:251

Cruse PJ, Foord R (1973) A five-year prospective study of 23,649 surgical wounds. Arch Surg 107:206

McIlrath DC et al. (1976) Closure of abdominal incisions with subcutaneous catheters. Surgery 80:411

Noon GP et al. (1967) Clinical evaluation of peritoneal irrigation with antibiotic solution. Surgery 62:73

Polk HC Jr, Lopez-Mayor JF (1967) Postoperative wound infection: a prospective study of determinant factors and prevention. Surgery 66:97

Schwab PM, Kelly KA (1974) Primary closure of the perineal wound after proctectomy. Mayo Clin Proc 49:176

Sindelar WF, Mason GR (1979) Irrigation of subcutaneous tissue with povidonedine solution for prevention of surgical wound infections. Surg Gynecol Obstet 148:227

3 Rational Use of Drains

Purpose of Drains

Drains permit the escape from the body of pus, blood, serum, lymph, bile, pancreatic juice, or intestinal contents. They form a walled-off passageway, from the source of pus or other undesirable collection, to the outside. This passageway or tract must persist for a period long enough to assure complete evacuation of the collection.

In the presence of a discrete abscess, the need for and purpose of a drain is obvious and noncontroversial, as its therapeutic benefits are clear. In most other situations, the drain acts as a prophylactic instrument to prevent the accumulation of undesirable products. Because it is a foreign body, the drain also has the paradoxical effect of potentiating infection, as Magee et al. have pointed out. When and how a drain should be used for prophylactic purposes has long been a source of controversy.

Pros and Cons of Various Drains

Latex and Cigarette (Penrose)

Perhaps the most widely used method of drainage in the United States, the soft latex drain of various dimensions, is generally made of a thin radiopaque sheet of rubber. It has the advantage of being inexpensive. It is also successful in encouraging fibrosis, so that it forms a well-established tract within 8–10 days.

However, there are many disadvantages. If the surgeon does not take pains to bring the drain out in a straight line without any wrinkles, stagnant pools of serum accumulate around the wrinkled areas of the drain. After the drain is removed, the patient may have a 24-hour increase in temperature of 2°–3°. More fundamentally, the latex drain does not really empty a cavity. It simply permits the secretions to overflow from the abdomen to the outside. It is not particularly effective in evacuating oozing blood before a clot forms. There is no method of irrigating the depth of the wound with this type of drain, as there is when a tube or sump type is used.

Finally, the most important objection to the latex drain arises from the fact that it requires a 1–2 cm stab wound in the abdominal wall. This permits the retrograde passage of pathogenic bacteria down into the drain tract, which accounts for the occurrence of staphylococcal infection in the drain site following an uncomplicated cholecystectomy and subphrenic abscess following an essentially sterile splenectomy. These problems have been described by Nora et al. and Cerise et al.

Tube Drain, Polyethylene or Rubber

Both of these substances establish tracts to the outside, as they are mildly irritating and stimulate adhesions. They are effective in evacuating air and serum from the pleural cavity and bile from the common bile duct. Drain-tract infection following the use of tube drains is rare, for reasons discussed below.

Among the disadvantages of rubber or polyethylene tubes is that they will clog up with clotted serum or blood unless they are a large size. However, large tubes are unsuitable for placement deep in the abdominal cavity for a period of more than a few days, as there is considerable danger of erosion through an adjacent segment of intestine, which results in intestinal fistula.

Tube Drain, Silicone

Silicone or Silastic tubes are less reactive than are other types of drains. They are less prone to plug up as a result of the clotting of serum. Because of the soft texture of silicone, erosion into the intestine is uncommon.

One disadvantage of silicone drains is that their lack of reactivity may result in the failure of tract formation. When a Silastic T-tube used in the common bile duct is removed, the patient may develop bile peritonitis, because a firm fibrous channel has not been established between the bile duct and the outside.

Sump Suction Drains

Generally constructed of polyethylene tubing, sump drains must be attached to a source of continuous suction.

They are quite effective in evacuating blood and serum, especially if suction is instituted in the operating room, so that the blood may be evacuated before it clots. Instillation of an antibiotic solution also is feasible when indicated. If used regularly, fluid instillation is also effective in preventing obstruction of the drain due to the coagulation of serum or secretions. Drain tract infections with sumps are uncommon even though unsterile, bacteria-laden air is drawn down into the depths of the patient's wound by the continuous suction. Baker and Borchardt have demonstrated this phenomenon and have noted it may be minimized by the low-volume suction provided by a Gomco pump. A major disadvantage of sump drains is the requirement that the patient be attached permanently to a suction device, thereby impairing mobility.

Closed-Suction Drain

This device consists of one or two multiperforated polyethylene catheters attached to a sterile plastic container, which is the source of continuous suction. This is a closed system; the catheters are brought out through puncture wounds. Morris has reported that the incidence of infection is lower than that encountered with other techniques. Patient mobility is unimpaired, for the plastic container is easily attached to the patient's attire. Irrigation of the depths of the wound with an antibiotic solution can be undertaken by disconnecting the catheter from the suction device and instilling the medication with a sterile syringe.

The closed-suction drain should not be left in the abdomen for more than 10 days as we know of cases where tissues have been sucked into the fenestrations of a Jackson-Pratt catheter so firmly that it was impossible to remove the catheter except by relaparotomy.

Gauze Packing

When a gauze pack is inserted into an abscess cavity and is brought to the outside, the gauze in effect serves as a drain. Unless the packing is changed frequently, this has the disadvantage of potentiating sepsis by providing a foreign body that protects bacteria from phagocytosis.

Prevention of Drain-Tract Infection

Retrograde transit of bacteria from the patient's skin down into the drain tract is a source of postoperative sepsis. As Nora et al. and Cerise et al. have reported, this problem occasionally follows clean operations such as elective cholecystectomy and splenectomy. An analogy can be drawn between an abdominal drain and an intravenous catheter placed in the superior vena cava for total parenteral nutrition. In the early days of this method, the intravenous catheter was a common cause of phlebitis and sepsis despite the sterile technique used to insert it. Two additional precautions, which were later instituted, helped eliminate these infections. These precautions were 1) suture-fixation of the catheter to its exit wound in the skin to eliminate any possibility of to-and-fro motion of the catheter through the puncture wound and 2) the addition of an antiseptic ointment like povidone-iodine to the skin wound every time the dressing is changed.

When a polyethylene sump or a silicone closed-suction catheter is brought through a puncture wound of the skin, it is easy to suture it in place, like the intravenous catheter. Daily application of povidone-iodine ointment and a sterile dressing is also a routine precaution. On the other hand, when a latex drain is brought out through a 1–2 cm stab wound in the abdominal wall, there is no possibility of eliminating to-and-fro motion of the drain or of retrograde passage of bacteria into the drain tract. Consequently, when latex or gauze drains must be used in cases of established abscesses, the surgeon must accept an added risk of retrograde contamination with bacteria, in spite of sterile technique when dressings are changed.

Management of Intraperitoneal Sepsis

A distinction must be made, in managing intraperitoneal sepsis, between an isolated abscess—for instance, around the appendix—and multiple abscesses involving the intestines, accompanied by generalized peritonitis. In treating peritoneal sepsis of the latter type, "decortication"—excision of the abscess and its surrounding fibrin—is the goal, just as decortication of an empyema cavity in the thorax is superior to simple drainage. The presence of fibrin and necrotic tissue prevents adequate phagocytosis and perpetuates sepsis. When peritoneal sepsis has progressed to the point at which multiple abscesses involve much of the small intestine, excising the abscesses by the technique described by Hudspeth, starting at the ligament of Treitz and continuing to the terminal ileum, serves simultaneously to eliminate the infection and correct the chronic intestinal obstruction.

When treating a solitary abscess in the periphery of the peritoneal cavity, such as in the pelvis, the subphrenic space, or the appendix, this radical type of operation is not necessary. *When the abscess has developed rigid walls that do not collapse after evacuation of the pus, large drains must be inserted* in order to establish a reliable tract to the outside. Sometimes 2 to 5 weeks may be required for a rigid abscess cavity to fill with granulation tissue. It is not safe to remove the drains until injecting the abscess with an aqueous iodinated contrast medium has produced an X ray that demonstrates the cavity is no longer significantly larger in diameter than the drainage tract. If this is not done, subphrenic or pelvic sepsis can recur readily. For rigid-walled abscesses of this type, several large latex drains should be inserted together with one or two sump drains. An additional straight 10F catheter should be inserted for intermittent instillation of an appropriate dilute antibiotic solution. At least one drain should be left in place until the sinogram X ray shows that the abscess cavity has essentially disappeared. Care should be taken that none of the rigid tubes comes into contact with the intestine or stomach, as intestinal fistula can be a serious complication.

Other Indications and Methods of Drainage

Abscess

In abscesses of the extremities, trunk, or perirectal area, the important step is to unroof the abscess by making a cruciate incision so that the tract will not close before all the pus has been evacuated. For superficial abscesses, an unroofing procedure is adequate, and any type of temporary drain is sufficient. When the danger exists that the superficial portion of the tract will close before deep healing takes place, insertion of gauze packing is indicated. This should be changed often enough to keep the packing from blocking the egress of pus.

Blood and Serum

The presence of blood, serum, or fibrin in a perfectly sterile area is not dangerous to the patient. However, following any major operation, the operative field is never completely sterile. For this reason postoperative puddles of blood or serum in combination with even a small number of bacteria, can result in abscess formation, because the red blood cell impairs antibacterial defenses, as Davis and Yull have stated. In the low colorectal anastomosis, accumulated serum or blood in the presacral space, together with secondary infection and abscess formation is probably a frequent cause of anastomotic leakage. For these reasons, during any abdominal operation strenuous efforts should be exerted to eliminate bleeding. If these efforts have to be supplemented by some type of drainage, the ideal method is to insert one or two multiperforated Silastic tubes, which are brought out through puncture wounds in the abdominal wall and attached to a closed-suction system. If it is important to keep this system functioning for more than 2 or 3 days, as it is in the low colorectal anastomosis, then tubes of large size—6 mm in external diameter—should be employed, and patency guaranteed by intermittent instillation of a dilute antibiotic solution.

Following radical mastectomy or regional lymph node dissections of the neck, axilla, or groin, closed-suction drainage is also extremely effective. Here, tubing of smaller diameter is acceptable. This technique has also been successfully employed following abdominoperineal proctectomy with primary closure of the perineal floor and skin.

Bile

Because bile has an extremely low surface tension, it will tend to leak through anastomoses by way of tiny defects or even via suture tracts. This is essentially harmless if a passageway to the outside is established. For this purpose either a sump drain or closed-suction system works nicely. Silastic tubes are contraindicated, as the formation of a fibrous tract to the outside for the bile is desirable. This is especially true in the use of a T-tube in the common bile duct. Following hepatic lobectomy, it is worthwhile to use several cigarette and sump drains, as there is a large empty space following resection.

Pancreatic Secretions

Pure pancreatic juice in the abdominal cavity is not dangerous. This is evident in patients who have pancreatic ascites or fistula. However, if the pancreatic secretion is activated by the presence of bile, duodenal contents, or pus, the trypsinogen is converted to trypsin and the adjacent tissues are subjected to a raging inflammatory reaction. Recently constructed adjacent anastomoses may be digested and destroyed. Eventually, hemorrhage from retroperitoneal blood vessels ensues. Consequently, it is important to evacuate bilious and pancreatic secretions completely, especially after Whipple pancreatic resection. This is accomplished by inserting a long plastic catheter into the pancreatic duct in the tail of the pancreas. The catheter is brought through the segment of jejunum to which the duct is anastomosed. Then it is brought through a jejunostomy opening to an outside drainage bag. Unless the tube is displaced accidentally, it will convey all the pancreatic secretions out of the abdominal cavity.

In addition, a sump suction catheter should be inserted in the vicinity of the anastomosis, between the tail of the pancreas and the jejunum. Daily irrigation with an antibiotic solution may be necessary to keep the drain functioning if it must remain in for more than a few days.

Duodenal Stump

Occasionally, after closing a difficult duodenal stump, the surgeon will have some doubt about the adequacy of the suture line. Under these conditions a 14F whistle-tip or Foley catheter should be inserted as a lateral duodenostomy to prevent the buildup of pressure in the duodenal stump (see Figs. 15–33 and 15–34). After a difficult duodenal resection, even if the closure appears to be satisfactory, some surgeons prefer to institute drainage in this area because there may have been trauma to the head of the pancreas. For this purpose a sump or latex drain is used, provided that it does not come into contact with the suture line. In general, it is preferable to use the lateral duodenostomy method or no drains at all.

Anastomosis

Placing a drain down to an anastomosis of the gastrointestinal tract because the surgeon has some doubt about its integrity makes little sense, according to Berliner et al. and Manz et al. If anastomotic breakdown occurs, the presence of a drain may not prevent generalized peritonitis. If the surgeon believes there is any significant risk of anastomotic failure, the anastomosis should be taken apart and be done over again, or else both ends should be exteriorized, to be reconnected at a second-stage operation. The surgeon must not fall into the trap of fuzzy thinking, which would permit the acceptance of an anastomosis that might be less than adequate, rather than reconstructing the anastomosis or eliminating it from this stage of the operation.

In treating some cases of Crohn's disease accompanied by extensive cellulitis, some surgeons believe the inflamed areas should be drained. In reality, cases of cellulitis or contamination, such as might follow a perforated duodenal ulcer, do not benefit from drainage. It is well established that the peritoneal cavity as a whole cannot be drained.

If complete hemostasis in the vicinity of an anastomosis cannot be achieved, there may be some merit to the insertion of a silicone closed-suction drain for a few days, provided it does not come into direct contact with the suture line.

References

Baker BH, Borchardt KA (1974) Sump drains and airborne bacteria as a cause of wound infections. J Surg Res 17:407

Berliner SD et al. (1964) Use and abuse of intraperitoneal drains in colon surgery. Arch Surg 89:686

Cerise EJ et al. (1970) Abdominal drains: their role as a source of infection following splenectomy. Ann Surg 171:764

Davis HJ, Yull AB (1964) A toxic factor in abdominal injury. II. The role of the red cell component. J Trauma 4:84

Hudspeth AS (1975) Radical surgical debridement in the treatment of advanced bacterial peritonitis. Arch Surg 110:1233

Magee C et al. (1976) Potentiation of wound infection by surgical drains. Am J Surg 131:547

Manz CW et al. (1970) The detrimental effects of drains on colonic anastomoses: an experimental study. Dis Colon Rectum 13:17

Morris AM (1973) A controlled trial of closed wound suction. Br J Surg 60:357

Nora PF et al. (1972) Prophylactic abdominal drains. Arch Surg 105:173

4 Surgical Stapling: Principles and Precautions

Principles of Stapling Gastric and Intestinal Anastomoses

Preserving Tissue Viability

Preserving the viability of the tissues distal to the line of staples is basic to the concept underlying the use of staples to perform a surgical anastomosis. The flow of blood penetrates the double staggered rows of staples that have been applied to the tissues. Unless the tissues are much too thick to be suitable for stapling, one will notice blood oozing through the staple line because the staples assume the configuration of a B when they are fired. Consequently, there is tissue along the staple line that completely escapes being enclosed by the staples, permitting the passage of blood to and beyond the stapled anastomosis. If the tissues being stapled are so thick that compression by the stapling device is likely to produce necrosis, this technique is contraindicated. On the other hand, if the tissues are so thin that the staples cannot provide a firm approximation, bleeding and anastomotic leakage may occur.

There is some leeway when approximating tissues of varying thickness. Staples of two sizes are available for use with the TA stapling devices. The 3.5 mm staple is 3.5 mm in leg length and 4.0 mm wide across the base. The 4.8 staple also is 4.0 mm wide across the base, but its leg length is 4.8 mm. When the TA device is compressed sufficiently so that the thin black band on its handle reaches the exact midpoint of the wide black band, the degree of compression, using the 3.5 mm staple, is approximately 1.5 mm. With the same technique, the 4.8 mm staple compresses the tissues to approximately 2 mm. An additional method of correcting for the thickness of tissues is to tighten the wing nut on the TA–55 device so that the thin black band comes to rest at a point proximal to the exact midpoint of the wide black band. This compresses the tissues to a width of 2.4 mm instead of 2.0 mm. With the GIA stapler, no adjustments can be made for tissues of varying thicknesses, as only one staple size is available. The GIA compresses tissues to a thickness of approximately 1.75 mm.

Stapling in Eversion

Even when tissues are stapled in eversion, with mucosa facing mucosa, satisfactory healing takes place. Ravitch et al. (1966) have demonstrated this phenomenon in anastomoses of the intestine. When a *sutured* anastomosis is performed with everting technique, the results are inferior to the inverted seromuscular anastomosis. On the other hand, the everted *stapled* anastomosis in experimental animals healed nicely with even less inflammation in the first 10–15 days than did the inverted sutured anastomosis. Extensive experience in humans, reported by Steichen and Ravitch, confirms the safety of mucosa-to-mucosa approximation when it is performed by stapling devices (see also Complications of Stapling Compared with Suturing, p. 25).

Instruments Used in Surgical Stapling

Stapling Devices Used for Gastrointestinal Tract Anastomosis

TA–55 and TA–90

The TA–55 applies a doubled staggered row of staples approximately 55 mm long; the TA–90 applies a doubled staggered row about 90 mm long. Each may be used with 3.5 mm or 4.8 mm staples, according to the principles described above. These devices are used to approximate the walls of stomach or intestine in an everting fashion. They find application in closure of the duodenal stump, of the gastric pouch in gastrectomy, and of the end of the colon when a side-to-end coloproctostomy is performed.

GIA

The GIA device creates a stapled anastomosis with the tissues in inversion. It applies two doubled staggered rows of staples while the knife in its assembly divides the tissue between the two double rows. It is used for side-to-side anastomoses, such as gastrojejunostomy, and "functional end-to-end" anastomoses.

EEA

The EEA device utilizes a circular anvil, a circular staple cartridge, and a circular knife to produce a doubled staggered row of staples that approximate two tubular structures in inversion while the knife cuts the tissue just inside the staple line. This creates an end-to-end anastomosis 21.4 mm in internal diameter. It compresses the tissues to a thickness of approximately 2.0 mm. While smaller cartridges that produce a circular anastomosis of smaller diameter are available, only one size of staple is obtainable. When the device is inserted through the anal canal, it is ideally suited for a low colorectal anastomosis.

Because the outside diameter of the cartridge is about 32.0 mm, the EEA device is not easily inserted into the esophagus for use in this application. Whether an anastomosis having an internal diameter of less than 21.4 mm will prove adequate for the passage of food remains to be seen. Until this question has been settled it may not be wise to use the EEA cartridges, which produce anastomoses with diameters smaller than this.

The EEA stapler has also been used successfully for the Billroth I gastroduodenal anastomosis.

Other Stapling Devices

LDS

The LDS device can apply two staples, which serve as ligatures, while it divides the tissue between these two staple-ligatures. Its principal application is in dividing the branches of the gastroepiploic vessels that supply the greater curvature of the stomach, a procedure carried out when the omentum is liberated during gastrectomy. Some surgeons also find it useful in dividing blood vessels in other parts of the abdomen.

Skin Stapler

All the instruments mentioned above are manufactured by the U. S. Surgical Corp., which along with the Ethicon Company also makes staplers for closing skin incisions. These staplers close skin incisions efficiently and rapidly, with satisfactory cosmetic results. Their major drawback is that staples are more expensive than sutures for this purpose.

Fascia Stapler

Since the fascia stapler violates the principles discussed in Chap. 5, we have not used it in our operations.

Indications for Stapling an Anastomosis

Stapled anastomoses, when constructed with proper technique, are no better and no worse than those done with sutures (see below). Stapling has the disadvantage of increased expense. It has the advantage of speed—a stapled anastomosis can generally be completed in 2–5 minutes—which is a tremendous benefit in the poor-risk patient who is critically ill and who may be undergoing an emergency operation. Even with the availability of skilled anesthesiologists, expert in the physiological support of the desperately ill patient, there is indubitably an advantage to completing the operation speedily.

Stapling technology is also an attractive option for the low anterior resection in patients who have lesions of the middle third of the rectum at 6–10 cm from the anal verge. Although there are many pitfalls of a technical nature in the use of the EEA device, after the technique has been mastered it seems to be superior to suturing in this location.

Contraindications

The use of staples is contraindicated under the same conditions that would make construction of a sutured anastomosis dangerous. There is no evidence that staples are safer than sutures, for instance, in the presence of advanced peritonitis.

Another contraindication is the presence of tissues that are too thick or too thin to meet the requirements for stapling, as discussed above.

There are occasional, although rare, instances in which the exposure does not allow enough room to insert a stapling instrument into a body cavity. If this is the case, it is contraindicated to apply traction to the tissues in order to permit the introduction of a stapling device.

Causes of Failure following Stapled Anastomosis

Quality of the Tissues

The blood supply of the bowel to be anastomosed must be vigorous when staples are used, just as it must be with sutures. Bowel that is not fit for suturing is not suitable for stapling.

When the GIA is used to anastomose the jejunum to the back wall of a gastric pouch (see Fig. 15–47), at least 2.0–2.5 cm of gastric wall should be left between the GIA staple line and the closed end of the gastric pouch. Otherwise, ischemia can develop in this strip of stomach between the two staple lines and produce anastomotic failure. Do not let the ease of inserting staples impair good judgment about the adequacy of tissue perfusion in the vicinity of any staple line. Always think of blood supply.

The stapling technique requires that the bowel be of such quality that it will remain viable when compressed to the thickness mentioned above during the process of constructing a stapled anastomosis. For example, when a chronic obstruction has caused the gastric wall to become hypertrophied to a thickness of 6–8 mm, compression by the TA–90 stapling device to a thickness of 2.0–2.4 mm may produce a linear tear in the serosa adjacent to the stapling device. Seeing this, the surgeon should invert the staple line with a layer of seromuscular Lembert sutures. Otherwise the staple line should be excised and the closure accomplished entirely with sutures. Although tissue thickness rarely is a contraindication to the use of staples, failure by the surgeon to identify those cases in which the tissues are unsuitable for reliance on stapling may lead to serious complications. On some occasions the tissues may be so thick that the TA instrument cannot be closed sufficiently to superimpose one black band upon the other. Obviously the stapling technique should be abandoned in these cases.

Linear tension that exerts a distracting force against a sutured anastomosis certainly is detrimental. In the stapled anastomosis this tension is even more undesirable. One should assume that the fine wire in the staples will tend to cut through tissues more readily than sutures, thereby producing a leaking anastomosis. This is a clinical impression unsupported by data, but we have observed a colostomy closure fail because of the postoperative dehiscence of the staple line. This occurred because the surgeon did not free enough proximal and distal colon from adhesions to the parietal peritoneum to relieve tension on the stapled closure. Other complications of this type are discussed in the section on staple complications (see below).

Instrument Failure

Misalignment of the GIA instrument may occur, especially if it has been dropped on a ceramic floor and the two forks of the instrument diverge instead of remaining parallel. In this case the increased distance between the cartridge and the anvil prevents the staples at the distal end of the instrument from closing properly. As a precaution, the *staple formation should be checked following the completion of each anastomosis.* In addition, when the GIA is used frequently it should be test-fired once a month on a latex drain or a sheet of plastic to check proper B formation.

Partial failure of the knife assembly in the GIA instrument may occur on rare occasions. When this happens the scalpel fails to make a complete incision between the two double rows of staples. If this is not detected by careful inspection, the resulting anastomosis will have an extremely narrow lumen.

Complete failure of the staple cartridge to discharge staples has been known to happen. An inattentive surgeon may not notice this, for pressure alone may hold the bowel walls in apposition temporarily. A cartridge will also fail to discharge staples if it has been spent and not replaced by a fresh cartridge before *each* application of the instrument.

If the staples do not close properly when the TA device is fired with the two black bands properly aligned, the cause probably is excessive wear and tear on the TA's component parts. Should this happen, return the instrument to the company for repair. When these devices are used often, they should be tested at regular intervals by firing them on a latex drain or a piece of plastic and inspecting the staples carefully. The B formation should resemble those in **Fig. 4–1a,b.**

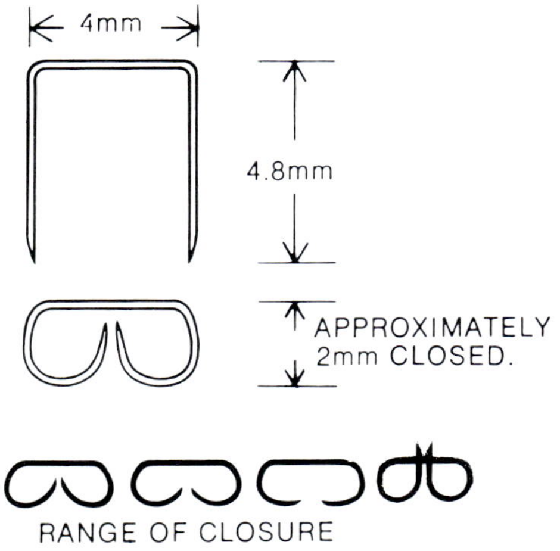

Fig. 4–1a. Dimensions of 4.8 staples.

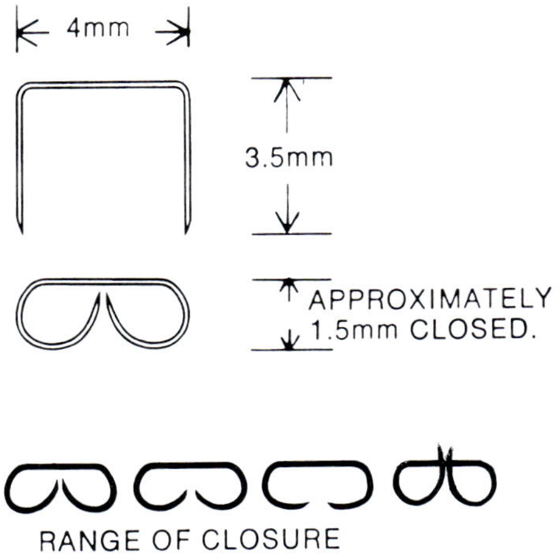

Fig. 4–1b. Dimensions of 3.5 staples.

Human Error—Instruments

If the operating room uses more than one GIA instrument, the two main components of each GIA *must not* be interchanged, as this may cause misalignment. The serial number on each component of each GIA should match.

In inserting the knife assembly of the GIA device, each of the three components of the knife assembly must be inserted in its own channel. Otherwise one whole line of staples may not be fired.

Occasionally, a novice at GIA stapling will fire the knife assembly, then withdraw the assembly and fire it a second time. This second firing of the spent GIA cartridge causes many small bits of plastic to be discharged into the lumen. These are the pusher components of the cartridge, which drive each staple out of the cartridge. Obviously, each cartridge should be fired only one time.

The GIA push-bar/knife assembly has a runner on its plastic handle. The runner goes into a slot on the cartridge fork; this aligns the knife assembly properly. If the knife assembly is fired with the runner out of its slot, its components get bent and jam, preventing the assembly from being withdrawn. If this happens, release the lock lever to partially separate the two forks while the GIA is still in the bowel lumen; then remove the device.

If the alignment pin of the TA–55 instrument is not pushed into the anvil, the staples will undergo improper closure, since the anvil and the cartridge may not be lined up in their proper positions. In the TA–90 device, the alignment pin consists of a screw, which serves the same purpose.

Never omit the insertion of the alignment pin. If the stomach is too wide to be encompassed by one application of the TA–90, do it in two steps. First, close the TA–90 over 90 mm of stomach. While the tissue is loosely in the jaws of the instrument, drive the alignment screw pin through the gastric walls into the anvil. Tighten the wing nut. Then fire the staples. Reapply the TA–90 with a fresh cartridge and anvil in such a direction that the gastric tissue damaged by the penetration of the alignment pin is included in the specimen. Fire the staples; the gastric wall will be stapled closed with complete safety.

Immediately after each use, discard both the spent staple cartridge and the anvil. This prevents the error of reusing a spent cartridge that no longer contains any staples.

If a TA instrument is not closed by turning the wing nut at the end of the handle to place the thin black band within the confines of the wide black band, then the distance between the cartridge and the anvil will be excessive and the staples will not close. This must be checked before any staple cartridge is fired.

In using the EEA device, be sure to tighten the screw on top of its anvil; this will avoid excessive space between the cartridge and the anvil when the device is fired.

Human Error—Judgment

A staple line should not cross the mesentery of bowel. If this happens, intramural hematomas may occur, which would interfere with proper healing. Also, mesenteric fat should not be included between the seromuscular layers of an anastomosis.

Whenever the GIA device is used on the gastric wall, carefully inspect the staple line for gastric bleeding. Transfix bleeding points with absorbable sutures. Occasionally an entire GIA staple line in the stomach bleeds excessively. If it does, the entire staple line should be oversewn with absorbable sutures inserted in the lumen of the stomach. Although it is preferable to insert sutures superficial to the staple line, with the GIA device there may not be sufficient tissue beyond the staples to accomplish this. On such occasions we have not had complications when 4–0 PG atraumatic sutures were inserted in the lumen of a GIA anastomosis and were passed deep to the staples. These sutures must not be tied with excessive tension. We have not observed significant bleeding following GIA stapling in organs other than stomach. Minor bleeding may be controlled by cautious electrocoagulation.

When an excessive amount of tissue is bunched up in the crotch of the GIA, firing the knife assembly may fail to incise the bowel between the two doubled rows of staples because the knife blade cannot penetrate the compressed tissue. As a result there will be narrowing or absence of an anastomotic lumen. Every GIA staple line must be inspected upon removing the instrument. If the incision between the staple lines has not been made by the GIA knife assembly, it should be accomplished with a straight scissors. Although this type of GIA failure is rare, its possibility should not be overlooked.

Occasionally the GIA is used to cut and staple across two layers of gastric wall, as in the Janeway gastrostomy (see Chap. 17) or the Collis gastroplasty (Vol. II). Because the two layers of stomach may be too thick for the GIA to compress them safely to a 1.75 mm width, these staple lines should be oversewn with sutures.

Multiple Allis clamps should be applied to the walls of intestine included in a TA staple line. This prevents the bowel from retracting out of the jaws of the instrument as the tissue is being compressed. If the tissue should retract from the jaws of the instrument, obviously the stapled closure would fail.

If an anastomosis constructed by the stapling technique has too small a lumen, this inadequate lumen probably will not dilate very much following the passage of stool or food, as it will if interrupted sutures have been used. If a stapled stoma is made too small, the two staggered rows of staples may keep it that way permanently after the anastomosis has been constructed. Consequently, more attention should be paid to the size of the lumen when constructing a stapled anastomosis than when constructing one by sutures. We have seen staples remain intact in anastomoses for as long as 5 years after surgery.

Avoid making a false intramural passage when inserting the forks of the GIA into stab wounds of the intestine or stomach, as this would prevent the formation of a proper anastomosis. Place each fork accurately in the lumen of the intestine or stomach.

The tissues of the bowel and esophagus should be in a relaxed position when a stapling device is applied to them. If excessive tension is applied to the tissue while the stapler is being fired, this tends to make the tissue too thin for proper purchase by the staples.

Special Precautions

1) After completing a stapled anastomosis, always inspect the entire circumference meticulously to ascertain that each staple has been formed into an adequate B. Test the lumen by invaginating the bowel wall with the index finger. Any point at which two or more staple lines cross should be carefully checked for possible leakage. Inspect the serosa for possible cracks or tears. If there is any doubt about the integrity of a stapled anastomosis, oversew it with a layer of interrupted seromuscular Lembert sutures. If the saving of time is a consideration, use a continuous Lembert suture of 4–0 atraumatic PG. Although the need to oversew the staple line will occur in no more than 1%–2% of the cases managed by a surgeon experienced in performing stapled anastomoses, oversewing can be an essential step in preventing leaks in some situations.

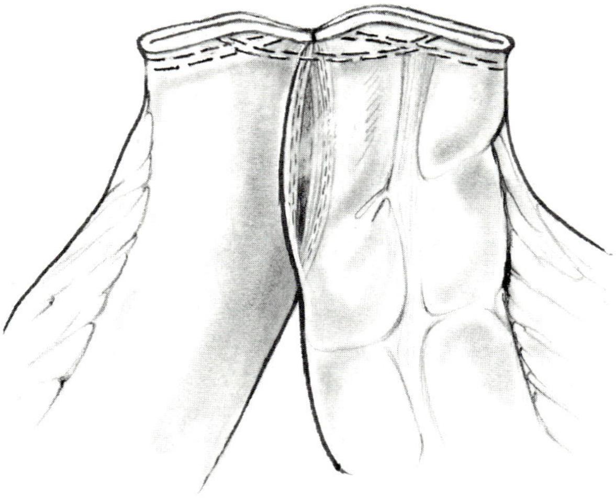

Fig. 4–2

A better way of avoiding this problem is to use our modification of the functional end-to-end anastomosis, as illustrated in Figs. 28–33, 28–34, 28–35, and 28–36.

3) Using the EEA for colorectal anastomosis is an excellent technique, provided that precautions are taken to avoid the many possible technical pitfalls. These are described in Chap. 30.

One general problem in inserting the EEA anvil into the colon or esophagus occurs when the lumen is too narrow to accommodate the anvil's 32 mm diameter.

2) In the last step of a functional end-to-end anastomosis, the defect is closed with a TA–55 device. If the two GIA staple lines (**Fig. 4–2**) are kept in perfect apposition during this maneuver, after the TA–55 is fired six rows of staples can be seen to come together at one point. We believe that such a point is weak and that it permits the development of an anastomotic leak, because the presence of many staples and much tissue in one spot results in the failure of proper closure. Occasionally this can be seen in the operating room when carefully inspecting the completed anastomosis. To prevent this weak point we have modified our technique by deliberately avoiding perfect apposition of the two GIA staple lines. Greater security will be achieved when applying the TA–55 if the bowel is aligned so that the GIA staple lines are not in exact apposition (**Figs. 4–3 and 4–4**).

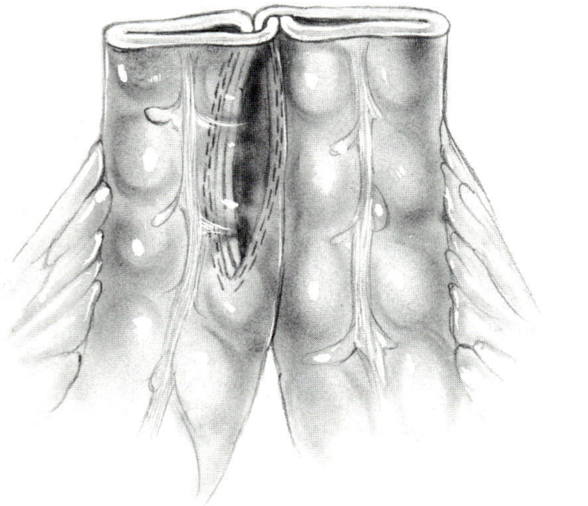

Fig. 4–3

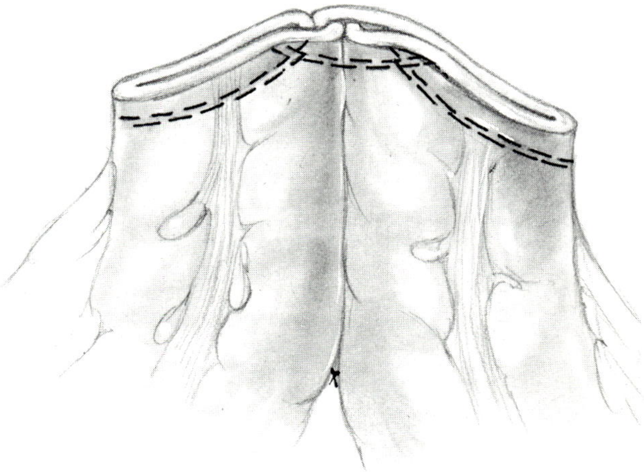

Fig. 4–4

This may result from muscle spasm, perhaps induced by narcotics such as fentanyl, which is commonly employed in the administration of "balanced" anesthesia. Excessively forceful dilatation tears the seromuscular coat of the colon. If dilating the bowel results in tissue too thin to hold staples firmly, stapling is contraindicated. We do not believe the smaller EEA cartridges should be used in either the esophagus or the rectum because the resulting stoma may be too small.

Complications of Stapling Compared with Suturing*

Although the first clinically useful stapling device was developed by DePetz in 1927, further progress was not remarkable until the early 1960's when the Institute for Experimental Apparatus and Instruments in Moscow developed a group of instruments capable of performing gastrointestinal tract anastomoses. Since these instruments were somewhat cumbersome and required that individual staples be inserted into the instrument by hand prior to each use, they did not receive widespread acceptance. Ravitch et al. (1959) were responsible for introducing a modified form of the Russian stapling device to this country. A great advance in the utility of the staplers was achieved with the development of instant loading with sterile cartridges, each containing as many as 33 staples. Ravitch and his associates also reported further studies in animals and humans and described techniques for the performance of gastrectomy as well as small bowel and colonic anastomoses.

It has been estimated, on the basis of staple sales, that several hundred thousand operations using Auto Suture stapling techniques were performed in the United States last year. Acceptance of staplers has largely bypassed the academic institutions where the necessity of teaching residents basic surgical techniques may have had a higher priority than study of the new technology.

Gritsman, one of the pioneers in the development of the Russian stapling apparatus, in 1966 reported a collective series of 1,663 stapled gastric resections performed by a large number of surgeons in the USSR, with a mortality rate of 2%. He compared these with a second series, which he collected from the world literature, of 52,886 gastrectomies done with suture technique by 62 surgeons, with a mortality rate of 4.4%. Steichen and Ravitch reported 147 of their own stapled gastrointestinal operations with 11 complications. Latimer and associates studied 112 stapled operative procedures with a stapler-related complication rate of 1.9%. Lawson and associates reported 122 operations on the alimentary canal done with stapling devices, accompanied by a 4.0% complication rate. No study has yet been reported comparing complications following stapled anastomoses with those following hand-sutured procedures performed by the same group of surgeons. In an effort to shed light on the relative merits of these two techniques, the authors are reporting a study of this type with reference to 812 consecutive gastrointestinal procedures.

Material and Methods

By reviewing the operating room log book of the Booth Memorial Medical Center for the period between July 1, 1973 and June 30, 1977, the names and chart numbers of all patients having gastrointestinal operations were obtained. These charts were then reviewed to determine the nature of each operative procedure, the technique of anastomosis and any complications which may have occurred during the course of hospitalization.

*From "The Stapled Gastrointestinal Tract Anastomosis: Incidence of Postoperative Complications Compared with the Sutured Anastomosis," by Jameson L. Chassin, M.D., Kenneth M. Rifkind, M.D., Barry Sussman, M.D., Barry Kassel, M.D., Arnold Fingaret, M.D., Sharon Drager, M.D., Pamela S. Chassin, in *Annals of Surgery*, Vol. 188, No. 5, November 1978. Copyright © 1978 by J.B. Lippincott Company. Reprinted by permission.

Classification of Complications

Complications of anastomoses were grouped in three categories: 1) If an enterocutaneous fistula, leak, hemorrhage, or obstruction occurred at the site of the anastomosis, this was obviously a "related" complication. Included also are cases of perianastomotic abscess and generalized peritonitis. 2) If the patient developed a subphrenic or pelvic abscess at a distance from the anastomosis with no direct contact, this was considered "possibly related," as was the development of intestinal obstruction due to adhesions not at the anastomotic site. 3) Complications were considered "unrelated" if the patient developed such conditions as myocardial infarction, atelectasis, cerebrovascular accident, or pulmonary embolism. A study of comparative wound infection rates is not included in this report even though the technique selected for anastomosis might indeed have influenced the incidence of infection in the incision. The reason for this omission stems from the fact that skin wounds, contaminated by the intra-abdominal procedure, were either left open, sutured closed, or drained according to the prejudices of the surgeon. Since there was no uniform pattern of wound management during the period under study, a statistical review of infected wounds as a "related" complication would prove meaningless.

Classification of Operative Procedures

Each gastrointestinal anastomosis was considered to be an operative procedure. Consequently, if a patient had both a small bowel resection with anastomosis and a colon resection with anastomosis, these were counted as two procedures. Billroth II subtotal gastrectomy, for the purpose of this study, was classified as two procedures: 1) duodenal stump closure and 2) gastroenterostomy. In this way it was possible to calculate the specific morbidity rate for each type of suture or staple procedure.

Anterior resections performed at or below the peritoneal reflection were classified as being done by suture if no staples were involved. These were all end-to-end anastomoses in this series. The Baker side-to-end colorectal anastomosis is a special case combining an everted stapled closure of the distal end of colon with suture anastomosis between the side of colon and the end of the rectal stump. In only two cases were low colorectal anastomoses done exclusively with staples. The new EEA stapling device, especially designed to perform this type of anastomosis, was not available during the time period of this study.

Surgical Technique

In each case the operative techniques were those described by Ravitch and Steichen. The everted stapled closures were not turned in with an additional layer of sutures in the cases included in this series. Ten attending surgeons and twelve surgical residents performed the operations, utilizing the Auto Suture TA–55, TA–90, and GIA stapling devices. When anastomoses were performed by hand suturing, standard techniques were utilized. In most cases involving either the small bowel or colon, open anastomoses were constructed using fine catgut for the mucosa and interrupted nonabsorbable sutures for the seromuscular layer, although occasionally a one-layer technique was used.

Case Selection

All gastrointestinal anastomoses done during the period under study were reviewed. Six patients were rejected because they died of unrelated causes, such as myocardial infarction, stroke, or preexisting sepsis, so soon after operation as not to allow sufficient time to elapse for an anastomotic complication to become manifest. All other cases were included in the study. Whether staples or sutures were to be utilized in any case was a decision left entirely to the judgment or personal preference of the operating surgeon.

Technical Training

Although a course of instruction in surgical stapling given at the University of Pittsburgh was attended by the senior author, much of the staff's early training in the application of the stapling devices was provided by representatives of the manufacturer.

Adverse Factor Analysis

Since this is a retrospective study, it is possible that a disproportionate number of patients with conditions having an adverse effect on anastomotic healing might have accumulated in one of the two groups under study, thus jeopardizing the validity of the comparison. Consequently, seven categories of adverse factors were selected: 1) emergent or urgent nature of the surgery; 2) peritonitis, gastrointestinal perforation, or intra-abdominal abscess; 3) gangrenous intestine; 4) gastric or intestinal obstruction; 5) Crohn's disease; 6) carcinoma, localized; 7) nonresectable carcinoma, liver metastases, or peritoneal carcinomatosis.

Most surgeons would agree from their personal experience that these factors do have an adverse effect on anastomotic healing, and statistical validation for most of the above items is evident in the report by Schrock et al. Charts of patients included in this study were reviewed for the presence of any of the above adverse factors. The incidence rate of each adverse factor was calculated individually for the various suture and staple techniques. Not subjected to this adverse factor analysis were colostomy closures and anterior resections because these cases were not done under emergency conditions and few of the other adverse factors were operative.

Results

Mean age of all patients having sutured anastomoses was 62.5 years compared to 63.3 for stapled cases. Analysis of the specific mean ages for each of the sutured and of the stapled operative procedures under study did not disclose any clinically significant differences.

Table 4–1 summarizes the incidence of factors having an adverse effect on anastomotic healing. It is obvious that with the exception of Crohn's disease, each of the adverse factors was more prevalent in patients undergoing stapled procedures. For example, 24% of 438 stapled anastomoses were done under emergency conditions compared to 9% of sutured procedures. Carcinomatosis, gastric or intestinal obstruction, gangrene of bowel, and infection were also more prevalent among the stapled cases.

Complications following each of the operative procedures under study are summarized in Table 4–2. There is no statistically significant difference in the incidence of "related" complications between the sutured and stapled groups when tested by the Chi-square method (3.0% vs 2.8%). The same is true of the incidence of "possibly related" complications for the two groups (1.4% vs 1.3%). It is interesting to note that of the 27 complications following those operative procedures of the types listed in Table 4–1, 22 occurred in patients having adverse factors. All of the complications are described in Tables 4–3 through 4–10.

As will be evident from a perusal of Tables 4–3 through 4–10, it is often difficult to ascertain whether a complication was related to the healing anastomosis or whether it was an inevitable result of the pathological process for which the operation was performed. In questionable cases the complications were included in our statistics as "possibly related."

Table 4–1. Incidence of Factors with Adverse Effect on Anastomotic Healing

	No.	Operations Nonelective	Perforation or Pus	Bowel Gangrene	Obstruction	Crohn's Disease	Carcinoma	Nonresectable CA or Metastases
Gastrojejunal								
sutured	32	19%	3%	0	26%	0	29%	23%
stapled	111	22%	5%	0	18%	1%	35%	24%
Duodenal stump								
sutured	31	13%	0	0	—[a]	0	13%	3%
stapled	68	28%	6%	0	—[a]	0	29%	3%
Ileocolonic								
sutured	57	7%	7%	5%	7%	14%	67%	9%
stapled	85	21%	20%	6%	15%	11%	71%	12%
Colocolonic								
sutured	71	6%	8%	4%	1%	1%	54%	8%
stapled	61	8%	8%	0	2%	2%	63%	33%
Small intestine								
sutured	30	30%	6%	3%	10%	0	30%	30%
stapled	106	39%	18%	20%	24%	3%	42%	27%
Esophagogastric								
sutured	4	0	0	0	0	0	100%	25%
stapled	6	0	0	0	0	0	100%	33%
Total								
sutured	224	9%	6%	3%	7%	4%	46%	13%
stapled	438	24%	11%	6%	14%	3%	47%	21%

[a]Not relevant.

Discussion

The incidence of anastomotic complications (Table 4–2) following stapled procedures was so nearly identical with that following hand-sutured operations as to be startling. Review of the data in Table 4–1 indicates that if there is any bias in this retrospective study, it heavily favors the sutured procedures. A much higher proportion of acutely ill patients undergoing emergency surgery had their anastomoses performed by the stapling technique in order to save operating time. Patients suffering from abdominal abscess, peritonitis, gangrenous bowel, intestinal obstruction, and peritoneal carcinomatosis underwent anastomoses by stapling far more frequently than by suturing. With respect to cases of small intestinal obstruction undergoing resection and anastomosis, of the 28 cases in this series, 25 were anastomosed with staples; of 22 with strangulation of small bowel, 21 had stapled procedures. It is notable that 69% of all 32 anastomotic complications occurred in patients with one or more adverse factors.

Schrock and his associates demonstrated that a marked increase in the incidence of clinically apparent anastomotic leakage followed ileocolonic and colonic resections if the operations were done under emergency conditions or were accompanied by bacterial or fecal contamination, operative hemorrhage, or shock. For example, when peritonitis, abscesses, or fistulae were encountered at operation, anastomoses leaked in 10.5% of cases, compared to 3.7% in the absence of infection. Emergent cases exhibited an 8.2%

Table 4–2. Complications following Sutured and Stapled Operative Procedures

		Complications	
	No.	Related	Possibly Related
Gastrojejunostomy			
sutured	32	0	1 (3%)
stapled	111	1 (1%)	3 (3%)
Duodenal stump closure			
sutured	31	2 (6%)	0
stapled	68	3 (4%)	0
Ileocolonic			
sutured	57	3 (5%)	2 (4%)
stapled	85	3 (4%)	2 (2%)
Colocolonic			
sutured	71	0	1 (1%)
stapled	61	0	0
Small intestine			
sutured	30	1 (3%)	0
stapled	105	4 (4%)	1 (1%)
Closure colostomy			
sutured	33	0	0
stapled	33	2 (6%)	0
Esophagogastric			
sutured	4	0	0
stapled	6	0	0
Anterior resection			
sutured	38	3 (8%)	0
Baker	44	0	0
stapled	2	0	0
Total			
sutured	296	9 (3.0%)	4 (1.4%)
stapled	472	13 (2.8%)	6 (1.3%)
Baker	44	0	0
Total	812		

leak rate. Even the presence of a localized colonic carcinoma resulted in a rate of clinical leakage twice that of operations performed for benign disease. Our study tends to confirm their findings with respect to both sutured and stapled anastomoses. Crohn's disease is included in our list of adverse factors due to the fact that most of our patients undergoing surgery for this condition had sustained one of the complications of the disease which produced some variety of intraperitoneal infection.

Although the procedure of right hemicolectomy with primary anastomosis has a reputation for successful healing even when performed under unfavorable conditions, Table 4–5 demonstrates that a number of anastomotic complications occurred following ileocolectomy performed in the presence of carcinomatosis, intestinal necrosis, peritonitis, or abscess. Welch and Donaldson noted a high mortality (18%) when right colectomy with anastomosis was performed for acute colonic obstruction, while Dutton et al. found that 36% of their patients died following emergency resection and anastomosis of the obstructed right colon.

In one patient a pelvic abscess followed subtotal colectomy and ileosigmoid stapled anastomosis done for an acutely obstructing carcinoma of the left colon. This is considered by the authors to be a case of poor surgical judgment, as results with preliminary colostomy followed by staged resection for left colon obstruction have been superior to one-stage resection (Dutton et al., 1976; Welch and Donaldson, 1974). In our series, closure of colostomy resulted in no deaths and only a 3% incidence of anastomotic complications.

Three cases of subhepatic or subphrenic abscess, cited in Table 4–3, followed gastrectomy either for carcinoma or

Table 4–3. Complications following Gastrojejunostomy

Sutured (32)
- Related—(0)
- Possibly related—(1)
  - Subhepatic abscess after gastrectomy for obstructing ulcer; relap.

Stapled (111)
- Related—(1)
  - Postoperative gastric hemorrhage, three units; no relap.; *technical error*
- Possibly related—(3)
  - Subhepatic abscess after gastrectomy for carcinoma; relap.
  - Subhepatic abscess after gastrectomy for carcinoma of residual gastric pouch; relap.
  - Obstruction due to fibrosis at efferent stoma after gastrojejunostomy for Crohn's duodenitis; relap.

obstruction. In each of these cases it is considered highly improbable that the infection resulted from any leak at the site of the gastrojejunostomy. Rather, contamination by virulent organisms present in the stomach appears to be the likely cause of these infections.

In the case of the postoperative gastric hemorrhage following a stapled gastrojejunostomy, this was considered to be a technical error. Performed early in our experience with stapling techniques, inadequate attention was paid to the oozing of blood from the gastrojejunal staple line. It is now known that it is imperative to correct this bleeding by means of electrocoagulation or suture ligation.

In reviewing duodenal stump closure it is notable that two of the five leaks occurred in patients with gastric carcinoma in whom the duodenum appeared to be free of pathology. The only fatal duodenal complication occurred in a patient in shock undergoing emergency gastrectomy for massive hemorrhage from a large posterior penetrating duodenal ulcer, in whom the precaution was taken of performing a tube duodenostomy at the time of gastrectomy. This was not successful in preventing duodenal fistula and peritonitis. In two stapled duodenal closures, minor leaks appeared along the drain tracts. In one patient, who was discharged from the hospital healed, a duodenal fistula occurred along the drain tract on the twenty-first postoperative day. Another patient with a duodenal leak following stapled closure underwent reoperation on the fourth postoperative day. No gross leak could be seen, but drains were inserted and the fistula persisted for three weeks. This complication was considered due to a technical error in that the duodenal stump was excessively scarred, making it too thick for proper closure by stapling. Since the stapling device will compress tissues to a thickness of 1 to 1.5 mm when using the 3.5 mm staple, it is important to remember that no tissue which may be necrotized by this degree of compression should be stapled. Vital to the success of any stapled closure is the viability of the tissue distal to the staple line. Stapling is not equivalent to a completely hemostatic ligature. One can uniformly observe a brief period of gentle oozing through the stapled closure. When tissue is too thick for this to occur, the technique is contraindicated. Some leeway in this area may be obtained by using the larger 4.8 mm staple, which will permit the closure of moderately thickened tissue. With the use of the larger staple, the tissue compression may be adjusted to a 2–2.4 mm thickness.

One of the technical failures following a stapled anastomosis occurred in a patient with a strangulating inguinal hernia requiring resection of the patient's

Table 4–4. Complications following Closure of Duodenal Stump

- Sutured (31)
  - Related—(2)
    - Duodenal fistula after gastrectomy for carcinoma; healed without relap.
    - Duodenal leak and peritonitis following suture closure of duodenum and tube duodenostomy during emergency gastrectomy for massive hemorrhage—fatal
- Stapled (68)
  - Related—(3)
    - Duodenal fistula healed in four weeks—minor; no relap.
    - Duodenal fistula along drain tract following gastrectomy for carcinoma appeared on p.o. 22, after discharge from hospital; healed in three weeks—minor; no relap.
    - Duodenal leak; reoperation p.o. 4 to insert tube duodenostomy; healed in two weeks; *technical error*—stump too thick for stapled technique

ileum. The resection and anastomosis was carried out in the inguinal incision after which the anastomosed segment was pushed through the fairly narrow hernial ring into the abdominal cavity. This complication was attributed to the technical error of applying excessive force to a fresh anastomosis. Another technical error was responsible for a large fecal fistula which followed stapled anastomosis for closure of a transverse colostomy. The operation was performed through a small incision with inadequate mobilization of colon from adjacent adhesions. This resulted in excessive tension on the stapled closure, with consequent leakage.

Needless to say, in an indeterminate number of additional cases, technical errors were detected and corrected during the course of stapling. Of course, this is also true of suture techniques, but surgeons spend five years in a residency program learning all the pitfalls of hand suturing. By contrast, the radically different technique of stapling is frequently applied with minimal preceptorship. Upon the completion of any stapling procedure, it behooves the surgeon to examine the entire anastomosis with meticulous care to seek out any possible imperfections. In the case of gastrojejunal anastomoses with the GIA device, complete hemostasis must be assured prior to completion of the procedure.

In our earlier application of stapled anastomoses to the small intestine, the authors felt some apprehension that the everted staple line might give rise to postoperative adhesions due to the rim of exposed mucosa. It was gratifying to observe that during the 4-year period of this study no patient returned with intestinal obstruction due to an adhesion involving one of these everted lines of staples. Since the period of observation is a brief one, some degree of apprehension remains and it may be advisable, when convenient, to cover the everted mucosa with adjacent mesentery or omentum.

Among the 32 complications related to anastomotic healing listed in Tables 4–3 through 4–10, there were only four fatalities from sepsis. This low rate is considered to be due to the emphasis in this institution upon prompt relaparotomy in all cases suspected of having anastomotic leakage. In these situations the anastomosis is generally divided and both limbs of intestine are exteriorized either as enterostomy or colostomy and mucous fistula.

Table 4–5. Complications following Ileocolonic Resection and Anastomosis

Sutured (57)
- Related—(3)
  - Perianastomotic abscess after palliative right colectomy in 75 year old patient with carcinomatosis; relap. p.o. 10
  - Obstruction, inflammation at anastomosis; relap. for bypass p.o. 15 (probable leak)
  - Death p.o. 11 of 90 year old following resection and jejunocaecostomy for gangrene of ileum; febrile p.o. course; no autopsy (suspected leak)
- Possibly related—(2)
  - Recurrent pelvic abscess after resection for perforated Crohn's ileitis with pelvic abscess and peritonitis; relap. p.o. 11
  - Transient small bowel obstruction in patient with peritoneal metastases; Cantor tube

Stapled (85)
- Related—(3)
  - Leak and peritonitis after subtotal colectomy and ileosigmoidostomy for Crohn's colitis; relap. p.o. 8
  - Subhepatic abscess adjoining anastomosis; patient readmitted for I. & D. p.o. 26
  - Obstruction due to kink, adhesions and small abscess at anastomosis in 90 year old; probable leak; relap. p.o. 9
- Possibly related—(2)
  - Small pelvic abscess noted at relap. for intestinal obstruction 15 days after emergency subtotal colectomy and ileosigmoid anastomosis for acutely obstructing carcinoma of left colon
  - RUQ abscess and infected ascites after resection right colon for necrotic tumor with peritoneal carcinomatosis; relap. p.o. 3. Died of pulmonary emboli p.o. 12

Table 4–6. Complications following Colon Resection and Colocolonic Anastomosis

Sutured (71)	
Related—(0)	
Possibly related—(0)	
	Postoperative small bowel obstruction successfully treated by Cantor tube
Stapled (61)	
No anastomotic complications	

The satisfactory results following stapling procedures in this series were not due to the efforts of a single experienced and skillful surgeon, but rather of a large number of staff surgeons and residents. It should be noted, however, that acquisition of experience and skill with these instruments was achieved in a gradual, organized fashion. No one inexperienced in the stapling technique performed an anastomosis without a preceptor being part of the operating team. Despite its apparent simplicity, there are just as many pitfalls to be avoided in learning stapling techniques as there are in learning how to sew. Once this technique is mastered, there appears to be no significant difference in results, comparing stapled and sutured anastomoses. Since the average stapled anastomosis takes no more than two to three minutes to perform, one reason for the increasing popularity of stapling is readily apparent. At present, approximately 60% of the anastomoses in our institution are done with stapling techniques. They are particularly appropriate in critically ill patients in whom curtailment of operating and anesthesia time may be important.

Table 4–7. Complications following Small Intestinal Anastomoses

Sutured (30)	
Related—(1)	
	Enterocutaneous fistula, 12 days duration, after side-to-side ileosigmoidostomy for carcinomatosis with obstruction
Stapled (105)	
Related—(4)	
	Leak following operation for strangulated hernia; resection done in groin and anastomosis forcibly reduced into abdominal cavity via hernial opening; relap. p.o. 7; *technical error*
	Enterocutaneous fistula following resection and anastomosis of multiple segments of small bowel for strangulating intestinal obstruction and abdominal abscesses, 10 days after hysterectomy; healed on hyperalimentation
	Enterocutaneous fistula following 2 small intestinal resections, sigmoid resection and drainage of abscesses for Crohn's enterocolitis and peritonitis; died of sepsis
	Enterocutaneous fistula following small bowel resection and resection enterovesical fistula in 71 year old with carcinomatosis and obstruction; died of sepsis
Possibly related—(1)	
	Relaparotomy, enterolysis for adhesive small bowel obstruction 30 days after resection of jejunal angiodysplasia; no leak

Table 4–8. Complications following Colostomy Closure

Sutured (33)	
No anastomotic complications	
Stapled (33)	
Related—(2)	
	Obstruction; perianastomotic inflammation; reresection p.o. 14
	Fecal fistula; stapled anastomosis constructed under tension; *technical error*

Table 4–9. Complications following Esophagogastrostomy

Sutured (4)
No anastomotic complications
Stapled (5)
No anastomotic complications

Table 4–10. Complications following Anterior Resection of Rectum

Sutured (38)	
Related (3)	
	Perianastomotic abscess; drained transrectally
	Fecal fistula; conservative treatment
	Localized leak in patient with gauze pack in place for 3 days due to presacral hemorrhage. No relap.
Sutured and stapled (Baker side-to-end) (44)	
No anastomotic complications	
Stapled (2)	
No anastomotic complications	

In conclusion, data presented in this study do not show any significant difference in the incidence of anastomotic complications when stapled anastomoses are compared with sutured procedures in the gastrointestinal tract.

References

DePetz AA (1927) Aseptic technique of stomach resection. Ann Surg 86:388

Dutton JW et al. (1976) Mortality and prognosis of obstructing carcinoma of the large bowel. Am J Surg 131:36

Gritsman JJ (1966) Mechanical suture by Soviet apparatus in gastric resection: use in 4,000 operations. Surgery 59:663

Latimer RG et al. (1975) Automatic staple suturing for gastrointestinal surgery. Am J Surg 130:766

Lawson WR et al. (1977) Mechanical suture methods in thoracic and abdominal surgery. Br J Surg 64:115

Ravitch MM et al. (1959) Experimental and clinical use of the Soviet bronchus stapling instruments. Surgery 46:1, 97

Ravitch MM et al. (1966) Closure of duodenal, gastric and intestinal stumps with wire staples: experimental and clinical studies. Ann Surg 163:573

Ravitch MM, Rivarola A (1966) Enteroanastomosis with an automatic stapling instrument. Surgery 59:270

Ravitch MM, Steichen FM (1972) Techniques of staple suturing in gastrointestinal tract. Ann Surg 175:815

Schrock TR et al. (1973) Factors contributing to leakage of colonic anastomoses. Ann Surg 177:513

Steichen FM, Ravitch MM (1973) Mechanical sutures in surgery. Br J Surg 70:191

Welch JP, Donaldson GA (1974) Management of severe obstruction of the large bowel due to malignant disease. Am J Surg 127:492

5 Incision, Exposure, and Closure

Achieving Exposure

Many dangerous surgical mishaps occur because the operative exposure is inadequate. The first step in obtaining good exposure is a well-planned incision of sufficient length.

The second step requires that the intestines be packed away from the area of operation. If a dissection requires the exposure of a large portion of the abdominal cavity, such as for left hemicolectomy or excision of an abdominal aortic aneurysm, the small intestine should be exteriorized into a sterile *plastic bag* for the duration of the dissection.

The third step is the retraction of the wound edges. This is accomplished by having an assistant apply a Richardson retractor to the abdominal wall, and deep retractors, such as the Harrington, to deeper structures. In some situations, a mechanical self-retaining retractor, such as the Balfour, may be inserted to separate the lips of a long abdominal incision. In the thoracoabdominal incision, a Finochietto retractor is excellent for separating the ribs.

One disadvantage of using a mechanical self-retaining retractor in the abdomen is that it may inflict trauma if intense pressure is exerted against the rectus muscles. This pressure can be lessened by using long incisions and by padding the musculature with moist gauze pads. If the Balfour retractor is not needed for exposure, it should not be used, as prolonged pressure, ischemia, and trauma of the abdominal muscles all encourage wound infection.

The *"chain" retractor* (**Fig. 5–1**), developed at the University of Alabama Medical School, as reported by Aldrete et al., is an inexpensive improvisation that permits the insertion of a retractor blade beneath the lower end of the sternum or beneath either costal margin. The retractor is attached to an ordinary link chain, which can be purchased in a hardware store for about $2.00. To the side rail at the head of the operating table the anesthesiologist attaches a curved steel post borrowed from the gynecological lithotomy stirrup set. When the post is adjusted to the proper height, the chain is fixed to a snap at the tip. By rotating the post in the proper direction, the lower end of the sternum and the thoracic cage can be retracted forcefully cephalad and anteriorly to elevate the sternum by as much as 8–10 cm.

This device is ideal for operations around the lower esophagus, such as a vagotomy or hiatus hernia repair. It does not require the purchase of new instruments other than 25–30 cm of chain. It may be installed when necessary, without preparation, even in the middle of an operation. It is also very helpful in liberating the splenic flexure of the colon. Here the device is placed on the left side of the operating table and the retractor is positioned to draw the left costal margin to the left, cephalad and anteriorly, thus improving exposure tremendously. Whenever exposure for operations on the biliary tract is difficult, application of the "chain" retractor to the right costal margin can be of great benefit.

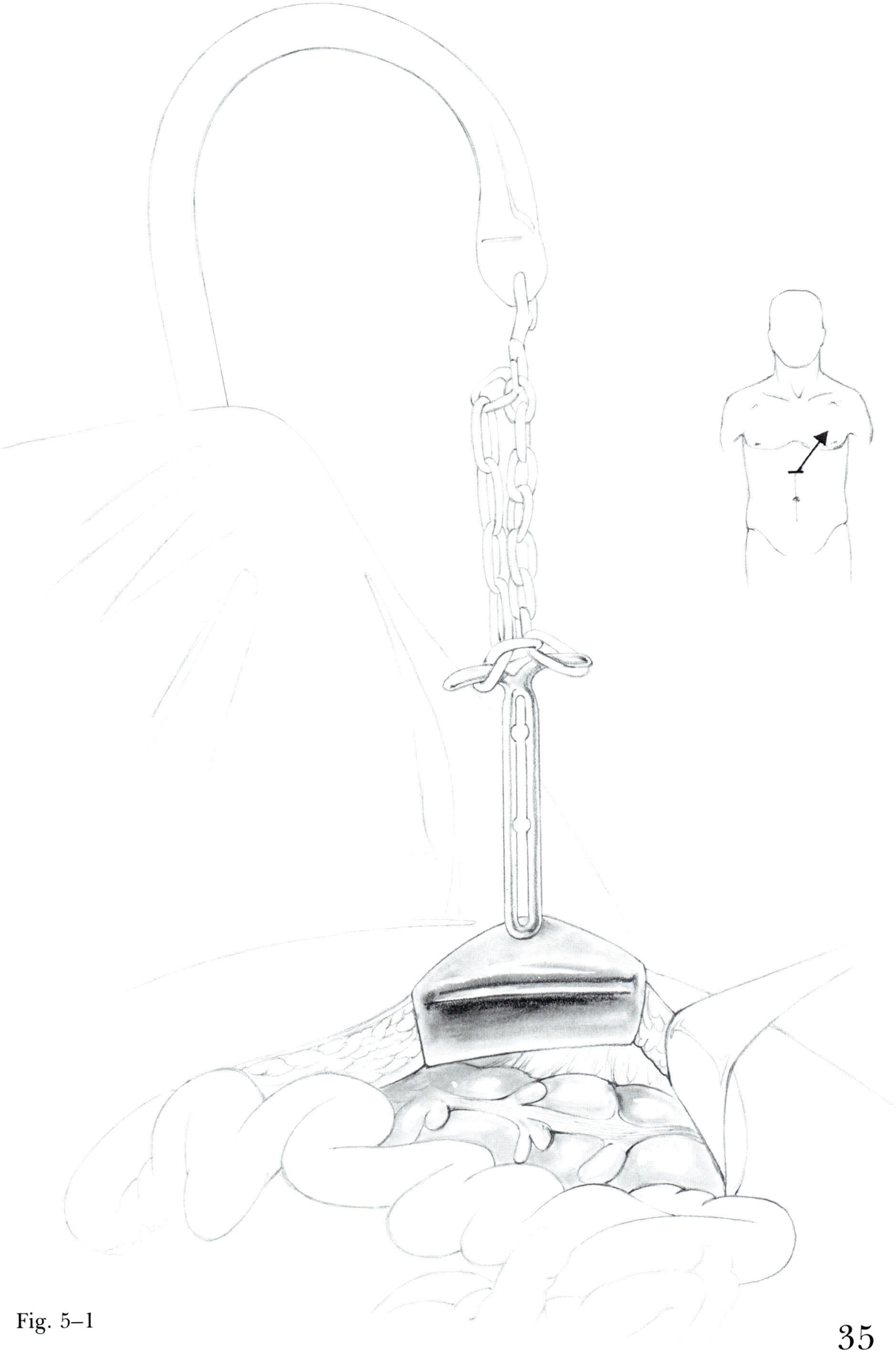

Fig. 5–1

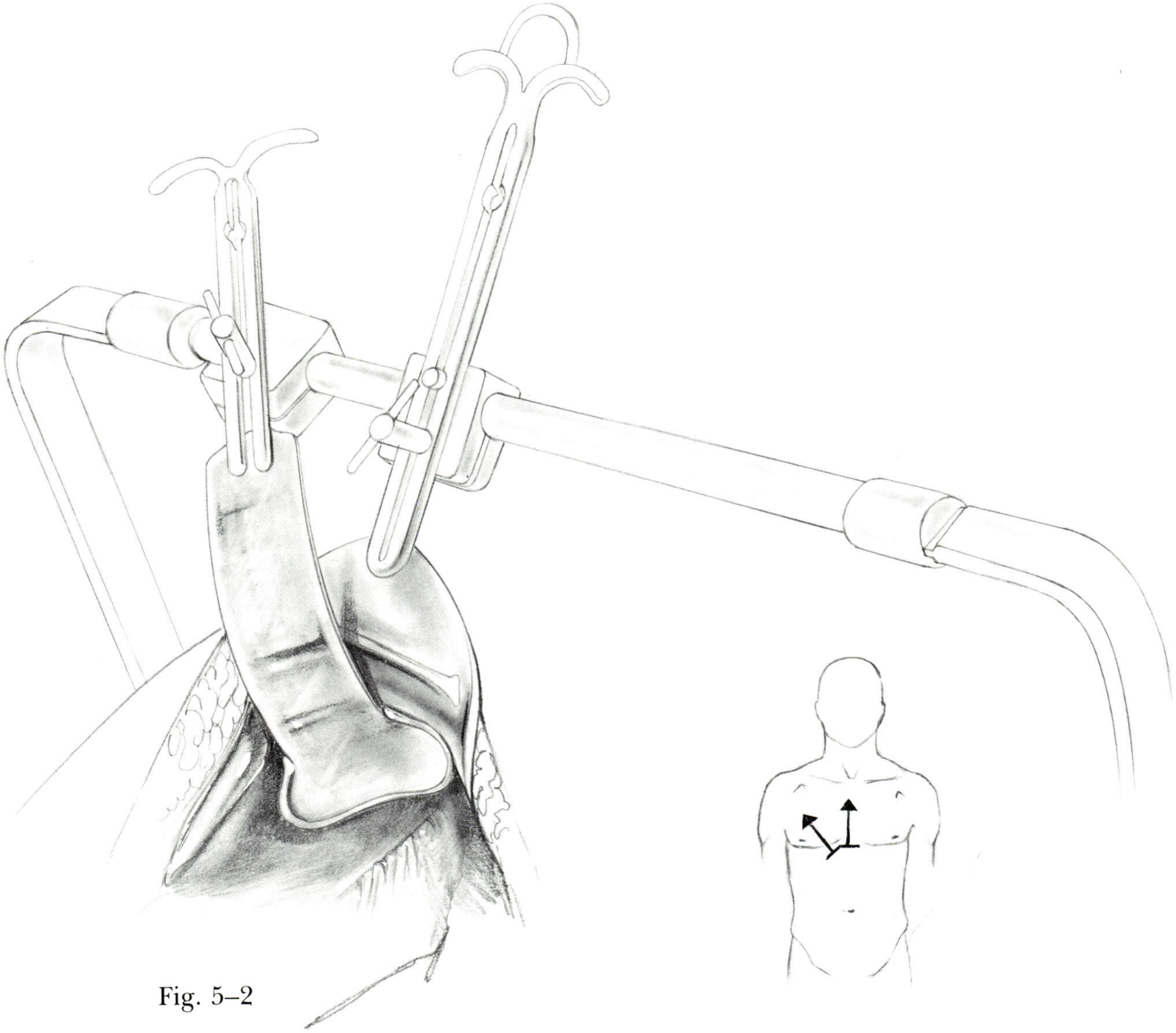

Fig. 5–2

Another mechanical retractor that is attached to the operating table to improve upper abdominal exposure is the *Upper Hand retractor* (**Fig. 5–2**) developed by Lally. This device is a steel bridge that is attached to both sides of the operating table and passes across the patient at the midsternal level. Its height is set at 4–10 cm above the sternum, depending upon the type of retraction desired. Two separate retractor blades can be attached to the steel bridge, one of which may be used to elevate the lower sternum in a manner similar to the "chain" retractor. A second blade may be attached to the bridge to retract the liver for biliary tract surgery; this method sometimes eliminates the need for a second assistant.

The primary aim of the "chain" and the Upper Hand retractors is not to reduce the number of assistants in the operating room, though. These devices are used because the exposure they provide in upper abdominal incisions cannot be duplicated by hand-held retractors.

Incisions for Abdominal Surgery

Although many surgeons have long believed that transverse incisions are stronger and have a lower incidence of dehiscence than midline incisions, this belief is false (see following section). Some think that the upper transverse incision interferes less with respiration than does the upper midline incision. Clinically, this does not appear to be important. A long, vertical *midline incision* gives excellent exposure for all parts of the abdomen. It also provides flexibility, since extensions in either direction are simple to execute. With the aid of either the "chain" or Upper Hand retractor, splenectomy, splenic flexure resection, hiatus hernia repair, vagotomy, pancreatectomy, and biliary tract surgery can easily be done. Whenever exposure in the upper abdomen by this technique is inadequate, it is a simple matter to extend the midline incision into a right or left *thoracoabdominal* approach by dividing the costal cartilage and intercostal muscles. Yet another advantage of midline incisions is the speed with which they can be opened and closed.

In spite of these advantages, we often use a *subcostal* approach for cholecystectomy because a shorter length of incision provides direct exposure of the gallbladder bed. If the gallbladder has already been removed, and if a secondary common duct exploration is necessary or a pancreaticoduodenectomy is contemplated, a midline incision extending 6–8 cm below the umbilicus provides excellent exposure and is preferred.

For the usual appendectomy, the traditional *McBurney* incision affords reasonable exposure, a strong abdominal wall, and a good cosmetic result. To accomplish the same exposure with a vertical incision would require either a long midline or paramedian incision or an incision along the lateral border of the rectus muscle, which might transect two intercostal nerves and produce some degree of abdominal weakness.

Avoiding Wound Dehiscence and Hernia

Although a number of reports have appeared in the literature specifying rates of dehiscence well under 1%, both Efron and a *Lancet* editorial reported that the incidence of abdominal wound disruption is more like 3%–5% throughout the world for "routine" surgery performed by surgeons who do not have a particular interest in avoiding this complication. As recently as 1975, Goligher et al. in a controlled study found a 10% incidence of wound dehiscence in 107 patients whose wounds had been closed in multiple layers, using chromic catgut, rather than with mass sutures. Because abdominal wound dehiscence has been followed by mortality rates as high as 35% and by a high incidence of large incisional hernias, the problem deserves close study.

The major causes of wound disruption are:

- Inadequate strength of suture material
- Rapid absorption of suture material, e.g., catgut
- Knots becoming untied, especially with some monofilaments like nylon and Prolene
- Sutures tearing through the tissue

All these causes except the last are self-explanatory; suture tear is poorly understood by the majority of surgeons. A stitch will tear through if it is tied too tightly or if it encompasses too small a mass of tissue. While it is true that in some patients there appears to be a diminution in the strength of the tissue and its resistance to tearing, especially in the aged and in extremely depleted individuals, this does not explain the fact that many wound disruptions occur in healthy patients.

Through extensive experience in the experimental laboratory with healing laparotomy wounds in normal and protein-depleted rats, we have compiled unpublished data demonstrating that as long as the incision is held together for a sufficient period of time, healing does occur. The rate of increase in the tensile strength of the healing wound is markedly depressed after an animal has lost 25% of its body weight, but 3 weeks following the laparotomy, satisfactory wound strength has developed. The problem, therefore, when collagen deposition takes place at a slow rate, is to support these wounds for a sufficient period of time to permit healing to occur. When a healthy, middle-aged patient with good muscular development disrupts the incision following an uncomplicated cholecystectomy, there must be a mechanical explanation. Invariably the surgeon has closed the wound with multiple small stitches of fine suture material. Under these circumstances, a healthy sneeze by a muscular individual tears the sutures out of the fascia and peritoneum because the muscle pull exceeds the combined suture-tissue strength.

If the problem, then, is to maintain tissue approximation during a sneeze or abdominal distension for a period of time sufficient for even the depleted patient to heal, what is the best technique to use? We now have adequate data to identify the principles that must be observed if the rate of dehiscence is to be reduced below 1%, especially in the poor-risk patient. 1) Jones et al., Sanders et al., Jenkins, and Spencer et al. found that proper technique demands that a large mass of tissue be included in the stitch. 2) According to Sanders et al., Jenkins, and Martyak and Curtis, the stitch must be tied in a relatively loose fashion so that approximation is achieved and not much more.

Although Jones used a near-and-far type stitch with monofilament wire, resulting in only one dehiscence in 197 cases, his description and illustrations seem to indicate that no more than 1 cm of tissue was included in the stitch on either side of the incision. Spencer used a bite of 3 cm on each side of the linea alba and placed his wire sutures 1 cm apart. He experienced one wound disruption in 293 patients. According to Tera and Alberg, a midline incision closed in this manner resists 3 times the bursting force of a paramedian incision closed in layers and 1.7 times that of a transverse incision, when tested in a cadaver.

In clinical trials Goligher et al. found that the use of a layer closure, supplemented by large and closely spaced retention sutures through all the layers of the abdominal wall and skin, can keep the wound dehiscence rate in the vicinity of 1%. However, these retention sutures have to be left in place for at least 2 weeks, which often results in pain and infection because they cut the skin. Also, if the patient develops a serious subcutaneous abscess, adequate drainage in the presence of retention sutures is quite difficult. The development of necrotizing fasciitis is much less likely if the skin can be laid open widely; this is not possible when retention sutures are used.

There is evidence that the mass closure of the midline incision need not be done exclusively with wire nor exclusively with interrupted sutures. Jenkins and Martyak and Curtis reported on studies in which the same large-size tissue bites using one continuous suture of No. 2 nylon were taken in the linea alba, resulting in a minimal number of wound disruptions.

Modified Smead-Jones Wire Closure of Midline Incisions

Since 1961 virtually all the abdominal surgery we have performed has been through midline incisions, which have been closed by the modified Smead-Jones technique described below. (Appendectomies were done by the McBurney incision and are not included in this series.) Most cholecystectomies have been performed through right subcostal incisions. From 1961 to 1970, because of the mistaken belief that the transverse incision was less prone to wound dehiscence, 478 of these subcostal incisions were closed with continuous catgut to the peritoneum and interrupted cotton sutures to the fascia. There were five wound disruptions in this group, for a 1% dehiscence rate.

Since 1970 over 300 subcostal incisions have been closed by the modified Smead-Jones technique, with no dehiscences noted. A retrospective study is under way of approximately 1500 midline and 300 subcostal incisions, performed by the author or residents under his supervision, that employed a modified Smead-Jones technique using monofilament wire. Preliminary results of this study reveal that 30% of the patients were operated upon for carcinoma and 30% underwent colon resection and anastomosis. The mean age of the patients was in the seventh decade. Many of the patients, encountered before parenteral hyperalimentation became available, were nutritionally depleted and seriously ill, including a number with abdominal sepsis. Incisions made through a previous scar in the abdominal wall were eliminated from the study. There was only one wound dehiscence in this group of 1800 cases. The patient was an 83-year-old debilitated man suffering from carcinomatosis. His dehiscence was due to a technical error: an inadequate bite of tissue was enclosed in the abdominal sutures, all of which cut through by the eighth postoperative day.

Although there was some trepidation at the onset of this study that the intra-abdominal loops of wire might trap intestine, it is striking that there were no cases of intestinal fistula or other evidence that the bowel was lacerated by a wire suture. In the 1800 abdominal closures, using probably 16,000 sutures, there were only three suture sinuses leading to a wire stitch. There were six instances in which the end of a broken wire had penetrated the skin, with no evidence of surrounding inflammation; this complication occurred in thin patients. In two cases, marked induration appeared for a distance of 2–3 cm at the fascial level of the wound. Upon exploration, a granuloma was found in each case. Since both of these granulomas were in contiguity with a wire suture, it was assumed that this represented a foreign-body reaction secondary to the wire knot.

While the above statistics reveal that complications from monofilament wire, used by the technique to be described, are astonishingly rare, wire does have one serious disadvantage. It appears to produce a higher incidence of pain in the incision than is seen with other types of suture material. It is estimated that 2%–4% of patients who undergo this type of abdominal closure require the removal of one or two of the wire sutures from the abdominal wall because of localized pain. This is generally performed as an office procedure, using local anesthesia. In six cases (0.3% of the series), because of the persistent complaint of incisional pain, which was not localized, general anesthesia was employed for the removal of all the wire sutures in the abdominal wall. One explanation for the pain is that after a period of 6–12 months, some of the steel wire sutures break, as revealed by X ray. It is remarkable that, as far as we know, none of these broken wires has given rise to any clinically evident intra-abdominal complication. One-third of the six patients continued to experience pain even after all the wires had been excised.

Although the incidence of complications accompanying this technique is minimal, nevertheless the complaint of pain is annoying to patient and surgeon alike. Consequently, other suture materials should be studied for use in abdominal closure. A brief trial of 0 Prolene using the same technique of closure revealed an excessive number of suture sinuses and incisional pain, probably because of the large number of knots required. Although we have not had any experience with it, there is also a technique that uses continuous No. 2 nylon in the abdominal wall, taking large bites of tissue, with the knots tied inside the abdominal cavity; Martyak and Curtis have reported it has produced no dehiscence in 280 operations.

A trial at Booth Memorial Hospital of 250 consecutive abdominal closures, using No. 1 synthetic absorbable polyglycolic (PG) sutures resulted in no wound disruptions, but one patient developed a large hernia around a colostomy that had been brought out through the midline section. In our series of 1800 wire closures, there were no massive incisional hernias, except in one patient who developed necrotizing fasciitis. When postoperative incisional hernias did appear, the diameter of the ring was almost always 1–3 cm, as though one wire had either broken or cut through. Often the location of the hernia was adjacent to the umbilicus, where special care should have been taken to avoid leaving a gap in the closure.

While the nature of suture material may change in the future, it seems clear that a mass closure of the midline incision, paying special attention not to tie the stitches too tightly, can virtually eliminate the problem of wound disruption. An absorbable suture, similar to the polyglycolic material, but that can remain strong for 1 or 2 months instead of only 2–3 weeks, would be the ideal stitch for abdominal closure.

Operative Technique for Midline Incision

Making the Incision

Hold a large gauze pad in the left hand and apply lateral traction on the skin, as the first assistant does the same on the opposite side of the incision. Use the scalpel with a firm sweep along the course of the incision (**Fig. 5–3**). The initial stroke should go well into the subcutaneous fat. Then reapply the gauze pads to provide lateral traction against the subcutaneous fat, and use the belly of the scalpel blade to carry the incision down to the linea alba, making as few knife strokes as possible. The linea alba can be identified in the upper abdomen by observing the decussation of fascial fibers. Confirm this by palpating the tip of the xiphoid, which indicates the midline.

The custom of discarding the scalpel used for the skin incision, in the belief that it has thereby incurred bacterial contamination, is not supported by data, as Jacobs has shown, or by logic; it need not be observed.

Whether towels or an adherent sheet of plastic (Vi-Drape) are affixed to the skin in an effort to prevent contamination

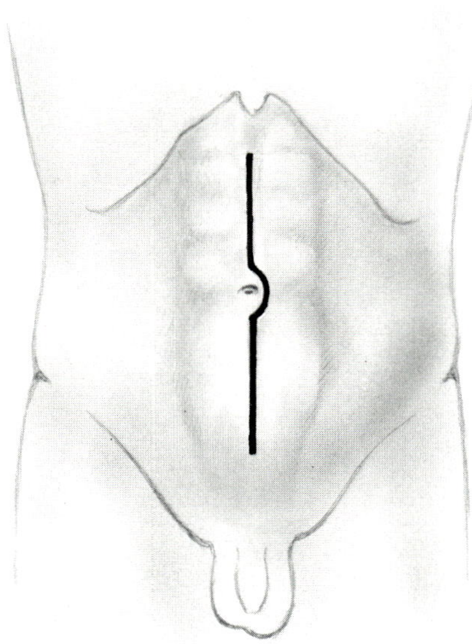

Fig. 5–3

from the skin into the incision is up to the surgeon. There does not appear to be any data proving the advantage in covering the skin with either material.

Because the subcutaneous fat seems to be the body tissue most susceptible to infection, every effort should be made to minimize trauma to this layer. Use as few hemostats and ligatures as possible; most bleeding points will stop spontaneously in a few minutes. If not, ligate small bites of tissue with 4–0 PG. Electrocoagulation of subcutaneous fat causes extensive trauma, which encourages wound infection. This modality should not be used in this layer.

Continuing lateral traction with gauze pads, divide the linea alba with the scalpel. If the incision is to be continued around and below the umbilicus, leave a 5–8 mm patch of linea alba attached to the umbilicus to permit purchase by a suture when the closure is being accomplished. Otherwise, a gap between sutures may appear at the umbilicus, leading to an incisional hernia.

As Martyak and Curtis have suggested, the peritoneum should be opened well to the left of the falciform ligament. When the peritoneum is opened close to its attachment to the undersurface of the left rectus muscle, virtually no blood vessels are encountered. Consequently, elevate the peritoneum between two forceps and incise it just above and to the left of the umbilicus. Using a Metzenbaum scissors, continue this incision in a cephalad direction until the upper pole of the incision is reached. If bleeding points are encountered here, grasp them with small hemostats and electrocoagulate or ligate them.

So as not to cut the bladder, be certain when opening the peritoneum in the lower abdomen to identify the prevesical fat and bladder. As the peritoneum approaches the prevesical region, the preperitoneal fat cannot be separated from the peritoneum and becomes somewhat thickened and more vascular. If there is any question about the location of the upper margin of the bladder, note that the balloon of the indwelling Foley catheter can be milked in a cephalad direction. It is easy to identify the upper extremity of the bladder this way. It is not necessary to open the peritoneum into prevesical fat, as this does not improve exposure. However, opening the fascial layer down to and beyond the pyramidalis muscles to the pubis does indeed improve exposure for low-lying pelvic pathology.

Closure of Midline Incision

This closure is almost identical with that reported by Spencer et al. in 1963. As mentioned above, we have modified the Smead-Jones technique by increasing the width of the tissue bite, which is in accord with the clinical data compiled by Sanders et al. and Jenkins indicating that the large bite and the loose suture are essential in preventing dehiscence. It is not necessary, in the upper abdomen, to include the peritoneum or falciform ligament in the suture, and this layer is generally ignored. Below the umbilicus there is no distinct linea alba, and the rectus muscle belly is exposed. In this region include the peritoneum in the stitch.

Apply Kocher clamps to the linea alba at the midpoint of the incision, one clamp on each side. Below the umbilicus the Kocher clamps should include a bite of peritoneum as well as of anterior fascia. With the suture of 2–0 monofilament stainless steel wire or No. 1 PG, encompass 3 cm of tissue on each side of the linea alba; then take a small bite of the linea alba, about 5 mm in width, on each side. This results in a small loop of wire within a large loop (**Fig. 5–4**). The purpose of the small loop is simply to orient the linea alba so that it will remain in apposition, rather than one side moving on top of the other. Place the small loop 5–10 mm below the main body of the suture to help eliminate the gap between adjacent sutures. Insert the next suture no more than 2 cm below the first. Large curved Ferguson needles are used for this procedure.

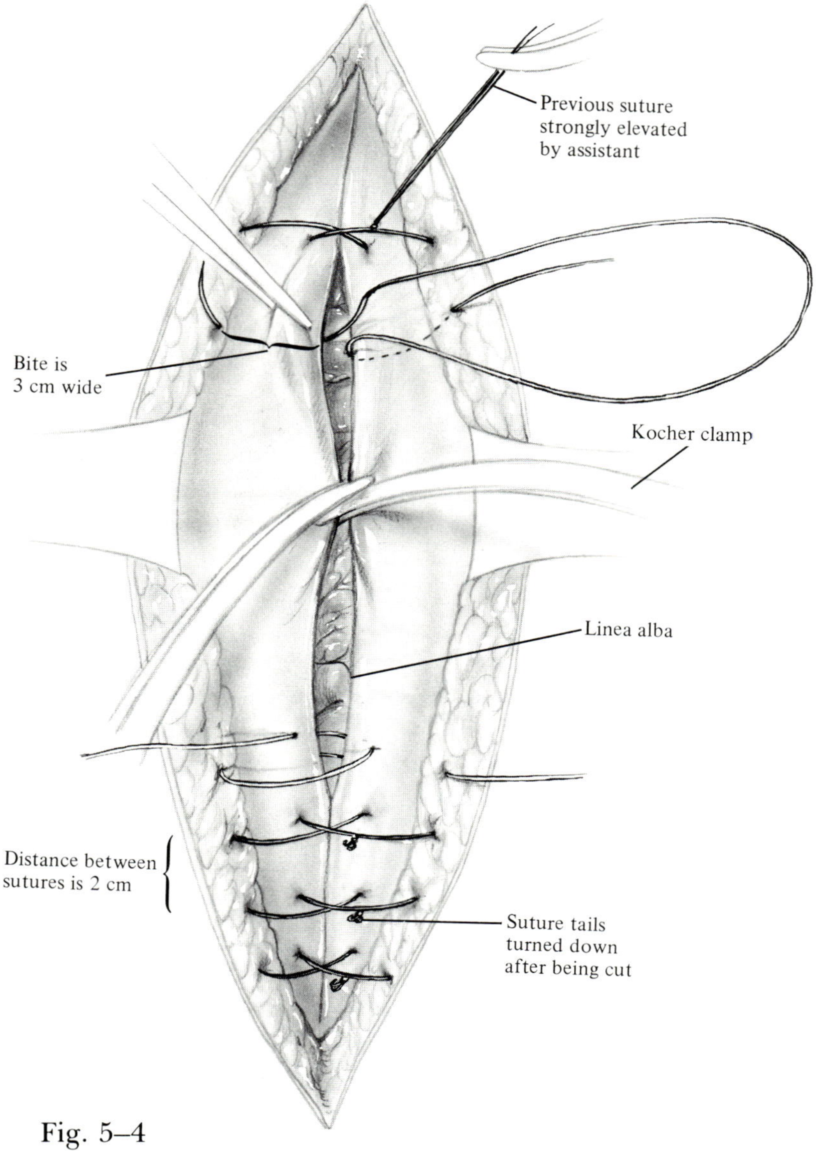

Fig. 5–4

To tie wire sutures properly, the wire *must* be entirely free of kinks. Accomplish a loose square throw and then pull the two wire ends in opposite directions until the knot has achieved adequate tension to approximate the tissue. *Avoid excessive tension*! Draw the two strands of wire sharply in an anterior direction. This maneuver sets the knot while the second square throw is being developed. Again draw the two ends of wire laterally to close the knot. Then apply a third square throw and tighten it. Grasp the two ends of the wire in a small hemostat. The assistant should apply skyward traction on this hemostat to elevate the abdominal wall and facilitate the insertion of the next stitch. If No. 1 PG is used, tie each suture with four square knots. When half the incision has been closed, start at the other end and approach the midpoint with successive sutures (Fig. 5–4). Do not tie the last few stitches, thus leaving enough space to insert the remaining stitch under direct vision. In no case should the surgeon insert a stitch without at all times seeing the point of the needle.

Then tie all the remaining sutures. Apply a straight Crile clamp to each stitch just above the knot, and use a wire scissors to cut the wires just adjacent to the straight clamp, which should be rotated to turn the

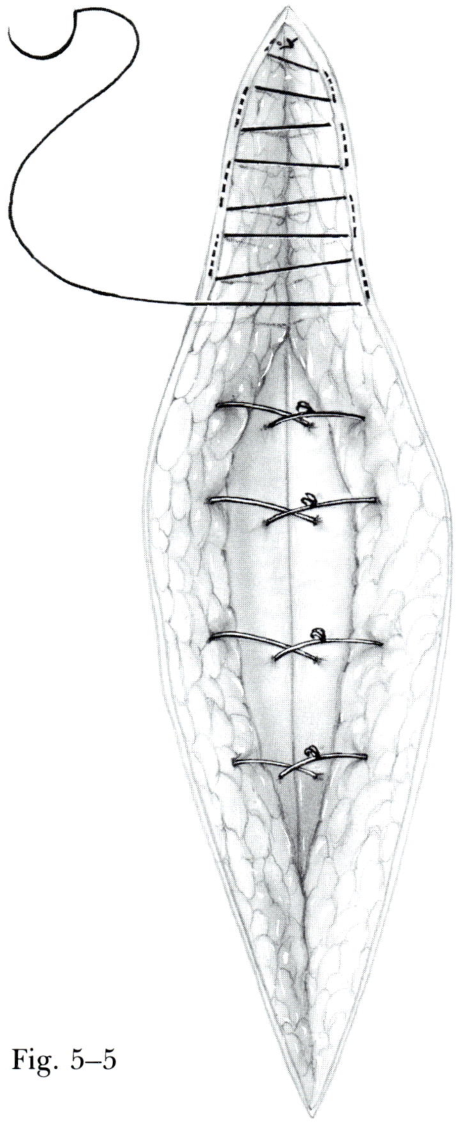

Fig. 5–5

short tails of the wire down toward the fascia. This helps prevent the sharp wire ends from irritating the subcuticular nerve endings (**Fig. 5–5**).

Accomplish skin closure by interrupted 4–0 nylon vertical mattress sutures, a continuous subcuticular suture of 4–0 PG, or staples.

A description of the *McBurney* incision is included in Chap. 24; the *Pfannenstiel* incision will be found in Chap. 42; and the *subcostal* incision under "Cholecystectomy" in Vol. II of this work.

References

Aldrete JS et al. (1977) Scientific exhibit at Clinical Congress Am Coll Surgeons. Dallas TX

Efron G (1965) Abdominal wound disruption. Lancet 1:1287

Goligher JC et al. (1975) A controlled clinical trial of three methods of closure of laparotomy wounds. Br J Surg 62:823

Jacobs HB (1974) Skin knife-deep knife: The ritual and practice of skin incisions. Ann Surg 179:102

Jenkins TPN (1976) The burst abdominal wound—a mechanical approach. Br J Surg 63:873

Jones TE et al. (1941) The use of alloy steel wire in the closure of abdominal wounds. Surg Gynecol Obstet 72:1056

Lally JJ (1967) New exposure instrument for the upper abdomen. Int Surg 47:396

Lancet Editorial (1977) Burst abdomen. Lancet 1:28

Malt RA (1977) Abdominal incisions, sutures and sacrilege. N Engl J Med 297:722

Martyak SN, Curtis LE (1976) Abdominal incision and closure. Am J Surg 131:476

Sanders RJ et al. (1977) Principles of abdominal wound closure—I. Animal studies. Arch Surg 112:1184

Spencer FC et al. (1963) Experiences with wire closure of abdominal incisions in 293 selected patients. Surg Gynecol Obstet 117:235

Tera H, Aberg C (1976) Tissue strength of structures involved in musculo-aponeurotic layer sutures in laparotomy incisions. Acta Chir Scand 142:349

Esophagus

6 Operations to Resect, Replace, or Bypass the Esophagus

Concept: Selection of Operation for Carcinoma near Esophagogastric Junction

A number of surgeons have asserted that resection of the lower esophagus and proximal stomach for lesions near the gastric cardia, followed by esophagogastric anastomosis, is an operation with a high mortality rate and a high incidence of reflux esophagitis. Moreover, some say this operation is no better from the nutritional point of view than total gastrectomy with esophagojejunostomy. Our experience is completely to the contrary. After total gastrectomy, dumping is common and nutritional rehabilitation is often difficult. On the other hand, we have observed that very few patients experience serious symptoms of reflux esophagitis following esophagogastrectomy with an end-to-side anastomosis. No dietary restrictions have been necessary. In 44 consecutive cases, among patients whose average age was over 70, we encountered (and reported) no clinical anastomotic leaks and no deaths.

If a tumor occupies a large segment of the gastric fundus, requiring more than 50% of the stomach to be removed for an adequate cancer operation, then total gastrectomy is indicated because the gastric remnant will be too small to permit construction of a proper end-to-side esophagogastric anastomosis. The end-to-end anastomosis results in an excessive number of leaks as well as reflux bile esophagitis. Otherwise, esophagogastrectomy properly performed is a safe operation with good nutritional and symptomatic results. There are no data as yet from follow-up studies comparing total gastrectomy with esophagogastrectomy, to indicate whether total gastrectomy results in longer survival in patients suffering from cancer of the gastric cardia or fundus.

For cancer of the distal 10–15 cm of the esophagus, we have found a *left* thoracoabdominal incision with esophagogastric resection and anastomosis to be extremely successful. If the tumor extends more proximally than was anticipated, we simply mobilize the esophagus above the arch of the aorta and perform a supra-aortic anastomosis.

Concept: Selection of Operation for Lesions of Mid- and Upper Esophagus

Except for lesions of the lower 10–15 cm of the esophagus, the operation of choice for carcinoma of the esophagus is subtotal resection by right thoracotomy, combined with mobilization of the stomach through a midline laparotomy. This should be followed by end-to-side esophagogastric anastomosis at the apex of the right chest or in the neck. With adequate preoperative preparation, this operation too can be done safely and result in good postoperative digestive function. In some institutions a course of preoperative radiation is given to these patients. Conclusive data to support this policy are not yet available.

As an alternative, it has been suggested that patients who have carcinoma of the midesophagus might undergo staged procedures. As the first stage the colon is interposed between the cervical esophagus and stomach through a substernal tunnel. This is followed by irradiation and then by removal of the thoracic esophagus. Because the majority of the patients who suffer from squamous cell carcinoma of the midesophagus have a limited life expectancy, and because a one-stage esophagogastrectomy can be done with a low mortality rate, this is the procedure of choice.

In those patients whose carcinoma is located in the neck or the upper thorax, the choice lies between an interposition of the left colon from the neck to the stomach or an esophagogastric anastomosis in the neck. Using stapled anastomoses to expedite the procedure, it is feasible in one stage to resect the esophagus and to complete a colon interposition operation. However, satisfactory results can also be obtained with cervical esophagogastrostomy.

Patients who suffer corrosive esophagitis (lye) and who require total esophagectomy or complete esophageal bypass are probably best handled by the interposition of the isoperistaltic left colon between the cervical esophagus or pharynx and stomach. This has been described by Belsey and by Glasgow et al. Similarly, for patients who have nonresectable carcinomas of the midesophagus, a colon bypass of the same type is preferred, although the reversed gastric tube advocated by Heimlich has some enthusiastic supporters. When using either the colon or a reversed gastric tube, it would appear preferable to make the proximal anastomosis in the cervical region, as there appears to be a small but significant incidence of leakage following anastomoses of these two types. If the leakage occurs in the neck, the resulting esophagocutaneous fistula is far less serious than from a similar leak in the thorax.

Concept: Colon or Jejunal Interposition following Resection of Lower Esophagus for Reflux Esophagitis

Almost all cases of stricture following reflux esophagitis can be managed by dilating the esophageal stricture, by lengthening the esophagus via a Collis gastroplasty, and by some type of fundoplication to eliminate reflux. On rare occasions intraoperative dilatation of the esophagus requires so much force that the esophageal wall bursts and must be resected. While it may be hypothesized that esophagogastric resection an end-to-side and anastomosis supplemented by a Nissen-type fundoplication might be successful in these cases, there has been an inadequate trial of this procedure to provide data in its support. On the other hand, Belsey, Glasgow et al., and others have demonstrated that the interposition of colon between the esophagus and stomach successfully prevents a recurrence of reflux esophagitis. The use of jejunal interposition, as described by Merendino, has achieved less popularity than colon interposition because it is more difficult to mobilize an adequate vascular pedicle in the jejunum than the colon. Consequently, following resection of the esophagus for the sequelae of reflux esophagitis, the interposition of a segment of left transverse colon, supported on a pedicle of left colic artery, seems preferable. The esophagocolonic anastomosis in these cases is performed end-to-end; the cologastric anastomosis is the end-to-side type. A modified fundoplication is constructed around the cologastric anastomosis. Operations for gastroesophageal reflux and its complications are described in Vol. II of this work.

References

Belsey R (1965) Reconstruction of the esophagus with left colon. J Thorac Cardiovasc Surg 49:33

Chassin JL (1978) Esophagogastrectomy: data favoring end-to-side anastomosis. Ann Surg 188:22

Glasgow JC et al. (1979) Colon interposition for benign esophageal disease. Am J Surg 137:175

Heimlich HJ (1972) Esophagoplasty with reversed gastric tube. Am J Surg 123:80

Merendino KA, Dillard DH (1955) The concept of sphincter substitution by an interposed jejunal segment for anatomic and physiologic abnormalities at the esophagogastric junction with special reference to reflux esophagitis, cardiospasm and esophageal varices. Ann Surg 142:486

7 Esophagectomy: Right Thoracotomy and Laparotomy

Indications

Esophagectomy via right thoracotomy is indicated in carcinoma of the esophagus, except for tumors of the distal 10–15 cm.

Preoperative Preparation

Institute nutritional rehabilitation, either by intravenous hyperalimentation or by nasogastric tube feeding, in patients who have lost more than 10 lbs. This is an important factor in lowering the mortality rate for this operation.

Perform preoperative esophagoscopy and biopsy.

Improve oral and dental hygiene, if necessary.

Stop patient from smoking.

Conduct a pulmonary function study.

Preoperative radiation therapy is a controversial issue. Until more data are accumulated as to the effect radiation has on postoperative survival, no definitive statement can be made.

Preoperative bronchoscopy is indicated in those patients whose lesion may have invaded the left main bronchus or trachea.

A nasogastric tube should be passed the morning of the operation.

Perioperative antibiotics should be administered.

Pitfalls and Danger Points

Hemorrhage from aorta

Perforation of trachea or bronchus

Anastomotic leak

Anastomotic stenosis

Inadvertent interruption of gastroepiploic arcade on greater curvature of stomach

Operative Strategy

When a tumor of the esophagus is densely adherent to the aortic arch, extreme caution is indicated. If the aorta is inadvertently perforated while the tumor is being removed from the arch, it will be extremely difficult to salvage the patient. If the surrounding aortic wall is indurated by fibrosis or tumor, this will make control of hemorrhage virtually impossible. Furthermore, it is doubtful that heroic measures for the resection of such invasive tumors will prove any more beneficial to the patient than would a palliative operation to bypass the lesion. The same is probably true of tumors that invade the right main bronchus. Long-term survival following the resection of a carcinoma of the middle esophagus is generally limited to those patients whose lesion is confined to the esophagus and shows no evidence of extrinsic invasion.

In favorable cases of this type, both Logan and Skinner have performed radical operations, including excision of the right and left mediastinal pleura, extensive mediastinal lymph node dissection, and thoracic duct dissection. Logan's mortality rate for these operations was over 20%, but modern postoperative care can lower this rate. Up to now the survival data are inadequate to prove that this procedure is effective.

Anastomotic leakage and postoperative stenosis have been minimized by the adoption of several techniques. Obviously it is important to maintain the blood supply to the stomach. This requires meticulous attention to the gastroepiploic arcade. The esophageal hiatus must be enlarged sufficiently to prevent any element of venous compression, as deficiency of the venous circulation is as detrimental as arterial ischemia. Also, as Chassin has pointed out, the use of an end-to-side esophagogastric anastomosis has markedly reduced the incidence of anastomotic leaks (see Chap. 8).

Since the submucosal spread of esophageal carcinoma has been observed by microscopy to extend a considerable distance cephalad from the visible carcinoma, a 10 cm margin of apparently normal esophagus should be removed with the specimen. The upper limit of the specimen should be checked by frozen section examination.

Operative Technique

Incision and Position

Use a small sandbag to elevate the patient's right side 30°, with the right arm abducted and suspended from the "ether screen" cephalad to the surgical field. Turn the patient's head to the left in case the right cervical region has to be exposed for the upper anastomosis. Prepare the right neck, the right hemithorax, and the abdomen. Rotate the operating table slightly so that the abdomen is parallel with the floor. Perform a midline upper abdominal incision for a preliminary exploration of the liver and lower esophagus to help determine whether an attempt should be made at resection. A moderate degree of hepatic metastasis does not contraindicate a palliative esophagectomy. Then make an incision along the course of the fourth intercostal space from the sternum to the posterior axillary line in men (**Fig. 7–1**). In women, make the skin incision in the inframammary fold. Incise

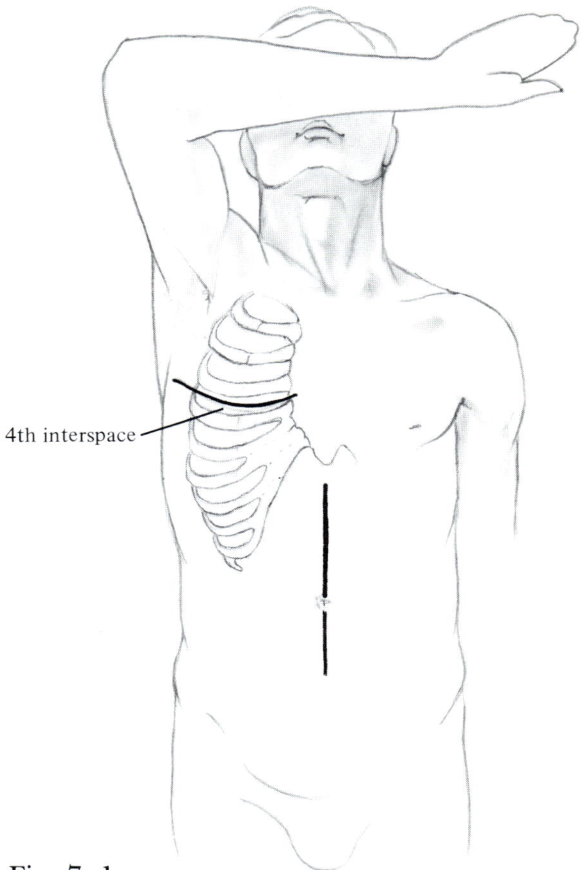

Fig. 7–1

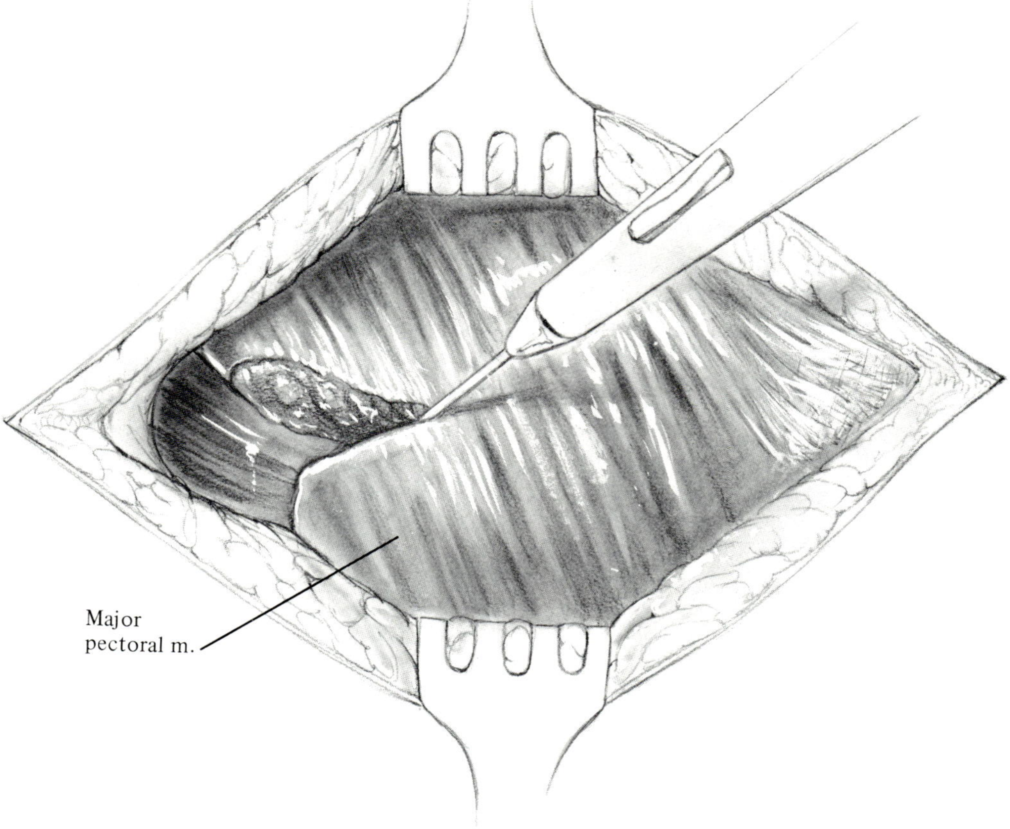

Fig. 7–2

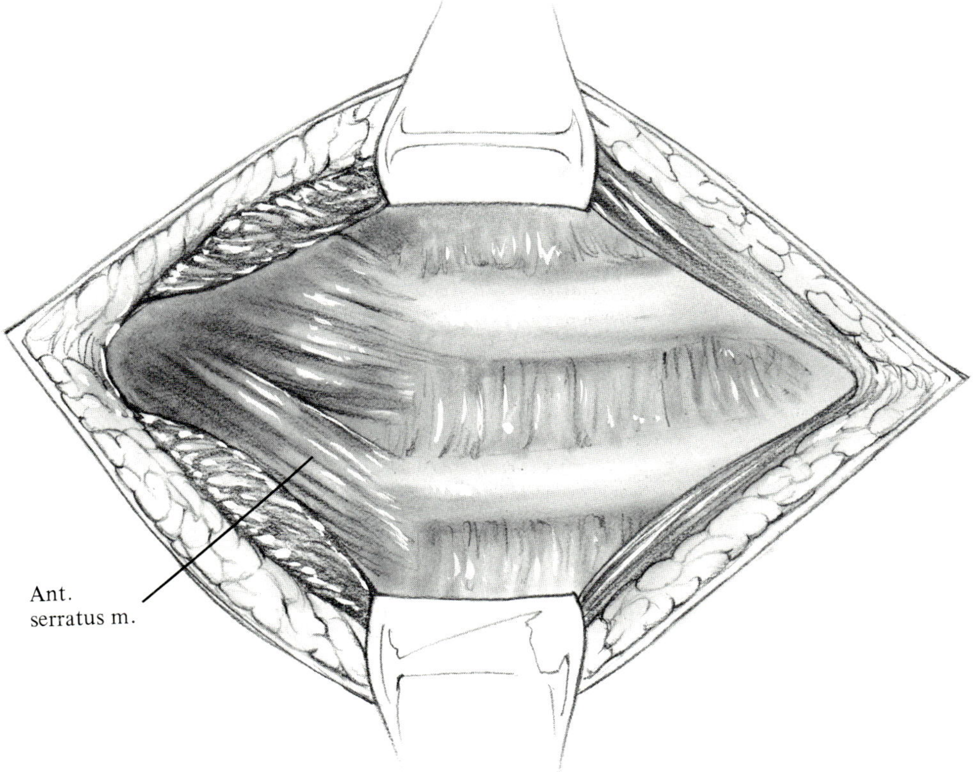

Fig. 7–3

the pectoral and anterior serratus muscles with the electrocoagulator along the fourth interspace (**Figs. 7–2 and 7–3**). Similarly incise the intercostal muscles along the upper border of the fifth rib. Identify the internal mammary artery near the sternal margin, where it is divided and occluded by ligature. Enter the pleura of the fourth intercostal space, and then divide the cartilaginous portion of the fourth rib near its articulation with the sternum (**Fig. 7–4**). Clamp the neurovascular bundle, divide it and ligate with 2–0 cotton (**Fig. 7–5**).

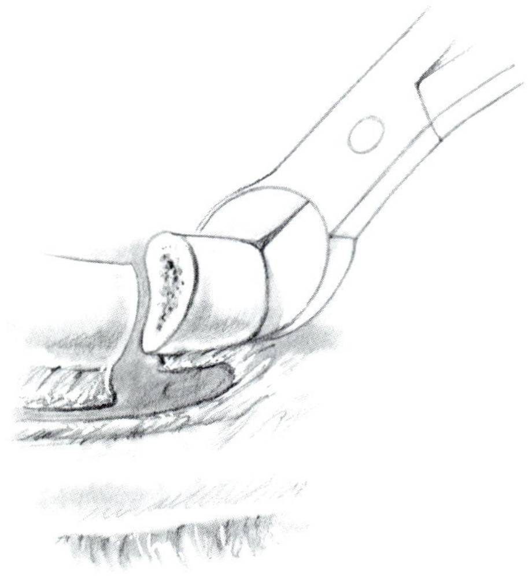

Fig. 7–4

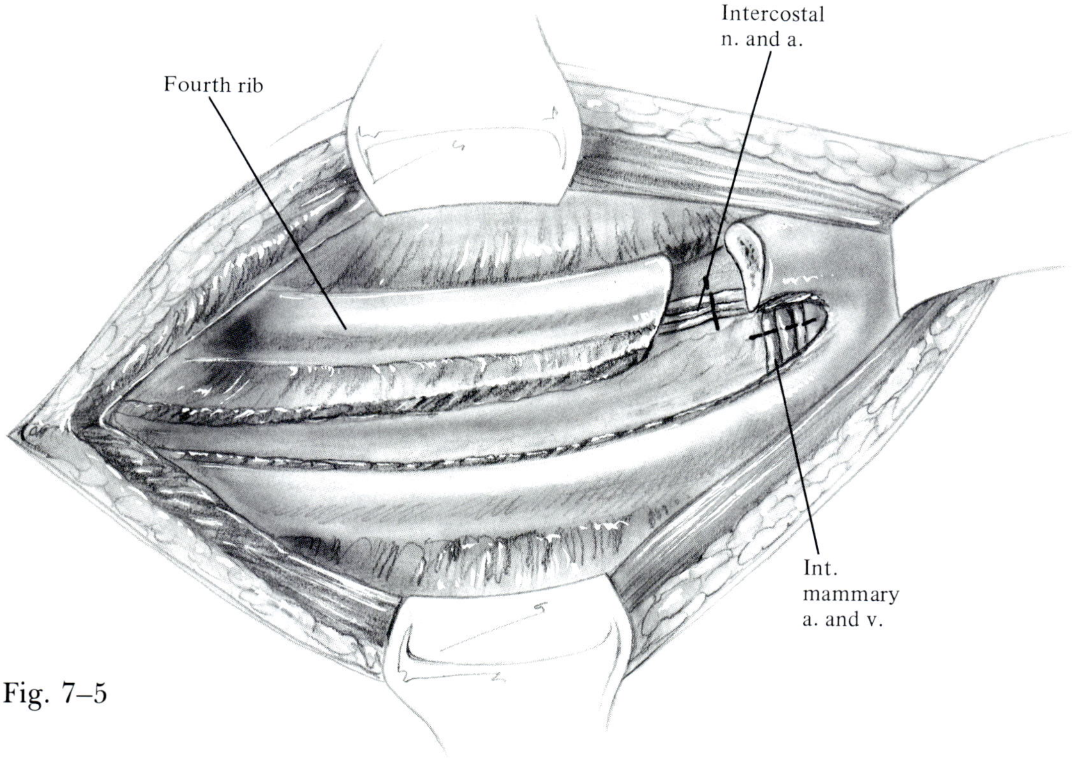

Fig. 7–5

Insert a Finochietto retractor over gauze pads and separate the ribs. If an additional costal cartilage requires division for adequate exposure, do not hesitate to perform this maneuver. Retract the lung anteriorly, cover it with gauze pads and hold it with Harrington retractors.

To perform this procedure, some geons prefer to make a complete posterolateral incision from the region of the paraspinal muscles to the sternum through the fourth or fifth interspace, but we have found the above exposure to be satisfactory. Also, using the anterior incision permits the placing of the patient in a position that is convenient for operating in the abdomen, in the thorax, and even in the neck, as necessary.

Mobilization of Esophagus

Make an incision in the mediastinal pleura, exposing the esophagus. The azygous vein should then be identified, skeletonized, divided, and ligated with 2–0 cotton (**Fig. 7–6**). Encircle the esophagus with the index finger at a point away from the tumor. Dissection will reveal several small arterial branches to the esophagus. Divide each branch between Hemoclips. Wherever the pericardium or pleura are adherent to the tumor, excise patches of these structures and leave them attached to the specimen. Also include adjacent mediastinal lymph nodes in the specimen. Dissect the esophagus from the apex of the chest to the diaphragmatic hiatus. This

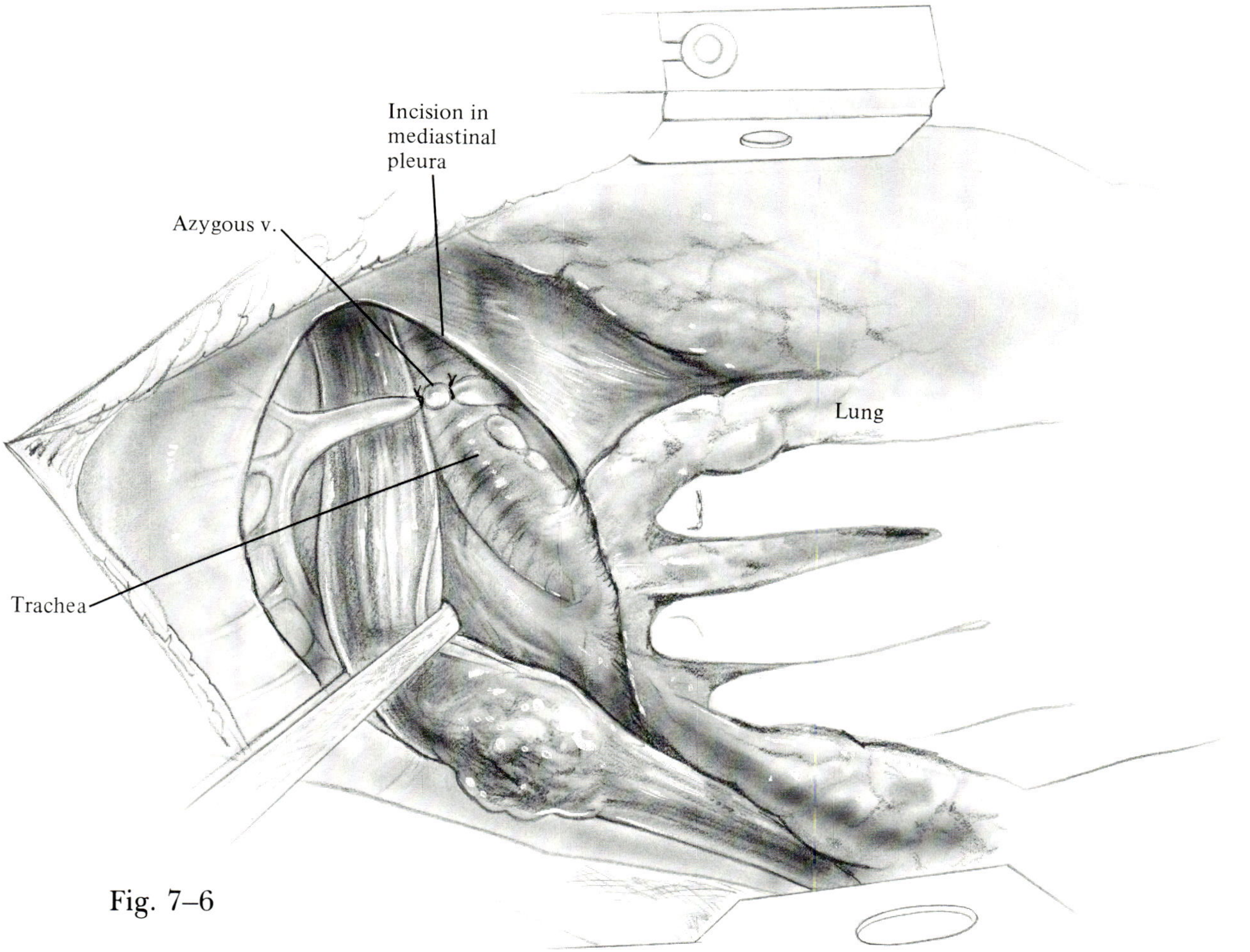

Fig. 7–6

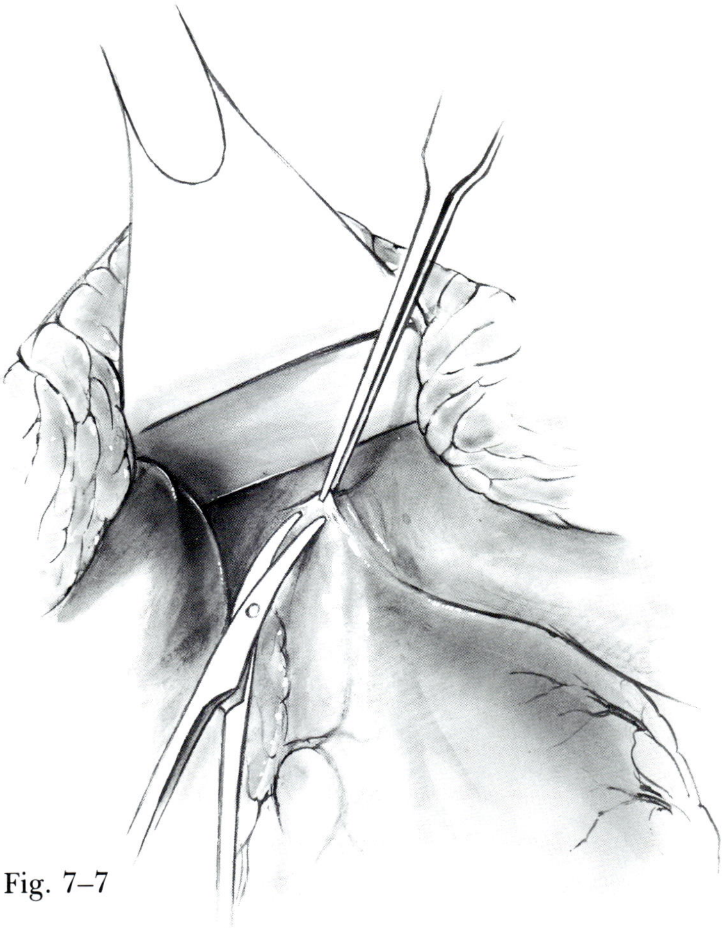

Fig. 7–7

will require the division of the proximal vagal trunks. In order to minimize the spillage of tumor cells, ligate the lumen of the esophagus proximal and distal to the tumor, utilizing narrow umbilical tapes or TA–55 surgical staples.

Remove the Harrington retractors and gauze pads permitting the right lung to expand. Cover the thoracic incision with a sterile towel.

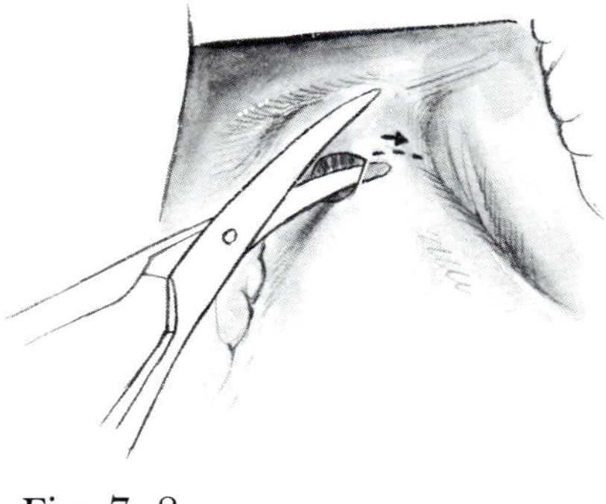

Fig. 7–8

Mobilization of Stomach

Expose the abdominal incision. Use a "chain" retractor to elevate the sternum. Elevate the left lobe of the liver in a cephalad direction with either a Harrington or Weinberg retractor and incise the peritoneum overlying the abdominal esophagus. Mobilize the lower esophagus as in performing a vagotomy and transect the vagal trunks and the surrounding phrenoesophageal ligaments (**Figs. 7–7, 7–8, and**

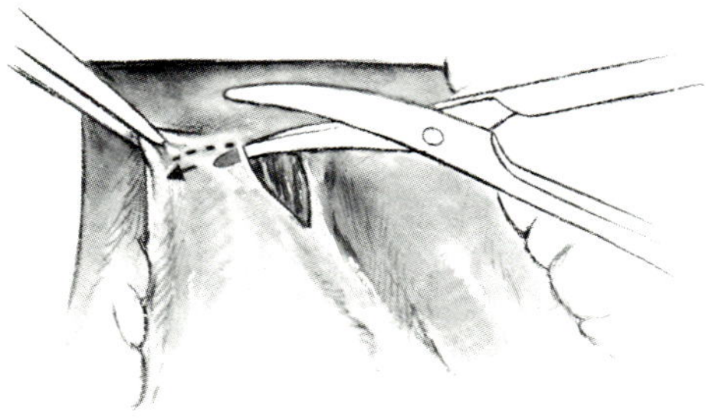

Fig. 7–9

7–9). The cephalad portion of the gastrohepatic ligament, generally containing an accessory left hepatic artery, should be doubly clamped, divided, and ligated with 2–0 cotton or Hemoclips (**Fig. 7–10**). Insert the left hand behind the esophagus and cardia of the stomach, elevate the gastrophrenic ligaments on the index finger and transect them (**Fig. 7–11**). This dissection will lead to the cephalad short gastric vessel; divide it between clamps and ligate it, along with the remaining short gastrics. The spleen need not be removed.

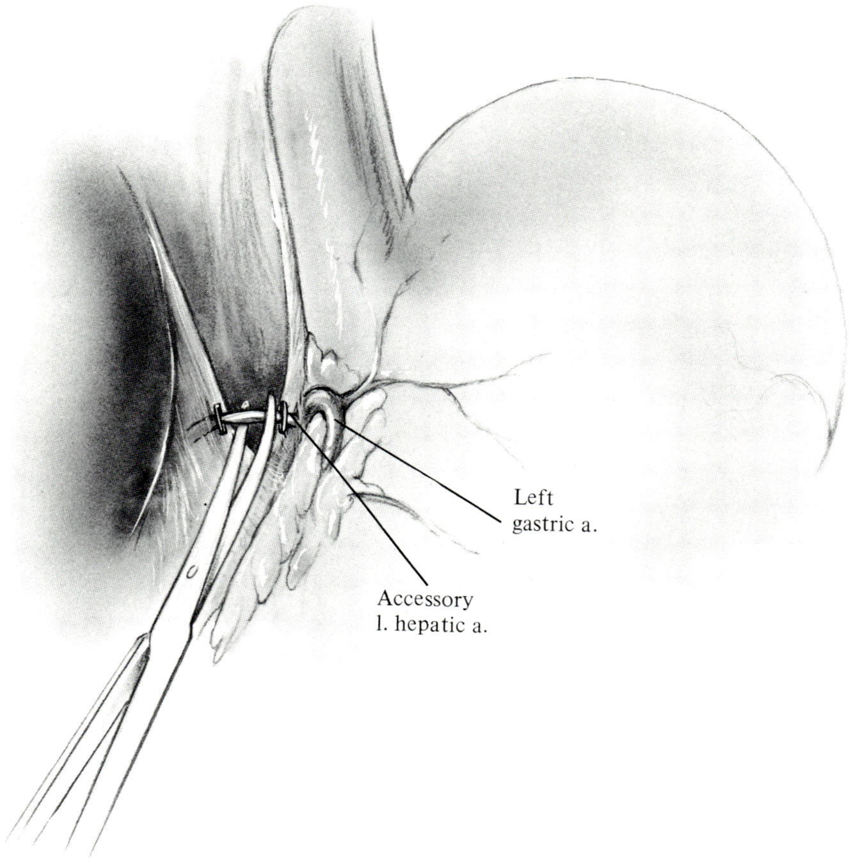

Fig. 7–10

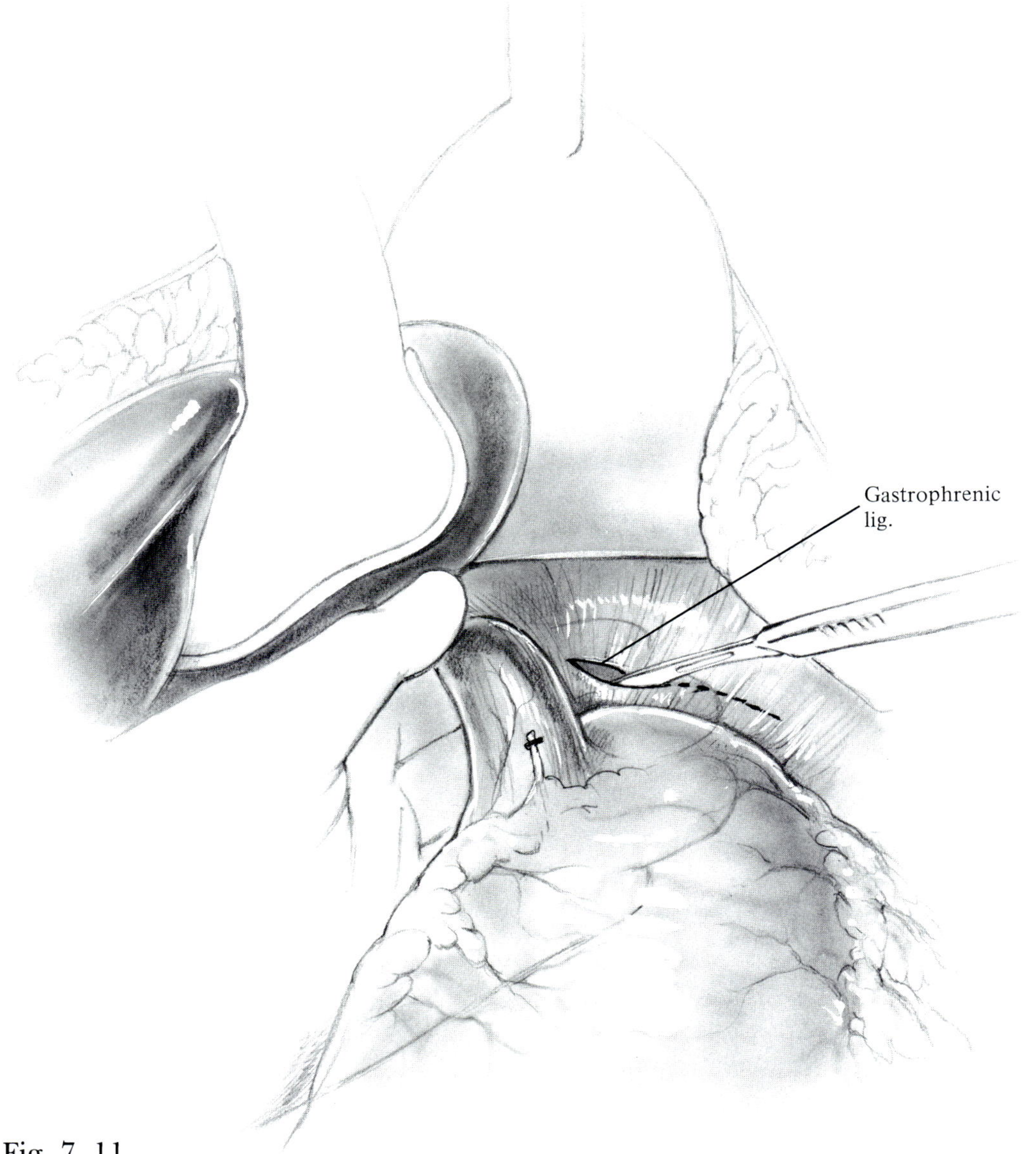

Fig. 7–11

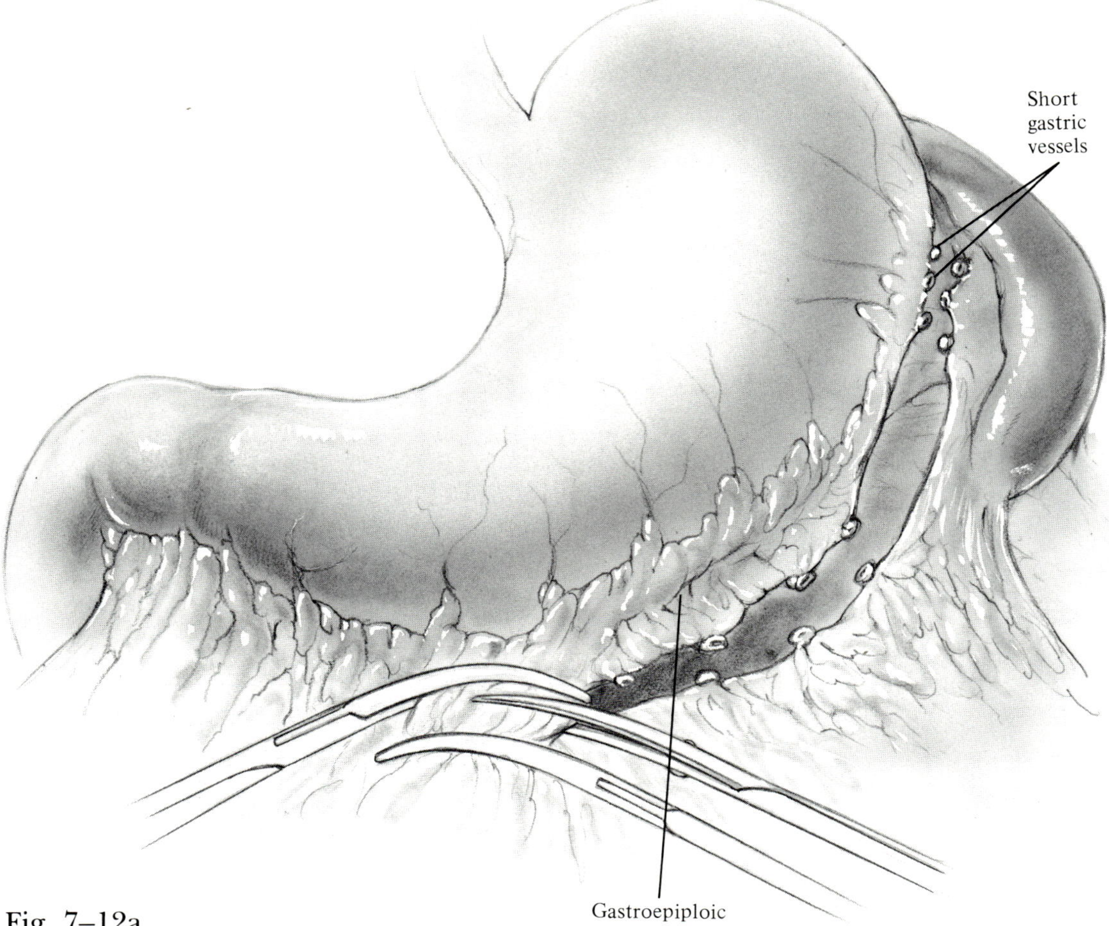

Fig. 7–12a

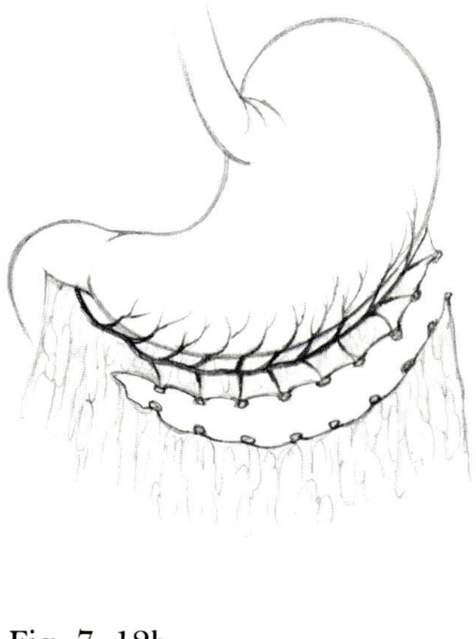

Fig. 7–12b

Divide and ligate the *left* gastroepiploic artery, but do the remainder of the dissection *outside* the gastroepiploic arcade, *which must be kept intact and free of trauma.* This is accomplished by dividing the greater omentum serially between Kelly clamps, leaving 3–5 cm of omentum attached to the arcade as a margin of safety. Discontinue this dissection 6–8 cm proximal to the pylorus (**Figs. 7–12a and 7–12b**).

With the greater curvature of the stomach elevated, use palpation to identify the origin of the left gastric artery at the celiac axis. The coronary vein is situated just caudal to the artery. Clear it and encircle it with a Mixter clamp and then divide it between 2–0 cotton ligatures. Skeletonize the left gastric artery (**Fig. 7–13**)

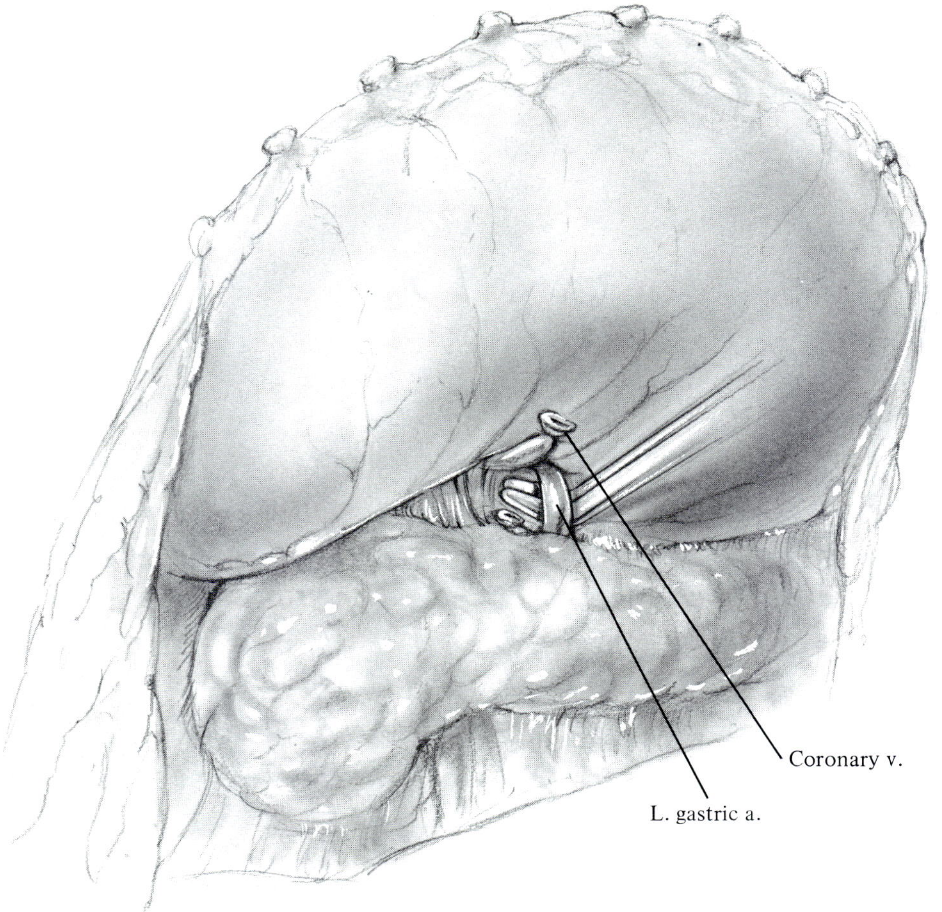

Fig. 7–13

so that two 2–0 cotton ligatures may be placed on the proximal portion of the artery and one on the specimen side. Transect the vessel. Follow this with an extensive Kocher maneuver.

Kocher Maneuver

Make an incision in the peritoneum lateral to the proximal duodenum (**Fig. 7–14**). Insert the left index finger behind the peritoneum and compress this tissue between fingertip and thumb, causing the retroperitoneal blood vessels and fat to fall away. Incise the peritoneum on the index finger with a scissors until the third portion of the duodenum is reached. Note that dividing the peritoneum alone is not sufficient to release the duodenum from its posterior attachments. There remains a ligamentous structure connecting the posterior duodenum to the region of Gerota's fascia.

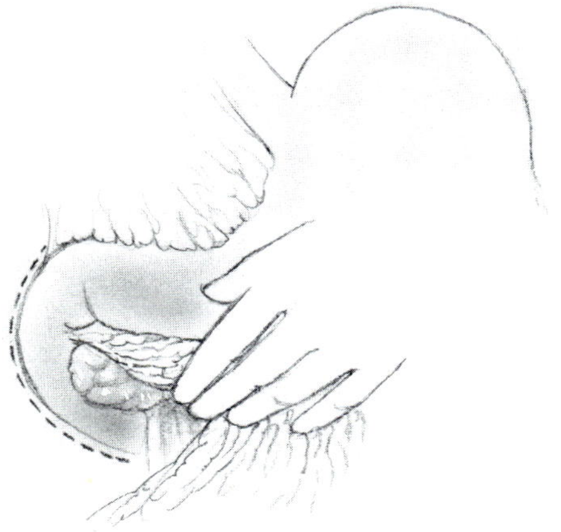

Fig. 7–14

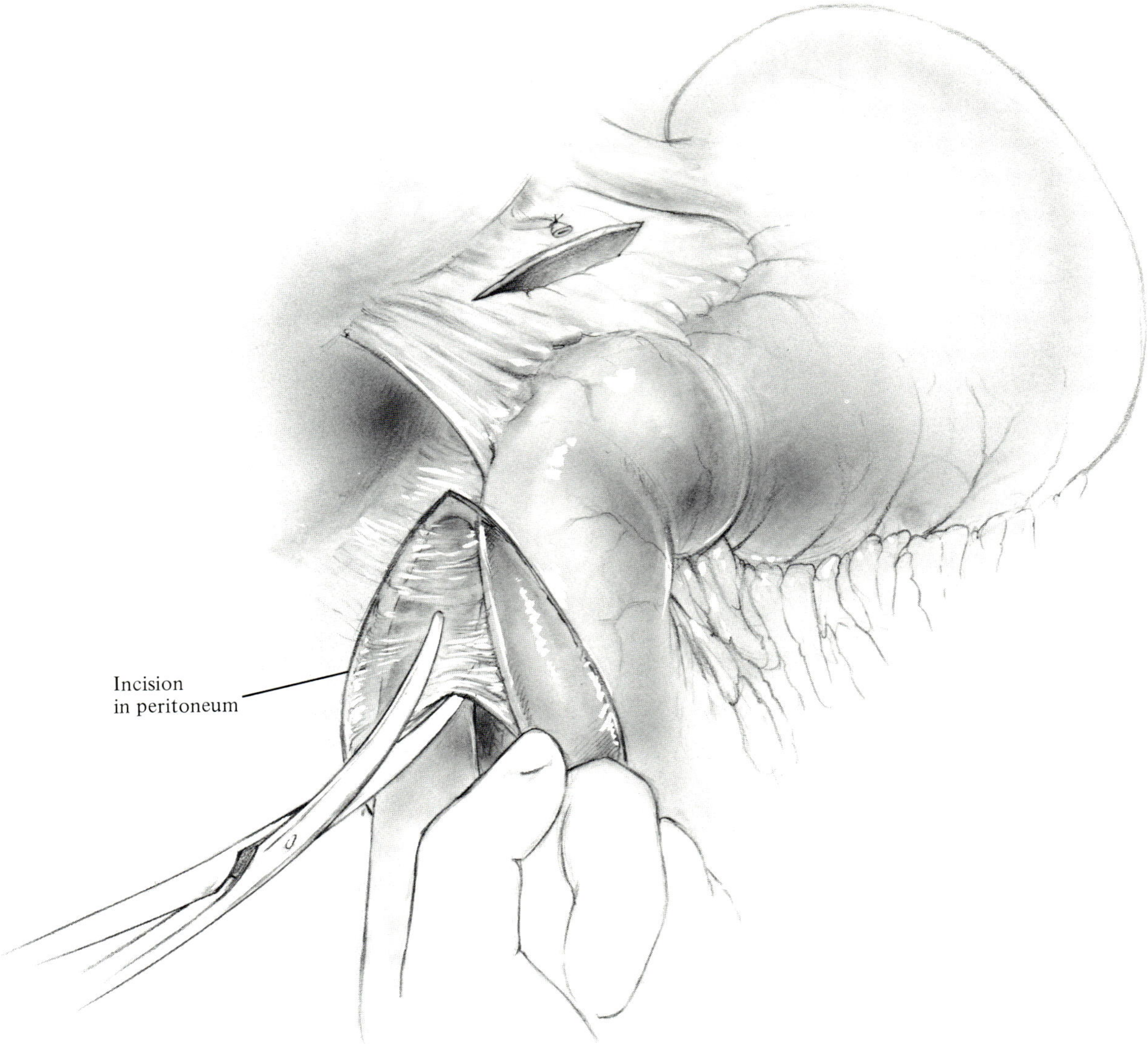

Fig. 7–15

This ligamentous structure is easily delineated by inserting the left index finger behind the pancreas. Move the finger laterally, exposing a lateral duodenal "ligament" behind the descending duodenum. Again, pinch the tissue between fingertip and thumb, which will leave vascular and fatty tissue behind, allowing this ligamentous structure to be divided. Incise it with a Metzenbaum scissors (**Fig. 7–15**). Repeat this maneuver, going around the second and third portions of duodenum (behind the hepatic flexure); this will lead to the point at which the superior mesenteric vein crosses over the duodenum. Be careful: excessive traction with the index finger may tear the branches of this vessel.

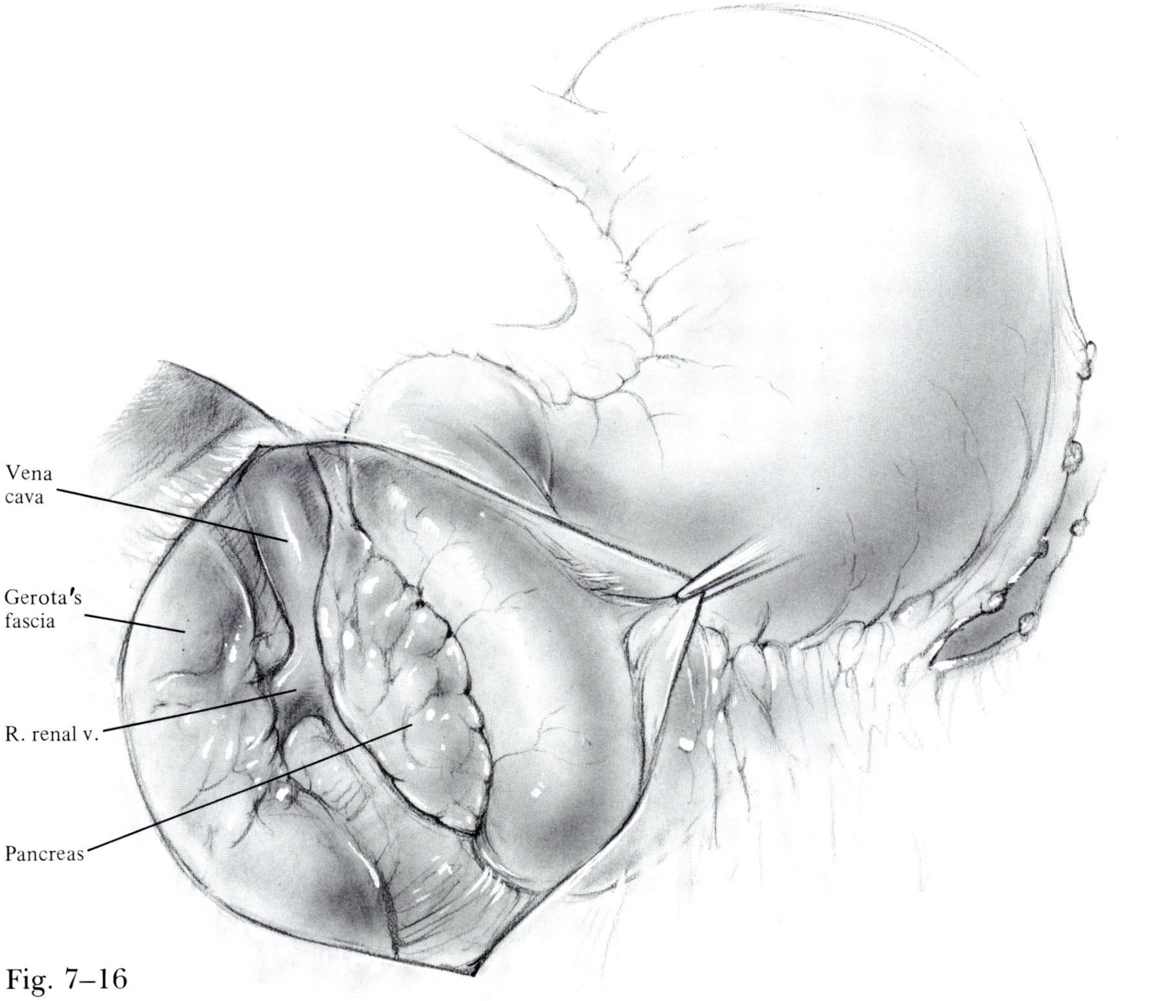

Fig. 7–16

For esophagogastric resection the Kocher maneuver need not be continued much beyond the junction of the second and third portions of the duodenum. At this point the left hand is easily passed behind the head of the pancreas, which should be elevated from the renal capsule, vena cava, and aorta (**Fig. 7–16**). This will permit the pyloroduodenal segment to be placed high in the abdomen, 8–10 cm from the esophageal hiatus, which in turn will permit the gastric fundus to reach the thoracic apex, or neck, without tension.

Pyloromyotomy

Although in many instances satisfactory results may be obtained without it, pyloromyotomy is generally performed at this point in order to prevent secondary operations for excessive gastric stasis due to vagotomy. Pyloromyotomy is accomplished by making a 1.5–2.0 cm incision across the anterior surface of the pyloric sphincter muscle (**Figs. 7–17, 7–18, 7–19**). It is difficult to do this in an adult who has normal muscle, but much easier in an infant who suffers hypertrophic pyloric stenosis. Frequently, sharp dissection with a No. 15 scalpel blade must be done through most of the circular muscle. Make a blunt separation of the muscle fibers with a hemostat until the mucosa bulges out. This procedure may be expedited by invaginating the anterior gastric wall into the pyloric sphincter with the index finger to divulse the few remaining circular muscle fibers. Exercise care not to perforate the mucosa; this is prone to occur at the duodenal end of the incision.

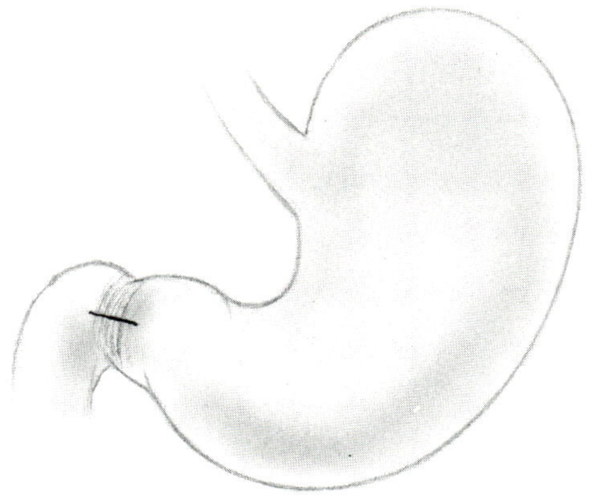

Fig. 7–17

Advancement of Stomach into Right Chest

Divide the right crux of the diaphragm transversely, using electrocautery (**Fig. 7–20**), and further dilate the esophageal hiatus manually. Advance the stomach into the right hemithorax, which should again be exposed by expanding the Finochietto retractor. There must be no constriction of the veins in the vascular pedicle of the stomach at the hiatus. Suture the wall of the stomach to the margins of the

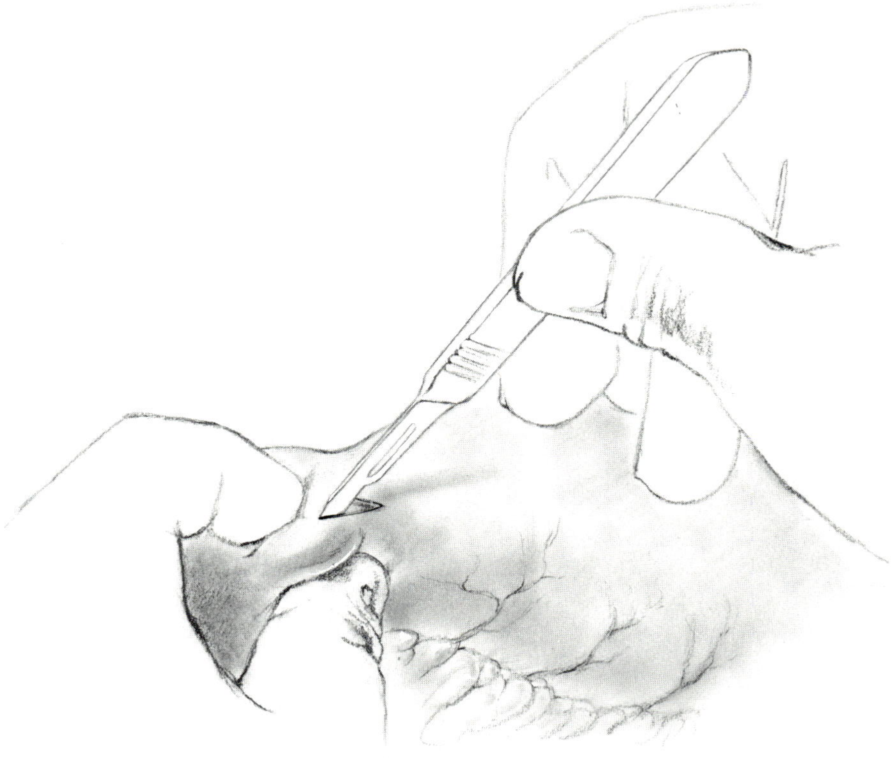

Fig. 7–18

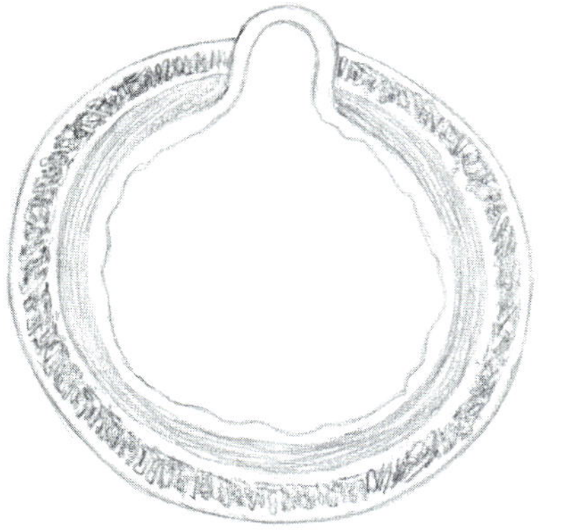

Fig. 7–19

hiatus by means of interrupted 3–0 cotton or Tevdek sutures spaced 2 cm apart in order to avoid postoperative herniation of bowel into the chest.

With the right lung retracted, expose the esophagogastric junction in the right chest. Generally, when the esophageal carcinoma is located in the middle or upper esophagus, it is not necessary to remove the lesser curvature of the stomach and the celiac lymph nodes.

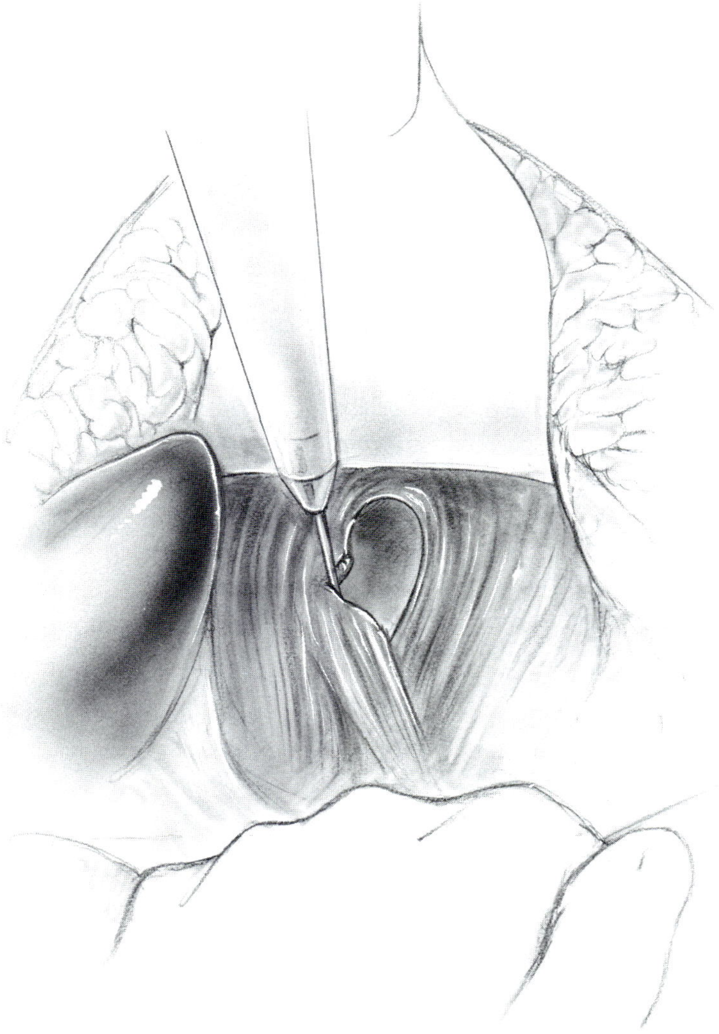

Fig. 7–20

After clearing the areolar tissue and the fat pad from the region of the esophagocardiac junction, apply a TA–55 stapler to the gastric side of this junction and fire the staples. Apply an Allen clamp to the esophagus, which should be transected flush with the TA–55 stapler. Place a rubber glove over the divided esophagus and fix it in place with a narrow tape ligature. Lightly electrocoagulate the everted gastric mucosa and remove the stapling device (**Fig. 7–21**). It is not necessary to invert this stapled closure with a layer of sutures; the fundus of the stomach reaches the apex of the thorax without tension. Take care to avoid twisting the stomach and its vascular pedicle.

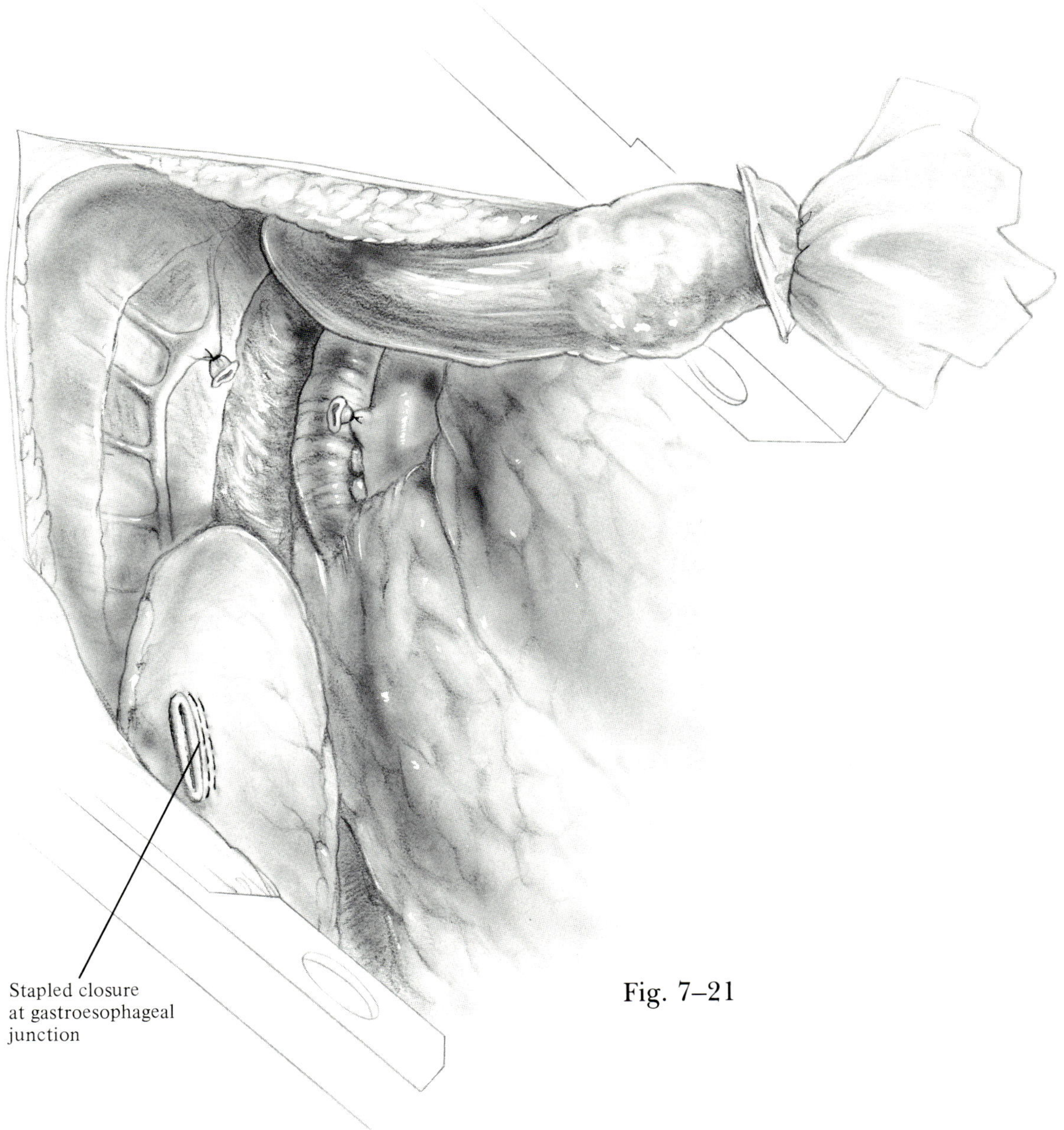

Fig. 7–21

Esophagogastric Anastomosis

Select a point on the proximal esophagus 10 cm above the tumor for the anastomosis. Before removing the specimen, insert the posterior layer of sutures to attach the posterior esophagus to the anterior seromuscular layer of the stomach at a point 6–7 cm from the cephalad end of the fundus (**Fig. 7–22**). The posterior layer should consist of about five interrupted atraumatic 4–0 cotton Cushing sutures. Each bite should be 5 mm in width and deep enough to catch submucosa. Using the Stratte needle-holder (see Glossary) often makes suturing the esophagus easier.

Transect the posterior wall of the esophagus with a scalpel at a point 6 mm beyond the first line of sutures. One can be certain that the esophageal mucosa has been transected when the nasogastric tube appears in the esophageal lumen. Now make a transverse incision in the stomach and control the bleeding points. This incision should be slightly longer than the diameter of the esophagus (Fig. 7–22).

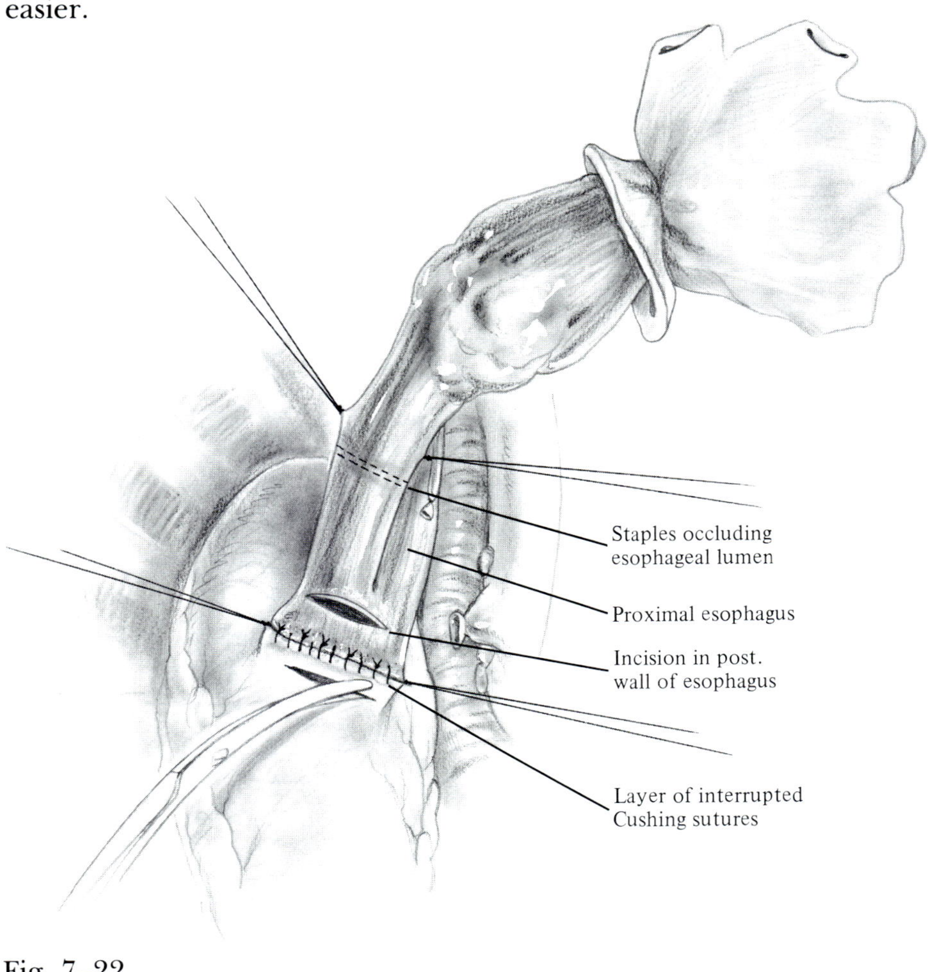

Fig. 7–22

Approximate the posterior mucosal layer by means of interrupted 4–0 atraumatic PG sutures, with the knots tied inside the lumen (**Fig. 7–23**). Then pass the nasogastric tube from the proximal esophagus through the anastomosis into the stomach.

In accordance with the suggestion of Fisher et al., detach the specimen by dividing the anterior wall of the esophagus with a scissors in such fashion as to leave the anterior wall of the esophagus 1 cm longer than the posterior (**Fig. 7–24**). This maneuver will enlarge the stoma if the incision in the stomach is large enough to match that of the elliptical esophageal lumen.

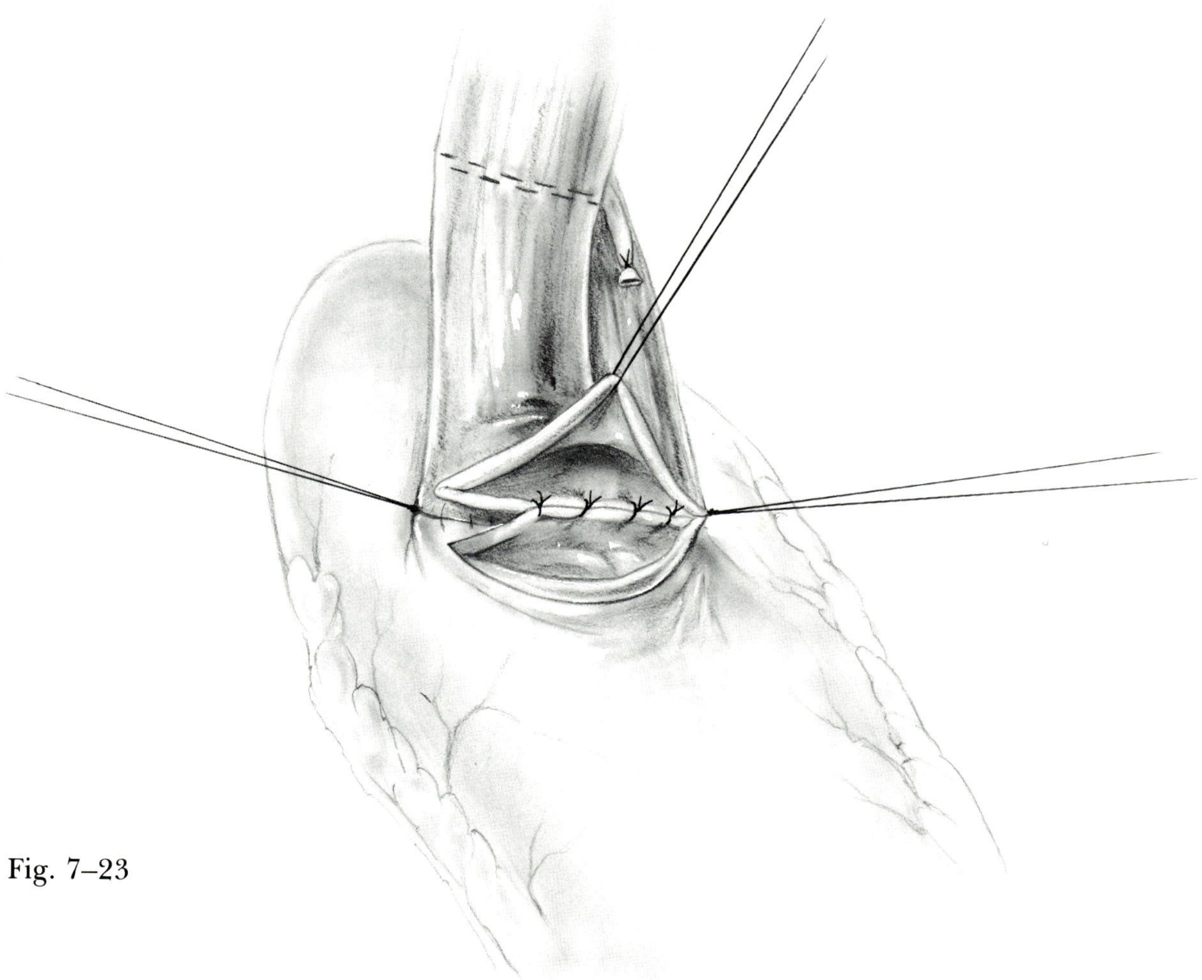

Fig. 7–23

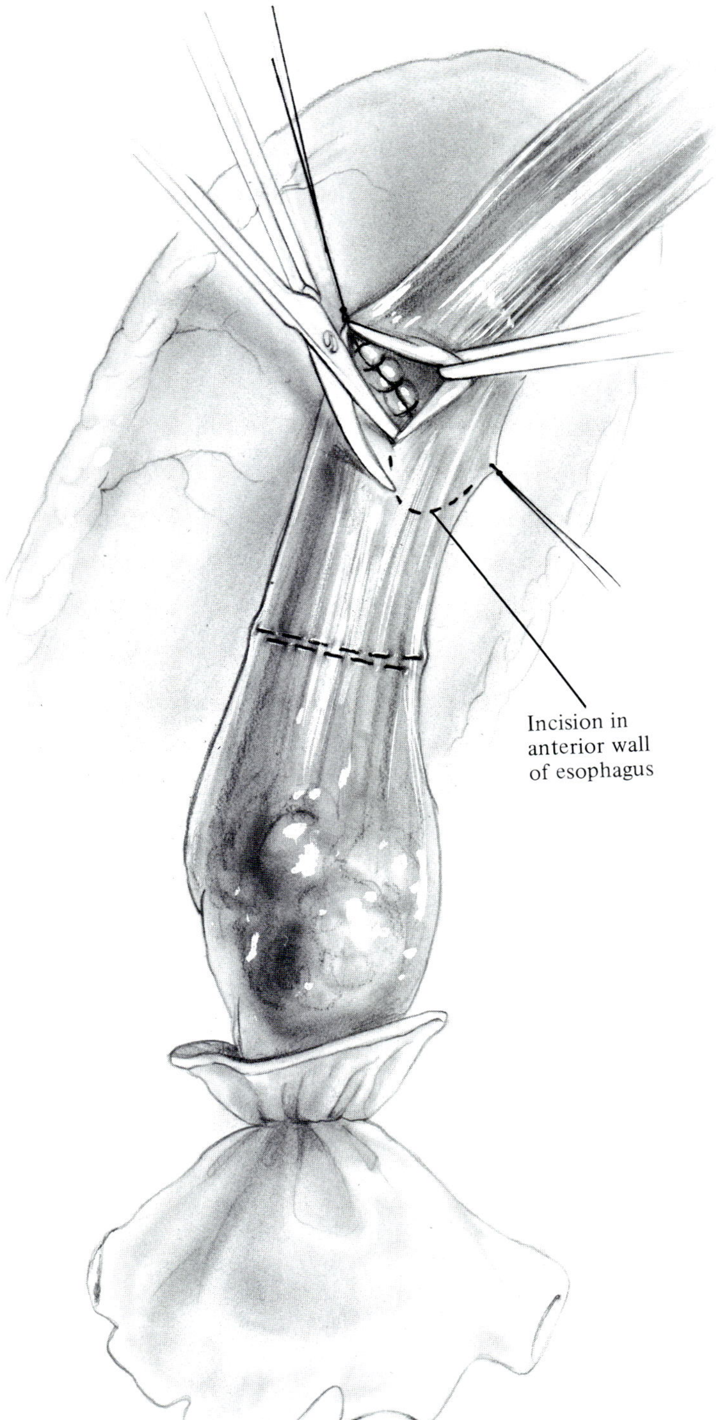

Fig. 7–24

Execute the anterior mucosal layer by means of interrupted sutures of 4–0 PG, with the knots tied inside the lumen, thus inverting the mucosa (**Fig. 7–25**). Accomplish the second anterior layer by means of interrupted Cushing sutures of 4–0 cotton (**Fig. 7–26**). The sutures must not be tied with excessive force.

At this point, some surgeons (Boyd et al.) prefer to perform a Nissen fundoplication, which can be done if there is enough loose gastric wall to permit a wraparound without constricting the esophagus. Otherwise, a partial fundoplication may be accomplished by inserting several sutures between the outer walls of the esophagus and adjacent stomach. We have observed that even if fundoplication is not performed, few patients develop reflux esophagitis following this operation—as long as end-to-side esophagogastric anastomosis has been accomplished 6 cm or more below the cephalad margin of the gastric remnant.

Surgeons who lack wide experience with this anastomosis might find it wise to inflate the gastric pouch with a solution of methylene blue, injected into the nasogastric tube by the anesthesiologist, in order to test the anastomosis for leakage.

As a final, essential step in this operation, prevent tension on the anastomosis by tacking the fundus of the stomach to the prevertebral fascia and mediastinal pleura at the apex of the thorax. Use interrupted sutures of 3–0 cotton or Tevdek for this purpose (Fig. 7–26). These sutures must not penetrate the lumen of the stomach, for as Fisher et al. have noted, a gastropleural fistula may result.

As soon as the specimen has been removed, examine the proximal end of the esophagus by frozen section to see if there has been submucosal extension of the cancer. If the pathologist notices tumor cells in the esophageal margin, more esophagus should be resected.

Stapled Esophagogastric Anastomosis

A stapling technique developed by Chassin for this anastomosis is described in Chap. 8.

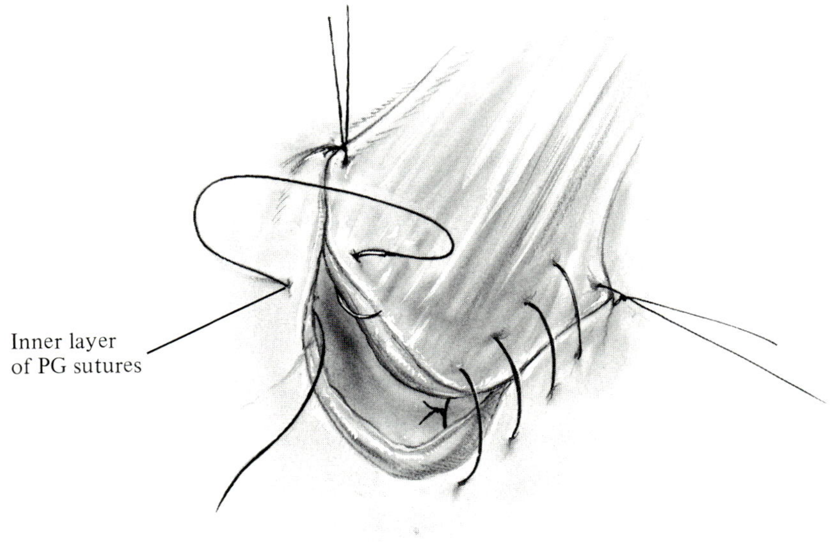

Fig. 7–25

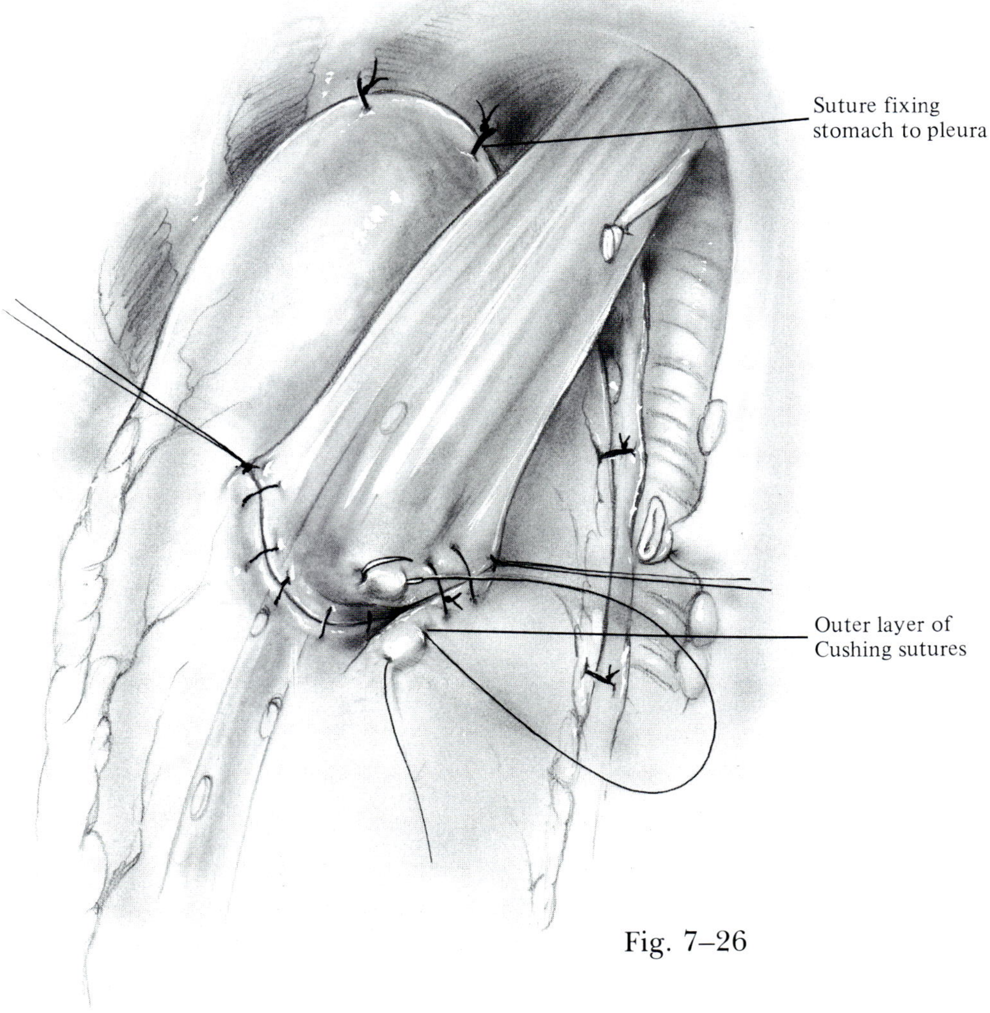

Fig. 7–26

Cervical Esophagogastric Anastomosis

In treating carcinoma of the mid-esophagus it is often necessary to resect the entire thoracic esophagus to obtain a sufficient margin of normal tissue above the tumor. This requires an esophagogastric reconstruction in the neck.

With the patient's head turned slightly to the left, make an oblique incision along the anterior border of the right sternomastoid muscle (**Fig. 7–27**). Carry the incision through the platysma. Identify (**Fig.**

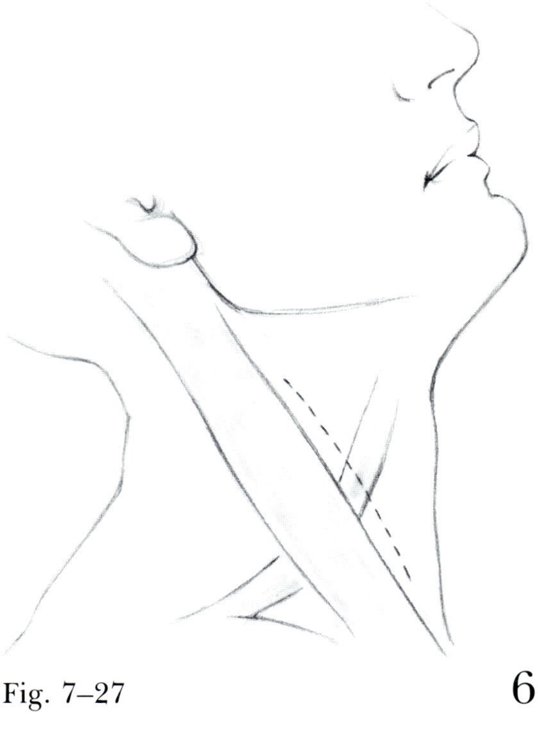

Fig. 7–27

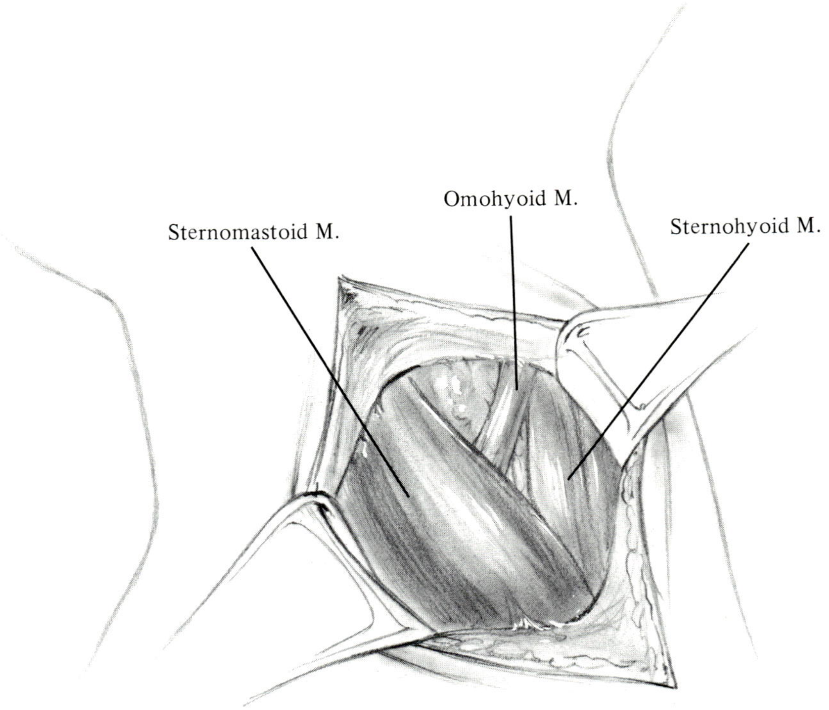

Fig. 7–28

7–28) and transect the omohyoid muscle. Retract the sternomastoid muscle and carotid sheath laterally and retract the prethyroid muscles medially, exposing the thyroid gland (**Fig. 7–29**). The middle thyroid vein, when present, should be doubly ligated and divided. Place the areolar tissue between the gland and the carotid

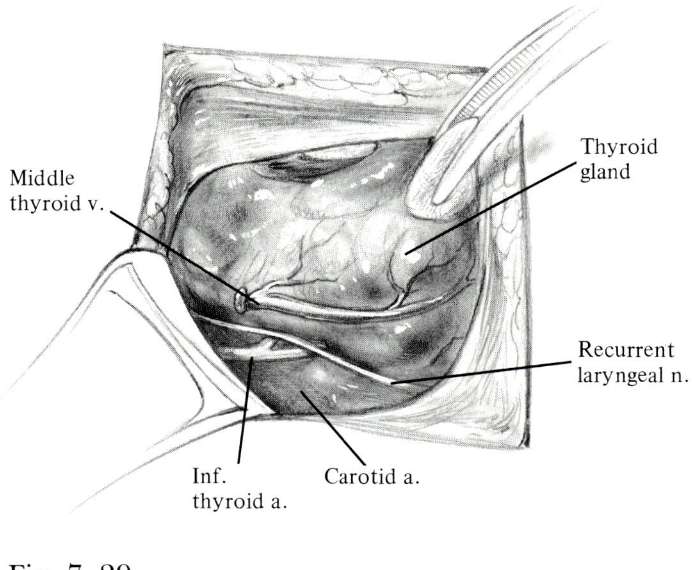

Fig. 7–29

sheath on stretch by upward and medial retraction of the thyroid. Identify and skeletonize the inferior thyroid artery, which crosses the lower third of the surgical field in a transverse direction, by a Metzenbaum dissection toward the prevertebral fascia. Dissect it toward the thyroid gland until the recurrent laryngeal nerve can be seen. Then dissect the nerve upward to achieve thorough exposure, so that it may be preserved (Fig. 7–29).

At this point the tracheoesophageal groove will be seen and the cervical esophagus can be encircled by the surgeon's index finger, which should be passed between the esophagus and the prevertebral fascia and then between the esophagus and trachea. The finger should stay close to the esophageal wall. Otherwise, the *left* recurrent laryngeal nerve may be avulsed during this dissection. Although the inferior thyroid artery generally will have to be ligated and divided before the esophagus is mobilized, in some cases its course is low enough in the neck so that it can be preserved.

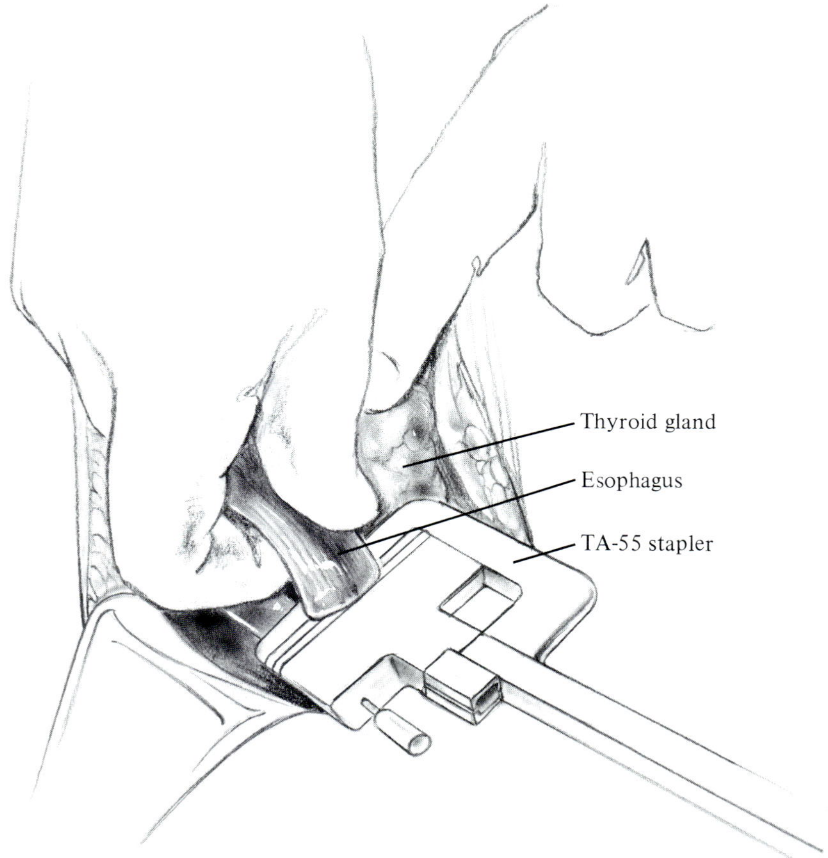

Fig. 7–30

Since the thoracic esophagus has been dissected up to the thoracic inlet, it is a simple matter to transect the esophagus low in the neck. When the proper point of transection of the esophagus has been selected, apply a TA–55 stapler to the specimen side (**Fig. 7–30**) and transect the esophagus flush with the stapler. Remove the specimen through the thoracic incision.

Now pass the fundus of the stomach, which has already been passed into the thorax, through the thoracic inlet into the cervical region. The fundus should reach the hypopharynx without tension. Anchor it to the prevertebral fascia with several 3–0 cotton sutures. Then construct an end-to-side anastomosis by the same technique described above (**Figs. 7–31, 7–32** and 7–25, 7–26).

We have not been impressed by the various stapling techniques recommended for the esophagogastric anastomosis in the neck.

Lavage the operative site with an antibiotic solution and initiate wound closure by inserting a layer of interrupted 4–0 PG sutures approximating the anterior border of the sternomastoid to the prethyroid strap muscles. Several similar sutures may

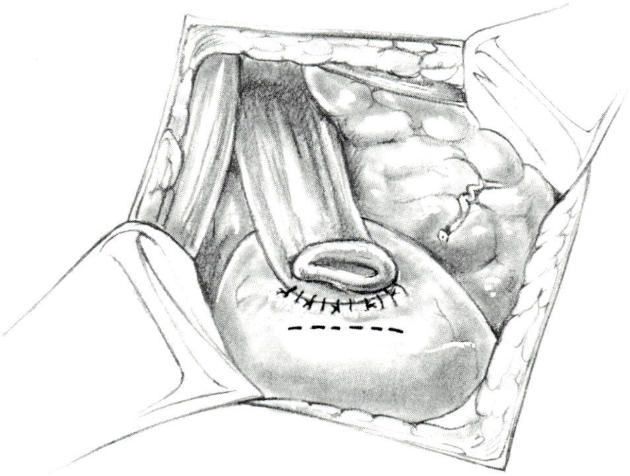

Fig. 7–31

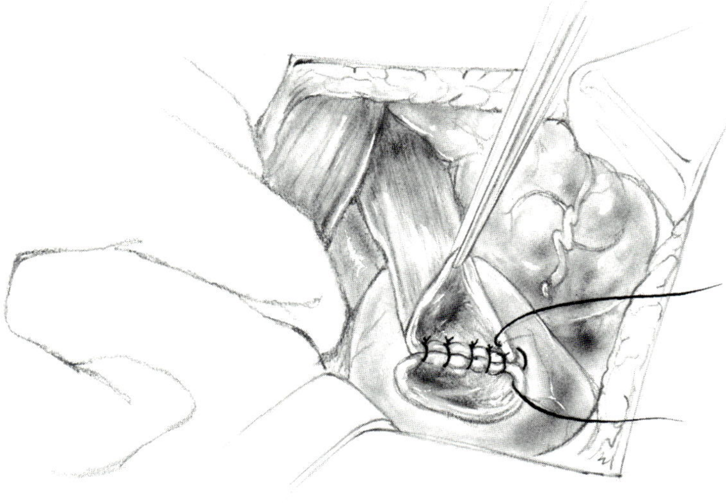

Fig. 7–32

be used loosely to approximate the platysma. Close the skin, generally by means of a continuous 4–0 PG subcuticular suture, leaving sufficient space to bring a latex drain out from the prevertebral region through the lower pole of the incision.

Closure

Make a stab wound in the ninth intercostal space. Insert a 36F multi-eyed plastic catheter through the stab wound and use 4–0 catgut to suture the catheter to the posterior pleura in the upper thorax. After thoroughly irrigating the thoracic and abdominal cavities with an antibiotic solution, approximate the ribs with four or five interrupted pericostal sutures of No. 1 PG and approximate the serratus and pectoral muscles in layers by means of continuous 2–0 atraumatic PG (**Figs. 7–33 and 7–34**). Close the skin with continuous 3–0 nylon or subcuticular 4–0 PG.

Close the abdominal wall in the usual fashion by means of interrupted 2–0 stainless steel wire sutures.

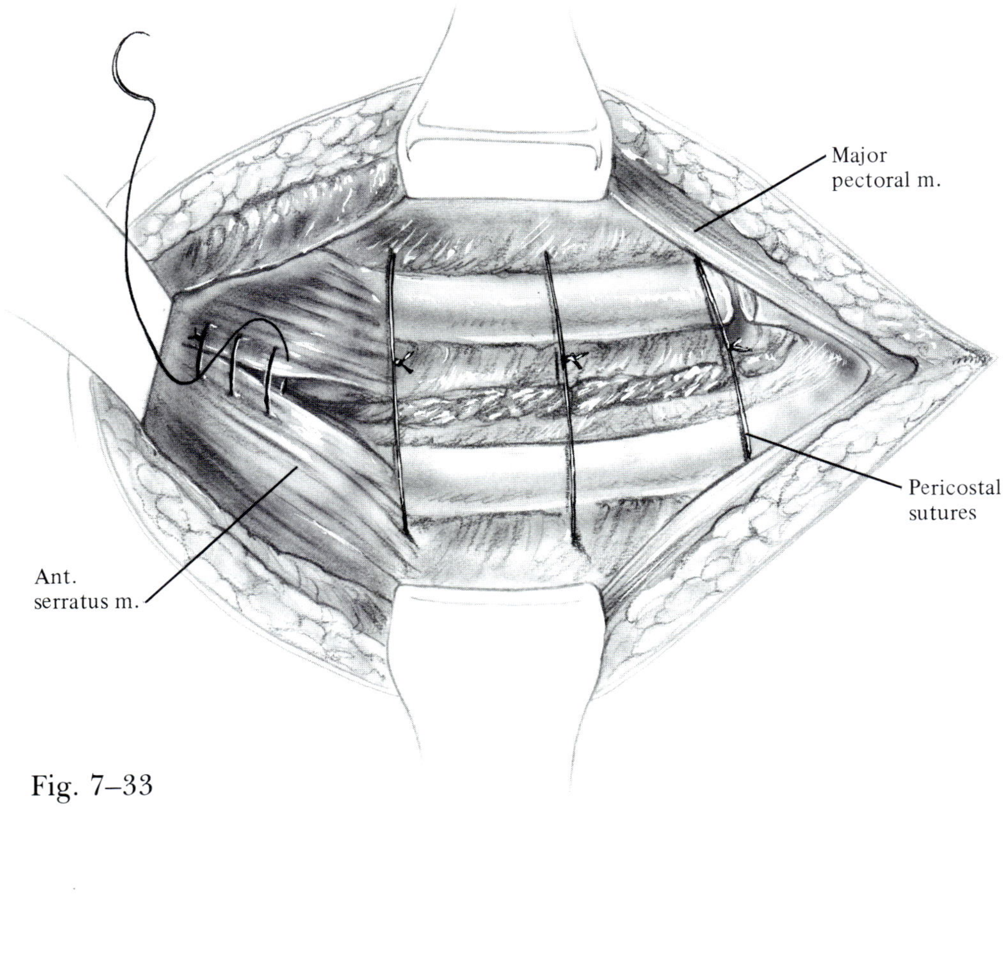

Fig. 7–33

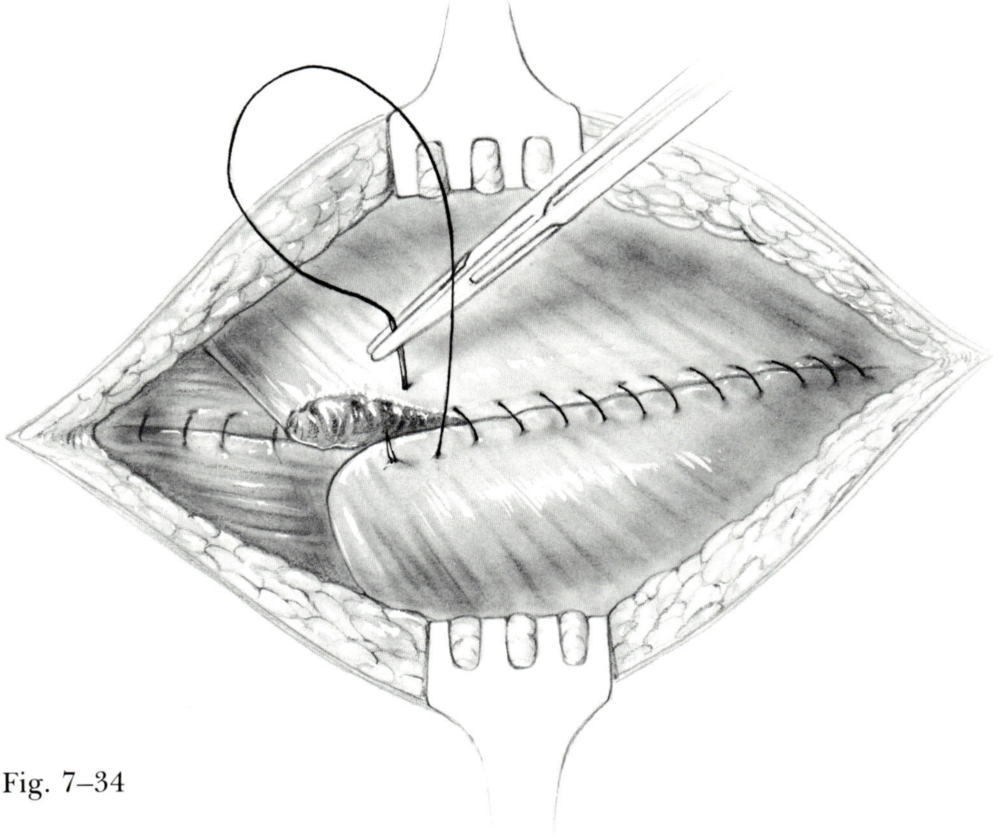

Fig. 7–34

Postoperative Care

Keep the nasogastric tube on low suction for 4–5 days. The patient should be permitted nothing by mouth until an esophagram with an aqueous contrast medium has been performed in the X-ray department on the seventh postoperative day to ascertain the integrity of the anastomosis. If no leak can be seen, the patient is given a liquid diet. This should be advanced to a full diet in 3–5 days.

The thoracic drainage tube is attached to Pleur-Evac underwater drainage for 4–5 days, and the routine steps for management of a postoperative thoracotomy patient are carried out, including frequent determination of arterial blood gases and pH. Tracheal suction is used with caution to avoid possible trauma to the anastomosis. Ventilatory support is employed when necessary.

Prophylactic antibiotics are continued until removal of the thoracotomy drainage tube.

Intravenous hyperalimentation is continued if the patient is malnourished.

Complications

Anastomotic leaks constitute by far the most important complication of this operation, but they are *preventable if proper surgical technique is used.* Over half the patients who develop clinical leakage die, according to the literature. Triggiani and Belsey have reported that unless the anastomosis is defunctionalized by cervical esophagostomy combined with adequate thoracic drainage, most patients will not survive an intrathoracic anastomotic leak. It is possible that reopening the thorax and wrapping the perforated anastomosis with a pedicled flap of parietal pleura, using Grillo's technique, may obviate the need for cervical esophagostomy in these cases.

On two occasions we have observed a small perianastomotic collection of contrast material in patients who were studied by X-ray esophagrams on the seventh postoperative day. In both cases there was absolutely no *clinical* evidence of leak. Both were treated conservatively, and oral feedings were instituted five days after the abnormal X-rays without ill effect. These were both end-to-end esophagogastric anastomoses, a technique now avoided whenever possible.

Fisher et al. have reported finding a gastropleural fistula following leakage from one of the sutures used to tack the stomach to the mediastinal pleura. This case proved fatal. As consultants we have seen one similar case involving a stitch between the gastric wall and the diaphragmatic hiatus. In this patient, bile-stained fluid appeared in the thoracic drainage tube on the second postoperative day. This was confirmed by the insertion into the nasogastric tube of methylene blue dye, which was recovered in the thoracic drainage. The problem was managed by prompt reopening of the thoracic incision and closure of the defect in the gastric wall by several inverting 4–0 cotton seromuscular sutures. The patient made an uneventful recovery.

A subphrenic or subhepatic abscess may follow an operation for an ulcerated malignancy because a necrotic tumor often harbors virulent organisms. The incidence of this complication can be reduced by antibiotic irrigation during the procedure and by administering prophylactic antibiotics before and during the operation. Treatment is by surgical drainage.

Pulmonary complications were common in the past, but their incidence has been minimized by proper postoperative pulmonary care. Whenever indicated by arterial oxygen and carbon dioxide determinations, postoperative ventilatory support should be utilized, especially in aged patients whose pulmonary reserve is diminished.

Cardiac failure and arrhythmia are not uncommon in patients who are in their seventh or eighth decade of life. Generally, with careful monitoring and early detection, these complications can be easily managed. This requires the use of a Swan-Ganz catheter for measurement of pulmonary wedge pressure and of cardiac output in some of these cases.

In the absence of recurrent mediastinal cancer, stenosis of the anastomosis has not occurred in any of the cases Chassin has managed and reported on. When this complication does occur, repeated passage of Maloney bougies may reverse the condition.

References

Boyd AD et al. (1975) Esophagogastrostomy: analysis of 55 cases. J Thorac Cardiovasc Surg 70:817

Chassin JL (1978) Esophagogastrectomy: data favoring end-to-side anastomosis. Ann Surg 188:22

Fisher RD et al. (1972) Esophagogastrostomy in the treatment of carcinoma of the distal two-thirds of the esophagus. Ann Thorac Surg 14:658

Grillo HC, Wilkins EW Jr (1975) Esophageal repair following late diagnosis of intrathoracic perforations. Ann Thorac Surg 20:387

Logan A (1963) The surgical treatment of carcinoma of the esophagus and cardia. J Thorac Cardiovasc Surg 46:150

Triggiani E, Belsey R (1977) Oesophageal trauma: incidence, diagnosis and management. Thorax 32:241

8 Esophagogastrectomy: Left Thoracoabdominal

Indications

Esophagogastrectomy by the left thoracoabdominal approach is indicated for malignant lesions of the distal 10–15 cm of the esophagus, of the esophagogastric junction, and of the gastric fundus.

Preoperative Care

In these cases nutritional rehabilitation is often the most important single preoperative measure. Also

- Cessation of smoking
- Pulmonary function studies
- Preoperative esophagoscopy and biopsy
- Perioperative antibiotics
- Nasogastric tube before the operation

Pitfalls and Danger Points

Anastomotic failure.

Vascularity of gastric pouch. Meticulous attention must be paid to preserving the entire arcade of right gastroepiploic artery and vein along greater curvature of stomach.

Hemorrhage. Occasionally, left gastric artery is imbedded in tumor by invasion from metastatic lymph nodes. Unless this vessel can be identified, transecting the artery through the tumor may produce hemorrhage that is difficult to control.

Pancreas. Trauma to tail of pancreas while spleen and gastric lesion are being removed may induce acute hemorrhagic pancreatitis.

Sepsis. Some malignancies in proximal portion of stomach are ulcerated and bulky with areas of necrosis that contain virulent bacteria. These may produce postoperative subhepatic or subphrenic abscesses by contaminating the operation even if there is no anastomotic leakage.

Inadequate cancer operation. Because gastric and esophageal malignancies can spread for some distance submucosally without being visible, frozen section studies of both proximal and distal margins of the excision are helpful.

Paralysis of the diaphragm.

Operative Strategy

Objectives of Esophagogastrectomy

In operations done for cure the objective is the wide removal of the primary tumor, along with a 6–10 cm margin of normal esophagus in a proximal direction and a 6 cm margin of normal stomach below. Even if the stomach is not involved, when the tumor is situated low in the esophagus, the proximal lesser curvature of the stomach should be included in order to remove the left gastric artery at its origin and to remove the celiac lymph nodes. Splenectomy and removal of the lymph nodes at the splenic hilus should be done for all lesions of the lower esophagus and proximal stomach. Any suspicious nodes along the superior border of the pancreas should be removed also.

Thoracoabdominal Incision with Preservation of Phrenic Nerve Function

When gastric cancer encroaches upon the gastroesophageal junction, an operation that is done by abdominal incision exclusively is contraindicated for several reasons. In the first place, this anastomosis will frequently require the surgeon's hand and the needle-holder to be in an awkward position, and may result in leakage. Furthermore, the abdominal incision makes it difficult to perform a wide excision of possible areas of invasion of the distal esophagus. Some upper gastric lesions we have seen have extended up into the esophagus as far as 10 cm.

The left thoracoabdominal incision, we have found, is both safe and efficacious. It is easy to divide all the muscles of the thoracic cage rapidly by electrocautery. Even patients in their eighties have tolerated this incision well when given adequate postoperative support.

The diaphragm should *not* be incised radially from the costal margin to the esophageal hiatus because this would transect the phrenic nerve and paralyze the left diaphragm. Many patients who require gastric surgery for cancer are aged and have limited pulmonary reserve, and as atelectasis is a common postoperative complication, it is better to make a circumferential incision in the periphery of the diaphragm so as to preserve phrenic nerve function and normal diaphragmatic motion.

Postoperative pain at the site of the divided costal margin has been alleged to be common following the thoracoabdominal incision. In our experience proper resuturing of the costal margin with monofilament steel wire results in solid healing of this area. Pain has *not* been a problem.

Anastomotic Leakage

Delicacy of suture technique and adequate exposure are very important in preventing anastomotic leaks. If a gastric or lower esophageal lesion has spread up the lower esophagus for a distance of more than 6–8 cm, the esophagogastric anastomosis should not be constructed high up under the aortic arch, as this is a hazardous technique. Instead, 1 cm posterior segments of two additional ribs should be resected, and the esophagus should be liberated behind the arch of the aorta and passed up to a supra-aortic position. This exposure permits the anastomosis to be done in a manner less traumatic to the tissues than an anastomosis constructed high up under the aortic arch. Otherwise, the surgeon's hand and wrist are situated in an awkward position, which makes smooth rotation of the wrist and needle-holder very difficult. Jerky suturing motions produce small tears in the esophagus, especially in the difficult posterior layer.

End-to-End versus End-to-Side Anastomosis

In a report published in the *Annals of Surgery,* we have shown that the end-to-end esophagogastric anastomosis carries with it a much higher rate of leakage as well as a higher mortality rate than the end-to-side. Explanations for the increased complication rate following end-to-end esophagogastrostomy are not hard to find:

It is necessary to close a portion of the end of the stomach because of the disparity between the lumen of the stomach and that of the esophagus. This increases the technical difficulty of doing the end-to-end anastomosis (**Figs. 8–1a and 8–1b**).

The blood supply of the gastric pouch at its proximal margin is inferior to that at the site of the end-to-side anastomosis.

Inserting the posterior layer of esophagogastric sutures may be difficult because traction is often being applied to the esophagus to improve exposure while the surgeon's hand and the needle-holder device may have to assume positions that are awkward for efficient and nontraumatic suturing. This produces imperfections in the suture line. As seen in **Fig. 8–2a,** protection from posterior leakage is achieved in the end-to-side cases by the buttress effect of a 6–7 cm segment of gastric wall behind the esophagus. In end-to-end operations, however, there is no second line of defense against technical error.

Although the anterior layer of either the end-to-end or the end-to-side esophagogastrostomy is much easier than the posterior layer to construct without technical defects, even here the end-to-side version offers advantages. **Fig. 8–2b** illustrates how the anterior wall of the esophagus invaginates itself into the stomach for

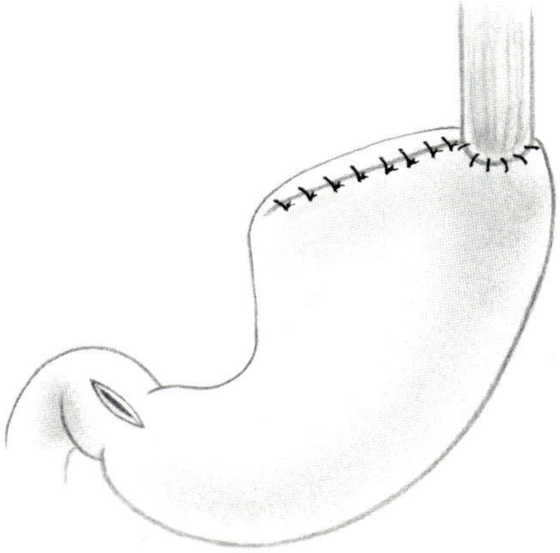

Fig. 8–1a

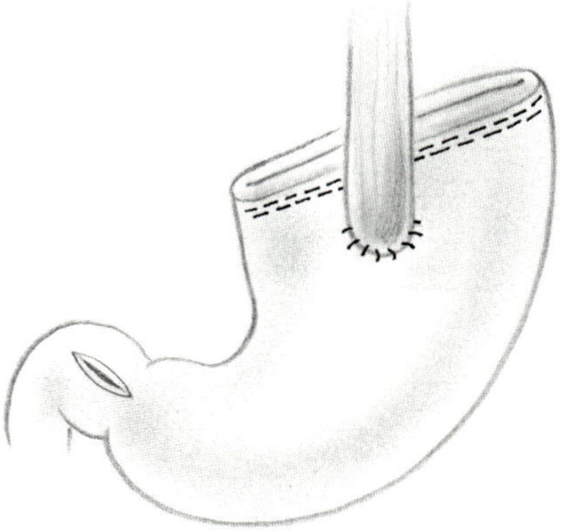

Fig. 8–2a

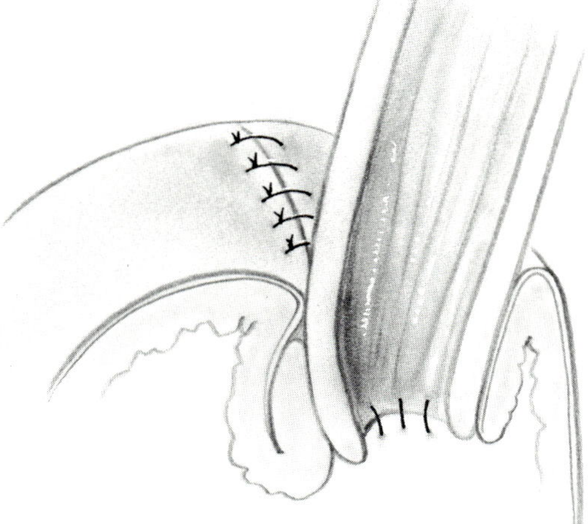

Fig. 8–1b

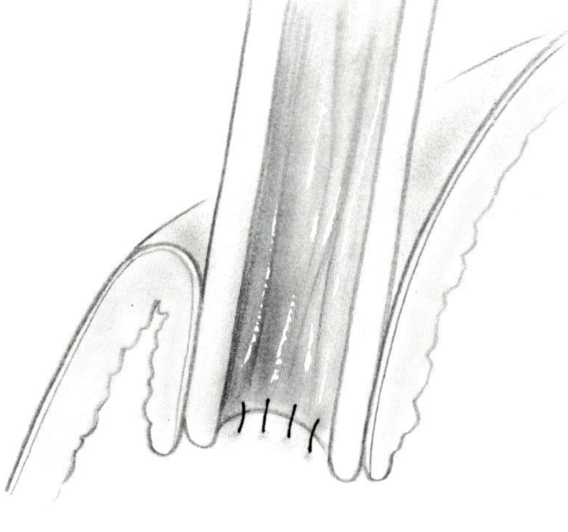

Fig. 8–2b

additional protection. If this were attempted with an end-to-end anastomosis, the large inverted cuff would produce stenosis at the stoma (Fig. 8–1b).

Additional protection against leakage from the anterior aspect of the end-to-side anastomosis can be achieved by performing a Nissen fundoplication around the anastomosis. This also helps prevent postoperative gastroesophageal reflux, but it requires the presence of a large gastric pouch and can not be performed, unless modified, when the proximal stomach has been resected.

Avoiding Postoperative Reflux Esophagitis

Another serious drawback of an end-to-end esophagogastric anastomosis is the occurrence of reflux esophagitis in patients who achieve long-term survival. This can be avoided by implanting the end of the esophagus end-to-side into the stomach at least 6 cm beyond the proximal margin of the gastric pouch. This type of construction functions as a valve, probably because air in the gastric pouch behind the distal esophagus compresses the overlying esophagus. This is fortunate, as there is rarely enough remaining stomach to fashion an adequate "fundoplication" when the gastric fundus has been resected.

When the anastomosis is performed by our stapling method, described below, there should preferably be a distance of 8 cm between the proximal gastric margin and the overlying esophagus because the stapled anastomotic stoma uses a slightly larger area of anterior gastric wall than does the suture technique.

Efficacy of Stapling Techniques for the Esophagogastric Anastomosis

We have developed and reported, in the *American Journal of Surgery,* a stapling technique for end-to-side esophagogastrostomy that has been used in 21 consecutive cases without evidence of leak, either on clinical grounds or when checked by routine esophagram X-rays on the seventh postoperative day. It can be done swiftly, and after a long and sometimes complicated dissection, an accurate anastomosis that takes only 2 or 3 minutes of operating time constitutes a welcome epilogue, especially when treating poor-risk patients.

Use of the recently introduced EEA stapling device, presents the surgeon with a serious dilemma. The EEA comes in large and small models. The large one has an external diameter of over 3 cm, which is much too big for the average esophagus. If a small model is used, the diameter of the resulting stoma may be too small to permit the passage of certain foods. In general, anastomoses made by staplers that produce two staggered rows of staples are quite difficult to stretch by bougienage. Until we have more data on the effects of the small EEA, its use is contraindicated. The diameter of the circle of staples laid down by the *large* EEA is only 2.2 cm, which is marginally acceptable.

Another drawback to the EEA technique is that it requires a 3 cm incision in the anterior gastric wall to introduce the device into the stomach. This incision, which must be closed after firing the EEA, may interfere with the blood supply to the anastomosis. General acceptance of the EEA technique for esophageal anastomoses awaits further data. Until this data becomes available we are continuing to use our method of esophagogastric stapling, which is faster and less prone to technical complications than is the EEA procedure. None of our 21 patients experienced any anastomotic leak, nor did any of them require postoperative bougienage for stricture.

Postoperative Sepsis

To prevent postoperative sepsis, be meticulous in avoiding spillage of the gastric content, which can contaminate the subhepatic or subcutaneous space. Any instruments that come in contact with the lumen of the stomach or esophagus should be treated as dirty, and the area should be walled off wherever possible. During the operation, the operative field should be irrigated frequently with a dilute antibiotic solution.

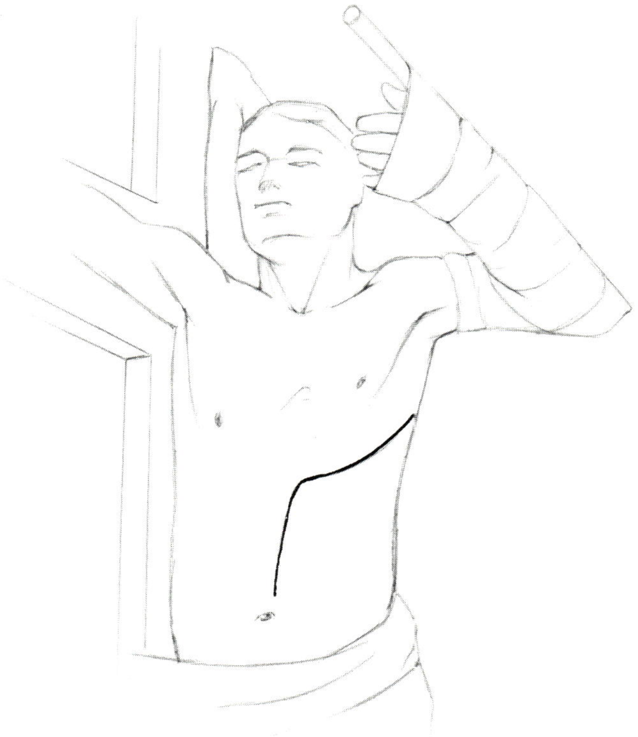

Fig. 8–3

Operative Technique

Incision and Position

With the aid of sandbags and wide adhesive tape across the patient's hips, elevate the patient's left side to a 60° angle. Pad the patient's left arm and suspend it in a forward position (**Fig. 8–3**).

Begin the incision at the umbilicus and continue it up the midline about halfway to the xiphoid. Then explore the abdomen. The presence of metastasis of a moderate degree to the celiac lymph nodes or to the liver does not constitute a contraindication to resection.

Redirect the incision to cross the costal margin into the sixth intercostal space and continue it to the region of the erector spinal muscle near the tip of the scapula. After the skin incision has been completed, use the coagulating current to divide the latissimus dorsi muscle in as caudal a location as possible (**Fig. 8–4**). The

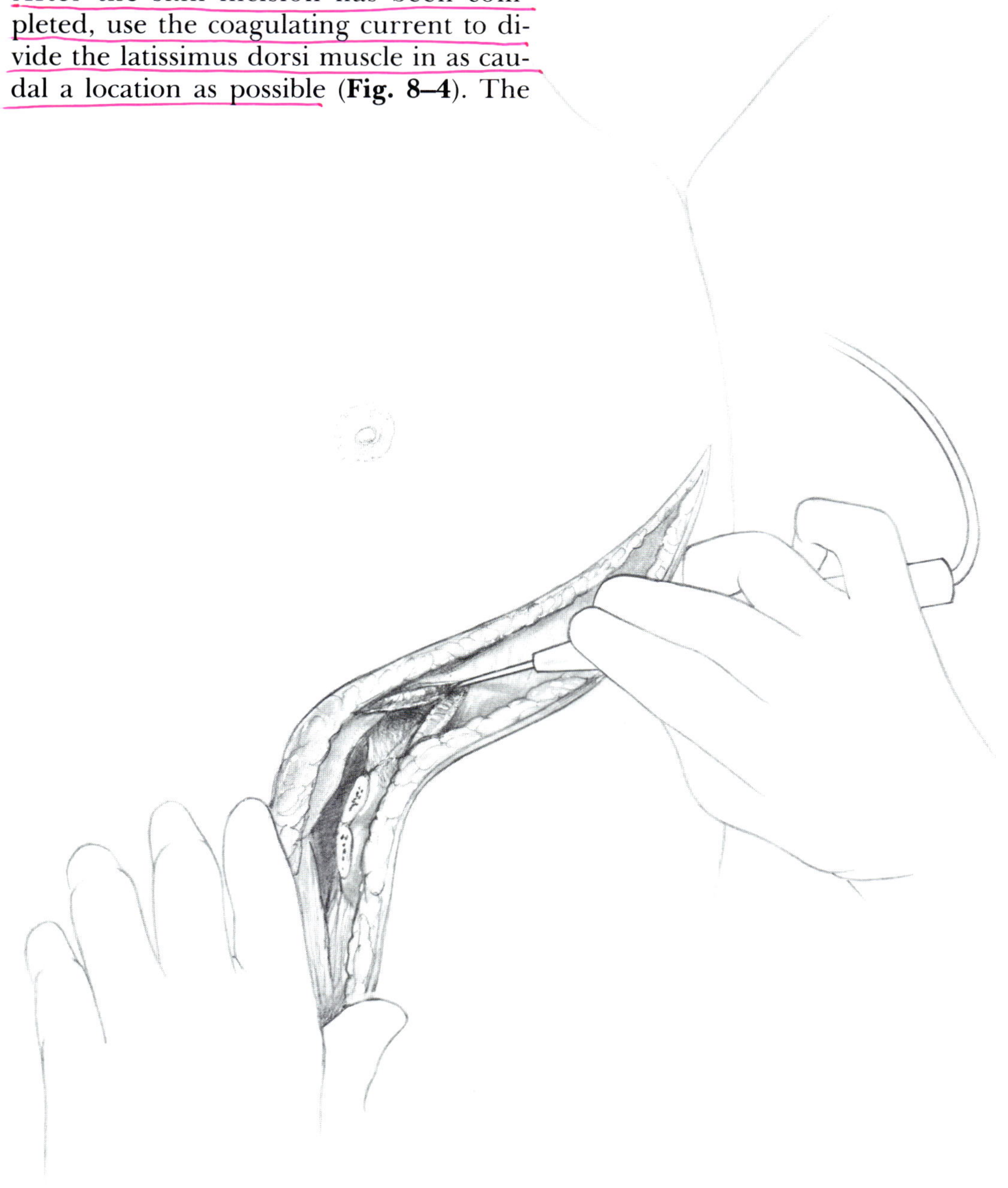

Fig. 8–4

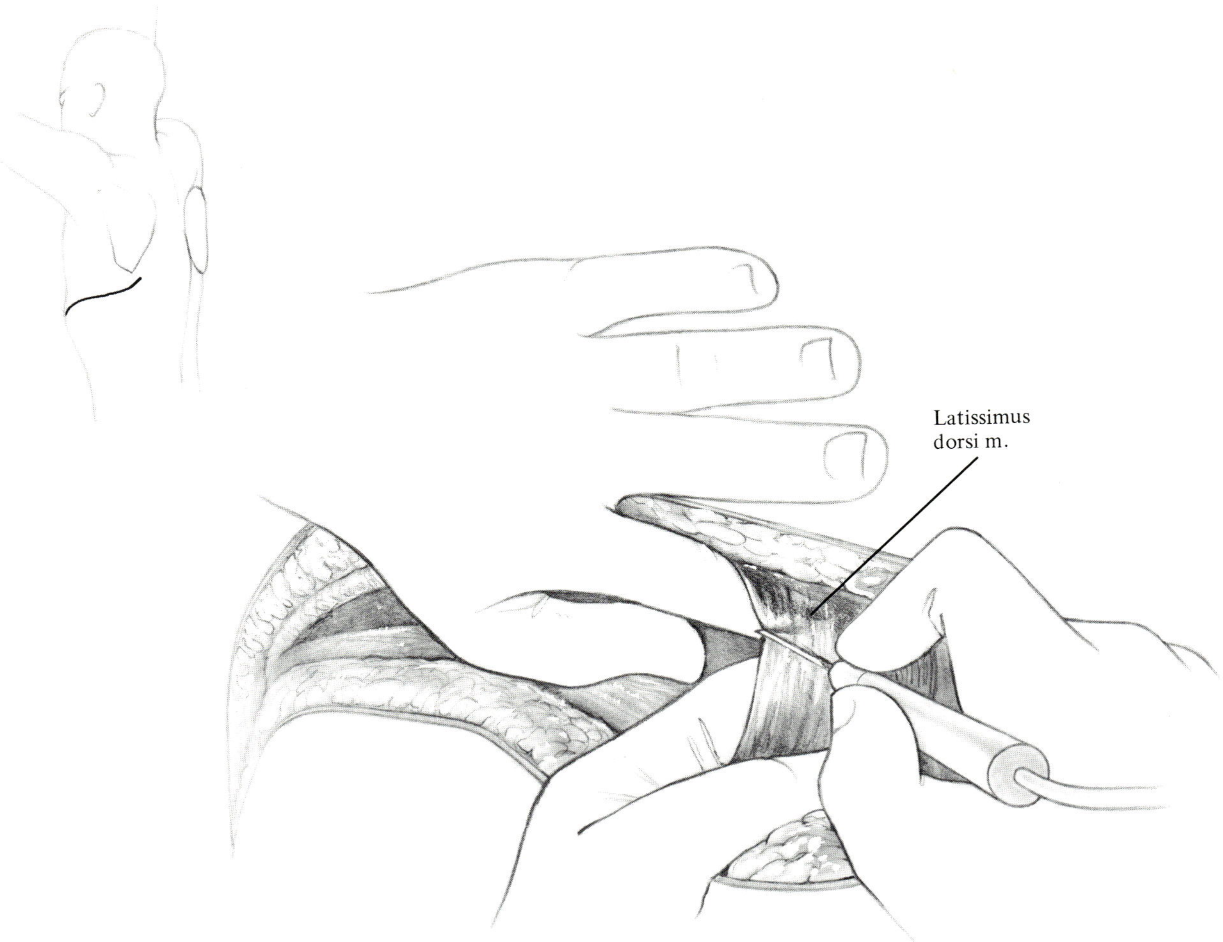

Fig. 8–5

index fingers of both the surgeon and first assistant should be inserted side by side beneath the latissimus muscle while the electrocoagulator divides the muscle (**Fig. 8–5**). A similar method should be applied to the division of the anterior serratus muscle. The rhomboid muscles medial to the scapula need not be divided unless a supra-aortic dissection proves necessary.

Next retract the scapula in a cephalad direction and count down the interspaces from the first rib to confirm the location of the sixth interspace. Divide the intercostal musculature by electrocautery along the superior surface of the seventh rib and enter the pleura (**Fig. 8–6**). Divide the costal margin with a scalpel or a rib cutter. Divide the internal mammary artery, deep and slightly lateral to the costal margin, and ligate or electrocoagulate it (**Fig. 8–7**).

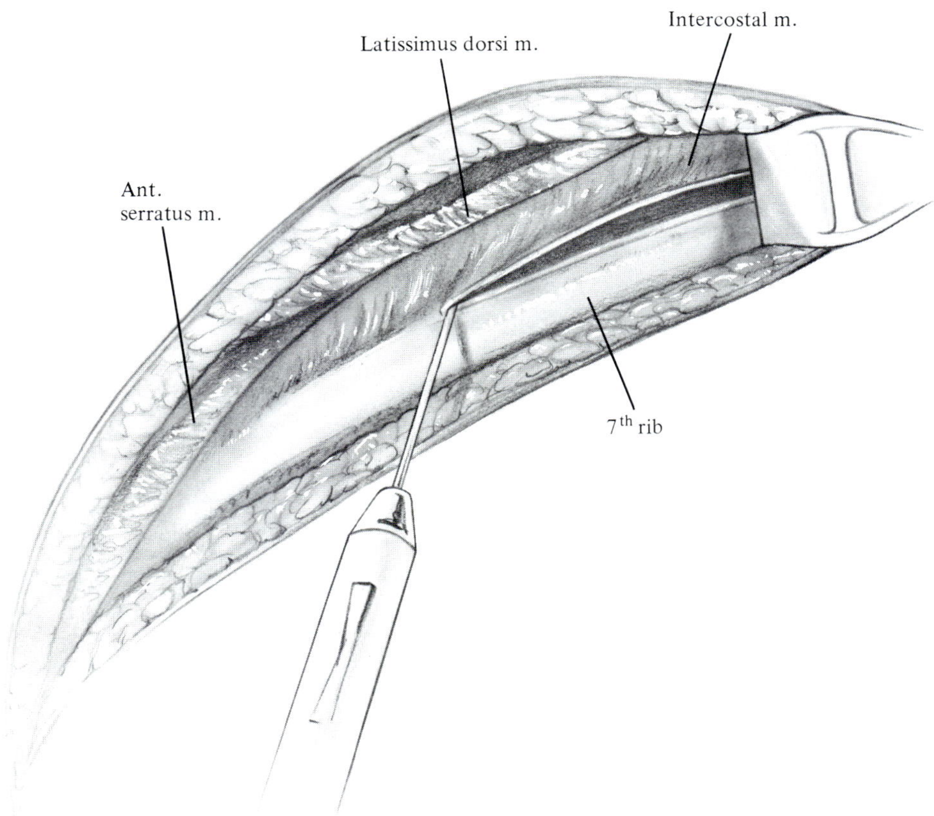

Fig. 8–6

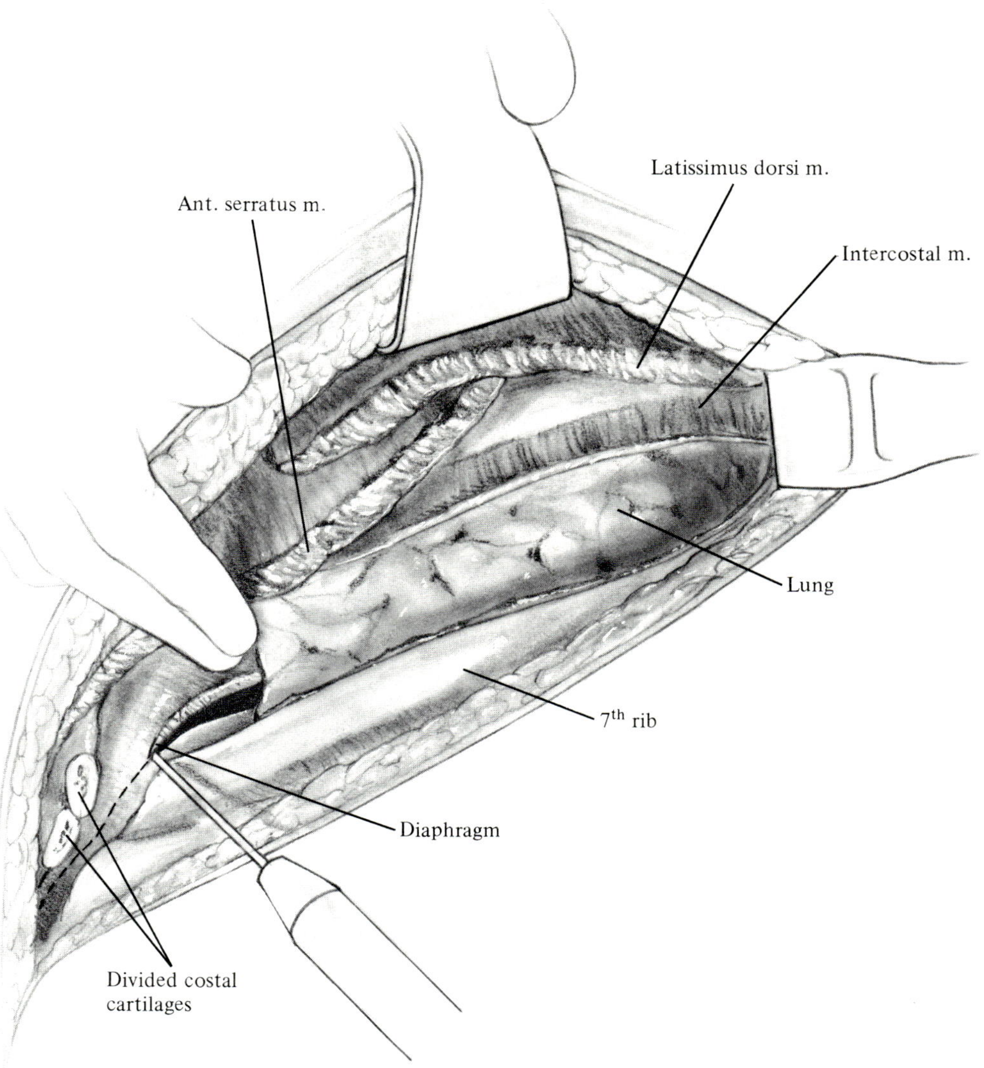

Fig. 8–7

Then incise the diaphragm in a circumferential fashion (**Figs. 8–7 and 8–8**) along a line 3–4 cm from its insertion into the rib cage. Use the electrocoagulator for this incision, which should extend laterally about 15–20 cm from the divided costal margin. Spread the intercostal incision by inserting a Finochietto retractor.

Liberation of Esophagus

Divide the inferior pulmonary ligament with long Metzenbaum scissors, going in a cephalad direction until the inferior pulmonary vein has been reached. Collapse the lung, cover it with moist gauze pads and retract it in a cephalad and anterior direction with Harrington retractors.

Incise the mediastinal pleura from the aorta to the hiatus, beginning at a point above the tumor (**Fig. 8–9**). Encircle

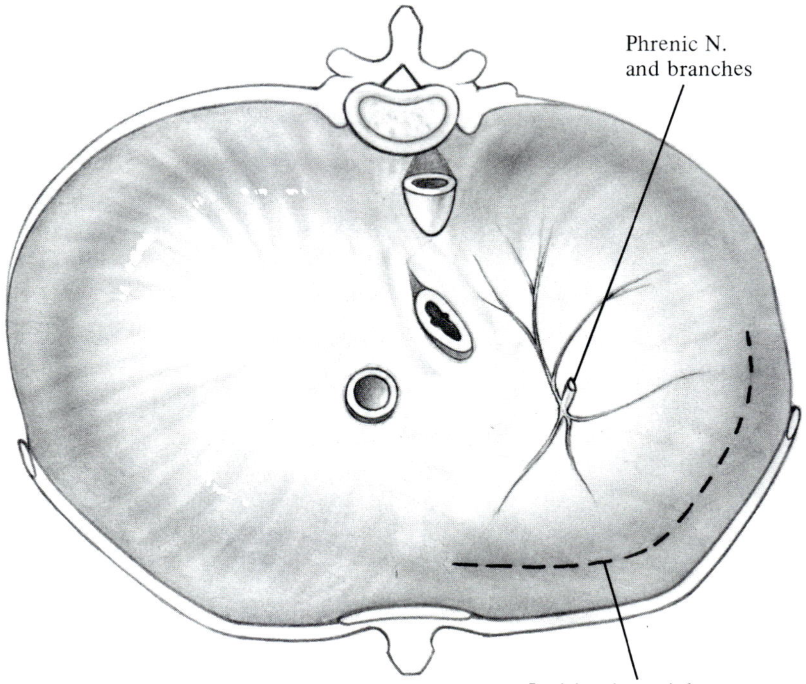
Phrenic N.
and branches
Incision in periphery
of diaphragm

Fig. 8–8

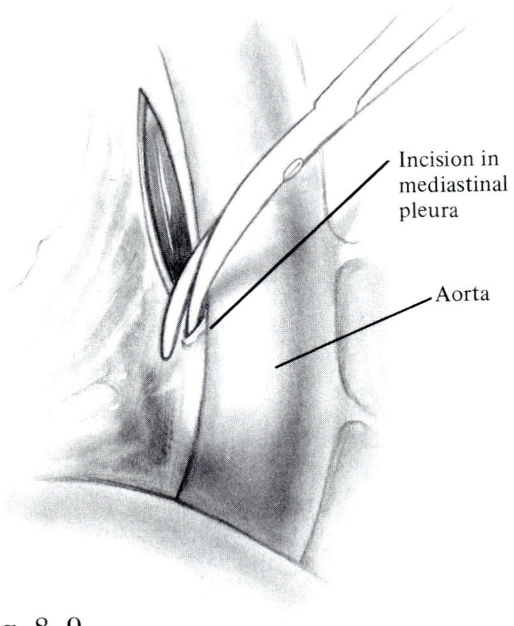
Incision in
mediastinal
pleura
Aorta

Fig. 8–9

the esophagus first with the index finger and then with a latex drain (**Fig. 8–10**). Divide the vagus nerves as they approach the esophagus from the hilus of the lung. Dissect the tumor and the attached vagus nerves away from the mediastinal structures. If the pleura of the right thoracic cavity or pericardium has been invaded by tumor, include it in the resection. The dissection of the esophagus should free this organ from the arch of the aorta down to the hiatus. Generally, only two or three branches of the descending aorta will join the esophagus. These should be occluded by Hemoclips and divided. Use an umbilical tape ligature or a row of 3.5 mm staples (TA–55) to occlude the lumen of the esophagus (above the tumor) in order to prevent the cephalad migration of the tumor cells (**Fig. 8–11**), but delay division of the esophagus until the stomach is mobilized.

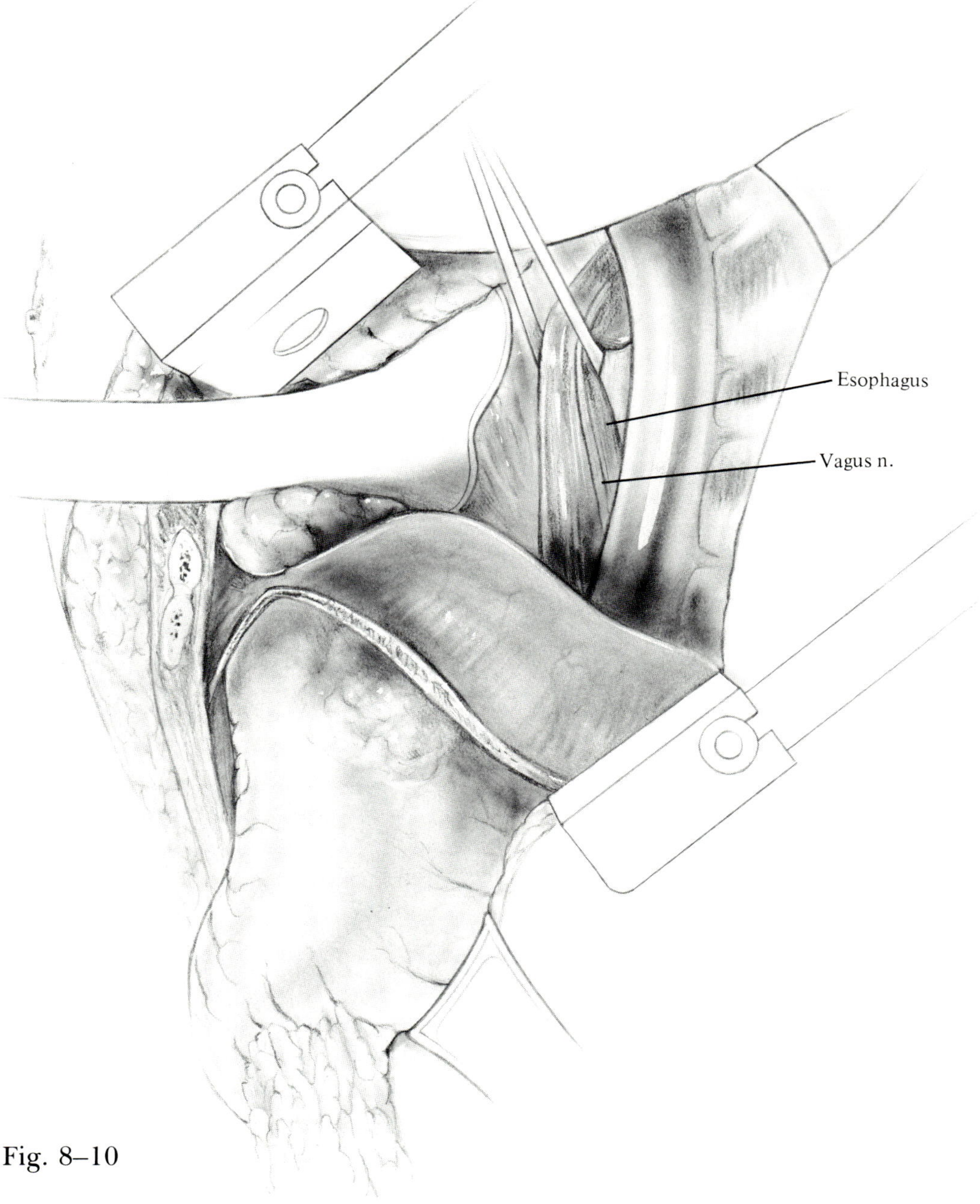

Fig. 8–10

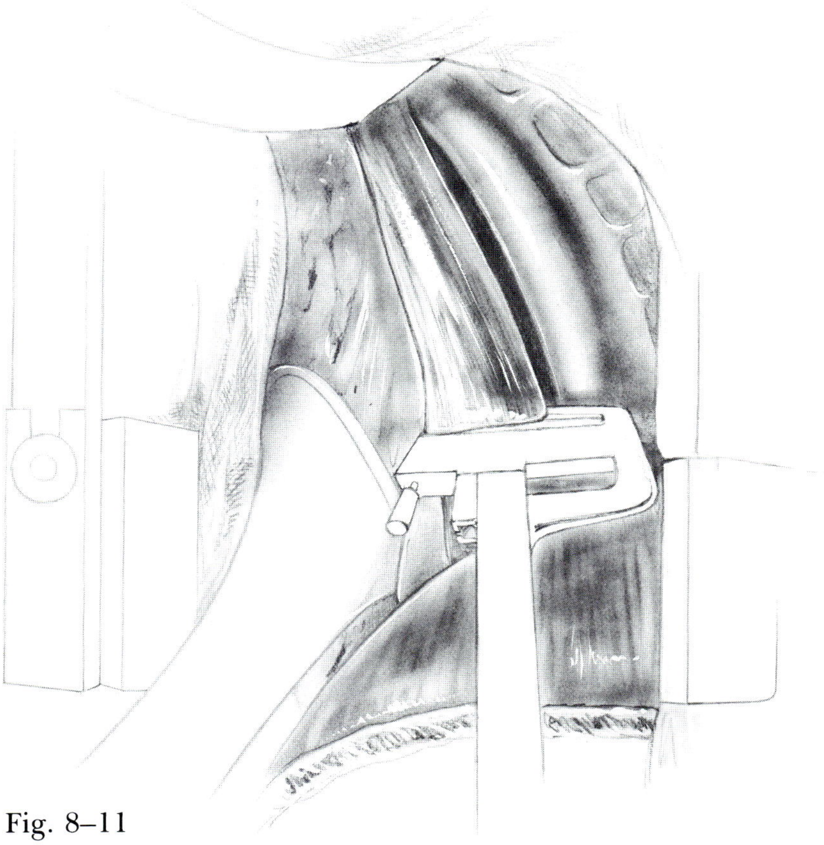

Fig. 8–11

Splenectomy

Retract the spleen medially and divide the lienophrenic ligament (**Fig. 8–12**). Gently elevate the spleen and tail of the pancreas from the retroperitoneal tissues by finger dissection. Divide the lienocolic ligament. Identify the splenic artery and vein on the posterior surface of the splenic hilus. Each should be divided and ligated with 2–0 cotton. It may be convenient to remove the spleen as a separate specimen after dividing each of the short gastric vessels. Do this on the anterior aspect of the stomach to visualize the greater curvature accurately, thereby avoiding any possibility of trauma to the stomach.

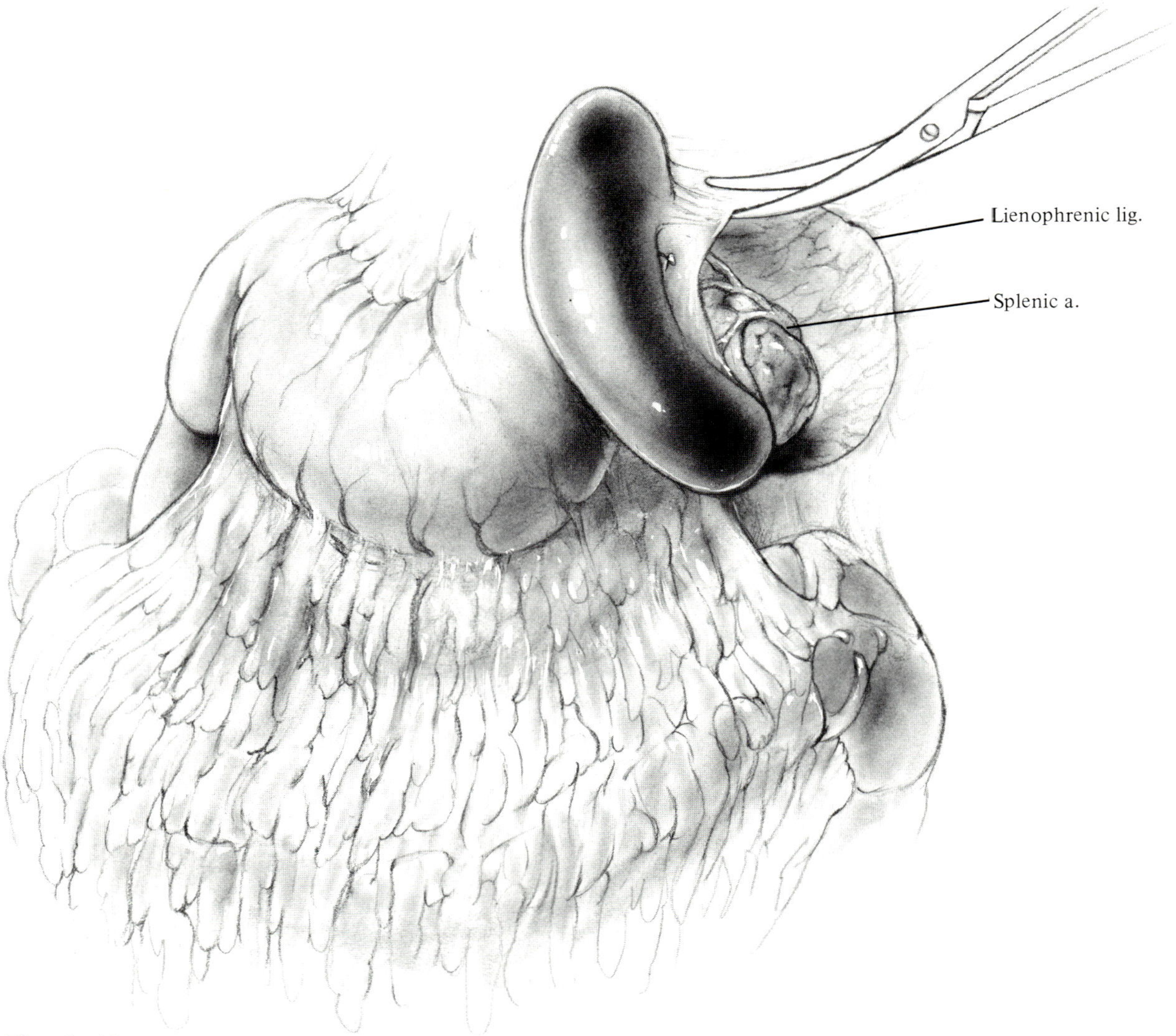

Fig. 8–12

Gastric Mobilization

The gastroepiploic arcade along the greater curvature of the stomach *must be preserved with compulsive attention to detail,* as the inadvertent occlusion of this vessel in a clamp or ligature will result in inadequate vascularity of the gastric pouch and anastomotic leakage. Preservation of the arcade is accomplished from above down by inserting the index finger behind the gastrocolic omentum, which is then divided between clamps. Be sure always to *leave 3–4 cm of redundant omentum attached* to the vascular arcade. Continue the dissection to a point 6–8 cm cephalad to the pylorus (**Figs. 8–13a and 8–13b**). The greater curvature now should be elevated. In order to accomplish this, incise its avascular attachments to the posterior parietal peritoneum at the pancreas.

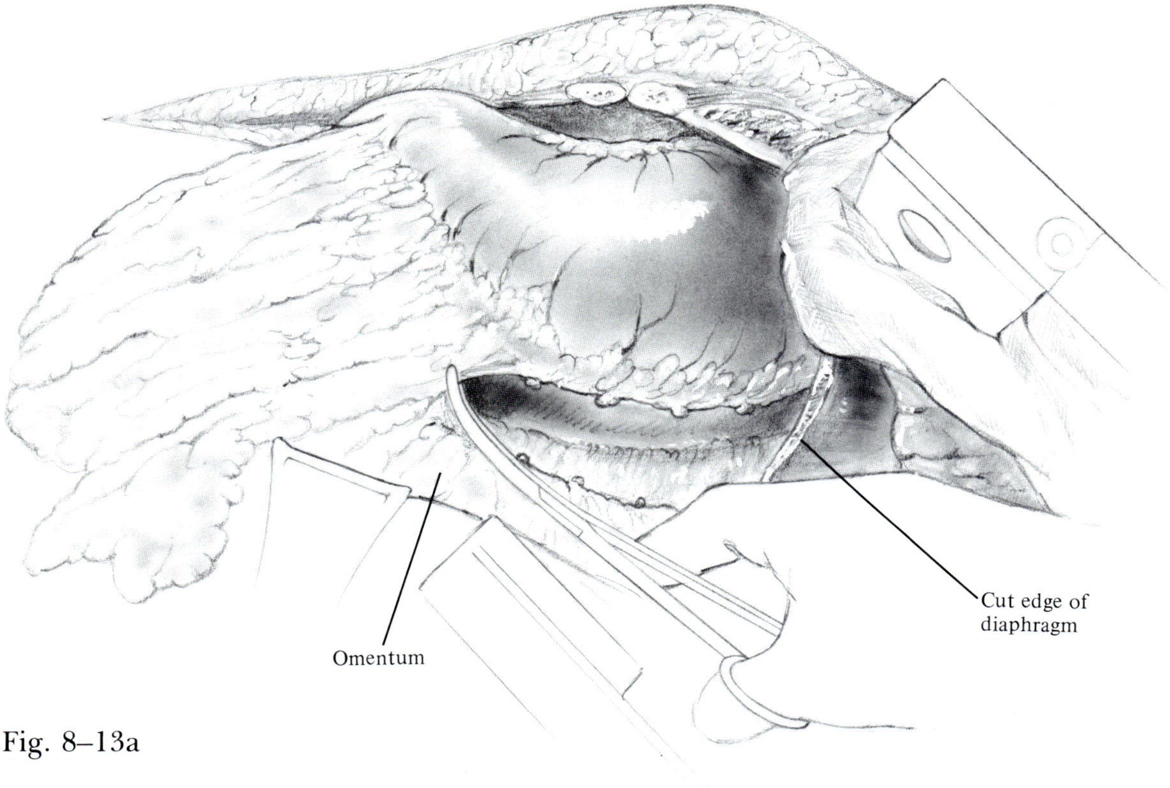

Fig. 8–13a

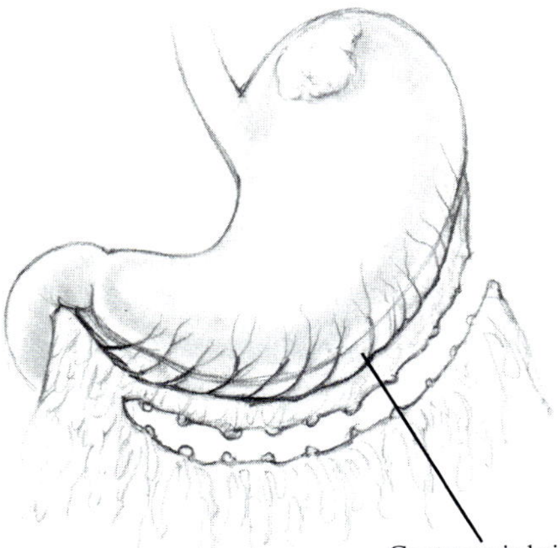

Fig. 8–13b

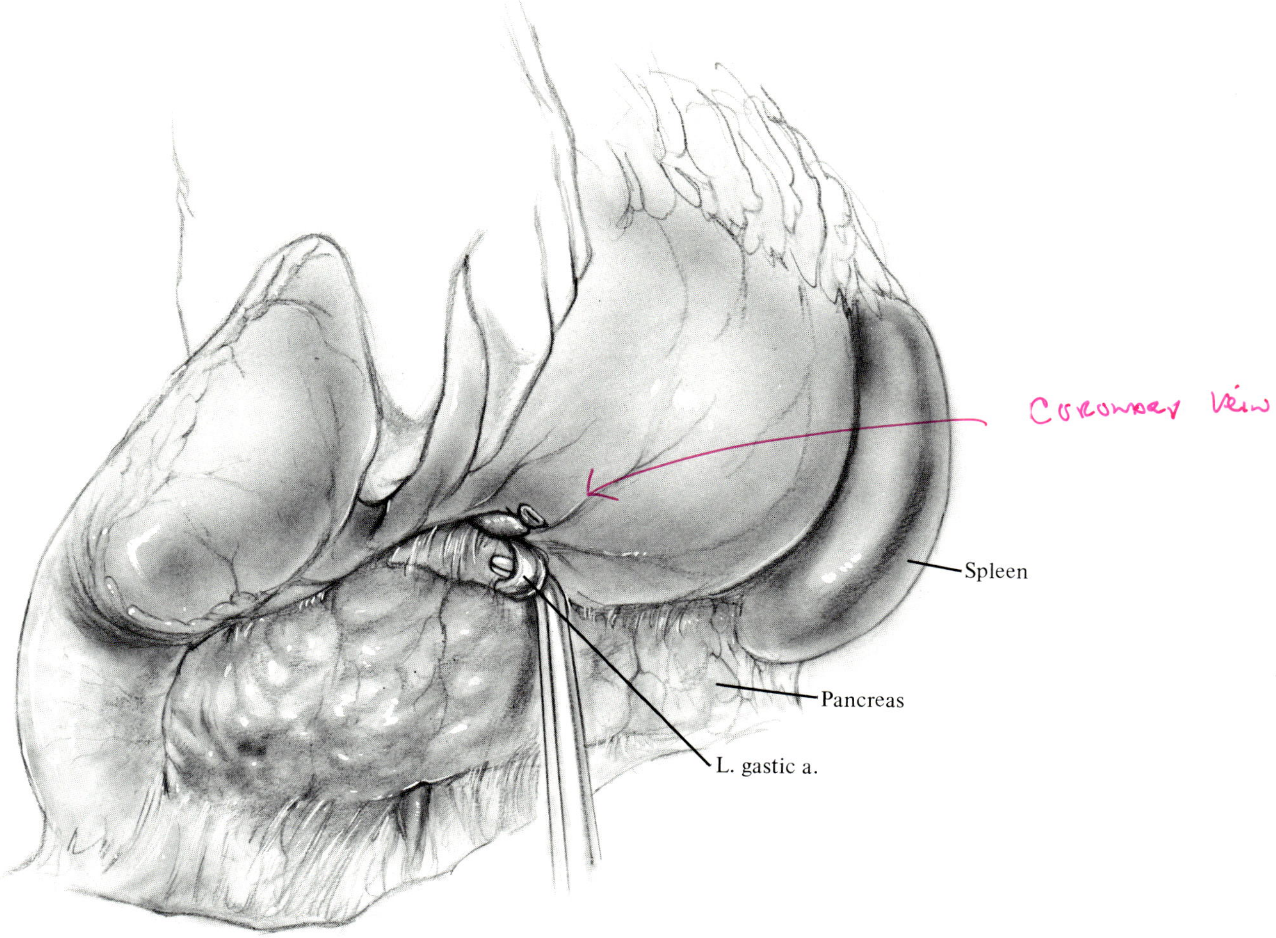

Fig. 8–14a

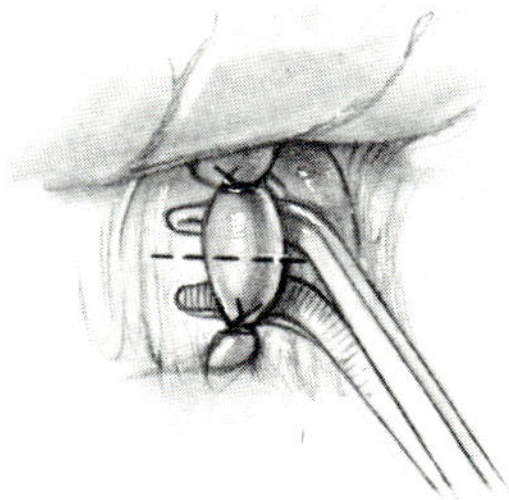

Fig. 8–14b

Identify the celiac axis by palpating the origins of the splenic, hepatic, and left gastric arteries. Dissect lymphatic and areolar tissues away from the celiac axis toward the specimen. Skeletonize the coronary vein, and divide and ligate it with 2–0 cotton. Immediately cephalad to this structure is the left gastric artery which should be doubly ligated with 2–0 cotton and divided (**Figs. 8–14a and 8–14b**). Incise the gastrohepatic ligament near its attachment to the liver (**Fig. 8–15**). An accessory left hepatic artery generally can be found in the cephalad portion of the gastrohepatic ligament. Divide this and ligate it with 2–0 cotton, and divide the remainder of the ligament and the peritoneum overlying the esophagus.

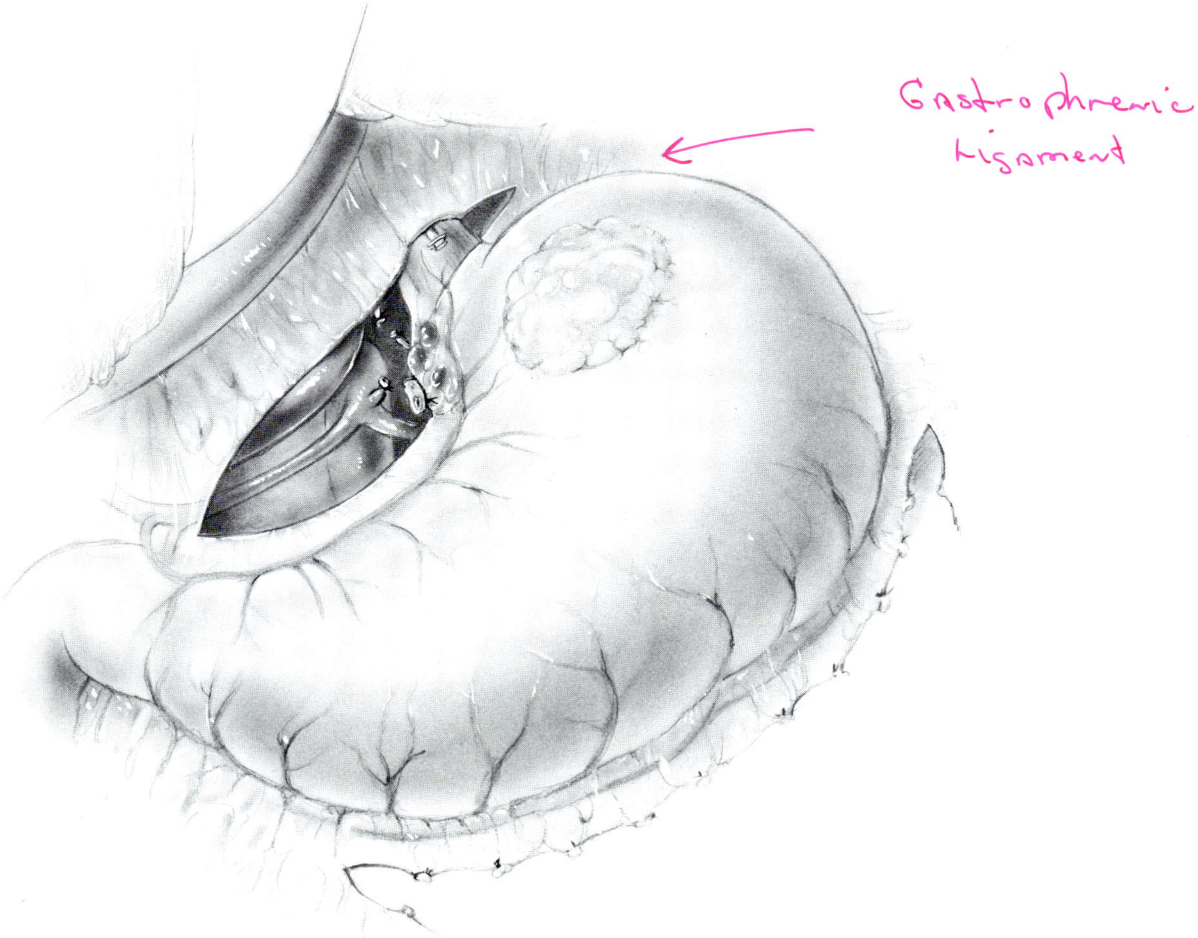

Fig. 8–15

Hiatal Dissection

A gastrophrenic ligament attaches the posterior aspect of the gastric fundus to the posterior diaphragm. Divide this, using the left index finger as a guide. If tumor has encroached upon the hiatus, leave crural musculature attached to the tumor and divide it from the surrounding diaphragm with the electrocautery. This may require division and ligature of the inferior phrenic artery. Divide the vagus

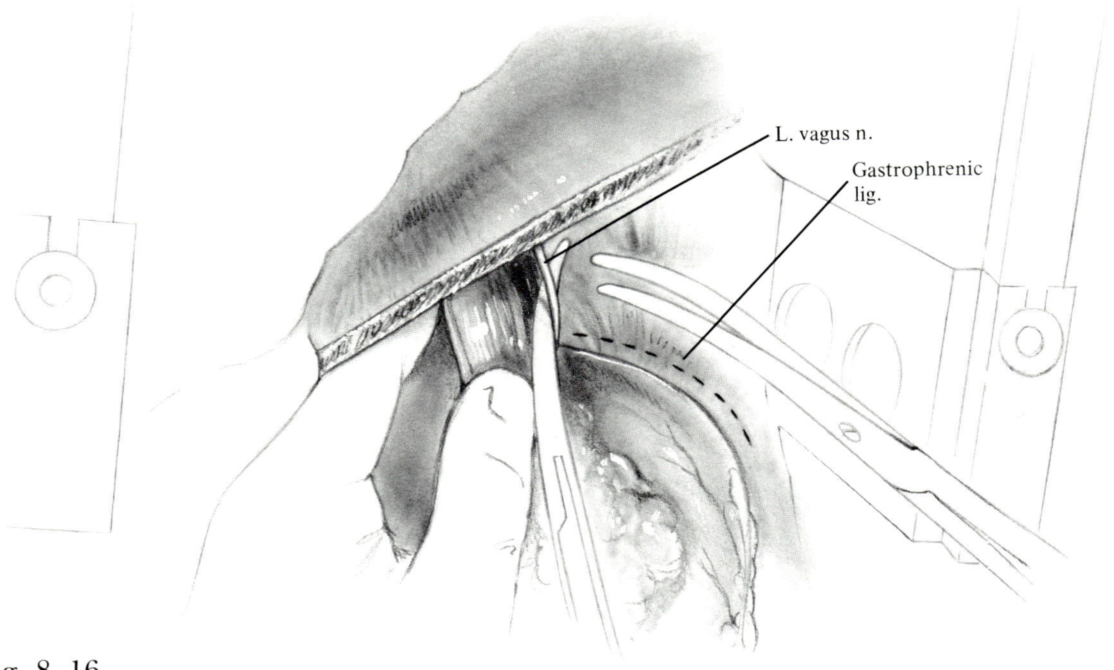

Fig. 8–16

nerves just below the hiatus (**Fig. 8–16**) and divide the phrenoesophageal ligaments; this frees the esophagus and stomach from the arch of the aorta down to the duodenum.

Kocher Maneuver

In order to achieve maximum upward mobility of the gastric pouch, divide the avascular lateral duodenal ligament and pass a hand behind the duodenum and the head of the pancreas (**Figs. 8–17 and 8–18**). If necessary, continue this Kocher maneuver along the duodenum as far distally as the superior mesenteric vein (see Figs. 7–15 and 7–16).

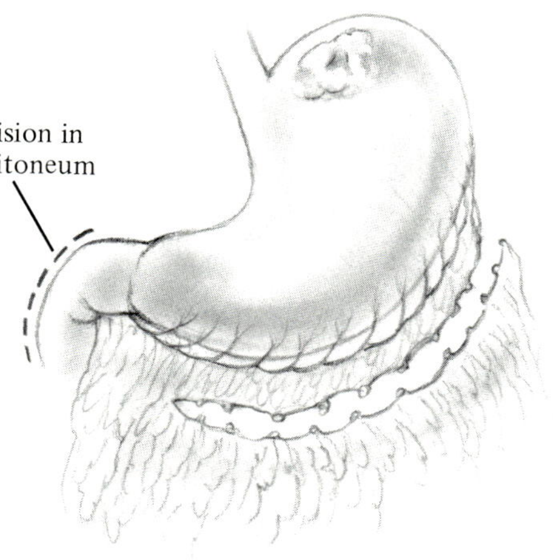

Fig. 8–17

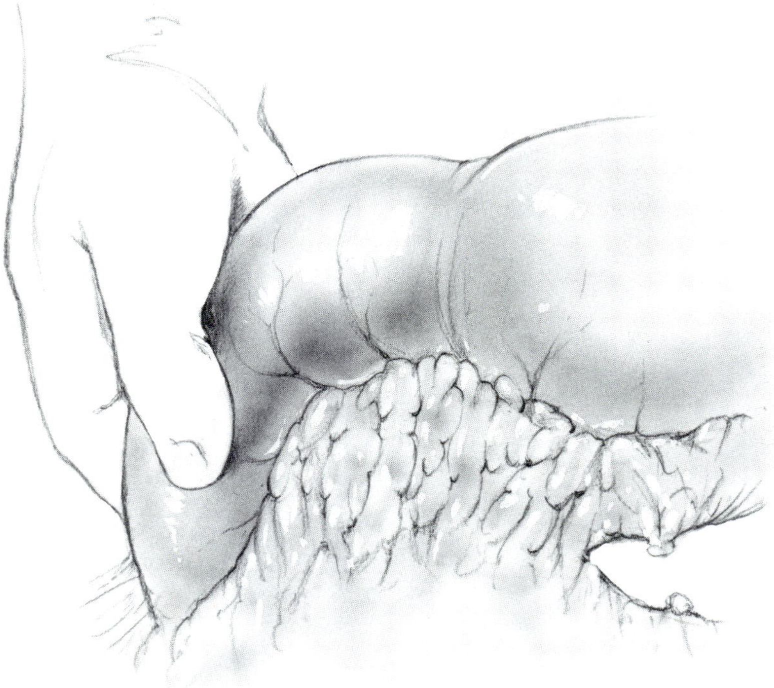

Fig. 8–18

Pyloromyotomy

Make a longitudinal incision 1.5–2.0 cm long across the anterior surface of the pylorus. Carefully deepen it, using the scalpel as well as blunt dissection, until the mucosa pouts out (**Figs. 8–19a, 8–19b, and**

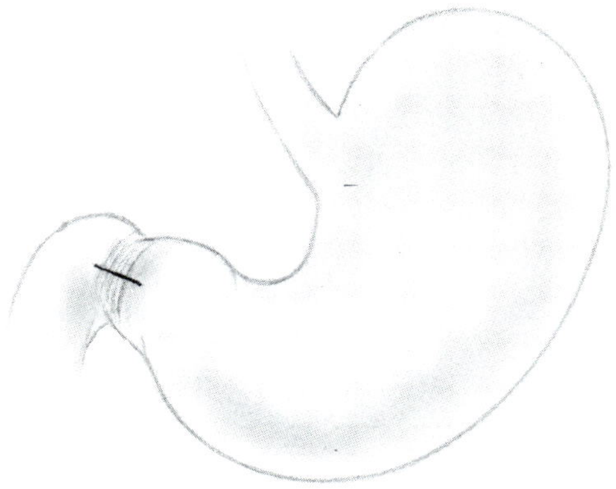

Fig. 8–19a

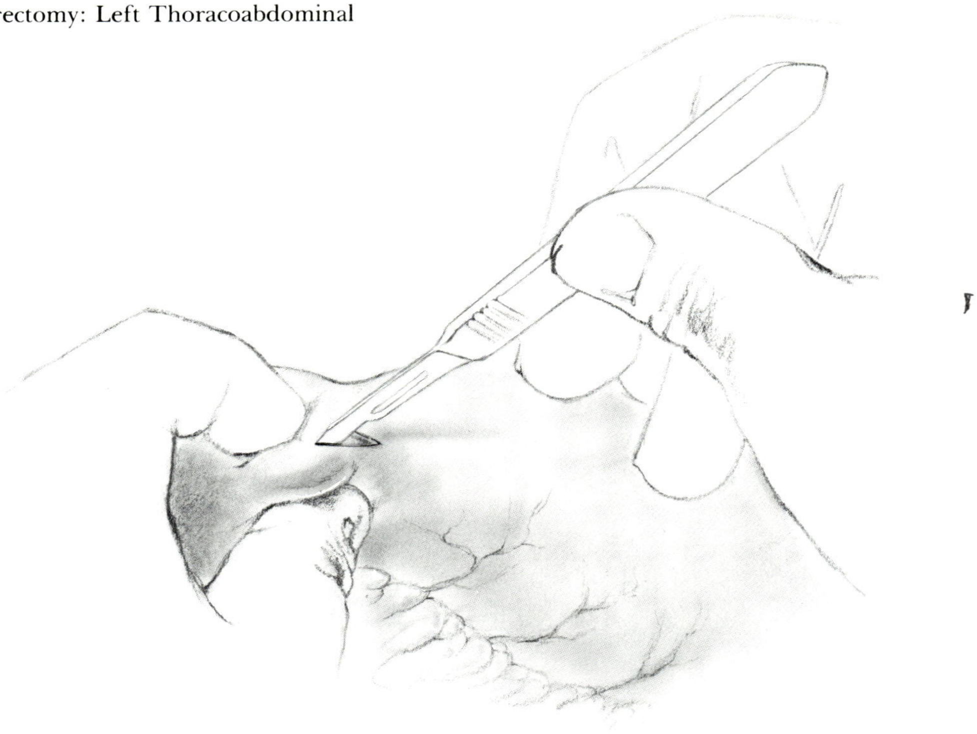

Fig. 8–19b

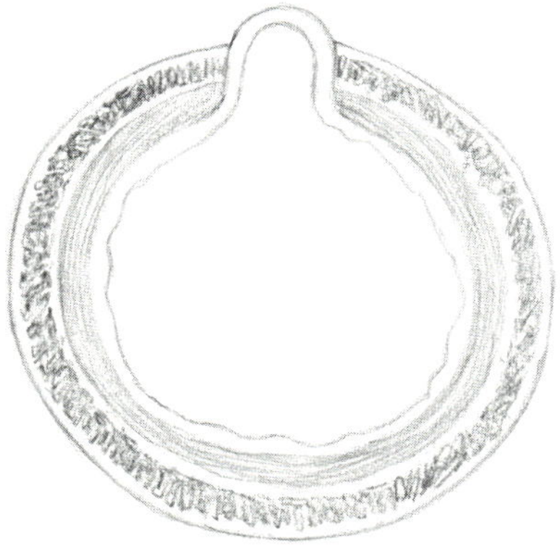

Fig. 8–19c

8–19c). Because the pyloric sphincter is not hypertrophied, as it is in infants who require this operation, it is easier to perforate the mucosa than it is in infants. The greatest danger of perforation is at the duodenal end of the pyloromyotomy. A tiny mucosal perforation may be repaired with 5–0 silk sutures and covered with omentum. A significant rent in the mucosa should be corrected by converting the pyloromyotomy into a Heineke-Mikulicz pyloroplasty. Pyloroplasty is a less desirable procedure than pyloromyotomy because it may impair the intramural flow of blood from the duodenum up into the gastric pouch. The objection may be merely theoretical, however, as many surgeons have used the pyloroplasty as a routine drainage procedure in esophagogastrectomy. Fisher et al. have been satisfied merely to dilate the pylorus by invaginating the anterior wall of the stomach forcibly into the pylorus, using a finger. We have successfully used this technique in a few patients.

Transection of Stomach and of Esophagus

To treat a primary tumor of the lower esophagus, apply the TA–90 Auto Suture stapler in an oblique fashion so as to remove the stump of the left gastric artery, the celiac lymph nodes on the lesser curvature of the stomach, and 5–6 cm of the greater curvature. To treat lesions of the proximal stomach, which is the operation illustrated in **Figs. 8–20a and 8–20b,** apply the stapler so that 5–6 cm of normal stomach distal to the lesion are removed.

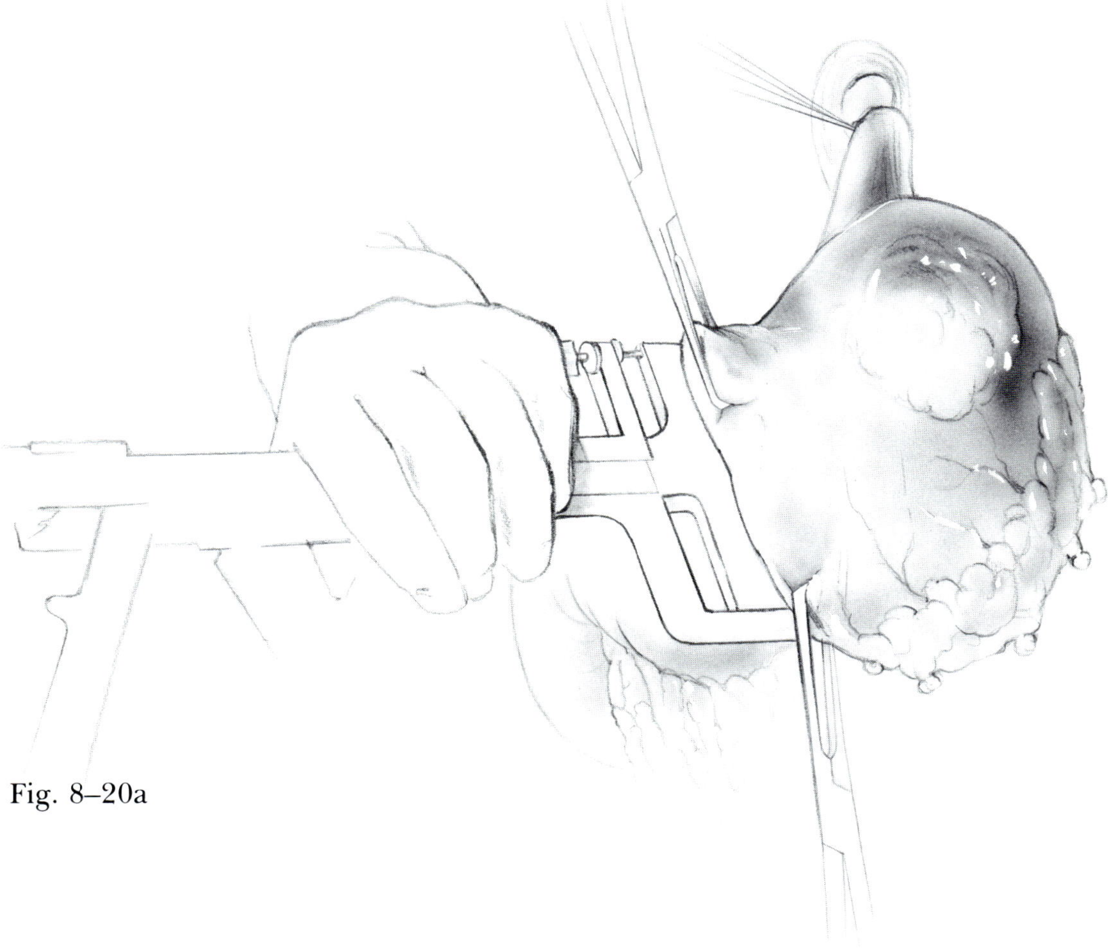

Fig. 8–20a

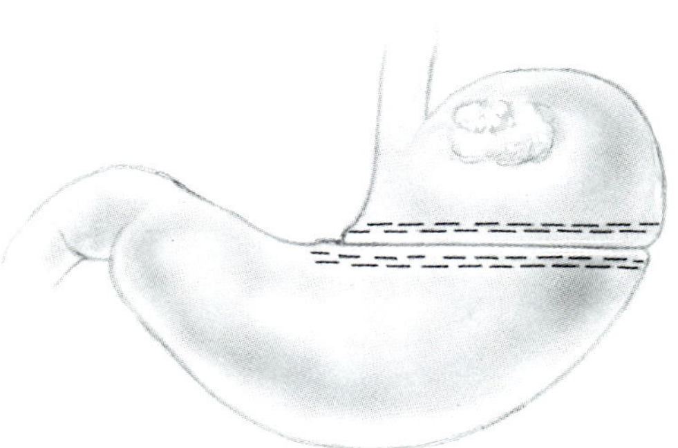

Fig. 8–20b

Divide the upper stomach between two TA–90 Auto Suture staplers. Make an incision with the scalpel flush with the stapler that is attached to the residual gastric pouch. If two TA–90 staplers are not available, the first stapler should be applied to the stomach, fired, and then reap-

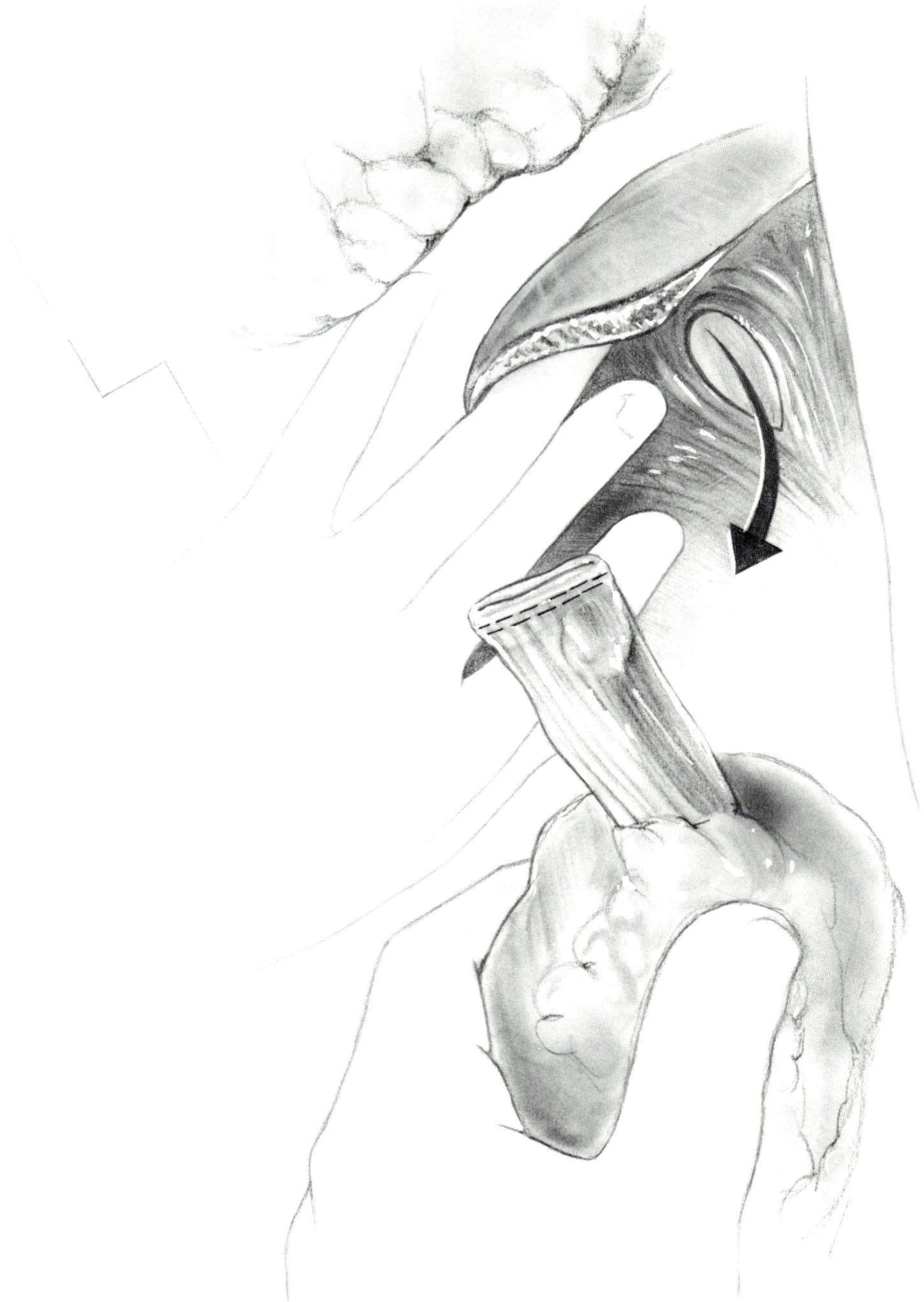

Fig. 8–21

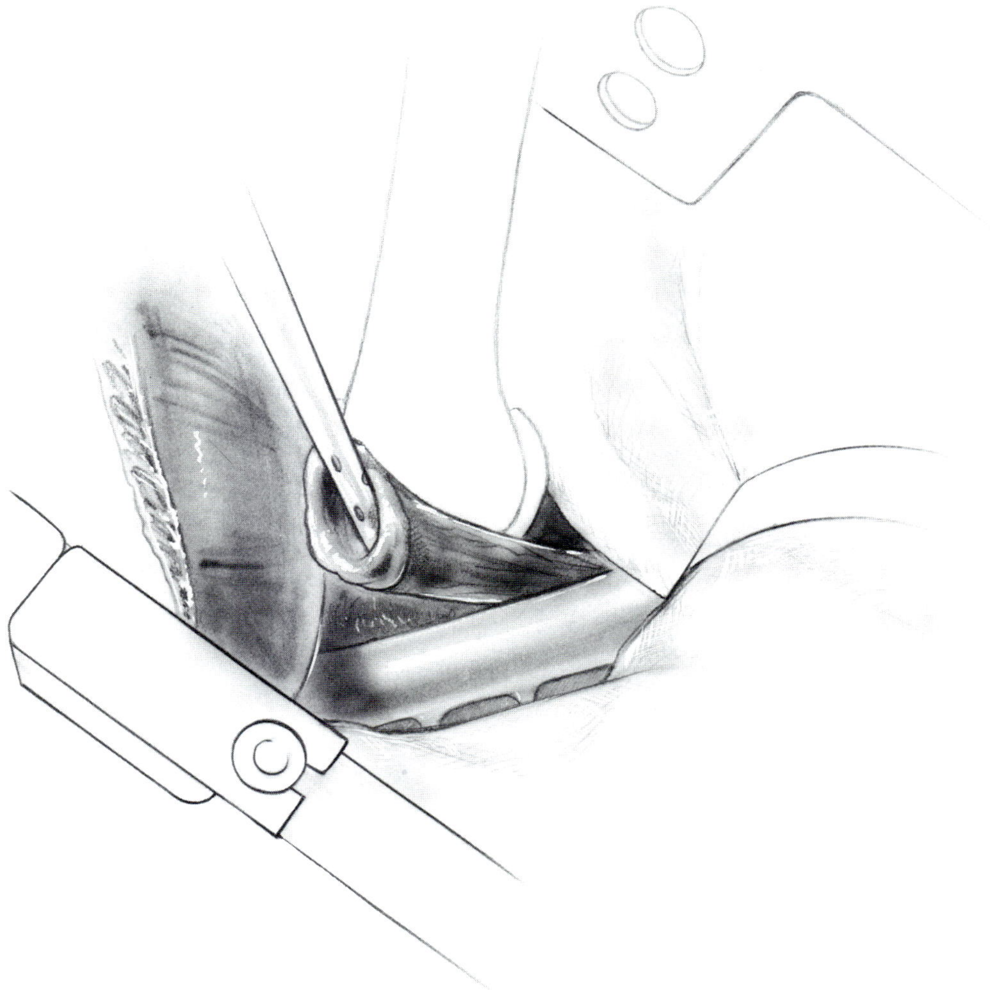

Fig. 8–22

plied 1 cm lower on the gastric wall. The transection should be made flush with the stapler on the gastric pouch. Sterilize the area by lightly running the electrocoagulator over the mucosa and remove the device. Before applying the stapling device, be certain that the nasogastric tube has been withdrawn, as transfixing the nasogastric tube with a row of staples can complicate the procedure considerably.

In a previous step the esophageal lumen proximal to the tumor was occluded with a row of staples (**Fig. 8–21**). Now transect the esophagus 8–10 cm proximal to the tumor and remove the specimen (**Fig. 8–22**). Submit the proximal and distal margins of the specimen to frozen section examination.

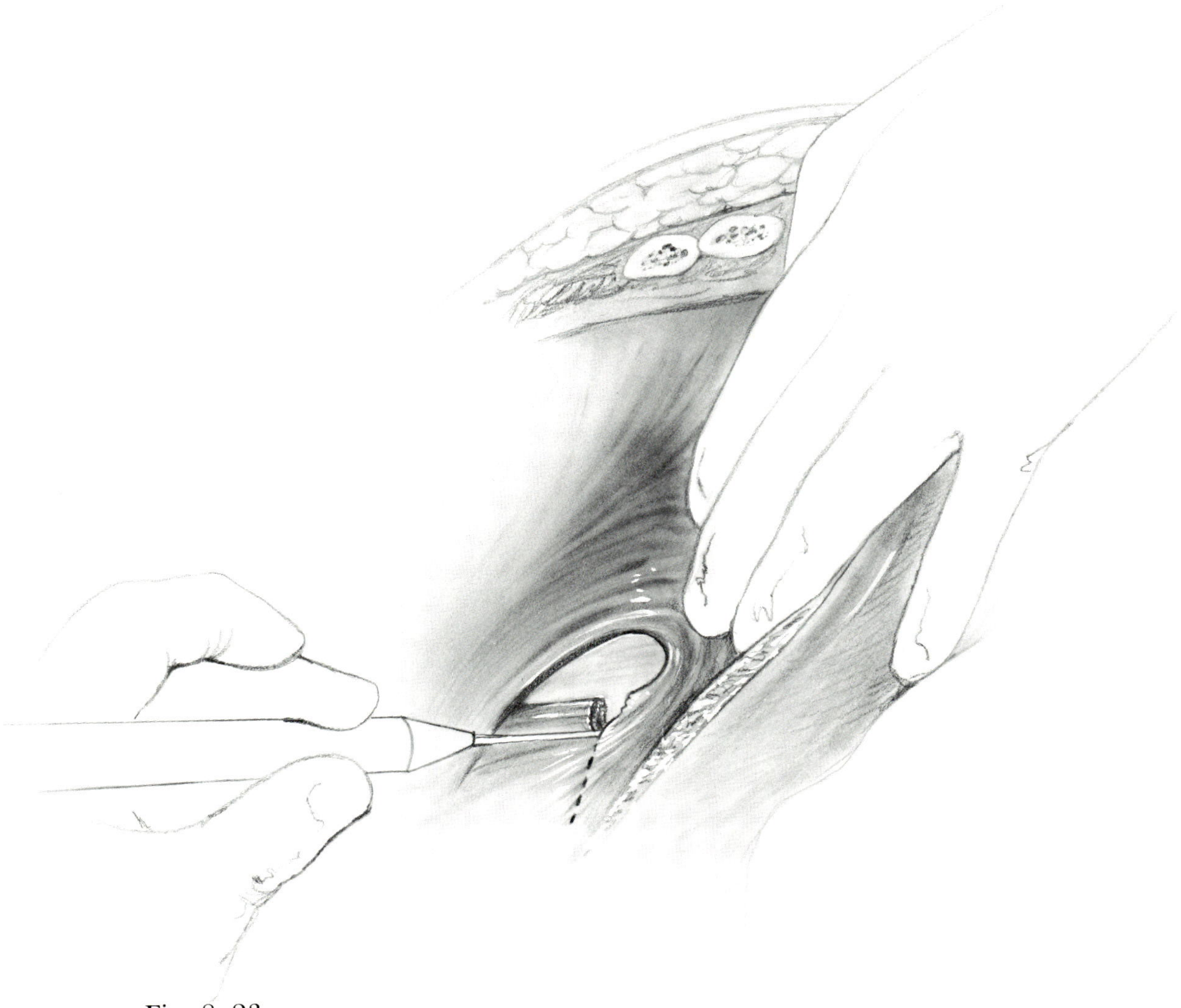

Fig. 8–23

Enlargement of Hiatus

Make a transverse incision by electrocautery in the left branch of the crux (**Fig. 8–23**). This should be of sufficient magnitude to allow the gastric pouch to pass into the mediastinum *without constriction* of its venous circulation.

Enlargement of Thoracic Incision if Supra-aortic Anastomosis Is Necessary

A properly fashioned end-to-side esophagogastric anastomosis requires the presence of at least 6–8 cm of esophagus below the aortic arch. If there is not 6–8 cm of esophagus below the aortic arch, the surgeon should not hesitate to enlarge the thoracic incision so that the esophagus can be passed behind the arch into a supra-aortic position. This will make the anastomosis far simpler and safer to perform, and requires only a few minutes to accomplish.

Now move to a position on the left side of the patient. Extend the skin incision up from the tip of the scapula in a cephalad direction between the scapula and the spine. With the electrocautery divide the rhomboid and trapezius muscles medial to the scapula. Retract the scapula in a cephalad direction and free the erector spinal muscle from the necks of the sixth and fifth ribs. Free a short (1 cm) segment of the sixth (and often of the fifth) rib of its surrounding periosteum and excise it (**Fig. 8–24**). Divide and either

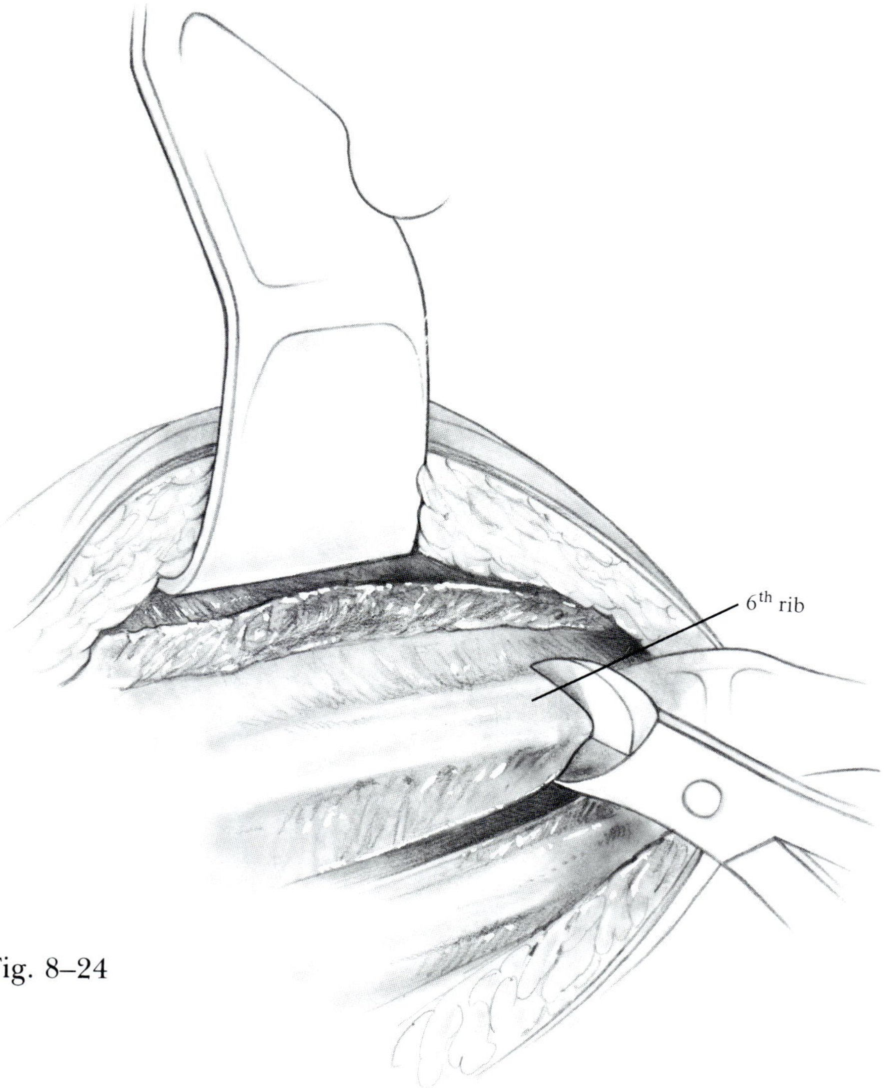

Fig. 8–24

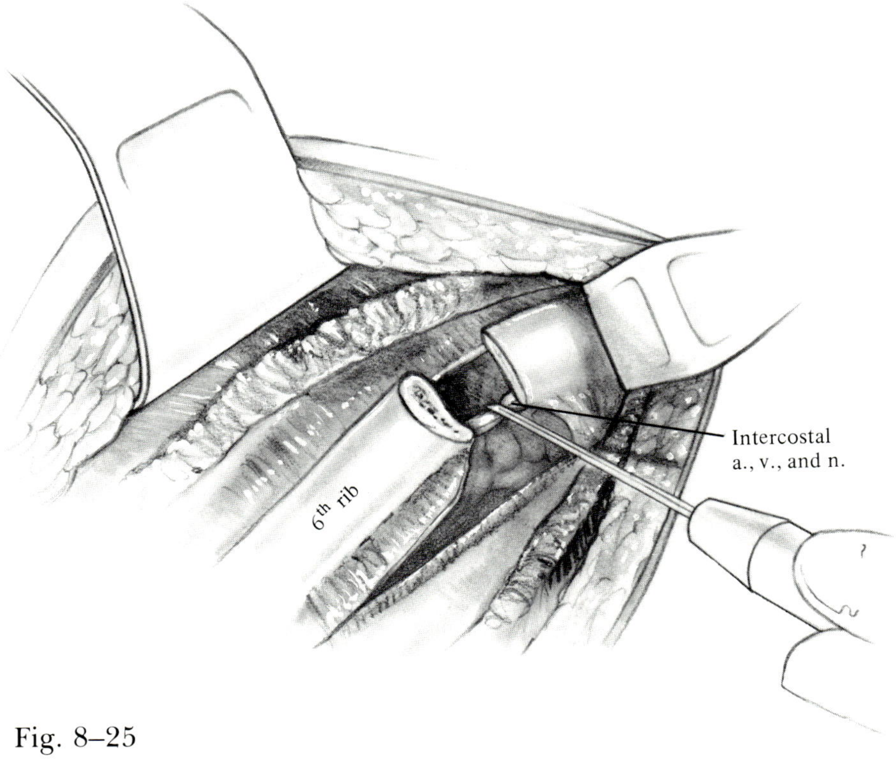

Fig. 8–25

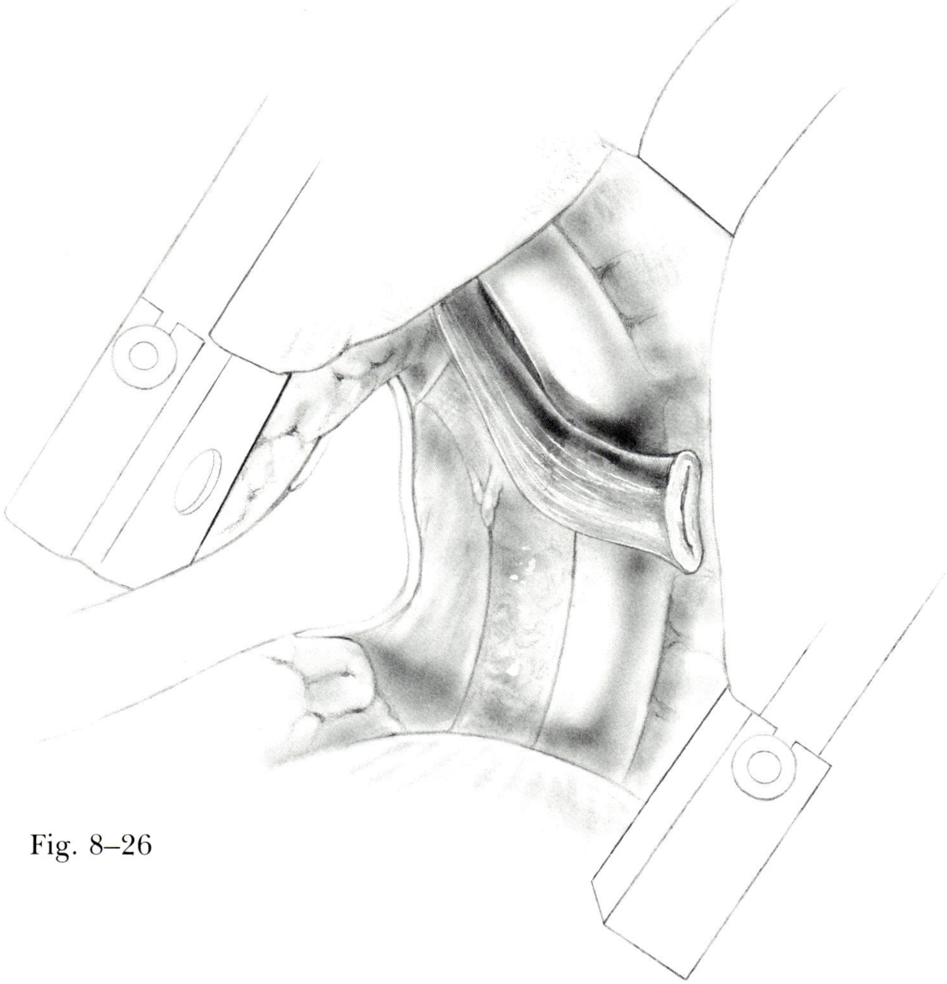

Fig. 8–26

ligate or electrocoagulate the intercostal nerves with their accompanying vessels (**Fig. 8–25**). Reinsert the Finochietto retractor (**Fig. 8–26**). If the exposure is still inadequate, a segment of the fourth rib may also be excised, but this has rarely been necessary.

Enter the space between the anterior wall of the esophagus and the aortic arch with the index finger (**Fig. 8–27a–c**). There are no vascular attachments in this area. The index finger will emerge cephalad to the aortic arch behind the mediastinal pleura. Incise the mediastinal pleura on

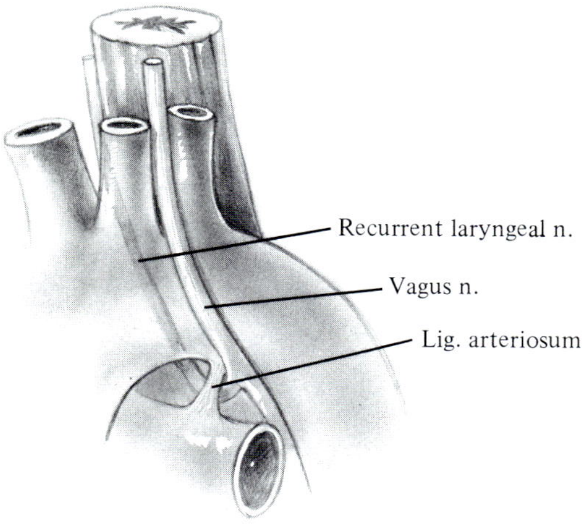

Fig. 8–27a

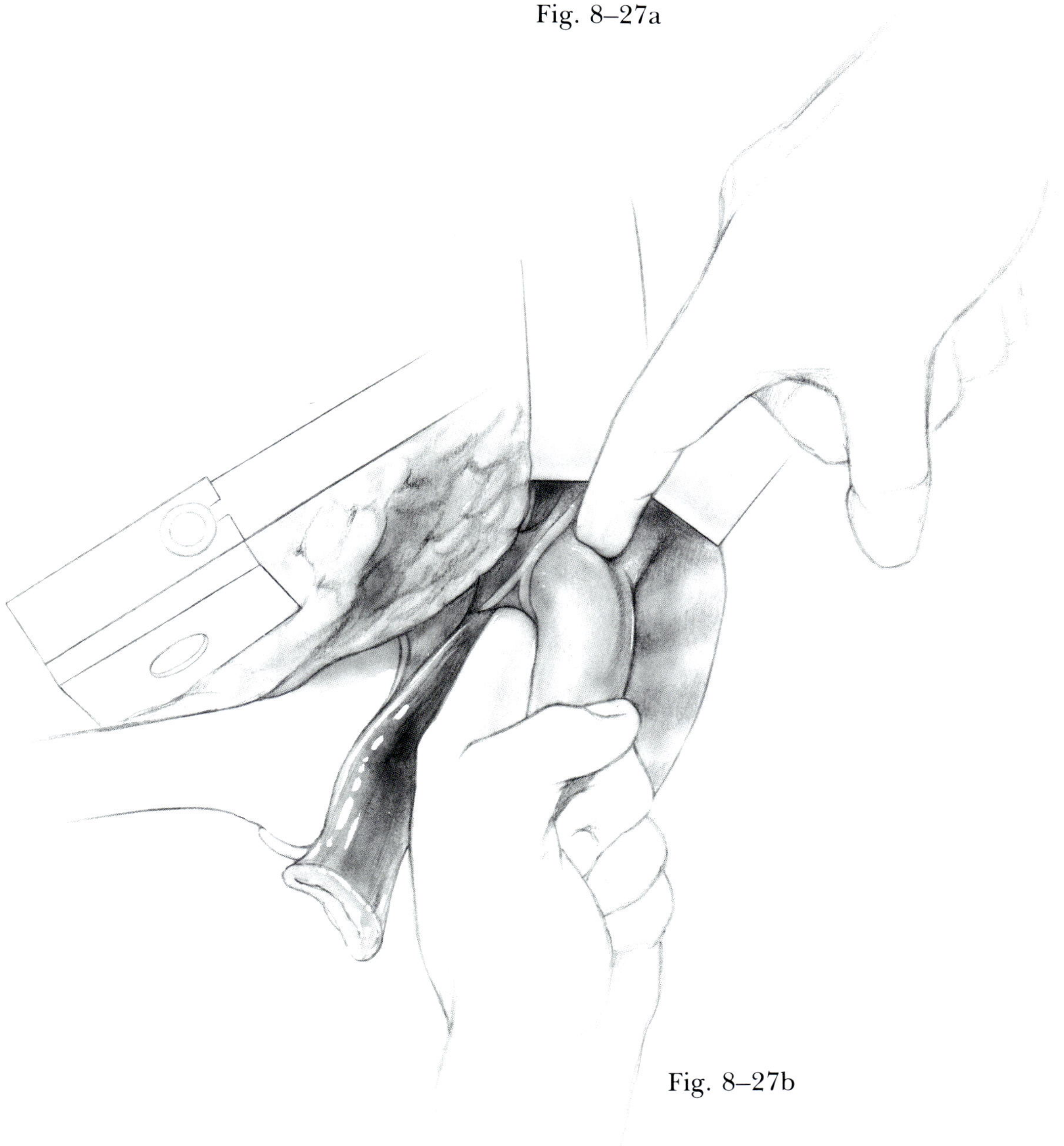

Fig. 8–27b

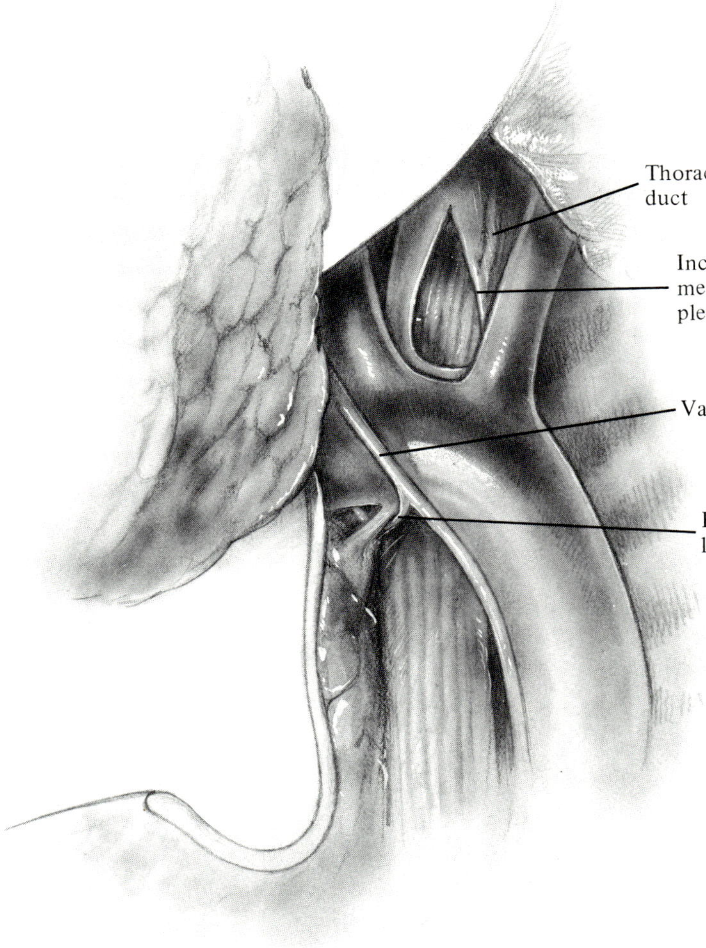

Fig. 8–27c

the index finger, making a window extending along the anterior surface of the esophagus up to the thoracic inlet. Now dissect the esophagus free of all its attachments in the mediastinum in the vicinity of the aortic arch. Avoid damage to the left recurrent laryngeal nerve, to the thoracic duct, and to the left vagus nerve located medial to the esophagus above the aortic arch. One or two vessels may have to be divided between Hemoclips.

Deliver the esophagus from behind the aortic arch up through the window in the pleura between the left carotid and subclavian arteries (**Fig. 8–28**). If the space between the carotid and subclavian arteries is narrow, bring the esophagus out through a pleural incision lateral to the subclavian artery. Irrigate the mediastinum and the esophageal lumen with antibiotic solution.

The esophagogastric anastomosis, as described below, should be constructed in a position lateral and anterior to the aortic arch. Exposure for the anastomosis in this

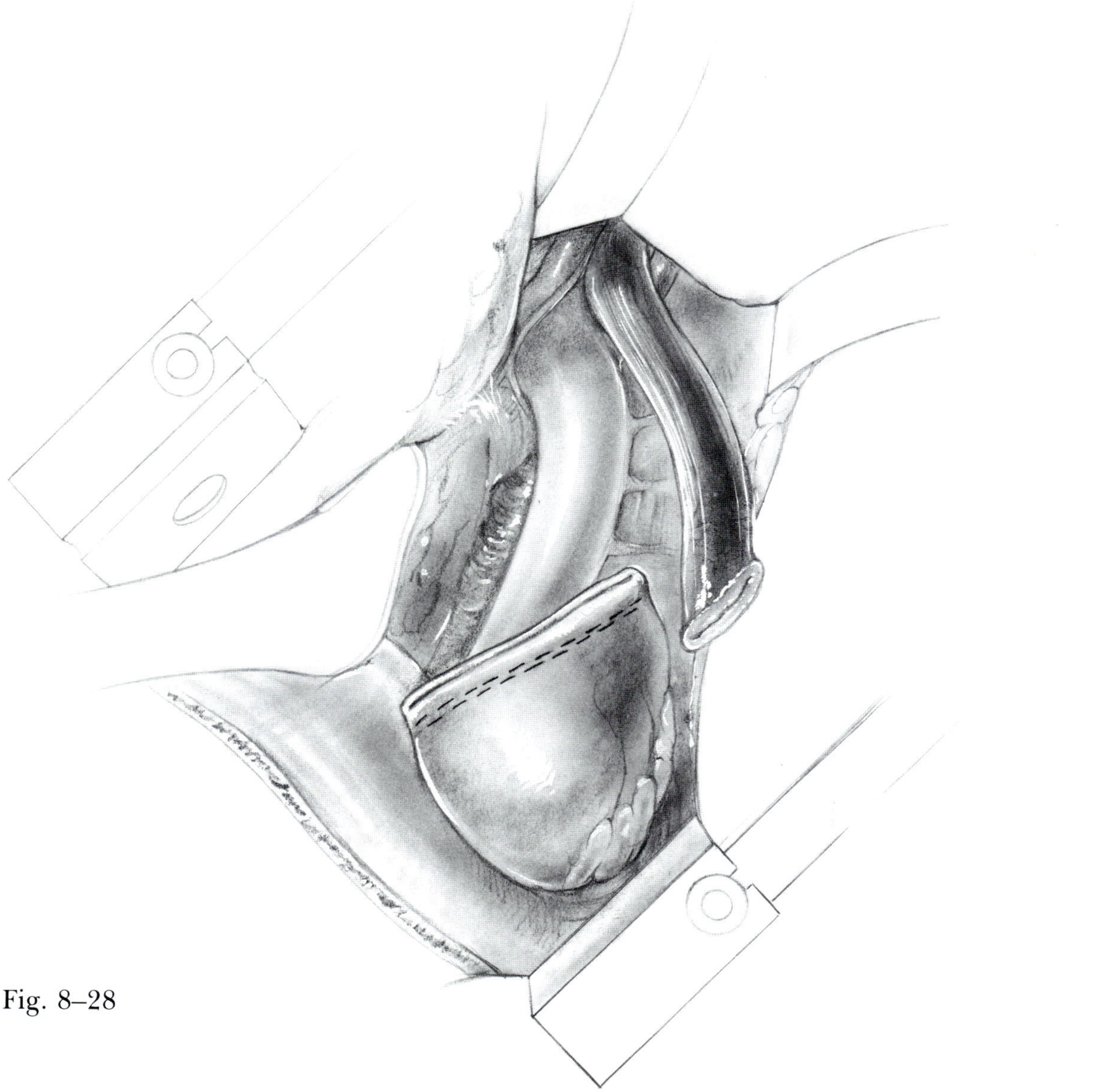

Fig. 8–28

location is excellent. Bring the esophagus down over the anterior wall of the stomach. An overlap of 6–7 cm is desirable. If the esophageal dissection has been carried out without undue trauma, the esophageal segment will have an excellent blood supply even though its distal 10 cm has been liberated from its bed in the mediastinum.

Esophagogastric Anastomosis, Sutured

The technique of sutured esophagogastric anastomosis is described and illustrated in Chap. 7.

Esophagogastric Anastomosis Performed by Stapling Technique

The stapling technique for esophagogastric anastomosis involves attaching the posterior aspect of the distal esophagus to the anterior wall of the stomach. It requires an overlap to enable 7–8 cm of the esophagus to lie freely over the front of the stomach. If a 7–8 cm overlap is not available, this stapling technique is contraindicated.

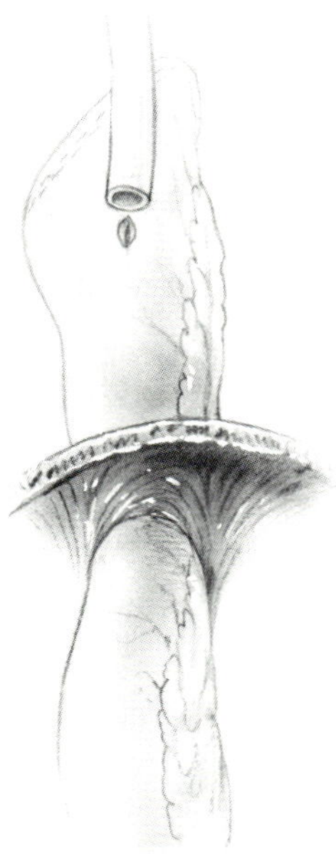

Fig. 8–29

Make a stab wound, 1.5 cm long, on the anterior wall of the gastric pouch at a point 7–8 cm from the cephalad margin of the stomach (**Fig. 8–29**). Insert one fork of the GIA stapling device through the stab wound into the stomach and the other fork into the open end of the overlying esophagus (**Fig. 8–30**). The GIA device should be inserted to a depth of 3.5–4.0 cm. Fire and remove the stapling device. This step will leave both the end of the esophagus and a large opening in the stomach unclosed (**Fig. 8–31**). The posterior layer of the anastomosis will already have been accomplished by the GIA de-

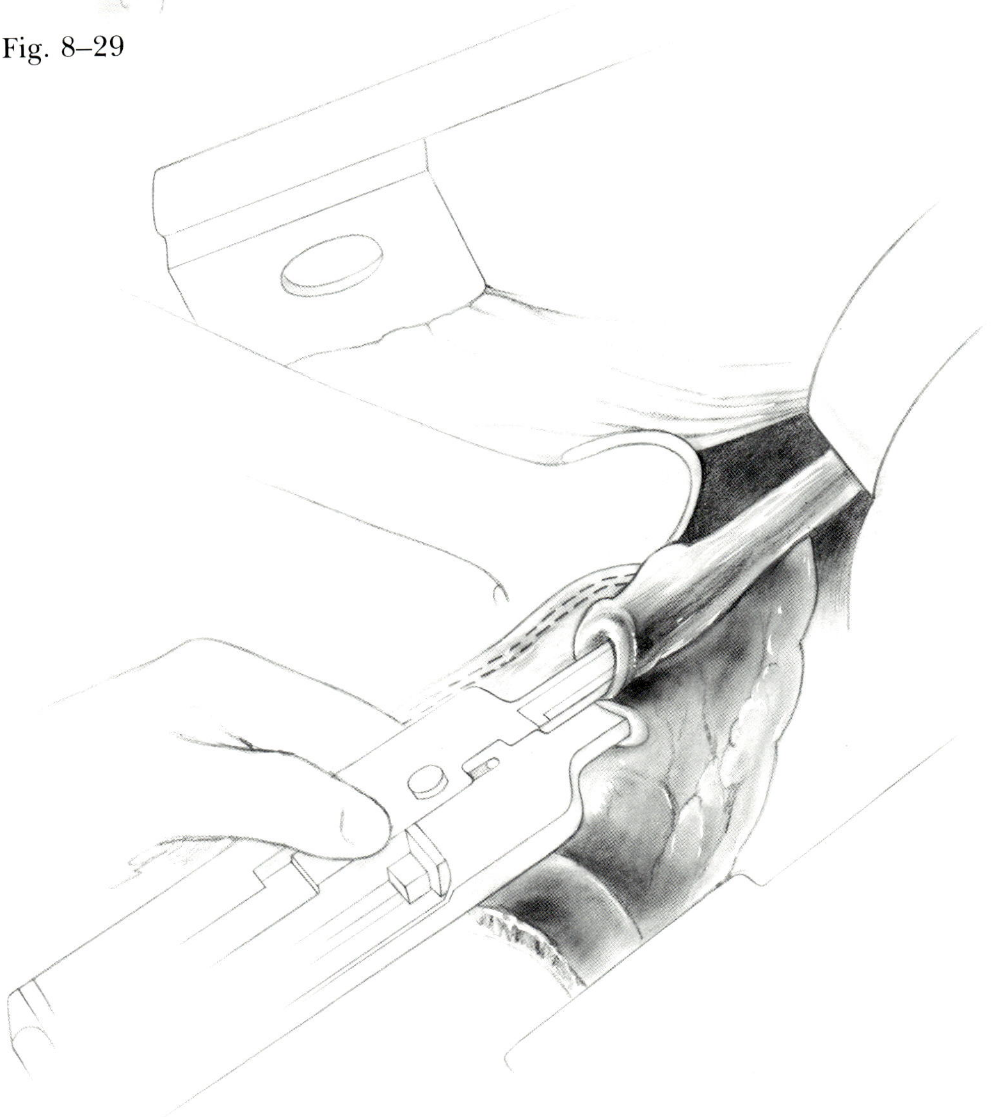

Fig. 8–30

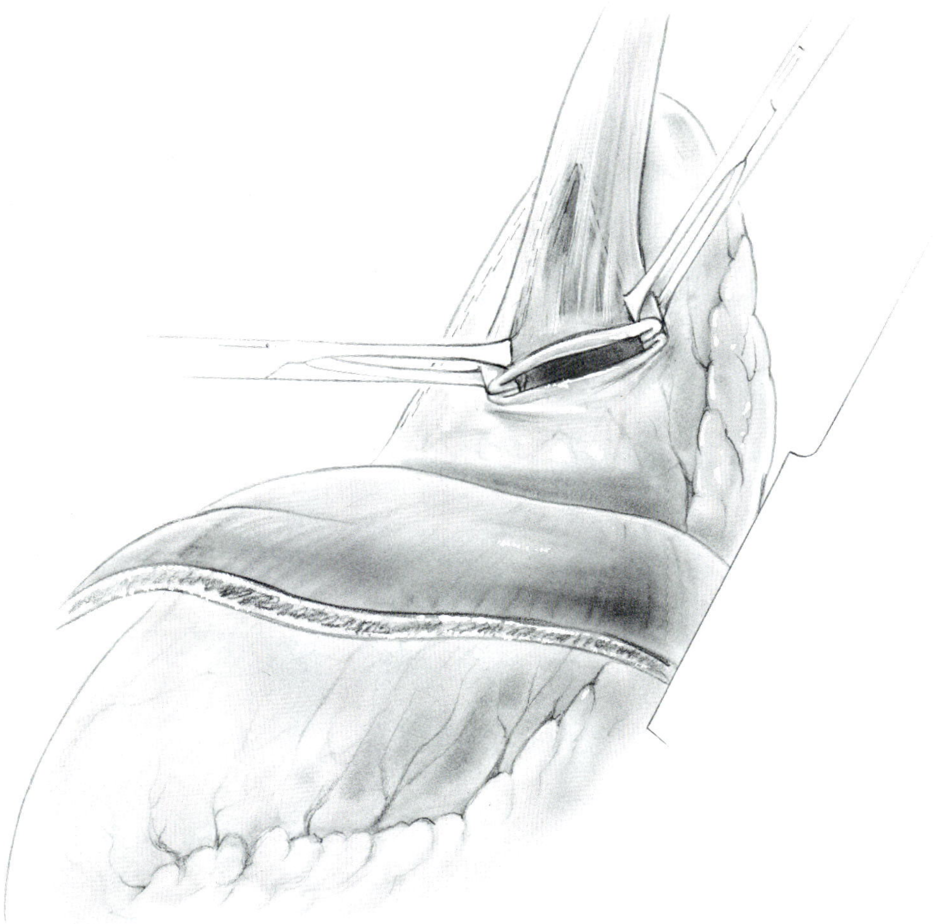

Fig. 8–31

vice. Complete the remainder of the anastomosis in an everting fashion by triangulation with two applications of the TA–55 stapler. To facilitate this, insert a 4–0 temporary guy suture through the full thickness of the anterior esophageal wall at its midpoint, carry the suture through the center of the remaining opening in the gastric wall (**Fig. 8–32**), and tie the suture. Apply Allis clamps to approximate the everted walls of the esophagus and stomach. Apply the first Allis clamp just behind the termination of the GIA staple line on the medial side. Hold the suture and the Allis clamps so that a

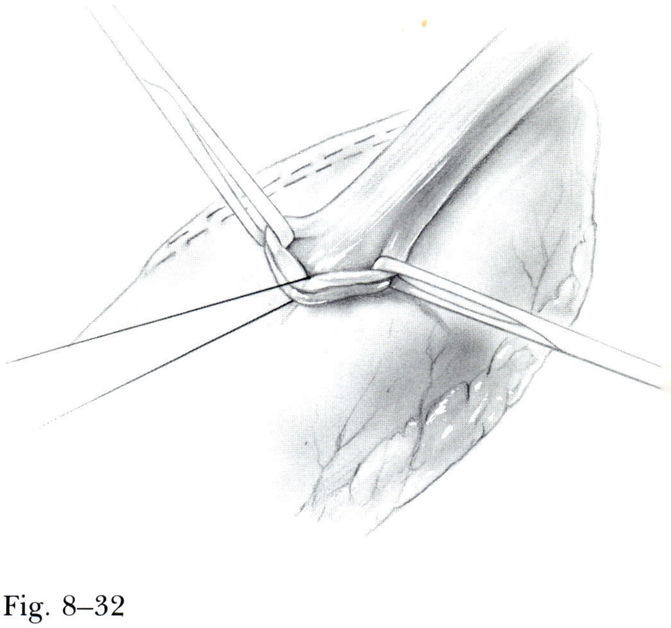

Fig. 8–32

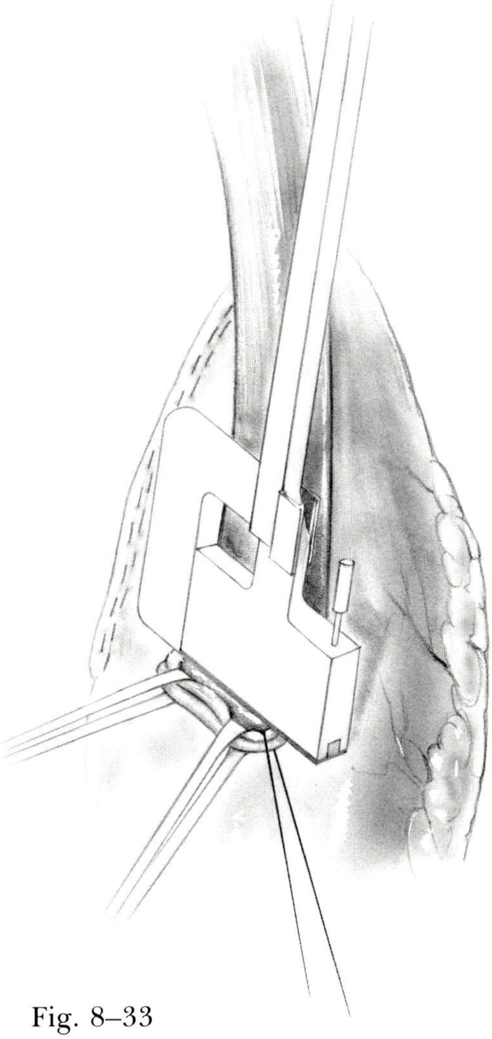

Fig. 8–33

TA–55 device can be applied just beneath the clamps and the suture (**Fig. 8–33**). Tighten and fire the stapling device. Excise the esophageal and gastric tissues flush with the stapling device with a Mayo scissors. Leave the guy suture intact.

Use an identical procedure to approximate the lateral side of the esophagogastric defect. Apply additional Allis clamps. Then place the TA–55 stapling device into position deep to the Allis clamps and the previously placed guy suture. Close and fire the stapler and remove the redundant tissue with the Mayo scissors (**Fig. 8–34**). It is essential that a small portion of the lateral termination of the GIA stapled anastomosis be included in the final TA–55 staple line. Include the guy suture also in this last application of

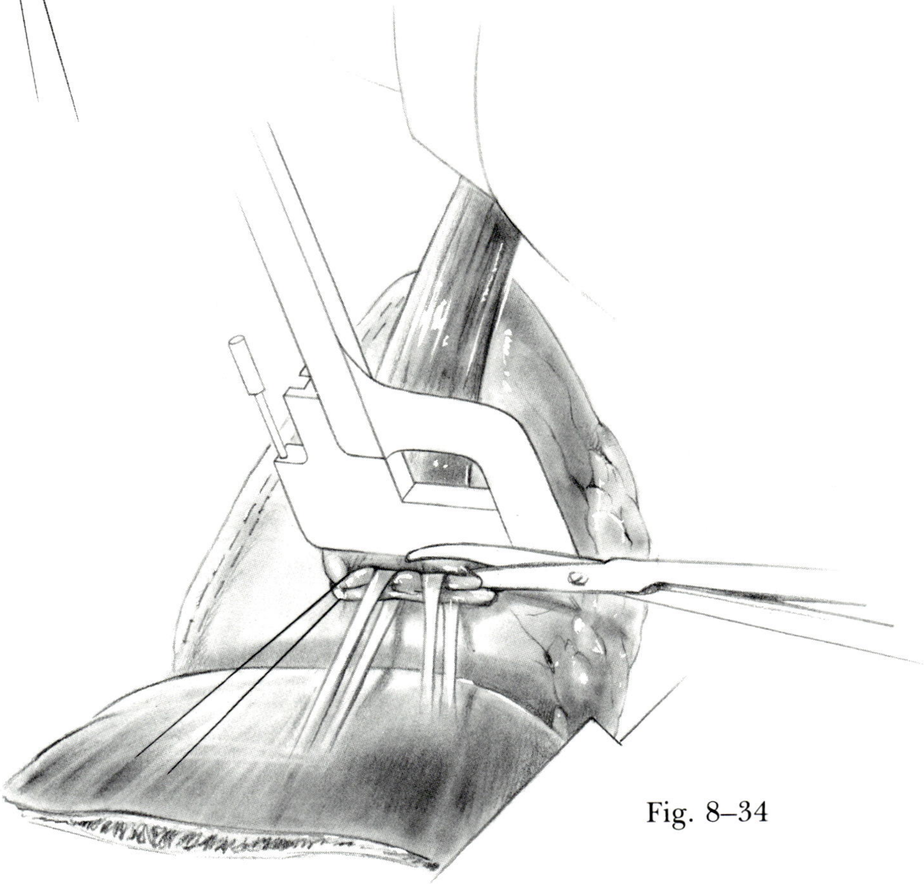

Fig. 8–34

the TA–55. These measures eliminate any possibility of leaving a gap between the various staple lines. The integrity of the anastomosis may be tested by inserting a sterile solution of methylene blue through the nasogastric tube into the gastric pouch. The appearance of the completed stapled anastomosis is shown in **Fig. 8–35**.

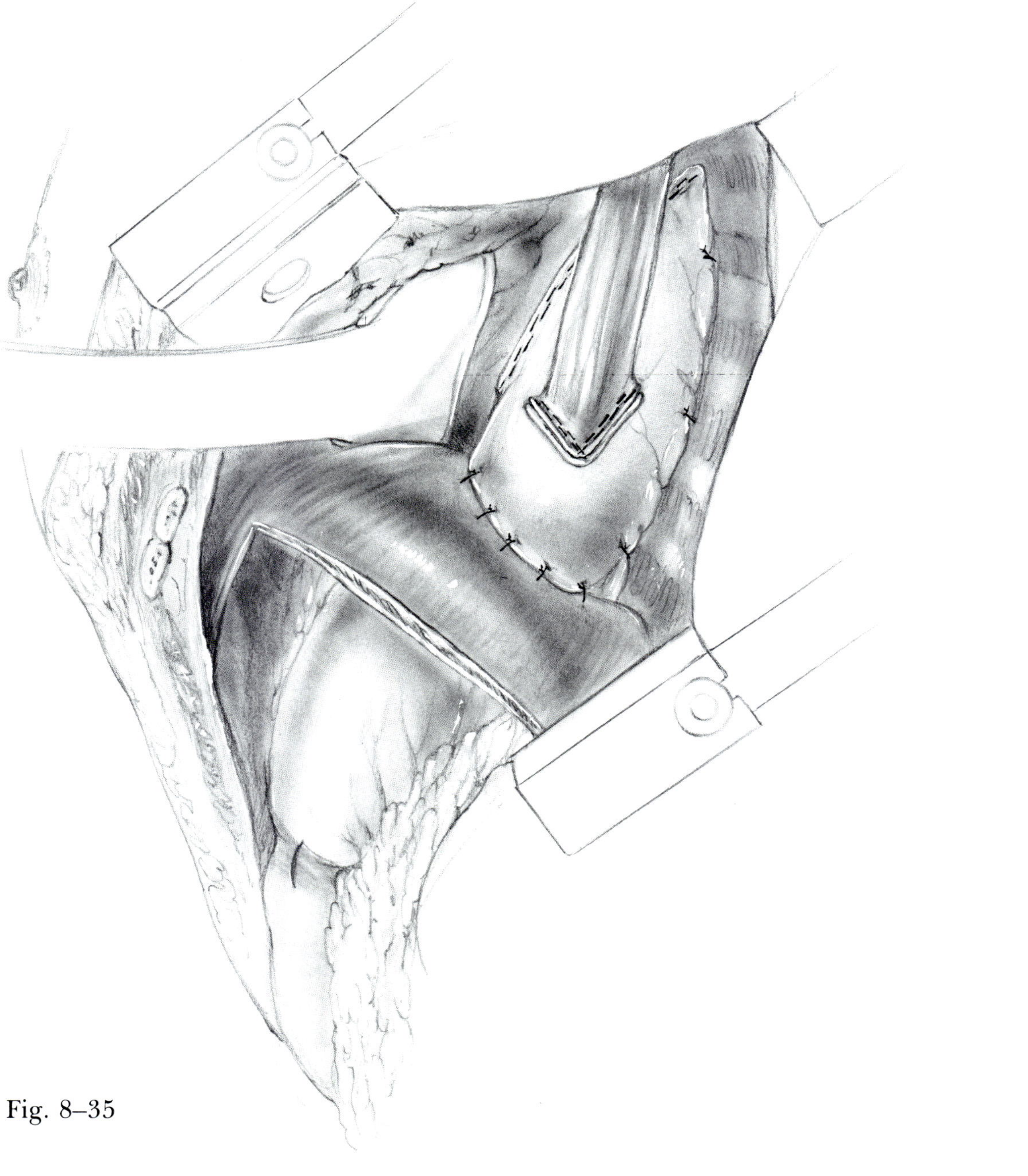

Fig. 8–35

Whether a Nissen fundoplication is to be constructed following this anastomosis depends upon the judgment of the surgeon and the availability of loose gastric wall. In some cases a partial fundoplication can be accomplished.

Stabilizing the Gastric Pouch

To prevent any gravity-induced tension on the anastomosis, the apex of the gastric pouch should be sutured to the mediastinal pleura or the prevertebral fascia with 3–0 cotton or Tevdek sutures.

The gastric pouch should then be fixed to the enlarged diaphragmatic hiatus with interrupted 3–0 cotton or Tevdek sutures, which attach the gastric wall to the margins of the hiatus (Fig. 8–35). These sutures should be 2 cm apart and should not penetrate the gastric mucosa, lest they induce a gastropleural fistula.

Closure

Irrigate the thoracic and abdominal cavities with an antibiotic solution. This should be suctioned off and the incision in the diaphragm closed with interrupted sutures of 2–0 cotton (**Fig. 8–36**). Take fairly large (1 cm) bites, as a dehiscence of

Interupttes stitches for Diaphragm

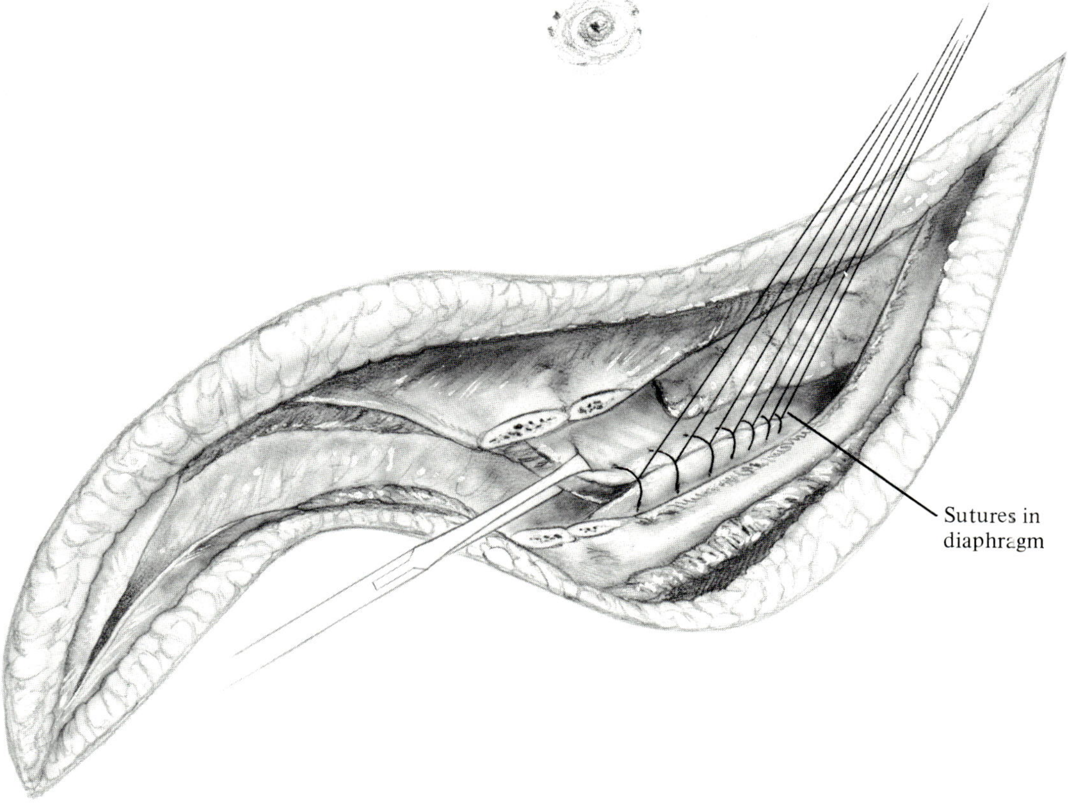

Fig. 8–36

this suture line can have serious consequences, such as herniation of small intestine into the chest.

Excise approximately 1 cm of cartilage from the costal margin to improve apposition (**Fig. 8–37**). Close the incision in the costal margin with one or two sutures of 2–0 monofilament stainless steel wire (**Fig. 8–38**). Insert four or five periocostal sutures of No. 2 PG to approxi-

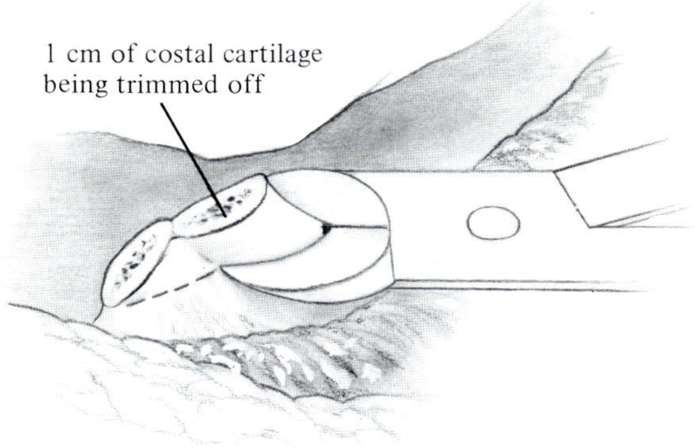

Fig. 8–37

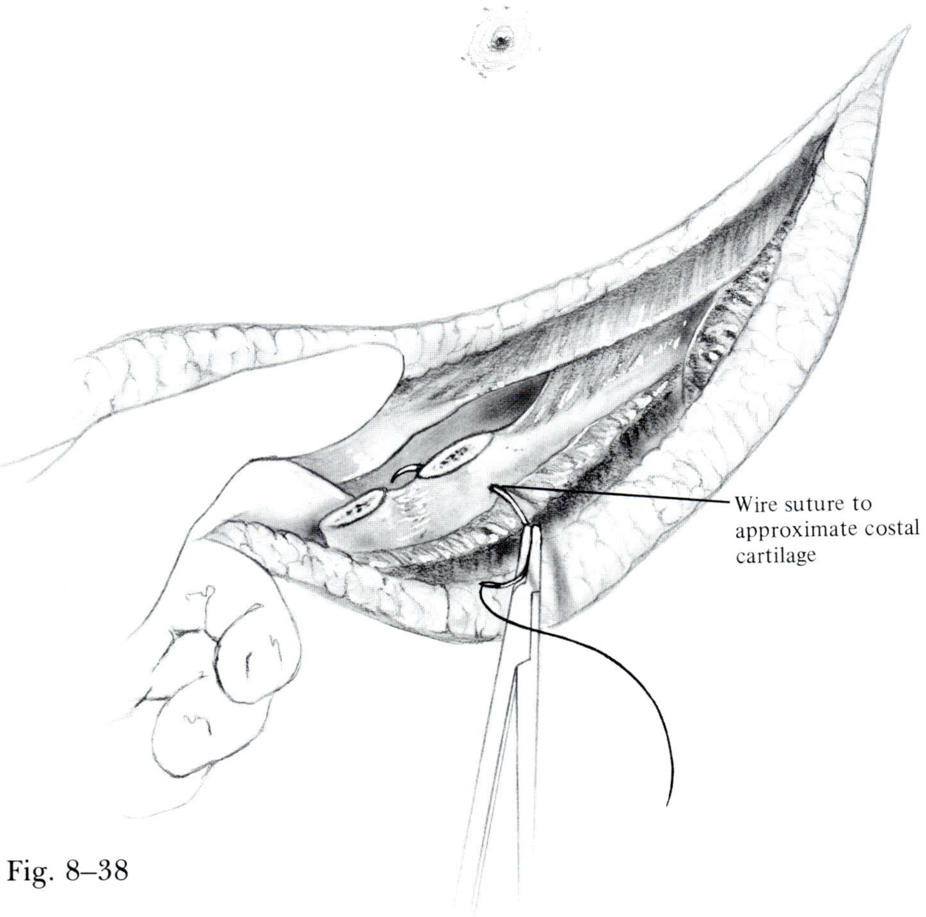

Fig. 8–38

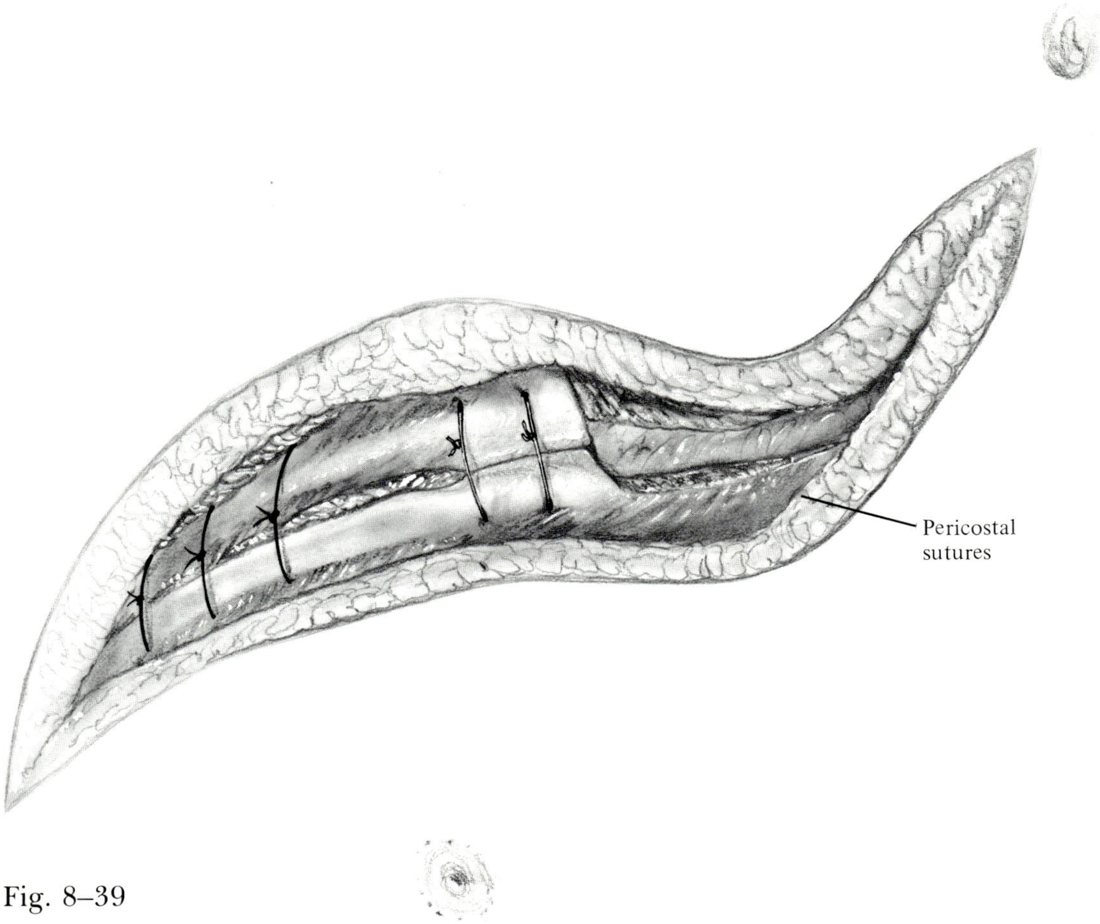

Fig. 8–39

mate the sixth and seventh ribs (**Fig. 8–39**). Bring a 30F plastic catheter through the ninth intercostal space in the anterior axillary line and carry it up to the level of the anastomosis. Suture it there to the parietal pleura posterior to the aorta, using 4–0 catgut. Inflate the lung to eliminate any atelectatic patches. If a significant number of air leaks from the lung are noted, pass a second chest catheter anterior to the lung up to the apex of the thorax. Tie the pericostal sutures and close the muscles in two layers with a continuous 2–0 PG atraumatic suture in each (**Figs. 8–40 and 8–41**).

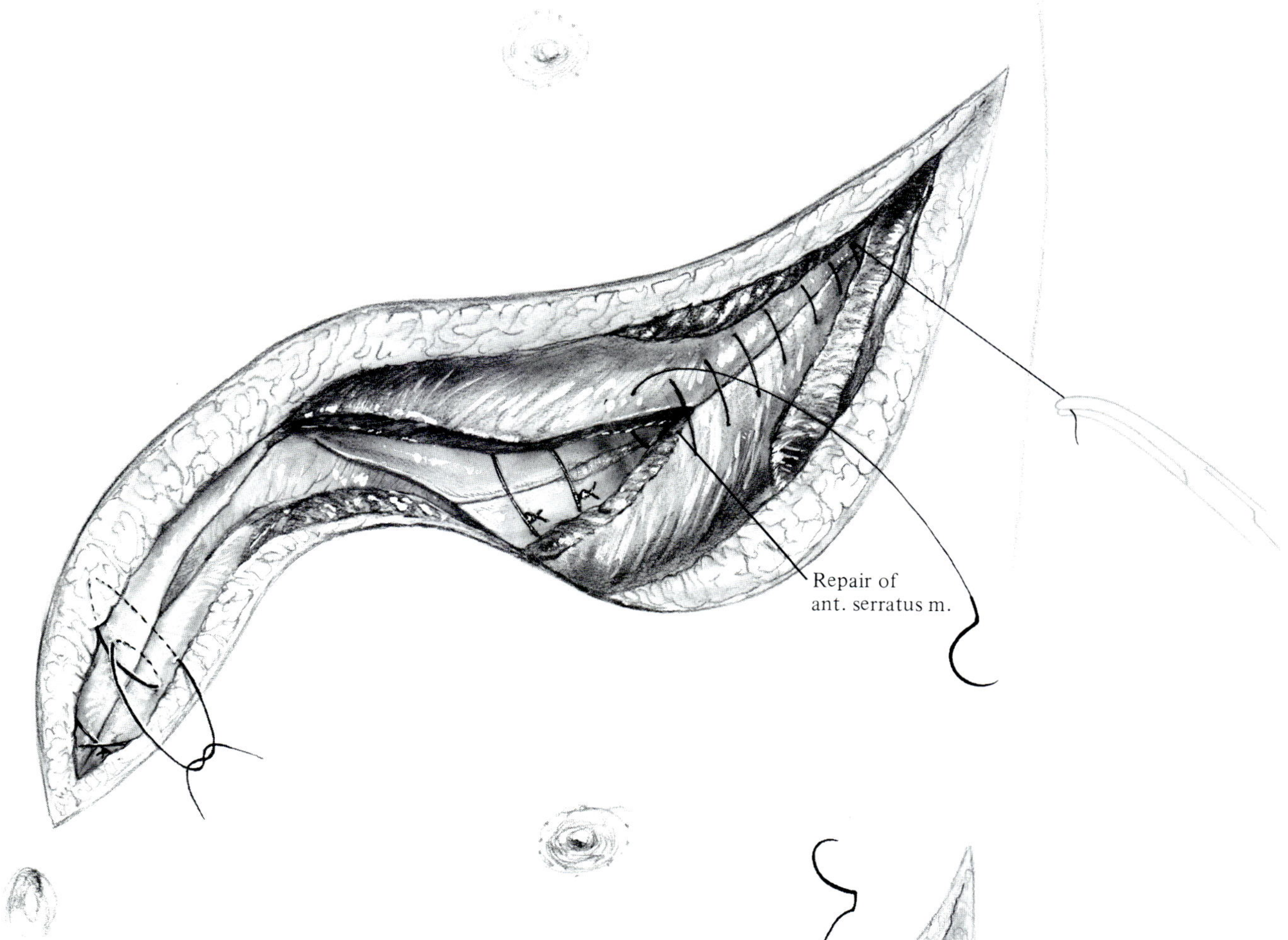

Fig. 8–40

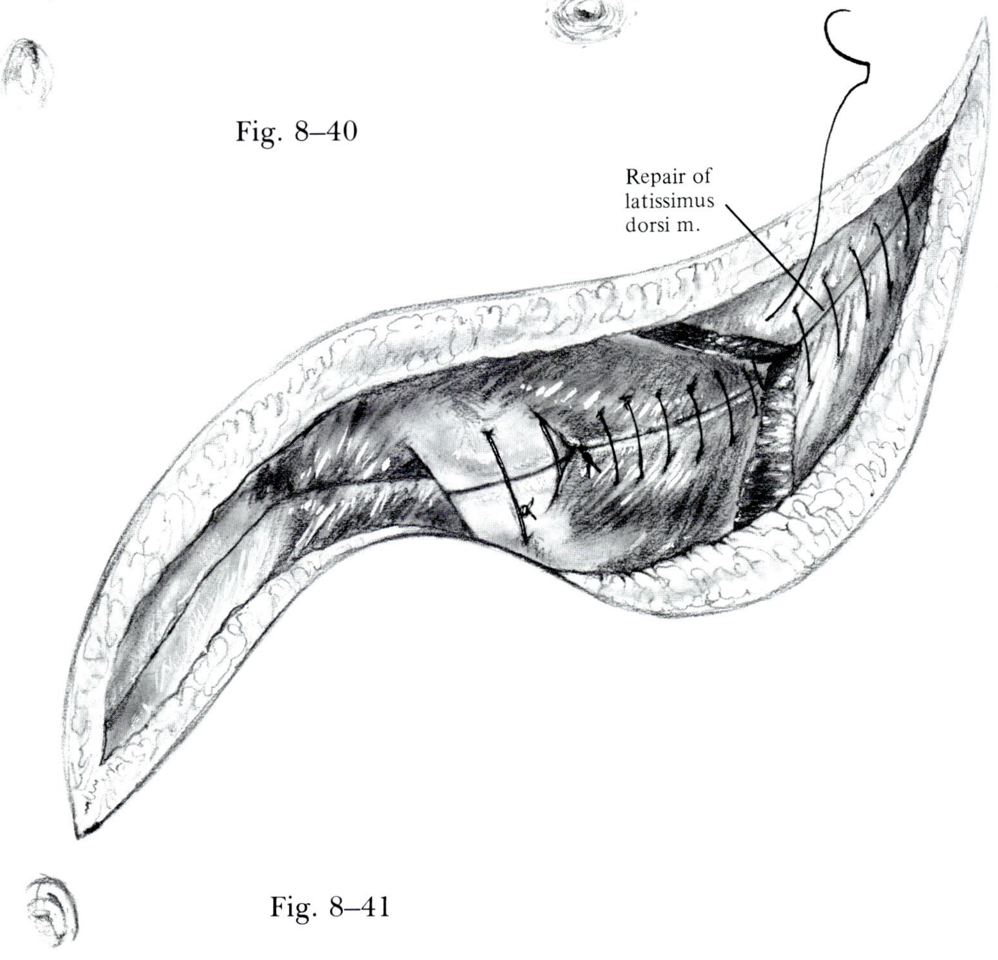

Fig. 8–41

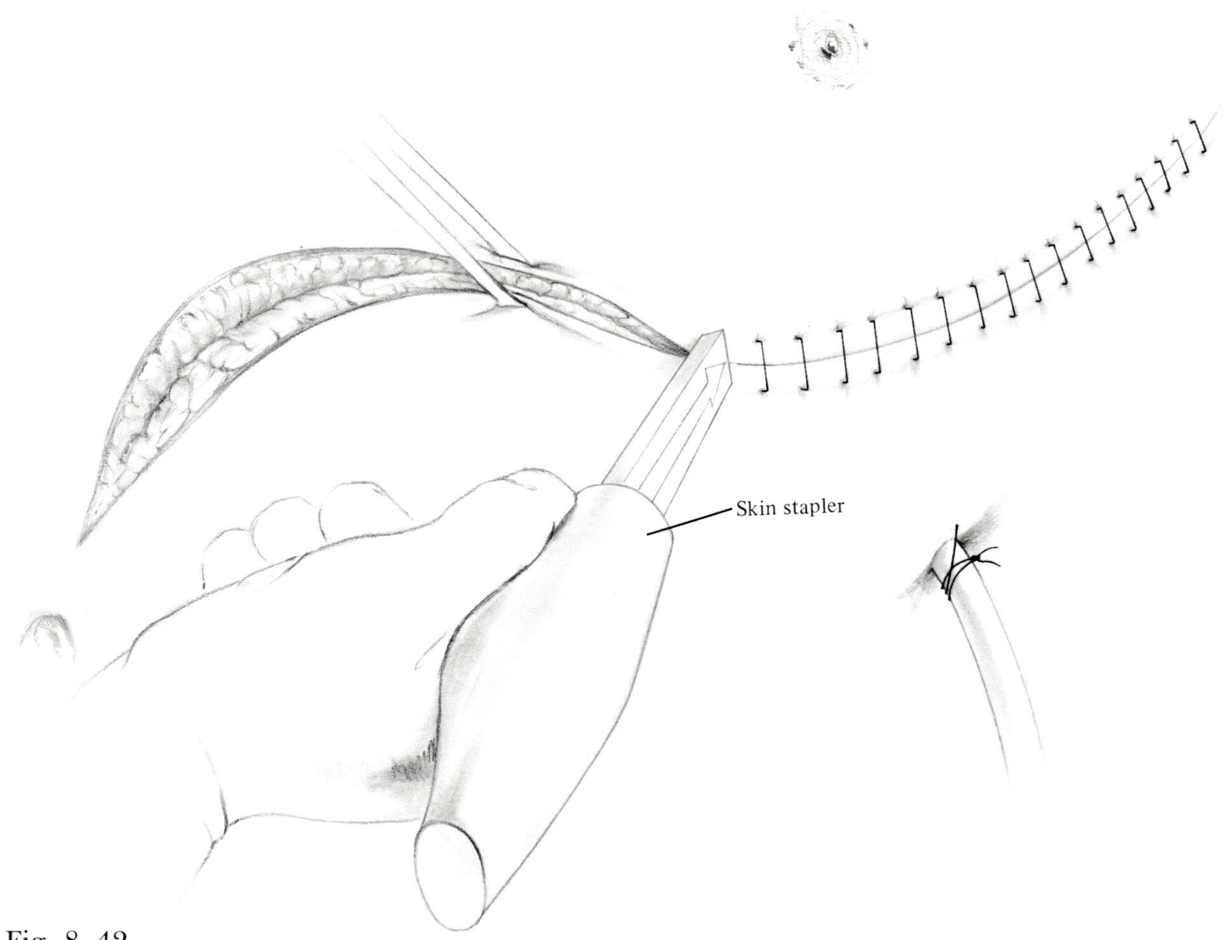

Fig. 8–42

Close the abdominal portion of the incision with interrupted 2–0 stainless steel wire Smead-Jones sutures as described in Chap. 5. Use staples or a subcuticular suture to close the skin (**Fig. 8–42**). No drains should be used in the abdominal cavity, but a subcutaneous suction catheter can be used if gastric contents have caused contamination (see Chap. 2).

Postoperative Care

(See Chap. 7.)

Complications

(See Chap. 7.)

References

Chassin JL (1978) Esophagogastrectomy: Data favoring end-to-side anastomosis. Ann Surg 188:22

Chassin JL (1978) Stapling technic for esophagogastrostomy after esophagogastric resection. Am J Surg 136:399

Fisher RD et al. (1972) Esophagogastrostomy in the treatment of carcinoma of the distal two-thirds of the esophagus. Ann Thorac Surg 14:658

Stomach

9 Operations for Peptic Ulcer

Selection of Operation for Duodenal Ulcer

Any peptic ulcer requires free acid to sustain it. Reducing the acid peptic content of gastric secretions cures the ulcer. This can be accomplished surgically by resecting three-quarters of the stomach to remove a large number of acid-secreting parietal cells. Unfortunately, such operations have produced a high incidence of undesirable postoperative symptoms. With the development of vagotomy, however, extensive resection of the stomach has become unnecessary. Vagotomy, then, should be routinely employed in surgery for duodenal ulcer. Which type of vagotomy, and which type of resection or drainage procedure should be employed, is a controversial question.

Antrectomy and Vagotomy

If removal of the gastrin-secreting antrum is combined with some form of gastric vagotomy, the postoperative secretion of free acid approaches zero levels. The chance of peptic ulcer recurring after this procedure is 0–2%. Counterbalancing this favorable aspect are studies by Goligher et al. (1979) and Herrington et al. that show an elective mortality rate of 0–2% when the patient is in expert hands, as well as a 3%–6% incidence of unsatisfactory results. Postgastrectomy fatalities generally follow a disruption of the duodenal suture line or acute necrotizing pancreatitis. Techniques aimed at preventing these two complications are discussed under "Operative Strategy" in Chap. 15.

Drainage Procedures and Vagotomy

According to Goligher et al. (1979), when pyloroplasty is combined with truncal vagotomy, the long-term recurrence rate of peptic ulcer is about 10% and the incidence of undesirable postoperative sequelae such as dumping or bile gastritis is not much different from that which follows antrectomy. On the other hand, the generally reported mortality rate for vagotomy and a drainage procedure performed under elective conditions is 0.5%. Because it is simple technically, this operation is often selected for the poor-risk patient, especially in cases of massive hemorrhage from a duodenal ulcer. Resection in these cases sometimes is difficult, and the reported operative mortality is high except when it is done by an expert.

Truncal versus Selective Vagotomy

The aim of selective vagotomy is to interrupt the vagal fibers going to the stomach while preserving the branches entering the liver and the celiac ganglion. The procedure was devised in the hope it would eliminate undesirable postvagotomy sequelae, such as diarrhea. The results of studies at Vanderbilt University by Sawyers et al. suggest that selective vagotomy reduces the incidence of incomplete gastric vagotomy. Since the incidence of significant postvagotomy diarrhea has in our experience been minimal and since selective vagotomy requires considerable operating time as well as the devascularization of the lesser curvature of the gastric pouch, this procedure has not achieved widespread popularity. If the additional dissection required for selective vagotomy is to be performed, the surgeon might well choose a proximal gastric vagotomy without a drainage procedure. In any case, anyone undertaking to perform gastric surgery should master the art of performing some type of vagotomy in a *complete* fashion.

Choice of Drainage Procedure

Unless there is edema of the duodenal bulb or extreme fibrosis, pyloroplasty is simpler than gastrojejunostomy. The Mikulicz pyloroplasty, the simplest of drainage procedures, is suitable for 90% of the patients who require drainage. On occasions when a markedly fibrotic pyloroduodenal area must be incised to control bleeding, the Finney pyloroplasty may be indicated, as it can compensate for a certain degree of rigidity of the tissues, which may make the Mikulicz technique inapplicable. Some surgeons believe that the Finney pyloroplasty, with its large stoma, is the technique of choice. It is interesting that Goligher's group (1979) found fewer undesirable long term sequelae after vagotomy and gastrojujunostomy than after vagotomy-pyloroplasty. As this part of their study was not done at random, its significance is not clear.

In comparing the Jaboulay gastroduodenostomy with the more traditional pyloroplasty techniques, there appears to be inadequate data to demonstrate any advantage.

Billroth I versus Billroth II Gastrectomy

There are now extensive data to demonstrate that the Billroth I operation, when combined with adequate vagotomy, produces as low an incidence of duodenal ulcer recurrence as the Billroth II. Billroth I has the advantage of eliminating afferent loop complications that occasionally follow the gastrojejunal type of reconstruction. Herrington, who has had vast experience with this procedure, believes that the gastroduodenal anastomosis is safe for most patients who suffer severe duodenal ulcer disease. In addition, White has pointed out that the incidence of postoperative steatorrhea is less after the Billroth I than after the Billroth II operation.

Proximal Gastric Vagotomy (Parietal Cell Vagotomy) without Drainage Procedure

History teaches us that early enthusiasm for new procedures in the treatment of duodenal ulcer is often followed by disappointment. Consequently, one must be skeptical until follow-up studies of 10–20 years' duration become available. Nevertheless, proximal gastric vagotomy is an operation that has many exciting features. First, it has the lowest mortality rate (0.3%) of all operations for duodenal ulcer, primarily because the gastrointestinal tract is not entered and there is no need for dissection in the region of the ulcer. While some experienced surgeons have reported a 2% ulcer recurrence rate, others have found recurrences in 20% of their cases. Unquestionably, the extension of the operation to encompass the lower 5–7 cm of the esophagus and the esophagogastric junction has improved the rate of success. The only reported fatal operative complication has been necrosis of the lesser curvature, which seems to occur less than once in a thousand cases, leading to speculation that it may be secondary to excessive operative trauma or hematoma.

Of all the operations being done for duodenal ulcer, proximal gastric vagotomy has by far the fewest undesirable postoperative digestive sequelae.

Another attractive feature of this operation is that in cases of recurrent ulcer, secondary antrectomy offers no great difficulty technically unless a splenectomy has been performed. In this instance, the blood supply to the residual gastric pouch, following antrectomy, proximal gastric vagotomy, and splenectomy would be precarious, as is evident from a study of the blood supply of the stomach (see Fig. 15–1). While it is still too early for a definitive decision, it appears likely that this procedure will replace most of the other alternatives.

Summary

When done by an expert, vagotomy and antrectomy can be accomplished with low mortality and will provide a long-term cure for duodenal ulcer in 99% of the patients operated on. Less experienced surgeons should heed Goligher's (1979) advice to avoid gastrectomy in the deeply penetrating posterior ulcer because "vagotomy and gastroenterostomy yield overall results not greatly inferior to those of resection" and "it would be preferable to have several recurrent ulcers, for which one can reoperate with a good chance of success, than to incur a single operative death." The same statement could probably apply to proximal gastric vagotomy if the surgeon has mastered the technique. Since 10- to 20-year follow-up data are not available, proximal gastric vagotomy cannot yet be named the operation of choice for duodenal ulcer.

One must be impressed by the 0% hospital mortality in 375 cases Goligher et al. subjected to gastrectomy (117), vagotomy-antrectomy (132), or vagotomy-gastrojejunostomy (126). They attribute the absence of fatalities among the 249 patients subjected to gastric resection to the good judgment exercised by the surgeons in rejecting for gastrectomy those patients for whom the duodenal dissection seemed hazardous. These patients underwent vagotomy and gastroenterostomy instead; they also had no mortality.

Concept: Selection of Operation for Gastric Ulcer

Most patients who have a duodenal ulcer display increased acid output, while gastric ulcer is often accompanied by below-average measurements of gastric acid secretion. The etiology of gastric ulcer is related to gastric stasis, which allows the acid to remain in contact with the mucosa for an abnormally long period of time. This situation is obvious in patients who have a chronic duodenal ulcer and a partial obstruction and then develop a secondary gastric ulcer. Another hypothesis for the pathogenesis of gastric ulcer is impairment of the mucosal resistance to acid. This permits back diffusion of the acid, which produces tissue destruction. Patients who have both duodenal and gastric ulcers should be treated by an operation designed to cure the duodenal ulcer. Patients who have ulcers in the pyloric channel or the immediate prepyloric region should also receive the same surgical management as is indicated for duodenal ulcer.

Gastric ulcer patients who have low gastric acidity and who do not fit into the above categories respond very nicely to conservative resection of the lower 40%–50% of the stomach, followed by gastroduodenal anastomosis without vagotomy. Following this procedure the rate of ulcers recurring is less than 1% according to a report by Davis et al. from the Mayo Clinic. There are inadequate data to demonstrate the need to add vagotomy to the resection in these cases. Tanner encountered one case of recurrent ulcer in 1,000 gastrectomies he performed for gastric ulcer. In the absence of cancer, the Billroth I type gastrectomy is preferred.

Because there is always the possibility of a malignancy in a chronic gastric ulcer, if feasible the ulcer itself should be included in the area of stomach to be resected. Cryostat frozen section examination of all gastric ulcers should be performed because if a carcinoma is diagnosed, this is an indication for a more extensive resection than would be necessary for the cure of a benign ulcer.

Occasionally a chronic, deeply penetrating ulcer is situated high on the lesser curvature of the stomach. If this can easily be encompassed by a Schoemaker-Hoffmeister type gastric resection without impinging on the esophagogastric junction, then this is the preferred method of management. If the ulcer is large, is surrounded by edema, and impinges on the esophagogastric junction, multiple quadrant biopsies for frozen section analysis should be taken through a gastrotomy incision. If the biopsies are negative, a 40% gastrectomy, including antrum and pylorus (Madlener operation), should be carried out without further disturbing the ulcer. If the ulcer is benign it should be completely healed by both X-ray and gastroscopy within 6 weeks after the Madelener operation.

Some surgeons advocate vagotomy and pyloroplasty for the definitive treatment of gastric ulcer if the biopsies are benign. Although good short term results have been reported with this technique, and although it may be suitable for the extremely poor-risk patient, extensive data support partial gastrectomy. When performed for gastric ulcer, gastrectomy is almost as safe a procedure as vagotomy and pyloroplasty. The latter operation is followed by an excessive number of recurrent ulcers within 5–10 years.

Still under study for the treatment of benign gastric ulcer is the use of proximal gastric vagotomy combined with local excision. It is too soon to make a definitive judgment on its value.

Indications

Hemorrhage of massive proportions or recurrent hemorrhage while patient is under treatment in hospital.

Perforation of ulcer. Plication is the treatment of choice for perforated duodenal ulcer, but there are a number of exceptions. In patients who have a prior history of symptoms, whose perforation has not been of long duration, and in whom massive contamination has not occurred, a definitive operation aimed at curing the ulcer is indicated. In the case of gastric ulcer the perforation is frequently quite large or may be located on the posterior wall of the antrum where plication with omentum can not be done satisfactorily. Under these conditions emergency gastrectomy is mandatory. Otherwise the incidence of reperforation will be frequent and often lethal. Because chronic gastric ulcer has a high recurrence rate, some surgeons believe that most gastric perforations should be resected, not plicated.

Gastric outlet obstruction. Definitive gastric surgery should be done following a period of nasogastric suction of sufficient duration to permit any edema in the hypertrophied gastric walls to recede. On the other hand a transient obstruction in a patient who does not have a previous history of ulcer may be managed by a trial of medical therapy.

Intractability. Medical management by means of frequent feedings, antacids, and cimetidine has been successful in managing over 90% of those patients who have duodenal ulcers. However, when a patient has experienced four or five recurrences of duodenal ulcer over a period of years, surgery is indicated. The recurrence rate of gastric ulcer following successful medical management is notoriously high. In a study by Littman, 42% of the patients suffering from gastric ulcers experienced a recurrence within 2 years of apparently successful medical management. Also, in the absence of duodenal pathology, the incidence of complications and fatalities following surgery for gastric ulcer is considerably lower than after surgery for duodenal ulcer. For these reasons definitive gastric ulcer surgery should be undertaken after only one or two recurrences.

Preoperative Preparation

Nasogastric suction for patients with pyloric obstruction; in other cases, passage of nasogastric tube morning of operation

Gastric analysis for determining basal and maximal acid output

Gastroscopy and biopsy of gastric ulcers

Serum gastrin determination in patients whose gastric analysis or clinical picture suggests multiple endocrine adenopathy

References

Davis Z et al. (1977) The surgically treated chronic gastric ulcer: an extended followup. Ann Surg 185:205

Goligher JC et al. (1964) Controlled trial of vagotomy and gastro-enterostomy, vagotomy and antrectomy and subtotal gastrectomy in elective treatment of duodenal ulcer: interim report. Br Med J 1:455

Goligher JC et al. (1979) Several standard elective operations for duodenal ulcer: ten to 16 year clinical results. Ann Surg 189:18

Herrington JL Jr et al. (1973) A 25 year experience with vagotomy–antrectomy. Arch Surg 106:469

Littman A (ed) (1971) Veterans Administration cooperative study on gastric ulcer: healing, recurrence, cancer. Gastroenterology 61:567

Sawyers JL et al. (1968) Comparative studies of the clinical effects of truncal and selective gastric vagotomy. Am J Surg 115:165

Tanner NC (1962) in Harkins HN, Nyhus LM, Surgery of the stomach and duodenum. Little, Brown, Boston p. 433

White TT, Harrison RC (1973) Reoperative gastrointestinal surgery. Little, Brown, Boston

10 Truncal Vagotomy

Indications

Patients who are having surgery for duodenal ulcer should generally undergo vagotomy as well (see also Chap. 9).

Preoperative Preparation

(See Chap. 9).

Pitfalls and Danger Points

- Esophageal trauma
- Splenic trauma
- Inadequate vagotomy
- Disruption of esophageal hiatus with postoperative hiatal hernia; gastroesophageal reflux

Operative Strategy

Esophageal Trauma

The best way to avoid trauma to the esophagus is by performing most of the esophageal dissection under *direct vision.* Forceful, blind, finger dissection can be dangerous. After the peritoneum overlying the abdominal esophagus is incised (**Figs. 10–1, 10–2, and 10–3**), the crural musculature should be clearly exposed. The next vital step in this sequence is to develop a groove between the esophagus and the adjoining crux on each side. This should be done under direct vision, using a peanut dissector (**Fig. 10–4**). Only after the anterior two-thirds of the esophagus has been exposed is it permissible to insert the index finger for encircling the esophagus.

Splenic Trauma

Splenic trauma can be prevented by avoiding any traction that will draw the stomach toward the patient's right. This may avulse the splenic capsule because of attachments between the omentum and the surface of the spleen. Consequently, all traction on the stomach should be applied on the lesser curvature side and directed toward the patient's feet. Avulsion of a portion of the splenic capsule, in the absence of gross disruption of the splenic pulp, does not require splenectomy. Application of Surgicel gauze, sutures, or in some cases Avitene powder may control bleeding satisfactorily.

Incomplete Vagotomy

In the majority of cases of recurrent marginal ulcer, it turns out the posterior vagal trunk has not been divided. This trunk is generally the largest encountered in the vagotomy operation. The surgeon's failure to locate the posterior vagus suggests an inadequate knowledge of the anatomy of the posterior vagus. The right (posterior) vagal trunk is frequently 2 cm or more distant from the right lateral wall of the esophagus. It is often not delivered into the field by the usual maneuver of

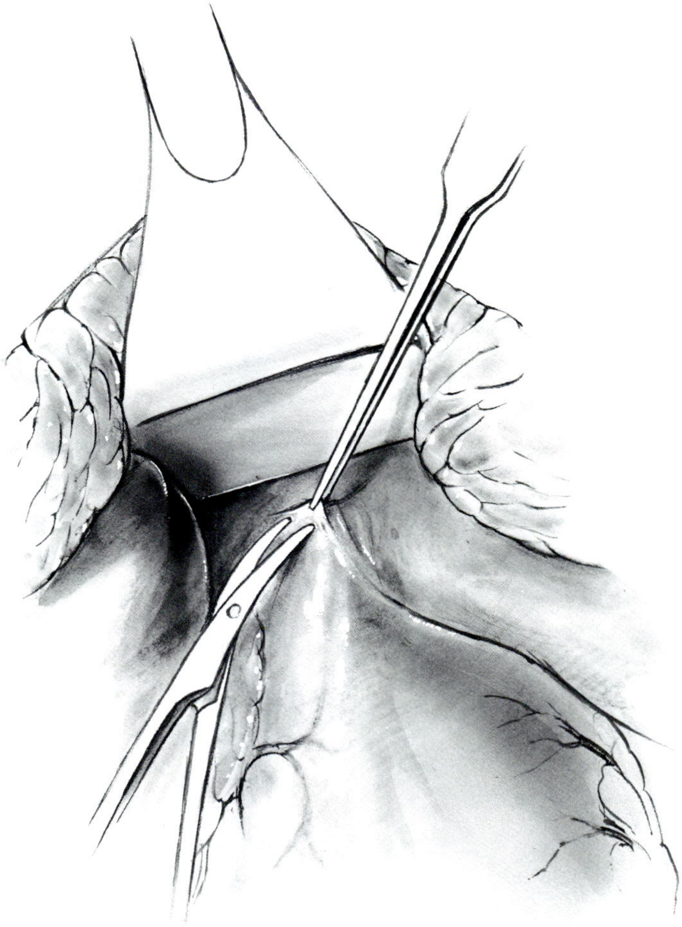

Fig. 10–1

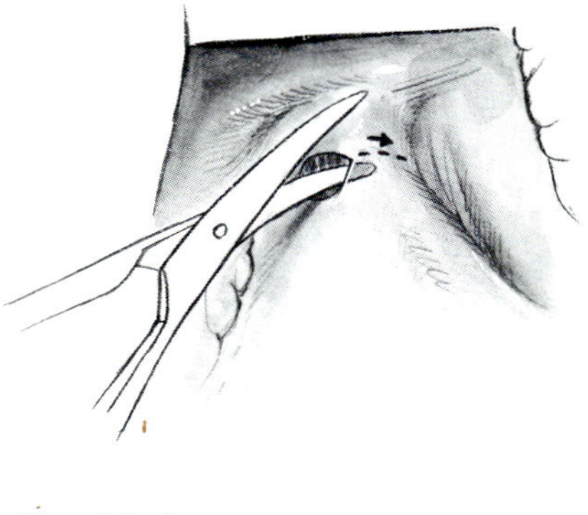

Fig. 10–2

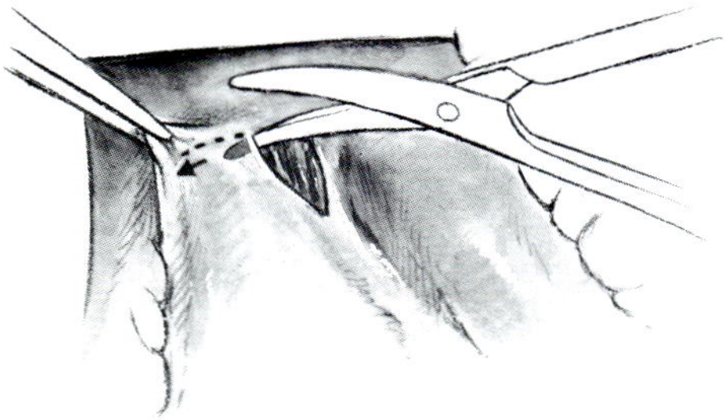

Fig. 10–3

encircling the esophagus with the index finger. If the technique described below is carefully followed, this trunk will rarely be overlooked.

To improve tissue-recognition skill the surgeon should place each nerve specimen removed from the vicinity of the esophagus into a separate bottle for histological examination. Each bottle should have a label indicating the anatomical area from which the nerve was removed. The pathological report that arrives several days after the operation will serve as a test of the surgeon's ability at visual nerve identification. The surgeon may be surprised to find that four or five separate specimens of nerve have been removed in a complete truncal vagotomy. Frozen section examination is helpful but not conclusive because it cannot prove that *all* the vagal nerve branches have been removed. The surgeon must gain sufficient skill at identifying nerve trunks in order to be certain that no significant nerve fiber remains.

Hiatus Hernia

Although significant hiatal hernia following vagotomy occurs in no more than 1%–2% of cases, this percentage can probably be reduced if the surgeon repairs any large defects seen in the hiatus after the dissection has been completed. It has been noted that the lower esophageal sphincter functions better when it rests upon a buttress of solid crural musculature. It may be weakened if there is a hiatal defect along its posterior margin.

Operative Technique

Incision and Exposure

Make a midline incision from the xiphoid to a point about 5 cm below the umbilicus. The incision can be extended into the xiphocostal junction if necessary. Elevate the sternum 8–10 cm by means of an Upper Hand or "chain" retractor. Elevate the upper half of the operating table about 10°. Retract the left lobe of the liver in a cephalad direction utilizing either Harrington or Weinberg retractors. In rare instances the triangular ligament has to be incised and the left lobe of the liver retracted to the patient's right for exposure.

Using long DeBakey forceps and long Metzenbaum scissors incise the peritoneum overlying the abdominal esophagus (**Figs. 10–1, 10–2, and 10–3**). Next, identify the muscles of the right and left branches of the crux. Use a peanut dissector to develop a groove between the esophagus and the adjacent crux, exposing the anterior two thirds of the esophagus (**Fig. 10–4**). At this point insert the right index finger gently behind the esophagus and encircle it.

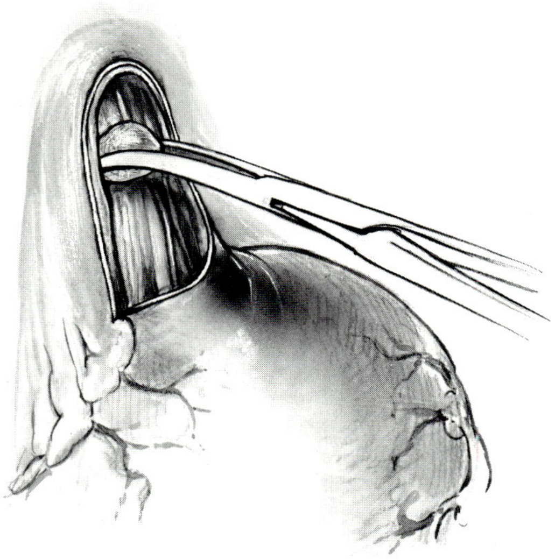

Fig. 10–4

Left (Anterior) Vagal Trunk

In our experience, whereas the posterior trunk often exists as a single structure in the abdomen, the anterior vagus divides into two *or more* trunks in over 50% of the cases. The main left trunk generally runs along the anterior wall of the lower esophagus, and the other branches may be closely applied to the longitudinal muscle of the anterior esophagus. The major nerve branches may be accentuated by caudal traction on the stomach, which will make the anterior nerves prominent against the esophagus. After applying Hemoclips remove segments from each of the anterior branches (**Fig. 10–5**). Any suspicious fibers should be removed with forceps and sent to the pathology laboratory for analysis.

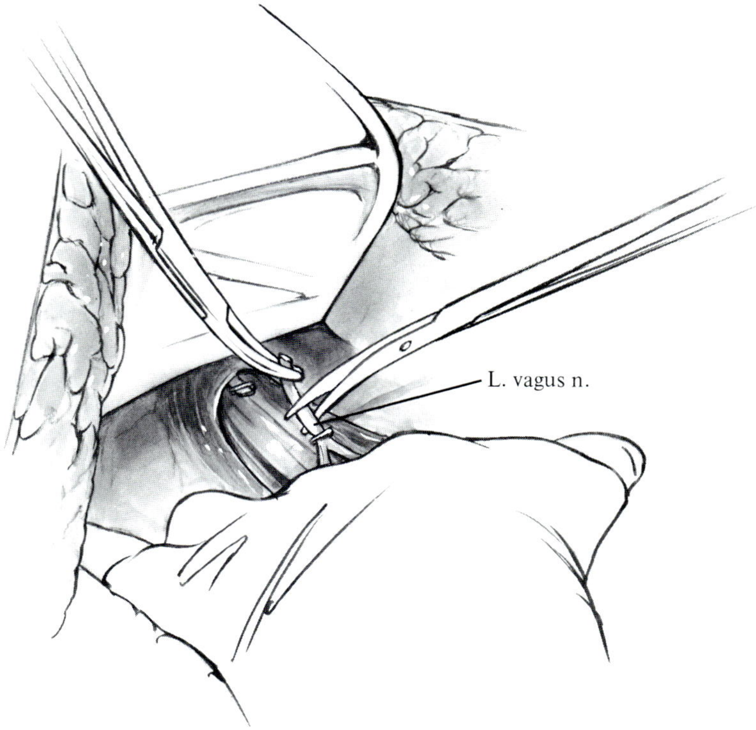

Fig. 10–5

Identification of the Right (Posterior) Vagus

The posterior vagal trunk often is situated 2 or 3 cm lateral and posterior to the right wall of the esophagus. Consequently, its identification requires that when the surgeon's right index finger encircles the lowermost esophagus, going from the patient's left to right, the fingernail should pass over the anterior aorta. The finger should then go a considerable distance toward the patient's right before the finger is flexed. Then the fingernail rolls against the *deep* aspect of the right branch of the crural muscle. When this maneuver is completed, the right trunk, a structure measuring 2–3 mm in diameter, is contained in the encircled finger to the right of the esophagus (**Fig. 10–6**). Its identification may be confirmed in two ways. First, look for a major branch going toward the celiac ganglion. Second, insert a finger above the left gastric artery near the lesser curvature of the stomach and draw the left gastric vessel in a caudal direction. This applies traction to the posterior vagus, which then stands out as a stout cord. The right trunk rarely divides in the abdomen above the level of the esophagogastric junction.

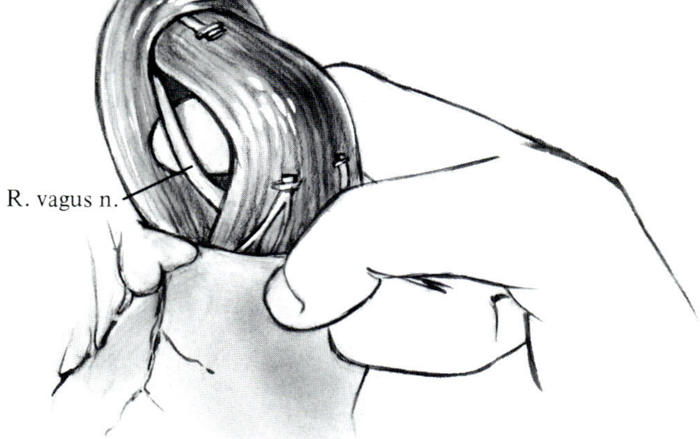

Fig. 10–6

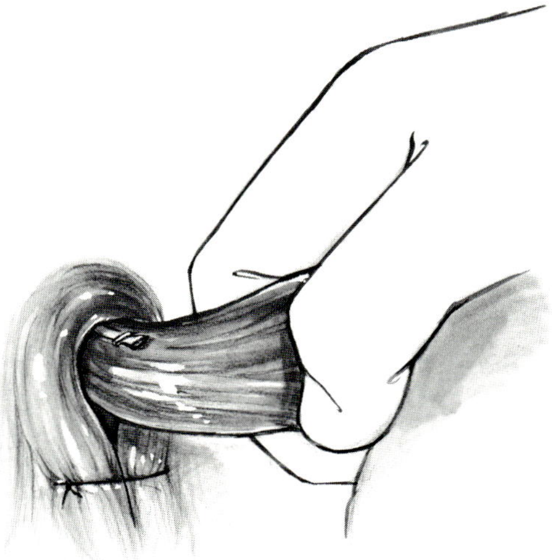

Fig. 10–7

Apply a long Mixter clamp to the nerve; place Hemoclips above and below the clamp; remove a 2–3 cm segment of nerve and submit for histological study.

Rotate the esophagus and inspect the posterior wall. At the conclusion of this step the lower 5 cm of esophagus should be cleared of all nerve fibers. One should see only longitudinal muscle throughout its entire circumference (**Fig. 10–7**).

Suture of Crural Musculature

At this time if the hiatus admits two or more fingers alongside the esophagus, one or two sutures of 0 cotton or Tevdek should be placed to approximate the muscle bundles behind the esophagus, taking care to leave a gap of one finger's breadth between the esophagus and the newly constructed hiatus. No attempt at fundoplication or any other antireflux procedure need be undertaken unless the patient had symptoms or other evidence of gastroesophageal reflux and esophagitis before the operation.

Hemostasis should be checked before going on to the gastric resection or drainage procedure.

Postoperative Care

(See Chaps. 12 and 13.)

Complications

Operative perforations of the esophagus must be carefully repaired with two layers of interrupted sutures. If additional exposure is needed, do not hesitate to extend the abdominal incision into the left sixth or seventh intercostal space. For additional security, cover the suture line with gastric wall by performing a Nissen fundoplication when repairing a low esophageal tear.

Postoperative gastric stasis

11 Proximal Gastric Vagotomy

Indications

Intractable Duodenal Ulcer

As mentioned in Chap. 9, proximal gastric vagotomy without a drainage procedure has the smallest number of undesirable postoperative sequelae and the lowest mortality rate of any operation for duodenal ulcer. On the other hand, the incidence of recurrent ulcer after this procedure may reach 10% over the course of a 5–10 year follow-up period. Because many of the complications following drainage procedures and gastric resection can be extremely unpleasant—such as dumping, weight loss, and malabsorption—it may prove worthwhile to assume the risk of a 10% recurrence rate to avert all these complications.

Duodenal Ulcer with Hemorrhage

When bleeding from a duodenal ulcer can be controlled by suture through a duodenotomy incision that does not transect the pylorus, proximal gastric vagotomy is an acceptable alternative to truncal vagotomy combined with either antrectomy or pyloroplasty.

Duodenal Ulcer with Perforation

In cases of early perforation, which can be easily controlled by plication, the addition of proximal gastric vagotomy helps assure the long-term cure of the ulcer.

Contraindications

Duodenal Ulcer with Obstruction

Although some surgeons have treated obstructing duodenal ulcers by performing proximal gastric vagotomy combined with forceful dilatation of the stricture, there are as yet inadequate data to support this combined procedure.

Preoperative Care

Gastrointestinal X rays

Gastric analysis

Gastroscopy when indicated

Nasogastric tube on morning of operation

Pitfalls and Danger Points

Hematoma of gastrohepatic ligament

Incomplete vagotomy

Damage to innervation of pyloric antrum

Injury to spleen

Operative Strategy

Exposure

Visibility of the area around the lower esophagus is greatly enhanced if either the "chain" or Upper Hand retractor is attached so that the blade underlying the lower border of the sternum elevates the sternum and also draws it in a cephalad direction.

Prevention of Hematoma and Injury to Gastric Lesser Curve

Hematomas in the region of the gastrohepatic ligament along the lesser curve of the stomach increase the difficulty of identifying the terminal branches of the nerve of Latarjet. Furthermore, rough dissection and hematomas in this area may damage the deserosalized muscle along the lesser curve to such an extent that necrosis may occur. Although this has been reported in less than 0.3% of the cases surveyed, it is probable that this complication, which is often fatal, can be prevented by gentle dissection and avoidance of hematomas. Resuturing the peritoneum produces inversion of the deserosalized portion of the lesser curve. This also helps prevent necrosis and perforation in this region.

Preserving Innervation of Antrum

Both the anterior and posterior nerves of Latarjet terminate in a configuration resembling the foot of a crow. As described below, the crow's-foot portion of these nerves maintains the innervation of the antrum and pylorus and ensures adequate emptying of the stomach.

Adequacy of Proximal Vagotomy

Hallenbeck et al. demonstrated that the incidence of recurrent postoperative ulcer dropped markedly when they extended the dissection so that the lower esophagus was completely freed of any vagal innervation. This required meticulous removal of all nerve branches reaching the lower 5–7 cm of the esophagus and the proximal stomach. Grassi noted that one reason the proximal vagotomy technique fails is that surgeons sometimes overlook a branch leading from the posterior vagus nerve to the posterior wall of the upper stomach. He named this the "criminal nerve." If all the vagal nerve branches that enter the distal esophagus or proximal stomach are divided, interruption of the criminal nerve will be included in the dissection.

Postoperative Gastroesophageal Reflux

Sanker et al. and Temple and McFarland have observed that the lower esophageal sphincter may become incompetent following proximal gastric vagotomy because of the extensive dissection that must be done in the region of the esophagogastric junction. To prevent postoperative gastroesophageal reflux, Sanker has recommended that posterior gastropexy be done routinely with proximal gastric vagotomy. Although we have not *routinely* added a step to the proximal gastric vagotomy operation aimed at preventing reflux, this step should certainly be included for those patients who have shown *preoperative* evidence of gastroesophageal reflux. Whether this step should be the modified posterior gastropexy recommended by Sanker or the operation developed by Hill or by Nissen depends on the operative findings and the experience of the surgeon.

Operative Technique

Incision and Exposure

With the patient supine, elevate the head of the operating table 10°–15°. Make a midline incision from the xiphoid to a point 5 cm below the umbilicus. Insert an Upper Hand or "chain" retractor to elevate the lower sternum about 8–10 cm. Insert a self-retaining retractor of the Balfour type without excessive tension to separate the margins of the incision. Depending on the patient's body habitus, use either a Weinberg or Harrington retractor to elevate the left lobe of the liver above the esophageal hiatus. On rare occasions this exposure may not be adequate, and the triangular ligament of the left lobe of the liver may have to be divided, with the left lobe retracted to the patient's right.

Identification of Right and Left Vagal Trunks

Expose the peritoneum overlying the abdominal esophagus and transect it transversely, using a long Metzenbaum scissors and DeBakey forceps. Extend the peritoneal incision to uncover the muscular fibers of the crura surrounding the esophageal hiatus (see Figs. 10–1, 10–2, and 10–3). Separate the anterior two-thirds of the circumference of the esophagus from the adjacent right and left crux of the diaphragm, using scissors and peanut-sponge dissection under direct vision (see Fig. 10–4). Thereupon, encircle the esophagus with the right index finger.

Because the right (posterior) vagus nerve is frequently 2 cm or more away from the esophagus, a special maneuver should be employed to insure that the index finger includes this vagal trunk in its encircling motion. In order to accomplish this, pass the right index finger behind the esophagus, beginning in the groove between the left branch of the crux and the left margin of the esophagus. Then pass the fingernail along the anterior wall of the aorta and curve it anteriorly along the posterior aspect of the right side of the diaphragmatic crux. The fingertip then enters the operative field adjacent to the right crux. As a result of this maneuver, the index finger almost invariably will contain both vagal trunks in addition to the esophagus. The right vagus generally is considerably larger than the left and is almost always a single trunk. Encircle it with narrow umbilical tape to which a hemostat is attached. The left (anterior) vagus can be identified generally at the right anterior surface of the *lower* esophagus. Encircle it in a similar fashion with narrow umbilical tape.

Identification of Crow's Foot

Pass the left index and middle fingers through an avascular area of the gastrohepatic omentum and enter the lesser sac. This enables the nerves and blood vessels along the lesser curvature of the stomach to be elevated and put on stretch. The anterior nerve of Latarjet, which is the termination of the left vagus trunk as it innervates the anterior gastric wall, can be seen through the transparent peritoneum adjacent to the lesser curvature of the stomach. It intermingles with terminal branches of the left gastric artery, which also go to the lesser curvature. As the nerve of Latarjet reaches its termination, it divides into four or five branches in a configuration that resembles a crow's foot. These terminal branches innervate the distal 6–7 cm of antrum and pylorus; they should be preserved (**Figs. 11–1 and 11–2a**).

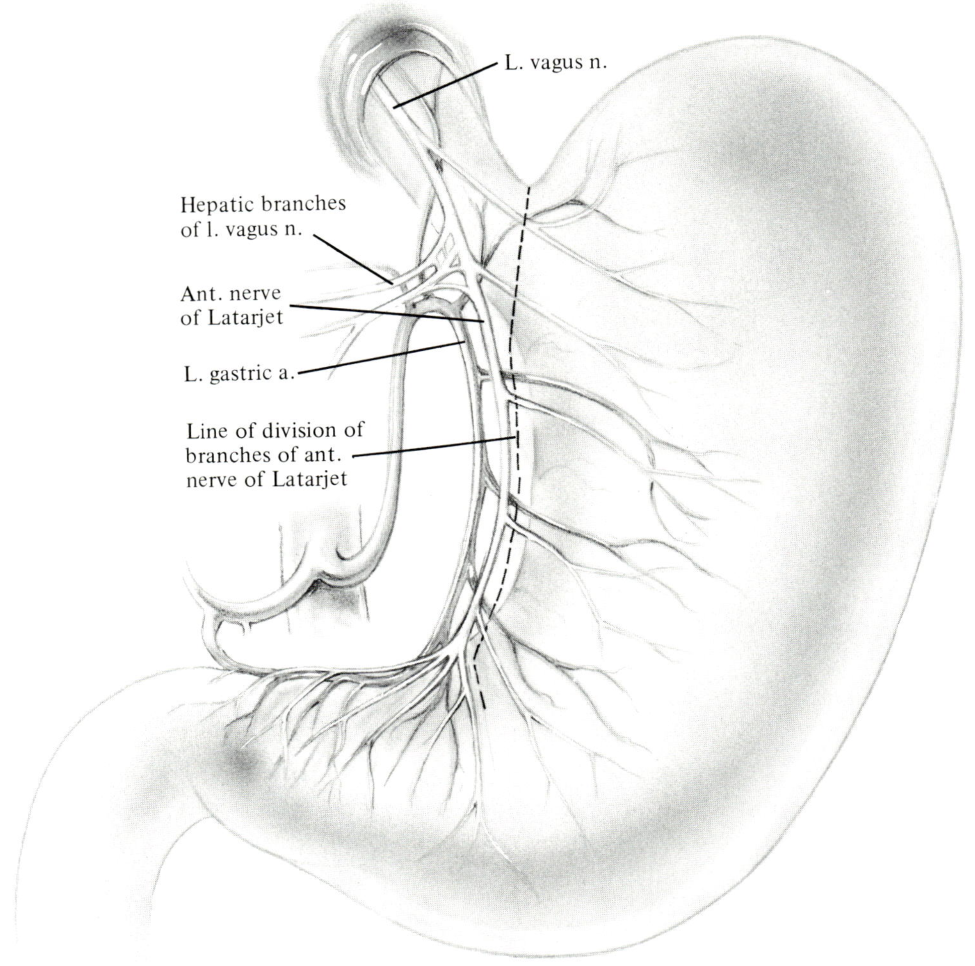

Fig. 11–1

Dissection of Anterior Nerve of Latarjet

After identifying the crow's foot, insert a Mixter right-angle clamp beneath the next cephalad branch of the nerve and the accompanying blood vessels (**Fig. 11–2b**). This branch is 6–7 cm cephalad to the pyloric muscle. After the clamp has broken through the peritoneum on both sides of these structures, divide them between Adson hemostats and carefully ligate with 4–0 cotton (**Fig. 11–2c**). Alternatively, each branch may be doubly ligated before being divided. Repeat the same maneuver many times, ascending the lesser curvature of the stomach and taking care not to include more than one branch in each hemostat. In order to preserve the innervation of the antrum, the hemostats must be applied close to the gastric wall so as not to injure the main trunk of the nerve of Latarjet. Great care should be taken not to tear any of these small blood vessels, as they tend to retract and form hematomata in the gastrohepatic ligament, obscuring the field of dissection. This is a particular hazard in obese patients. Trauma to the musculature of the gastric wall should be avoided, as this area of lesser curvature is not protected by a layer of serosa.

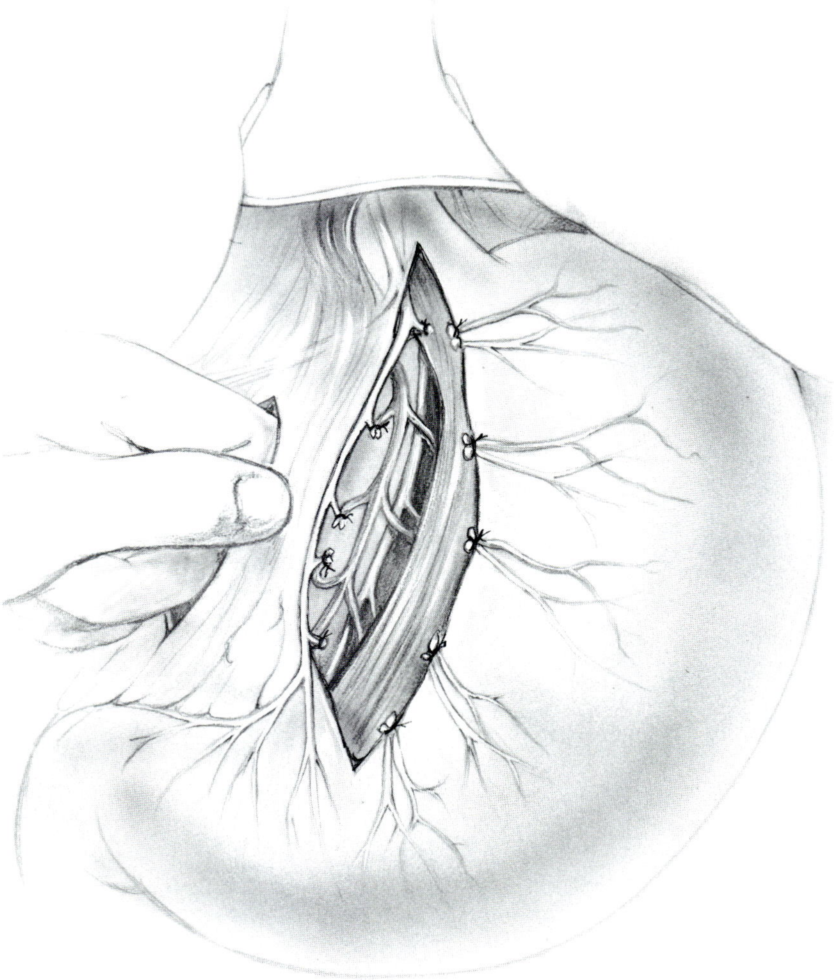

Fig. 11–2a

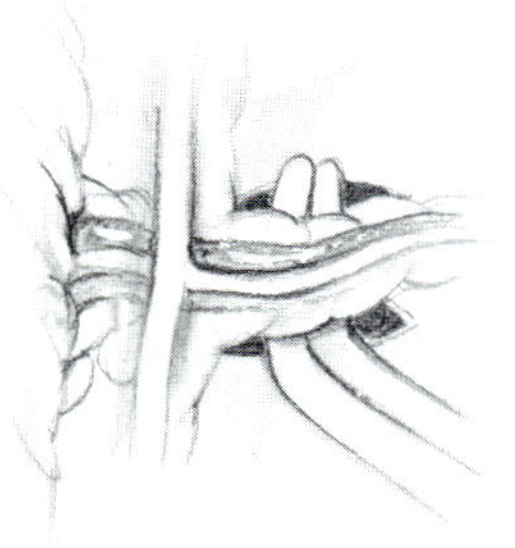

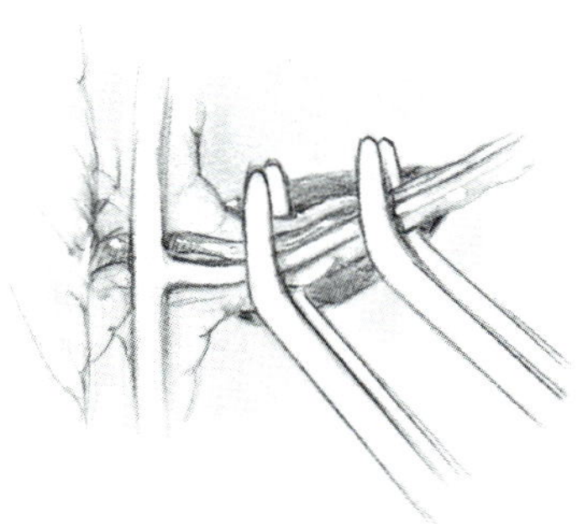

Fig. 11–2b Fig. 11–2c

Continue the dissection of the anterior layer of the gastrohepatic ligament until the main trunk of the left vagus nerve is reached. Retract this trunk toward the patient's right by means of the umbilical tape. At the conclusion of the dissection, the left vagus nerve should be completely separated from the wall of the esophagus for a distance of 6–7 cm above the esophagogastric junction. Any small

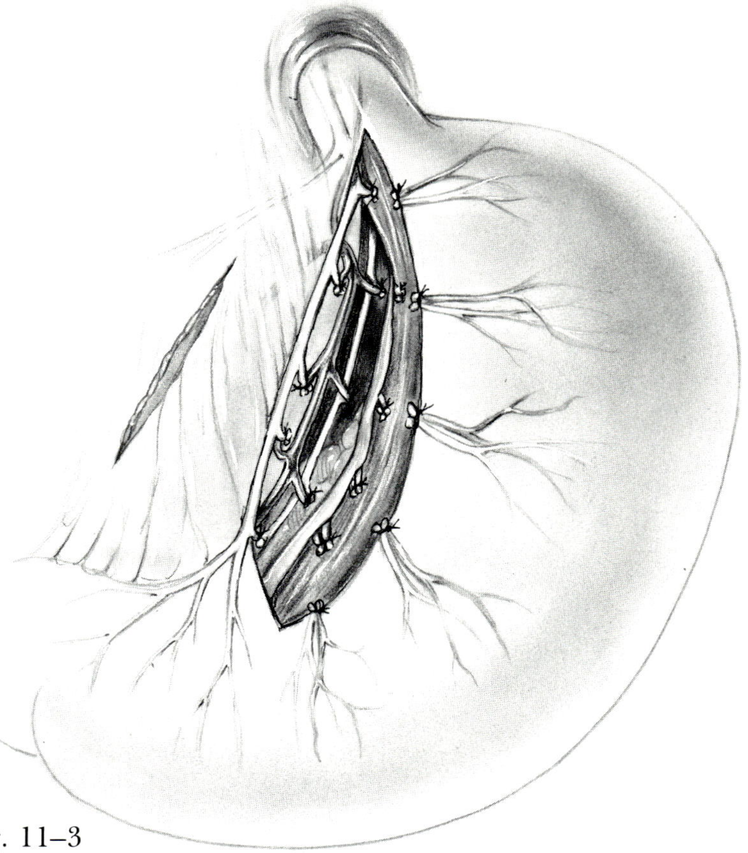

Fig. 11–3

nerve branching from the vagus nerve to this portion of the esophagus should be divided. In this fashion all the branches from the left vagus to the stomach are interrupted, with the exception of those innervating the distal antrum and pylorus. Preserve the hepatic branch of the vagus trunk also, for it leaves the left vagus and goes to the patient's right on its way to the liver.

Dissection of Posterior Nerve of Latarjet

Now delineate the posterior leaflet of the gastrohepatic omentum as it attaches to the posterior aspect of the lesser curvature of the stomach. Again, the crow's foot should be identified and preserved. Each branch of the left gastric artery and vein, together with each terminal branch of the *posterior* nerve of Latarjet, should be individually isolated, doubly clamped, divided, and ligated (**Fig. 11–3**). Take care to make this division close to the gastric wall in order to preserve the main nerve of Latarjet. Continue this dissection in a cephalad direction until the previously identified right vagal trunk can be seen alongside the distal esophagus. When this dissection has been properly completed, it will be evident that the right vagus nerve and the gastrohepatic ligament are situated far to the right of the completely bare lesser curvature. Now dissect away the posterior aspect of the esophagus from the posterior vagus nerve for a distance of 7 cm above the esophagogastric junction so that no branches from this trunk may reach the stomach by way of the distal esophagus.

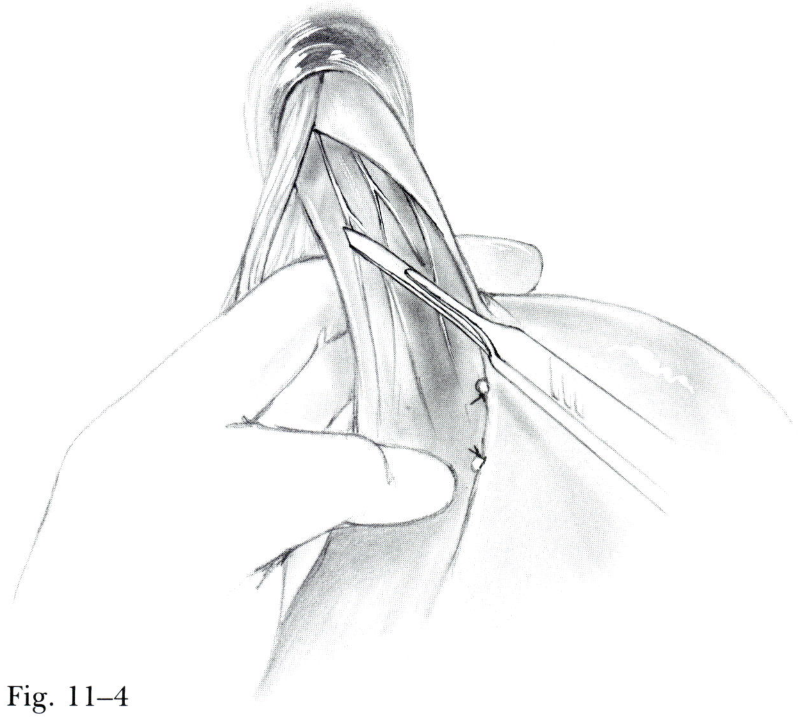

Fig. 11–4

Pay special attention to the criminal nerve described by Grassi, which is a branch of the posterior vagal trunk passing behind the esophagus to the posterior wall of the gastric cardia. If the surgeon's left hand can be passed between the freed vagal trunks and the distal esophagus as well as the gastric fundus, this would help insure that the extent of the dissection has been adequate. In addition, carefully inspect the longitudinal muscle fibers of the distal esophagus. Any tiny fibers resembling nerve tissue should be divided or avulsed from the musculature throughout the circumference of the lower 7 cm of esophagus (**Fig. 11–4**).

Repair of Lesser Curvature

Repair the deserosalized portion of the lesser curvature using interrupted 4–0 cotton sutures to approximate the peritoneum over the denuded gastric musculature (**Fig. 11–5**).

Close the abdominal incision in the usual fashion, without drainage.

Postoperative Care

Continue nasogastric suction and intravenous fluids for 48 hours. At the end of this time the patient generally is able to tolerate the postgastrectomy type of diet. Usually the postoperative course is uneventful, and undesirable postoperative gastric sequelae, such as dumping, are distincly uncommon.

Complications

One complication, which seems to be unique to proximal gastric vagotomy, is necrosis of the lesser curvature. Although

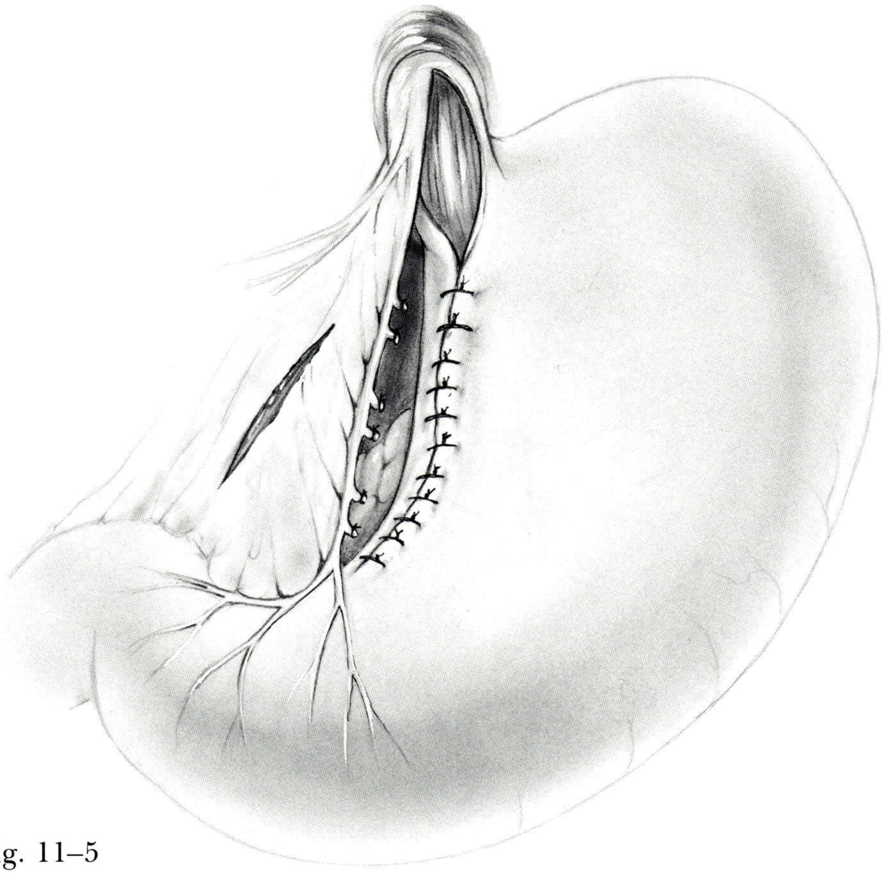

Fig. 11–5

this is quite rare (0.3% of all proximal gastric vagotomy operations), it is often fatal when it occurs. It probably results from trauma or hematoma of the gastric wall in an area that lacks serosa. Prevention requires accurate dissection. It is hoped that reperitonealization of the lesser curvature by suturing (Fig. 11–5) will also help avoid this complication. Treatment requires early diagnosis and resection.

References

Grassi G (1977) in Nyhus LM, Wastell C Surgery of the stomach and duodenum. Little Brown, Boston, p. 61

Hallenbeck GA et al. (1976) Proximal gastric vagotomy: effects of two operative techniques on clinical and gastric secretory results. Ann Surg 184:435

Sanker MY et al. (1976) The advantages of combining posterior gastropexy with proximal gastrectomy. Chir Gastroent (Surg Gastroent) 10:389

Temple MB, McFarland J (1975) Gastroesophageal reflux complicating highly selective vagotomy. Br J Surg 2:168

12 Pyloroplasty, Heineke-Mikulicz

Indications

This operation is generally performed for the surgical treatment of duodenal ulcer in the poor-risk patient, especially one undergoing emergency surgery for massive hemorrhage (see Chap. 9).

Preoperative Preparation

(See Chap. 9.)

Pitfalls and Danger Points

Suture line leak
Inadequate lumen

Operative Strategy

Even if fibrosis and inflammation of the duodenum are present, as they may be in severe ulcer disease, in most cases a Heineke-Mikulicz pyloroplasty is feasible. When the duodenum appears too inflexible to allow the performance of this procedure, the Finney pyloroplasty or gastrojejunostomy should be elected. These latter two operations, although slightly more complicated than the Heineke-Mikulicz, give assurance of producing an adequate lumen for gastric drainage.

Another method of assuring an adequate lumen in the pyloroplasty is to use a one-layer suture line for the Heineke-Mikulicz pyloroplasty. This prevents the inversion of an excessive amount of tissue.

Covering the pyloroplasty suture line with omentum is important for two reasons: 1) This step helps prevent leakage from the one-layer suture line. 2) Adhesions between the suture line and the under surface of the liver may cause angulation and partial obstruction unless omentum is used to separate these two structures.

Operative Technique

Kocher Maneuver

In the majority of cases a pyloroplasty requires a Kocher maneuver to provide maneuverability of the tissues. This is accomplished by grasping the peritoneum lateral to the duodenum with forceps and making an incision in this peritoneal layer. Alternatively, in many patients the surgeon's index finger may be insinuated behind the common bile duct and portal vein, pointing towards the ampulla of Vater. The finger then slides toward the patient's right. Overlying the fingertip is not only a thin layer of peritoneum but also an avascular lateral duodenal ligament that attaches the duodenum to the underlying retroperitoneal structures. Incise the peritoneal layer either with scissors or electrocautery, then stretch the lateral duodenal ligament with the fingertip and

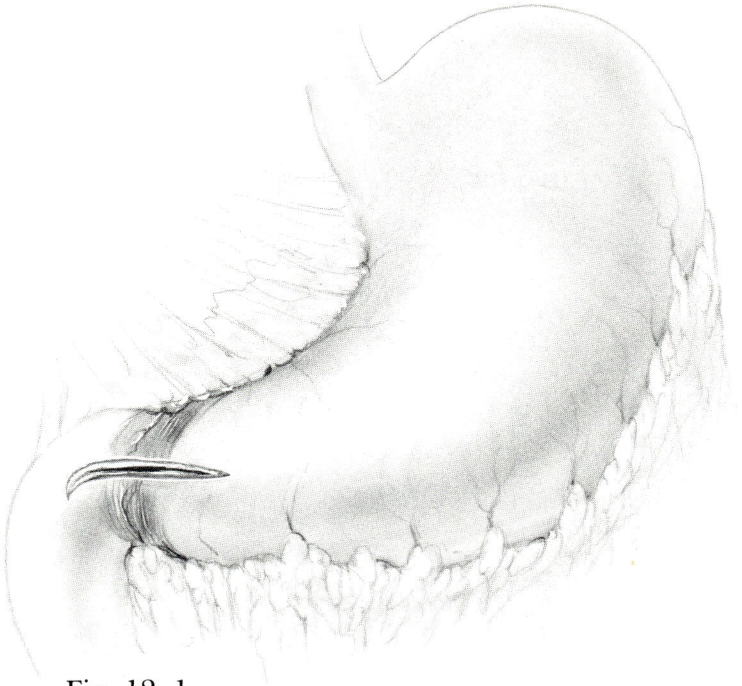

Fig. 12–1

divide it similarly. It is rarely necessary to mobilize the hepatic flexure to perform a complete Kocher maneuver (see Figs. 7–14, 7–15, and 7–16).

Pyloroduodenal Incision

Make a 5 cm incision across the lower antrum, the pyloric sphincter, and the proximal duodenum, with the incision centered on the pyloric muscle (**Fig. 12–1**). Apply a Babcock clamp to the cephalad and one to the caudal cut ends of the pyloric sphincter and draw apart the two Babcock clamps. Transfix any bleeding points either with 4–0 chromic catgut suture-ligatures or with careful electrocoagulation. Close the incision transversely, which will provide a patulous lumen for gastric drainage.

Suture of Pyloroplasty

Use one layer of sutures to prevent excessive tissue inversion. Most techniques call for a through-and-through suture. As the gastric wall is much thicker than the duodenal, it is difficult with this type of technique to prevent eversion of mucosa between the sutures. Consequently, we prefer either a deep "seromucosal" (see Fig. B–16) or interrupted Lembert sutures of 4–0 cotton. Insert the first suture at the midpoint of the suture line (**Fig. 12–2**).

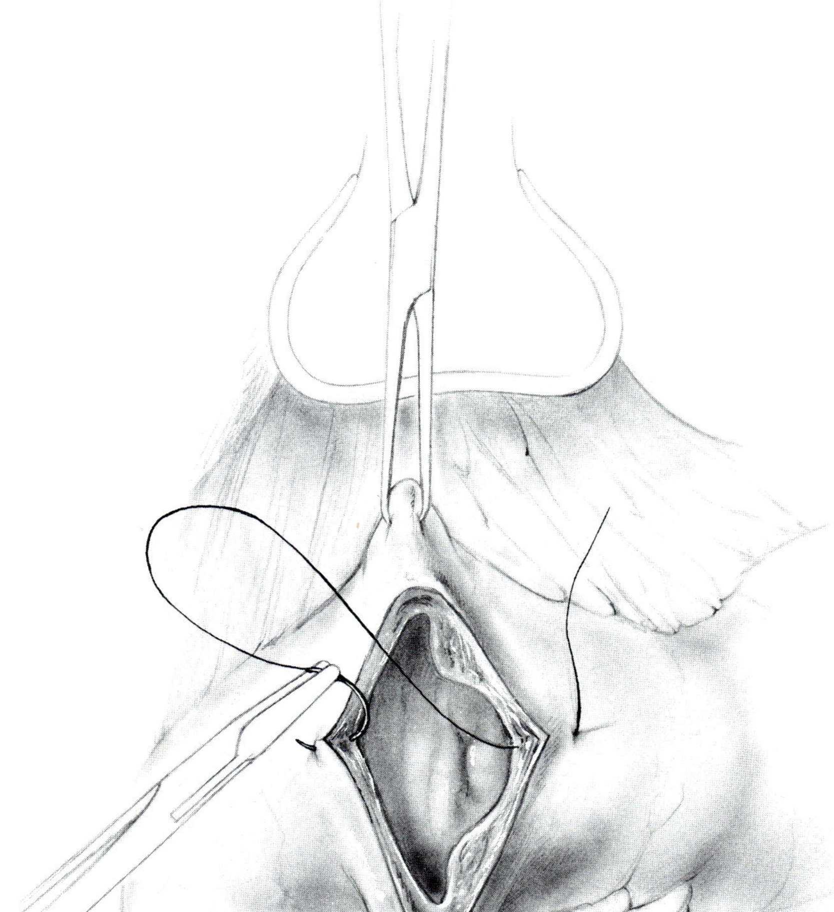

Fig. 12–2

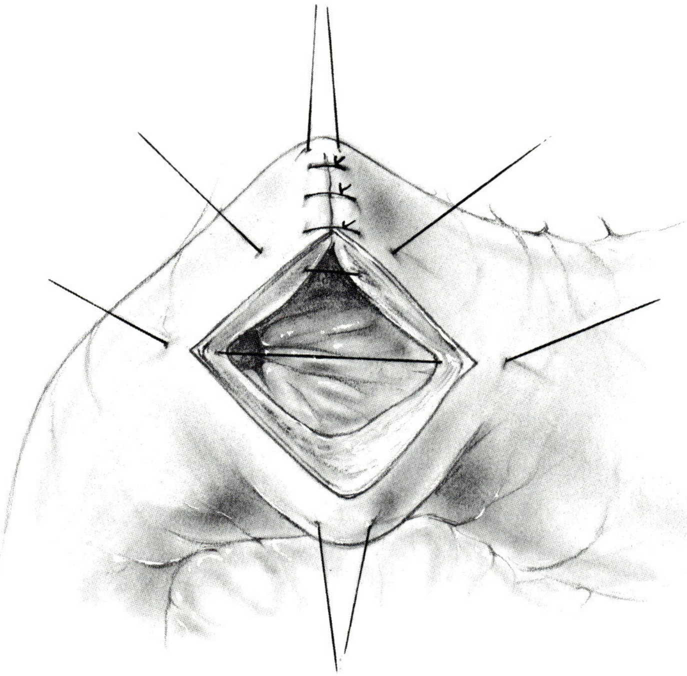

Fig. 12–3

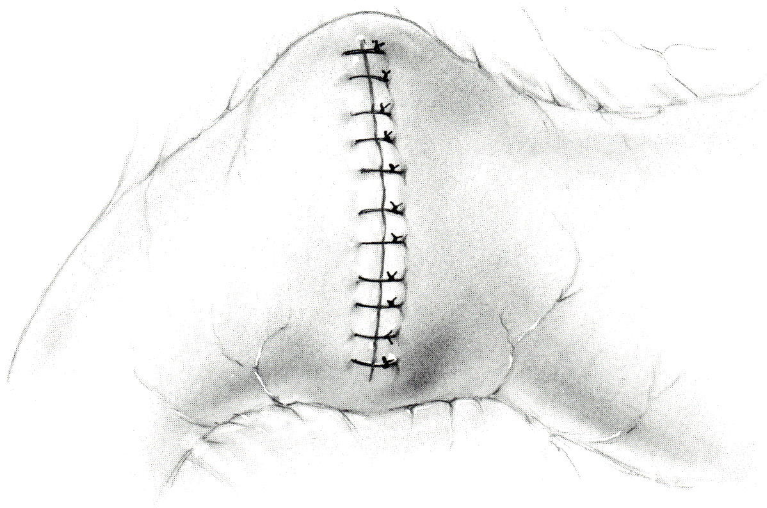

Fig. 12–4

Proceed with the closure from one corner to the midpoint and then from the other corner to the midpoint, inverting just enough of the seromuscular coat to prevent any outpouching of mucosa between the sutures (**Figs. 12–3 and 12–4**).

Then suture omentum loosely over the pyloroplasty to prevent adhesions to the undersurface of the liver.

Stapling of Pyloroplasty

Instead of suturing the pyloroplasty incision as described above, apply Allis clamps to the incision, approximating the tissues in eversion, mucosa to mucosa. Then apply the TA–55 device to the everted tissues just deep to the line of Allis clamps (**Fig. 12–5**). It should be loaded with 4.8 mm staples in most cases. Drive home the alignment pin, tighten the device, and fire the staples. Excise redundant tissue with a scalpel and lightly electrocoagulate the everted mucosa, and remove the TA–55 instrument. Carefully inspect the staple line to be sure satisfactory "B" staple formation is carried out (**Fig. 12–6**). Bleeding points may be controlled by conservative electrocoagulation or sutures of 4–0 PG. Place omentum over this stapled closure.

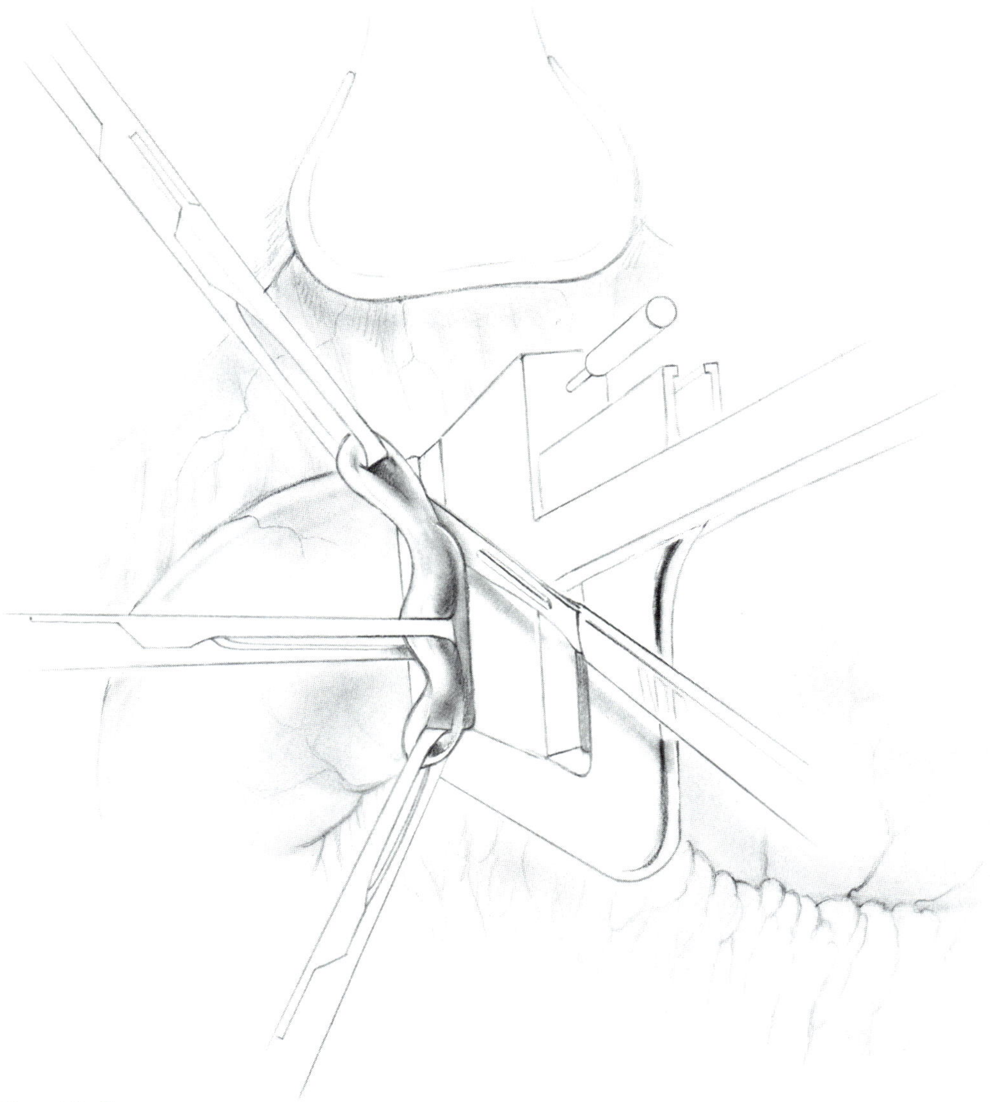

Fig. 12–5

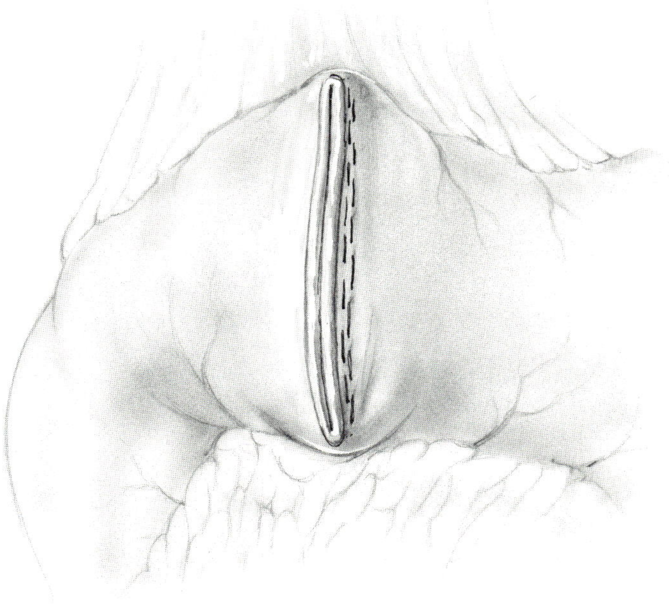

Fig. 12–6

Postoperative Care

Administer nasogastric suction until gastric and bowel function resume.

Complications

Complications following this operation are rare, although delayed gastric emptying occurs occasionally, as does suture-line leakage.

13 Pyloroplasty, Finney

Indications

Pyloroplasty is performed to provide gastric drainage following vagotomy.

Preoperative Preparation

(See Chap. 9.)

Operative Strategy

Unlike the gastroduodenotomy incision made for the Heineke-Mikulicz pyloroplasty, which is in the anterior midline, for the Finney pyloroplasty the gastroduodenal incision is kept close to the greater curvature side of the stomach and the pancreatic side of the proximal duodenum (Fig. 13–1). If the incision is not made in this manner, there will be excessive tension on the anterior suture line.

Operative Technique

Kocher Maneuver

Make a Kocher maneuver to mobilize the first and second portions of the duodenum.

Pyloroduodenal Incision

Insert a layer of interrupted 4–0 cotton Lembert sutures to approximate the greater curvature of the stomach to the superior portion of the proximal duodenum. These sutures should be inserted fairly close to the greater curvature of the stomach and fairly close to the junction of the duodenum and pancreas. Continue this suture line for a distance of 5–6 cm from the pylorus (**Fig. 13–1**).

When the sutures have been tied, make an inverted "U"-shaped incision along a line 5–6 mm superficial to the suture line (Fig. 13–1). Carry this incision through the full thickness of the pyloric sphincter. After the incision has been made the mucosal surface of both the gastric antrum and duodenum can easily be seen.

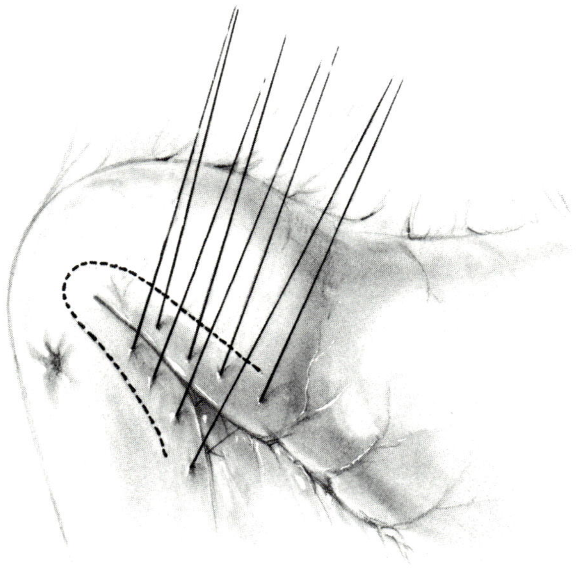

Fig. 13–1

Completion of Suture Line

Begin the mucosal suture at the inferior surface of the divided pyloric sphincter. Pass a needle armed with 3–0 atraumatic PG through the full thickness of stomach and duodenum at the pyloric sphincter and tie it (**Fig. 13–2**). Continue the suture in a caudal direction as a continuous locked stitch until the lowermost portion of the incision is reached. Then pass the needle from inside out on the stomach side. Approximate the anterior mucosal layer by means of a continuous

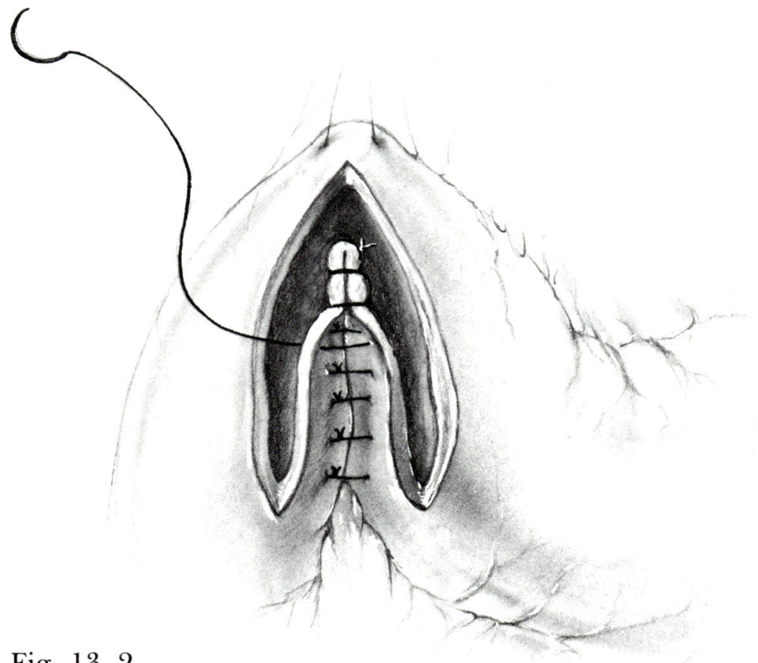

Fig. 13–2

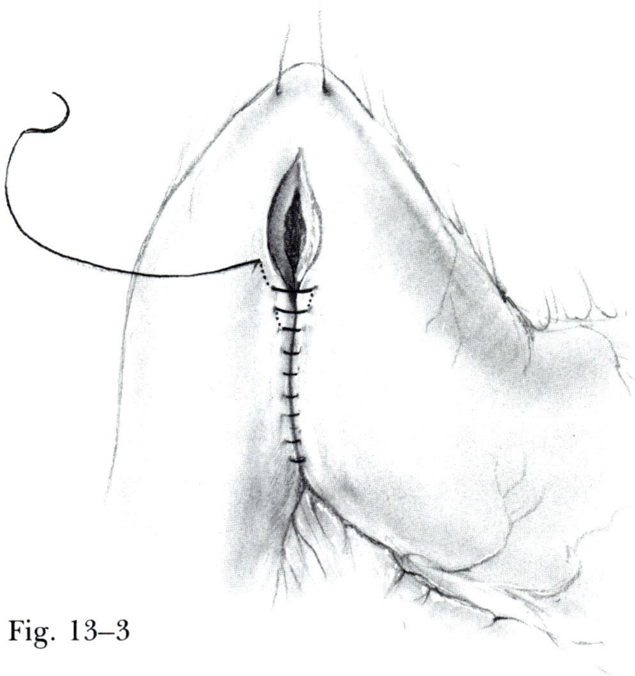

Fig. 13–3

Connell or continuous Cushing suture (**Fig. 13–3**), which should be terminated when the cephalad end of the incision is reached. Close the anterior seromuscular layer by means of interrupted 4–0 cotton Lembert sutures (**Fig. 13–4**). At the conclusion the lumen should admit two fingers.

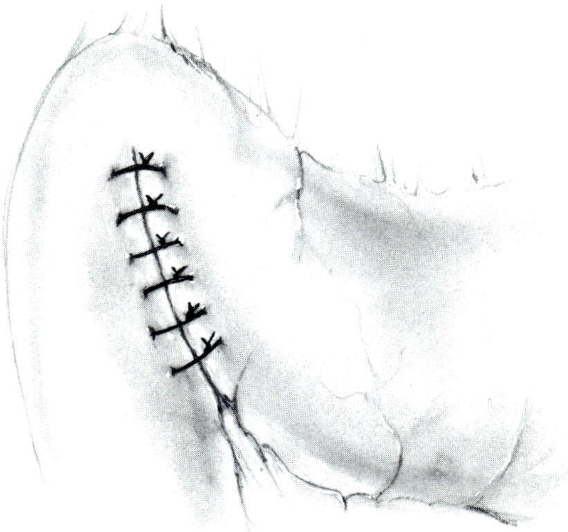

Fig. 13–4

Postoperative Care

Same as for Heineke-Mikulicz pyloroplasty (see Chap. 12).

Complications

Same as for Heineke-Mikulicz pyloroplasty (see Chap. 12).

14 Gastrojejunostomy

Indications

Gastrojejunostomy is performed to assure gastric drainage following vagotomy, when the duodenum is too inflamed or fibrotic to permit a pyloroplasty.

In patients who have inoperable carcinoma of the pancreas that occludes the duodenum, gastrojejunostomy will successfully bypass the obstruction. Routine vagotomy is not necessary, as these patients have a short life expectancy, and marginal ulcers do not seem to occur following gastrojejunostomy for pancreatic carcinoma.

Preoperative Preparation

(See Chap. 9.)

Pitfalls and Danger Points

Postoperative gastric bleeding
Anastomotic obstruction

Operative Strategy

Traditionally, gastrojejunal anastomoses have been placed on the posterior wall of the antrum in the hope they will improve drainage. Posterior drainage is dependent drainage only when the patient is lying in bed flat on his or her back. It is questionable, however, whether the average patient spends enough hours in this position during sleep to warrant the additional difficulty of placing the gastrojejunostomy in posterior location. We prefer to do an anterior gastrojejunostomy along the greater curvature of the antrum, situated no more than 5–7 cm from the pylorus.

Operative Technique

Incision

Make a midline incision from the xiphoid to the umbilicus. In cases of duodenal ulcer, carry out vagotomy as described above.

Freeing the Greater Curvature

Beginning at a point about 5 cm proximal to the pylorus, doubly clamp, divide, and individually ligate the branches of the gastroepiploic vessels on the greater curvature of the stomach, separating the greater omentum from the greater curvature of the stomach for a distance of 6–8 cm.

Gastrojejunal Anastomosis

Identify the ligament of Treitz and bring the jejunum in an antecolonic fashion, going from the patient's left to right. Make a longitudinal scratch mark with the back of a scalpel blade on the antimesenteric border of the jejunum, beginning at a point no more than 12–15 cm from the ligament of Treitz. The scratch mark should be 4 cm in length. This will mark the eventual incision into the jejunum for the anastomosis.

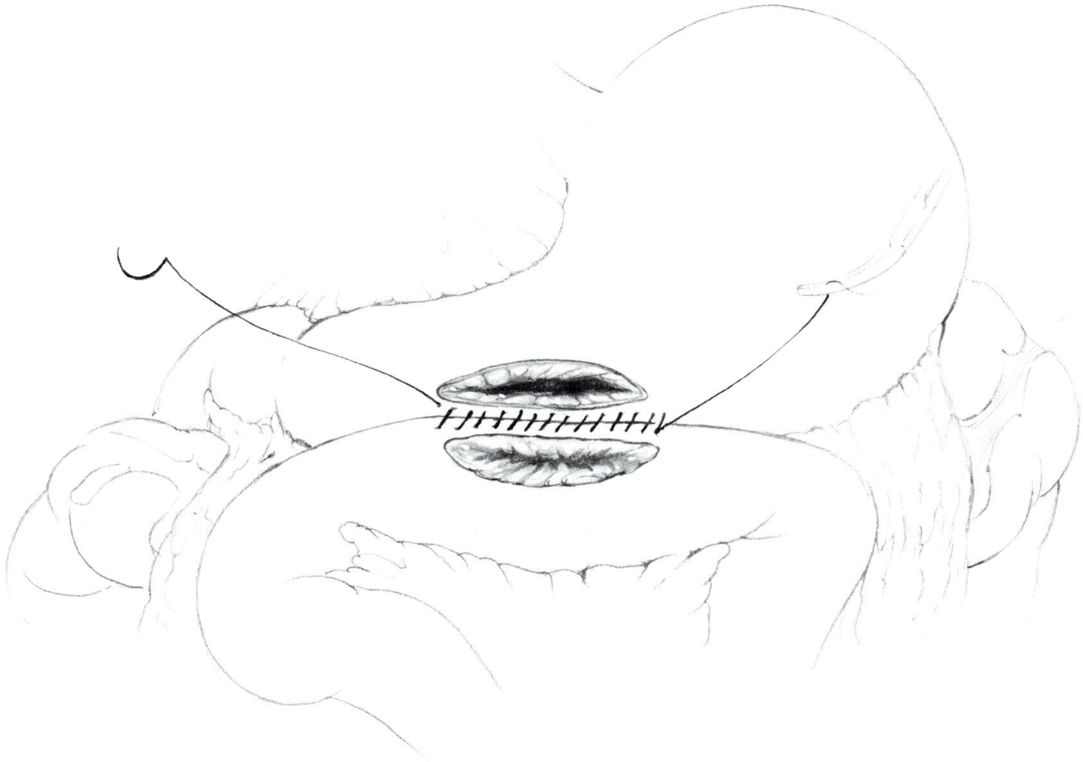

Fig. 14–1

Because of the large size of the anastomosis, continuous suture material is quite satisfactory in this situation. After freeing a 6 cm segment of greater curvature from omentum, initiate (close to the greater curve) a continuous Lembert suture of atraumatic 3–0 PG on the left side of the anastomosis and approximate the seromuscular coats of the stomach and jejunum for a distance of about 5 cm (**Fig. 14–1**). Lock the last posterior Lembert suture. Then make incisions, 4 cm long, on the antimesenteric border of the jejunum and along the greater curvature of the stomach. Begin approximating the posterior mucosal layer at the midpoint of the incision, utilizing 3–0 PG doubly armed with straight needles. Insert and tie the first suture. Continue the suture toward the patient's left as a continuous locked suture, penetrating both mucosal and seromuscular coats. Terminate it at the left lateral margin of the incision. At this time, with the second needle initiate a similar type stitch from the midpoint to the right lateral margin of the incision (**Figs. 14–2a and 14–2b**). Approximate the anterior mucosal layer by means of a continuous Connell or continuous Cushing-type stitch. The two sutures should meet anteriorly near the midline and be tied to each other.

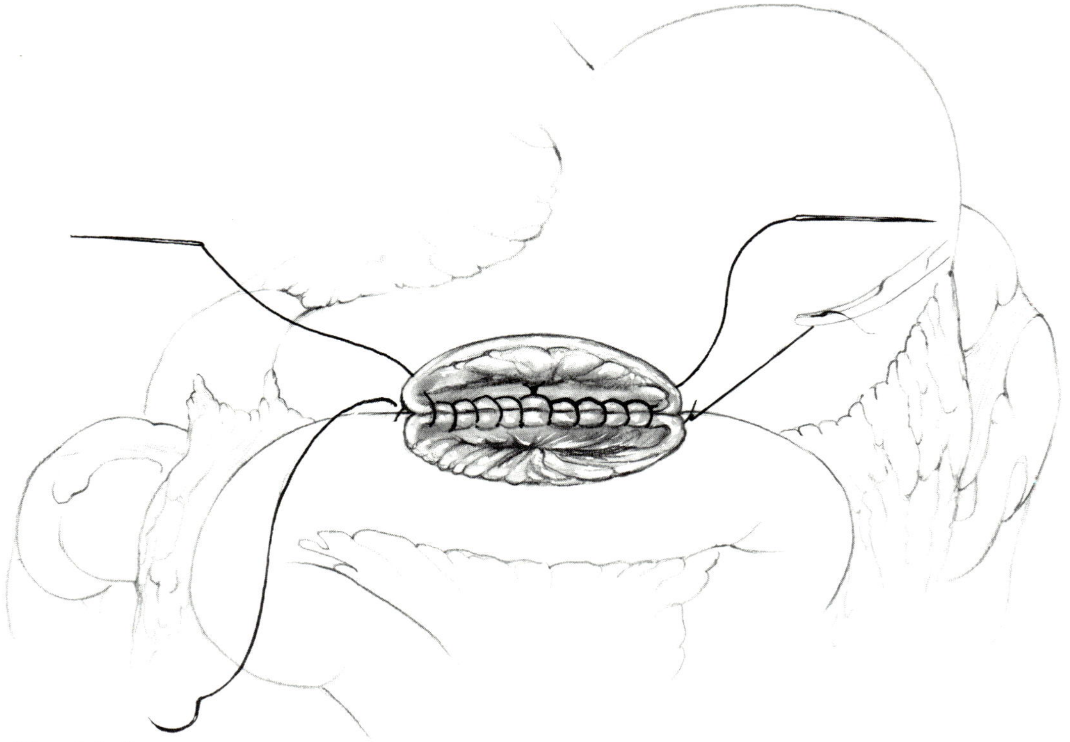

Fig. 14–2a

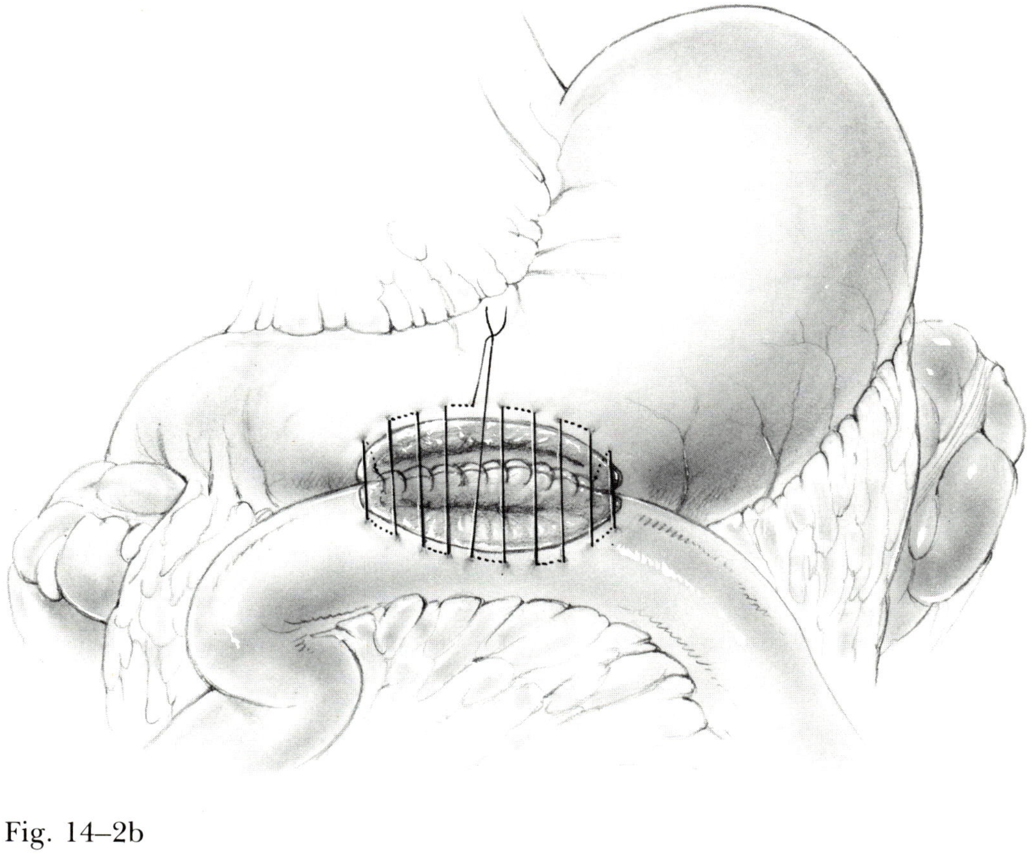

Fig. 14–2b

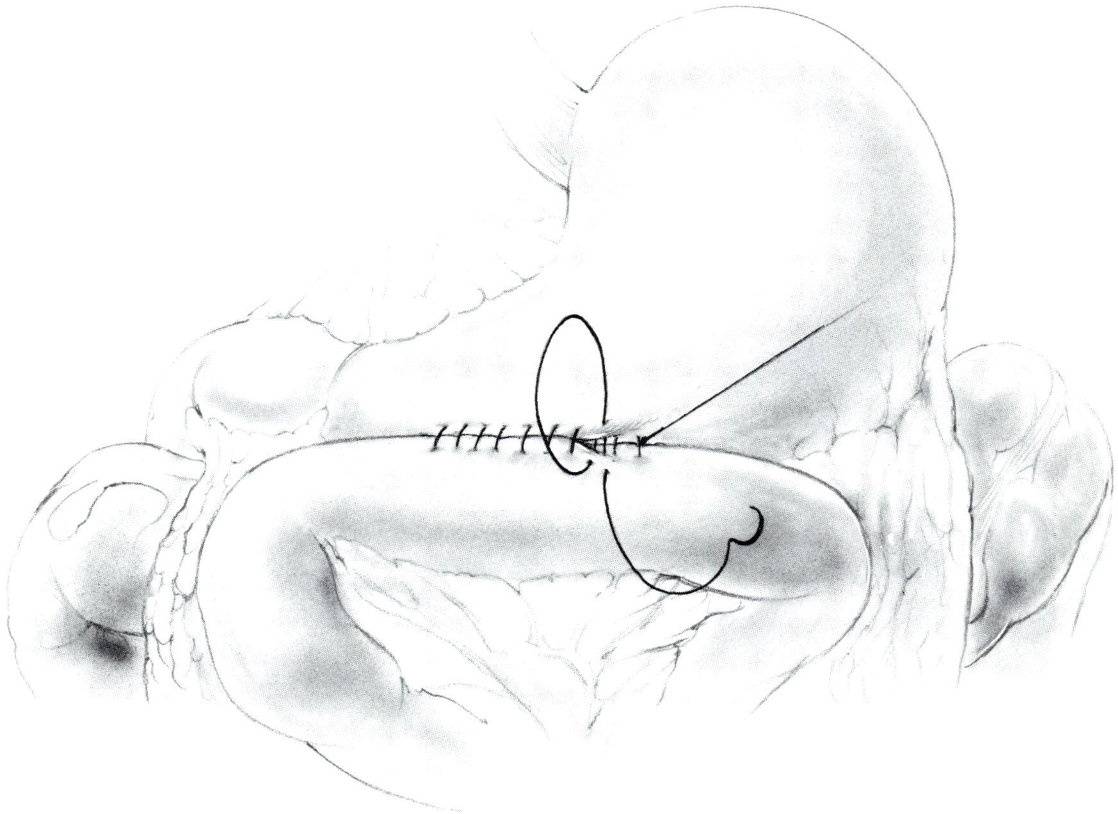

Fig. 14–3

Close the anterior seromuscular layer with the same curved needle that was utilized for the posterior layer. This should progress as a continuous Lembert suture (**Fig. 14–3**) from the right lateral margin of the anastomosis toward the left lateral margin. Terminate the suture by tying it to itself (**Fig. 14–4**). The anastomosis should admit two fingers.

Operative Technique: Gastrojejunostomy by Stapling

Clearing the Greater Curvature of the Stomach

Clear the greater curvature of the stomach by dissecting away the omentum as described above.

Application of the GIA

Identify the proximal jejunum and bring it to an antecolonic position as described above. With the electrocautery make a stab wound on the antimesenteric side of jejunum at a point 12–15 cm from the ligament of Treitz. Make a second stab wound along the greater curvature of the stomach at a point about 10 cm from the pylorus. Insert one fork of the GIA device

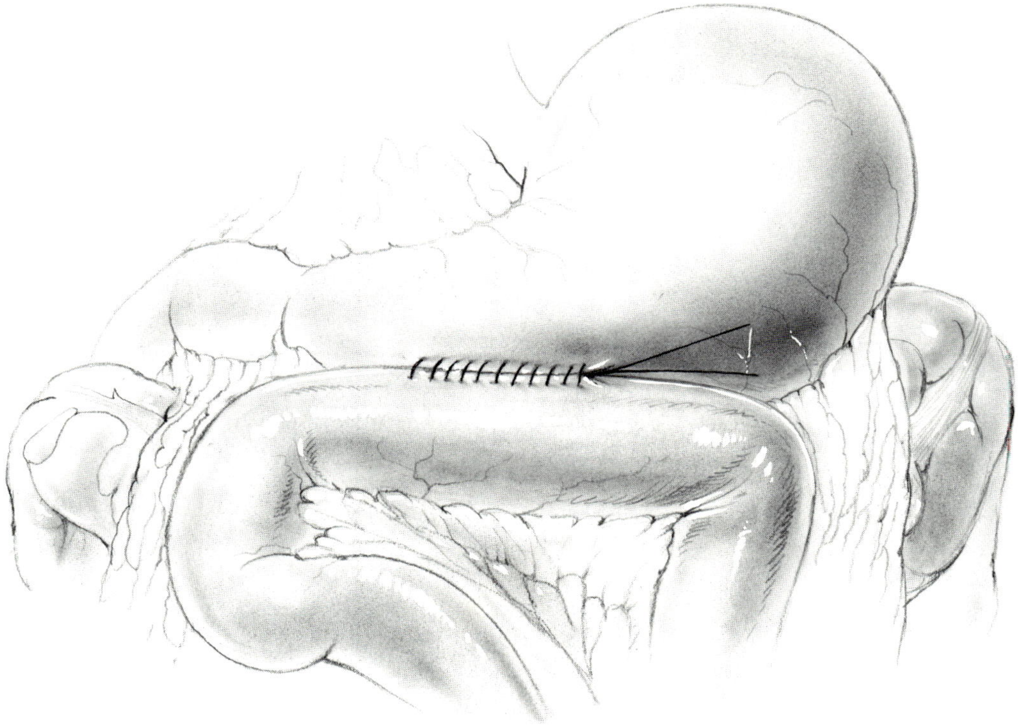

Fig. 14–4

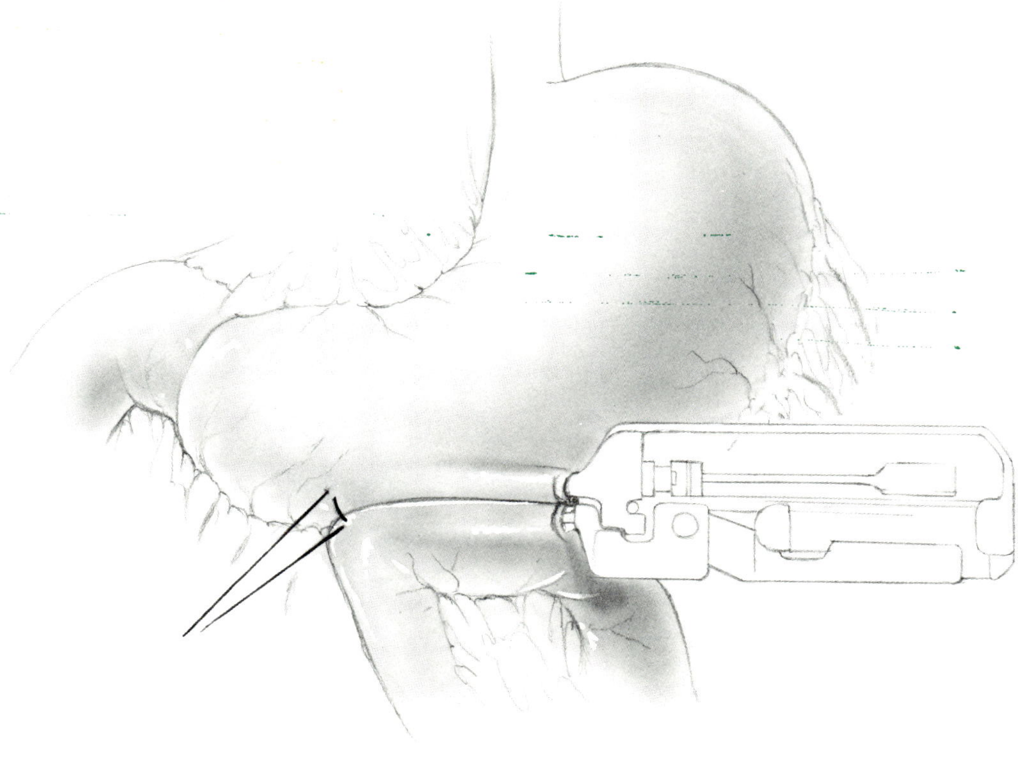

Fig. 14–5

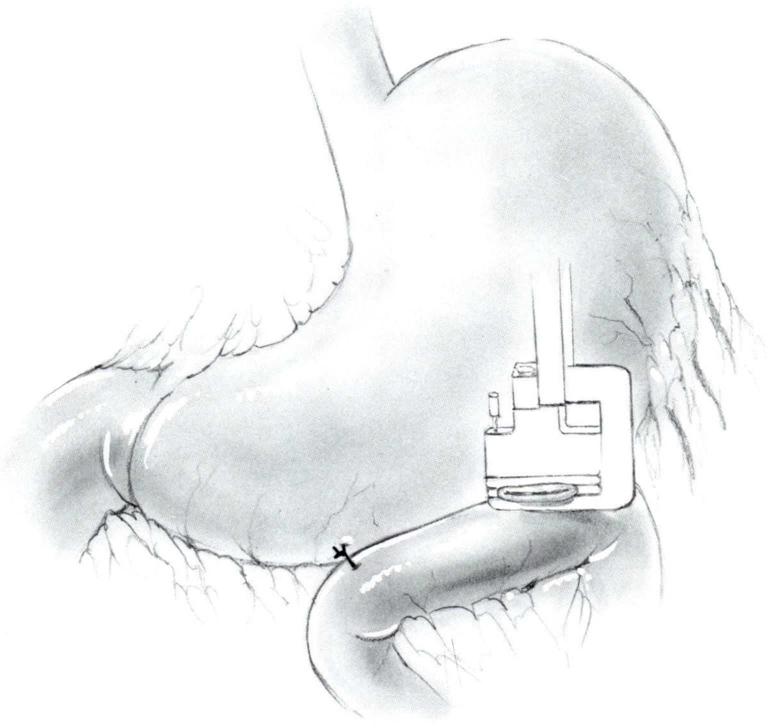

Fig. 14–6

into the jejunum and one fork into the stomach (**Fig. 14–5**). Align the jejunum so that its antimesenteric border is parallel to the fork of the GIA and lock the device. Check the proposed gastrojejunal staple line to insure that the forks of the GIA include no tissue other than stomach and jejunum. Now fire the GIA and remove it.

Apply an Allis clamp to the anterior termination of the GIA staple line. Apply a second Allis clamp to the posterior termination of the GIA staple line. Inspect the GIA staple line carefully for bleeding. Control any bleeding point, either by cautious electrocoagulation or by the insertion of 4–0 PG atraumatic suture-ligatures.

Closure of Stab Wound

Approximate the remaining defect in the anastomosis in an everting fashion by applying several Allis clamps. Apply the TA–55 stapler deep to the Allis clamps and push the alignment into place. If the gastric wall is of average thickness use 3.5 mm staples; otherwise, the larger size will be necessary. Fire the TA–55 stapler and excise the redundant tissue with a Mayo scissors (**Fig. 14–6**). Lightly electrocoagu-

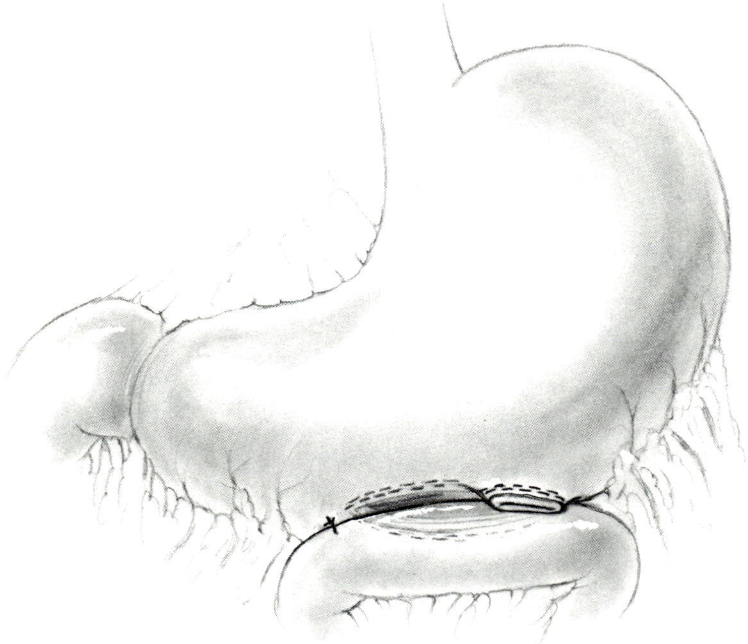

Fig. 14–7

late the everted mucosa and remove the stapling device. The lumen should admit two fingers without difficulty. Place a 4–0 seromuscular Lembert suture to fix the stomach to the jejunum on the right lateral margin of the newly stapled anastomosis (**Fig. 14–7**).

Postoperative Care

Administer nasogastric suction until there is evidence that gastric and bowel function have resumed.

Complications

Gastric bleeding is a rare complication, occurring in 1%–2% of the cases. Anastomotic leakage and obstruction are even less common than gastric bleeding.

15 Gastrectomy for Peptic Ulcer

Indications

(See Chap. 9.)

Preoperative Preparation

(See Chap. 9.)

Pitfalls and Danger Points

Inadequate duodenal stump closure

Trauma to pancreas resulting in postoperative acute pancreatitis

Incomplete removal of distal antrum

Splenic trauma

Laceration of common bile duct or ampulla of Vater during ulcer dissection

Inadequate lumen in gastroduodenal anastomosis (Billroth I) with postoperative obstruction

Inadvertent gastroileostomy (Billroth II)

Excessive length of afferent limb (Billroth II)

Operative Strategy

Duodenal Stump

Most of the serious postoperative complications of gastric surgery involve a failure of the duodenal stump closure. This leads to disruption and duodenal fistula or trauma to the pancreas, which results in acute pancreatitis. Because these complications result from persistent efforts to dissect the duodenum away from the pancreas when there is advanced fibrosis surrounding a penetrating duodenal ulcer, the simplest means of preventing trouble is for the surgeon to become aware early in the operation that the duodenal dissection is fraught with danger. When the difficult duodenum is identified early in the course of operation, either vagotomy with drainage procedure or proximal gastric vagotomy should be performed. If as a result of poor judgment the surgeon gets into difficulty after having broken into a posterior penetrating duodenal ulcer, he or she should be aware of the Nissen technique and the Cooper modification of it, as well as the procedure of catheter duodenostomy. These procedures, described below, can prove to be lifesaving. A successful Nissen maneuver, however, requires that the anterolateral wall of the duodenum be pliable and of fairly normal thickness. If this wall is shrunken and contracted with fibrosis or acutely inflamed, it may not be suitable for inversion into the pancreas by the Nissen-Cooper method.

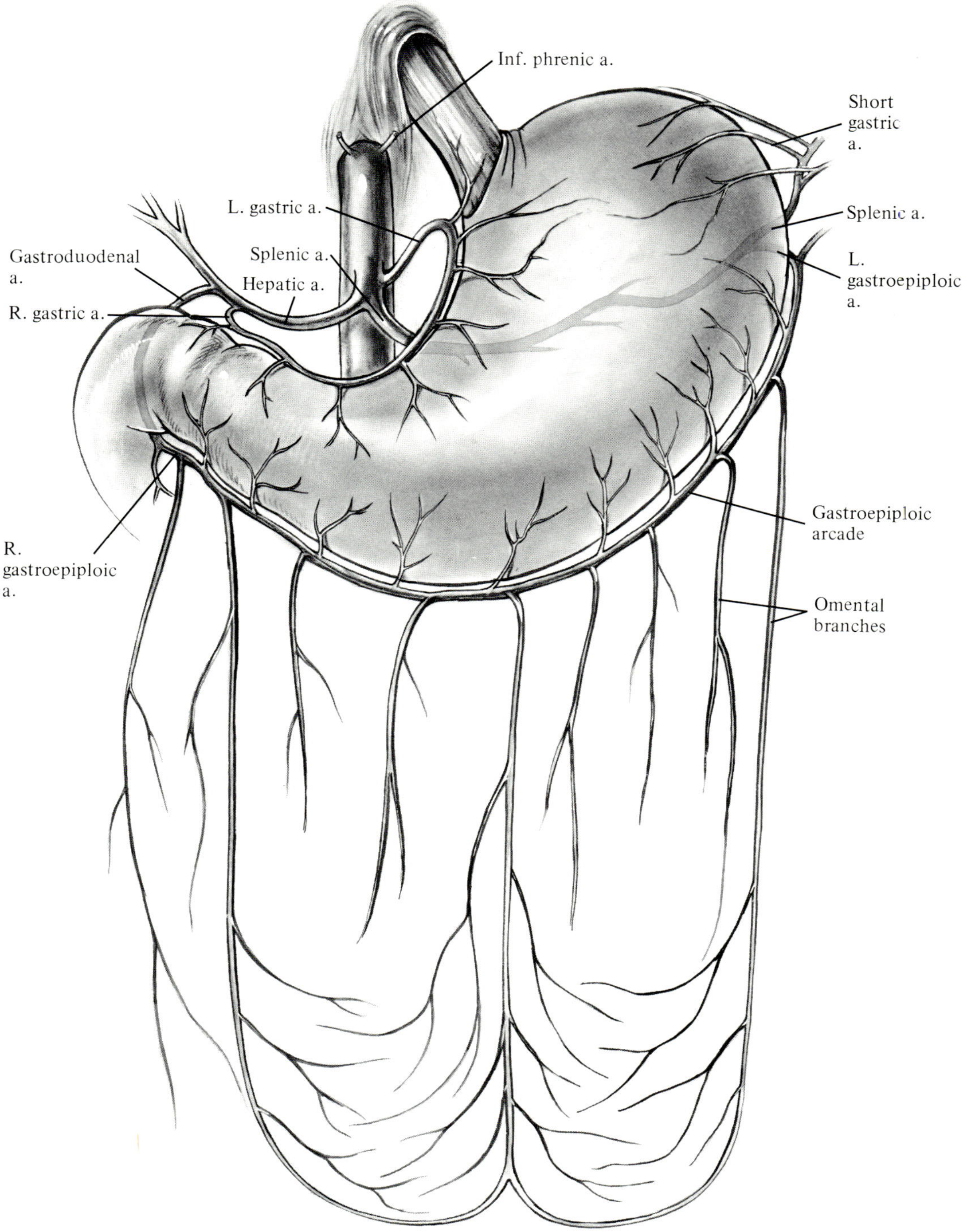
Inf. phrenic a.
Short gastric a.
L. gastric a.
Splenic a.
Gastroduodenal a.
Splenic a.
L. gastroepiploic a.
Hepatic a.
R. gastric a.
Gastroepiploic arcade
R. gastroepiploic a.
Omental branches

Fig. 15–1

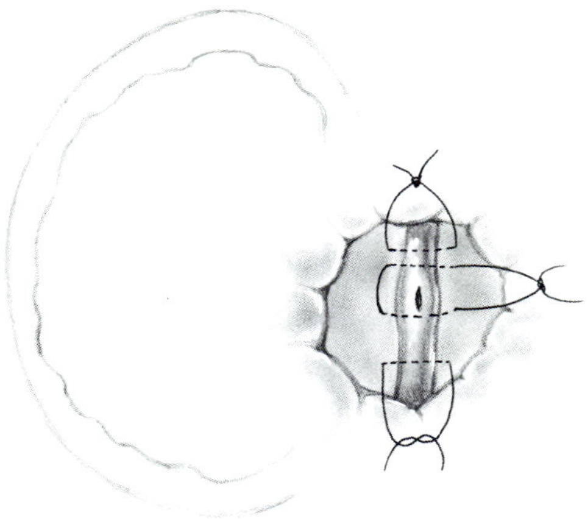

Fig. 15–2

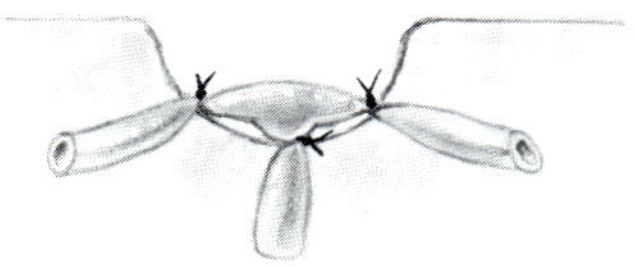

Fig. 15–3

Catheter Duodenostomy

In any case, a surgeon who doubts the security of the suture line after having closed the duodenal stump should insert a catheter into the duodenum for postoperative decompression. This provides a valuable safety valve and prevents disruption of the duodenal suture line in most instances.

Marginal Ulcer

Among the causes of postoperative marginal ulcer is the erroneous transection of the antrum proximal to the pylorus, thereby leaving antral mucosa in contact with the alkaline bilious secretions. Although an error of this type is not committed in the presence of normal anatomy, this mistake is indeed possible when the area is obscured by inflammation and fibrosis. When the landmarks of the pyloric sphincter are obscured, the surgeon should use frozen section biopsy to confirm the absence of antral mucosa at the cut end of the duodenal stump. If the line of transection is indeed in the duodenum, Brunner's glands will be seen by the pathologist.

Splenic Trauma

Hemorrhage from the spleen is most frequently the result of traction along the greater curvature of the stomach. This results in avulsion of a portion of the splenic capsule adherent to the greater omentum. If downward traction is necessary, it should be applied to the lesser curvature. We have reported that when a portion of splenic capsule has been avulsed, it can generally be managed by direct pressure over a sheet of Surgicel gauze.

Ligating the Bleeding Point in Duodenal Ulcer

The most common source of bleeding in patients who undergo emergency surgery for massive hemorrhage is a posterior duodenal ulcer eroding into the gastroduodenal artery. When the defect in this artery is identified, it should be closed by inserting three mattress sutures of 2–0 cotton. This should be done so as to interrupt the artery proximal, distal, and deep to the bleeding point. The arterial anatomy of the stomach and the proper ligation of a bleeding point in the gastroduodenal artery is illustrated in **Figs. 15–1, 15–2, and 15–3.**

Avoiding Postoperative Wound Infection

Patients who undergo resective procedures for ulcer in the presence of chronic obstruction or massive hemorrhage are more prone to develop postoperative wound infection than are patients who undergo elective surgery for duodenal ulcer. The former group should receive perioperative systemic antibiotics and antibiotic irrigation of the abdominal cavity and the wound at the conclusion of the anastomotic procedure. The skin of the abdominal wound in such cases should be managed as a contaminated incision (see Chap. 2).

Operative Techniques: Billroth I and II

Incision

The incision should be midline, from the xiphoid to a point 5 cm below the umbilicus. Use an Upper Hand or "chain" retractor to elevate the lower margin of the sternum and a Harrington to elevate the lower surface of the liver. Perform a vagotomy when indicated (see Chap. 10).

Evaluation of Duodenal Pathology; Control of Bleeding Ulcer

In many cases, characteristic findings from the patient's history and radiographic studies, as well as preoperative endoscopic visualization of the duodenum, make it unnecessary to open the duodenum to confirm the accuracy of the diagnosis of ulcer.

In the presence of active ulcer bleeding, a longitudinal incision across the pylorus and into the proximal 3 cm of the duodenum will generally provide good visualization of a posterior ulcer that is penetrating into the gastroduodenal artery. This artery should be transfixed with sutures of 2–0 cotton proximal and distal to the bleeding point. In addition, a suture should be placed deep to the bleeding point (**Fig. 15–3**) in order to occlude a hidden posterior branch of the gastroduodenal artery. This branch, generally the transverse pancreatic artery, may produce retrograde bleeding following an apparently successful proximal and distal ligation of the gastroduodenal artery. According to Berne and Rosoff, the failure to include all the branches in the operative ligatures will not become apparent unless the surgeon plucks the thrombus out of the lumen of the ulcerated artery to determine whether control of hemorrhage is complete.

It is not easy, when viewing the duodenum from its anterior aspect, to evaluate the potential difficulty of dissecting the posterior wall of the duodenum off the pancreas. Just how difficult the procedure may be will not be known until the posterior dissection is initiated. One should pay attention, however, to the quality and flexibility of the anterior wall of the duodenum. If the wall is soft and maneuverable, it will be useful should a Nissen-type stump closure become necessary. A markedly fibrotic, rigid, or edematous anterior wall indicates that closing the stump will be difficult. Marked edema or scarring in the region of the pylorus, pancreas, and hepatoduodenal ligaments is a relative contraindication to gastrectomy.

When the surgeon is uncertain of the nature of the pathology, a short incision may be made in the proximal duodenum in order to visualize the ulcer pathology. This will enable the surgeon to make a more accurate estimate of the technical expertise required to perform the resection. When in doubt, it is better to perform a vagotomy and a drainage procedure or proximal gastric vagotomy rather than a heroic duodenal dissection, for fatal duodenal leakage or acute pancreatitis may follow the dissection.

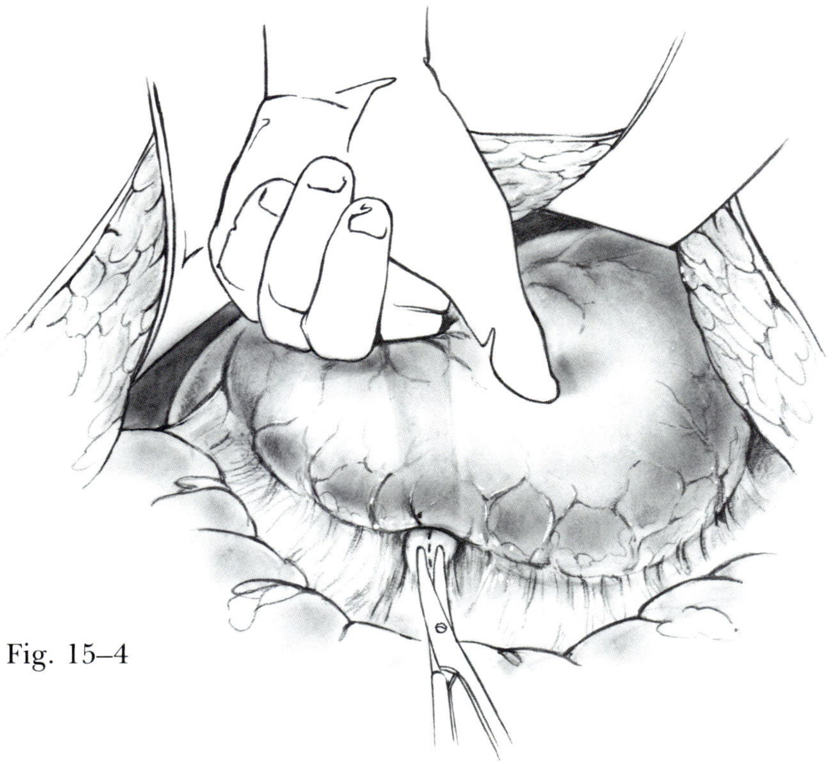

Fig. 15–4

Dissection of Greater Curvature

Incise the avascular portion of the gastrohepatic ligament to the right of the lesser curvature and pass the left hand behind the lesser curvature and antrum of the stomach, emerging deep to the gastroepiploic arcade along the greater curvature of the stomach (**Fig. 15–4**). This manuever serves to elevate the greater omentum from the underlying mesocolon, which contains the middle colic artery. Isolate the branches going from the gastroepiploic arcade to the greater curvature of the stomach, then doubly clamp and divide each. Continue this process up along the greater curve of the stomach until the halfway point between the pylorus and the diaphragm is reached (**Fig. 15–5**).

Next dissect the distal segment of the gastroepiploic arcade from the antrum. The distal 4 cm of this dissection should be done with care, as a number of fragile veins in the vicinity of the origin of the right gastroepiploic vessels may easily be torn. While the dissection of the greater curvature is under way, it is important simultaneously to divide the congenital avascular attachments between the back wall of the antrum and the pancreas. The completion of this dissection frees the entire distal half of the gastric greater curvature.

Division of Left Gastric Vessels

Select a point on the lesser curvature about halfway between the esophagogastric junction and the pylorus. This serves as a reasonably good approximation of the upper margin of the antral mucosa. Insert a large hemostat between the lesser curvature and the adjacent vascular bundle,

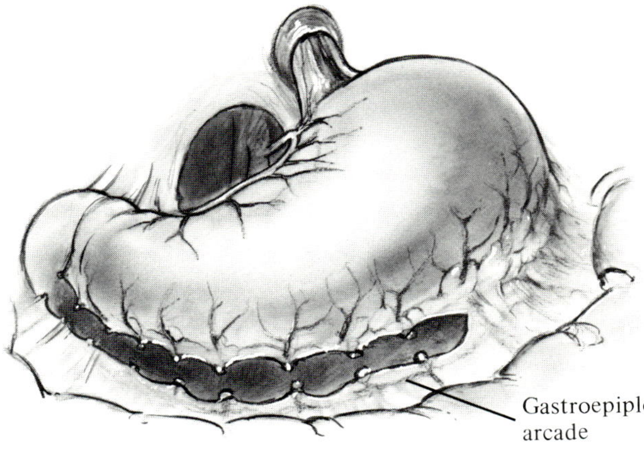

Fig. 15–5

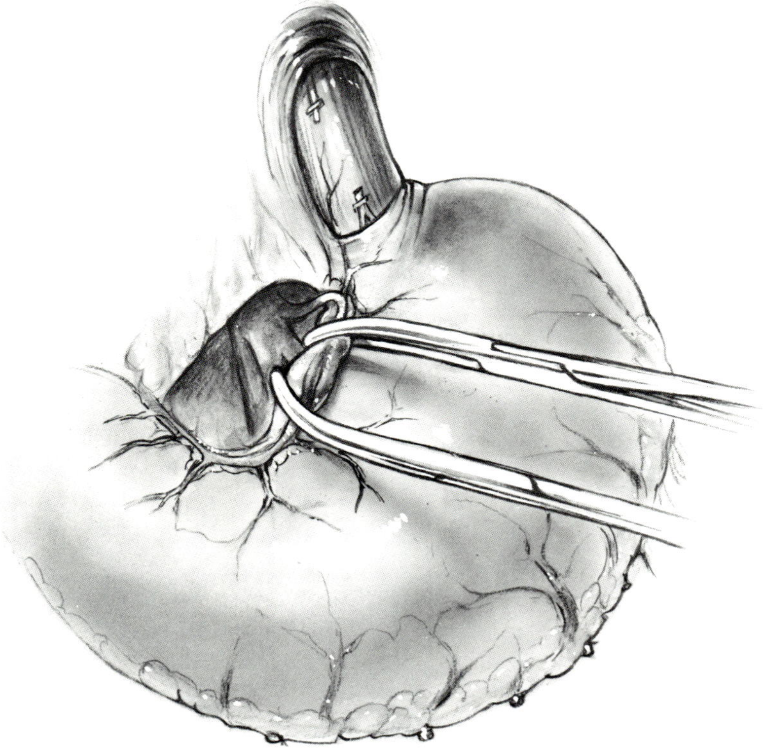

Fig. 15–6a

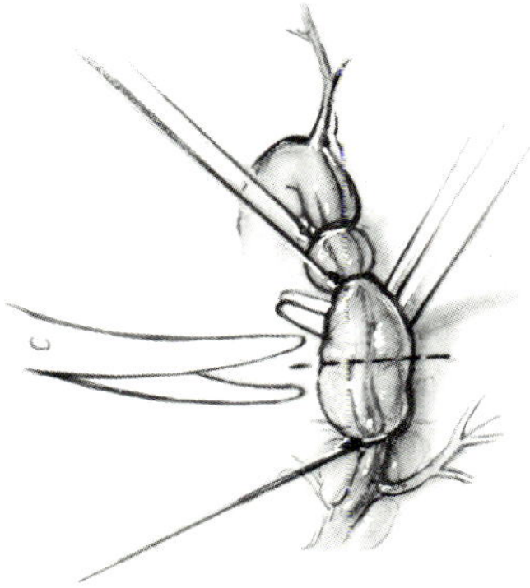

Fig. 15–6b

which should be divided between additional hemostats. Place two ligatures, consisting of either 0 cotton or a double strand of 2–0 cotton, on the proximal side and another one on the specimen side (**Figs. 15–6a and 15–6b**). Preferably there will be at least a 1 cm stump of left gastric artery beyond the cotton ties. This ligated pedicle should be carefully inspected for hemostasis, as occasionally the bulky nature of the ligature permits a trickle of blood to continue through the lumen of the artery. Several additional small venous branches to the lesser curvature may require individual ligatures, as they may get torn during the insertion of the mass ligatures.

Division of Stomach

If vagotomy is adequate, no more than 50% of the stomach need be removed (**Fig. 15–7**). This is accomplished by applying Allen clamps for a distance of 3 or 4 cm, at an angle 90° to the greater curvature of the stomach. The amount of stomach in the Allen clamp should equal the width of the gastrojejunal or gastroduodenal anastomosis that will be performed in a subsequent step.

After the gastric wall has been incised midway between these two clamps, apply a TA–90 Auto Suture stapler at a somewhat cephalad angle to close the lesser curvature portion of the residual gastric pouch (**Fig. 15–8**). Now fire the stapler.

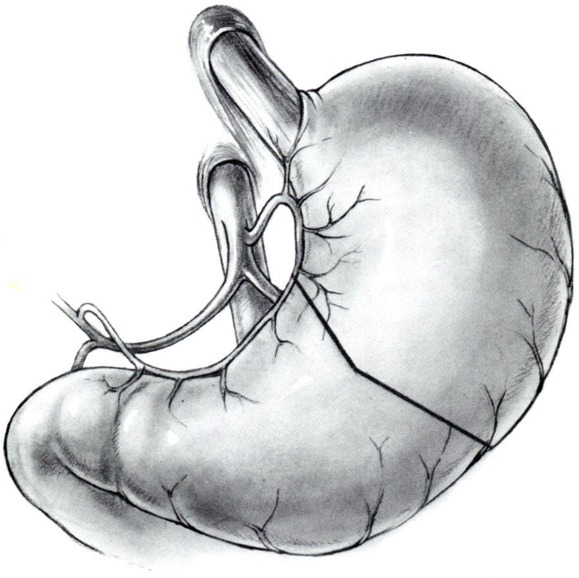

Fig. 15–7

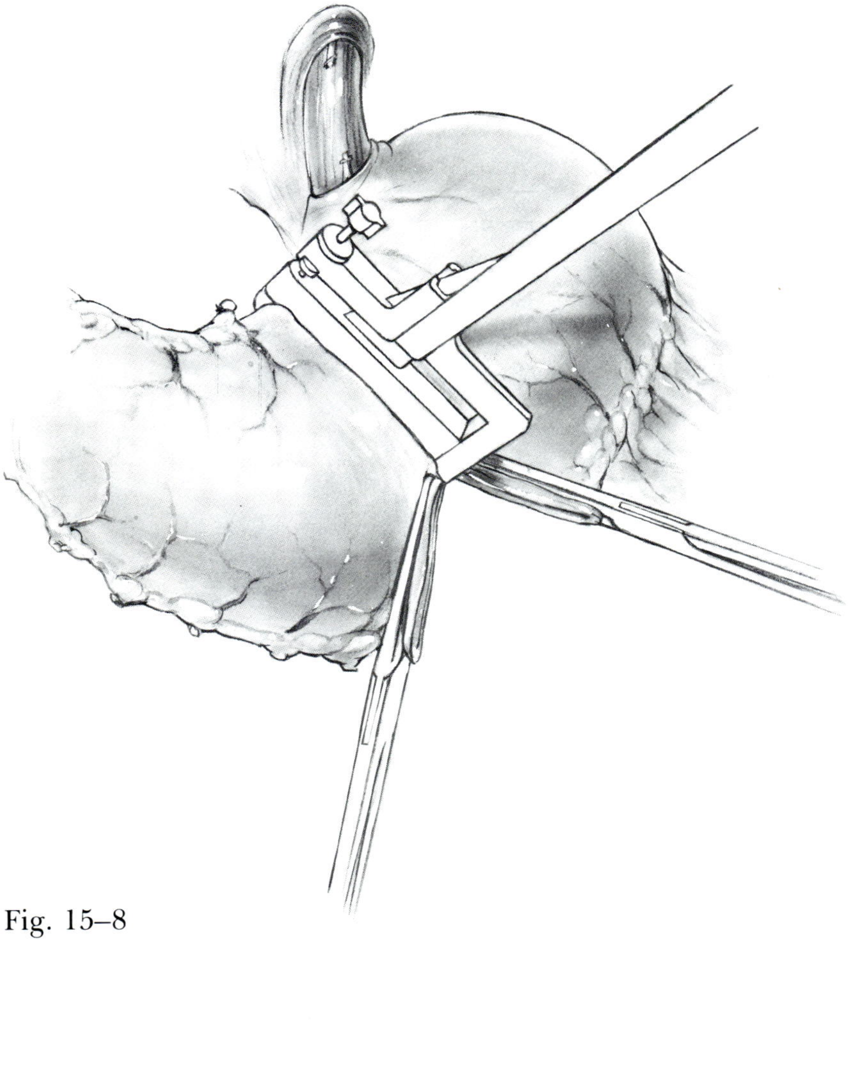

Fig. 15–8

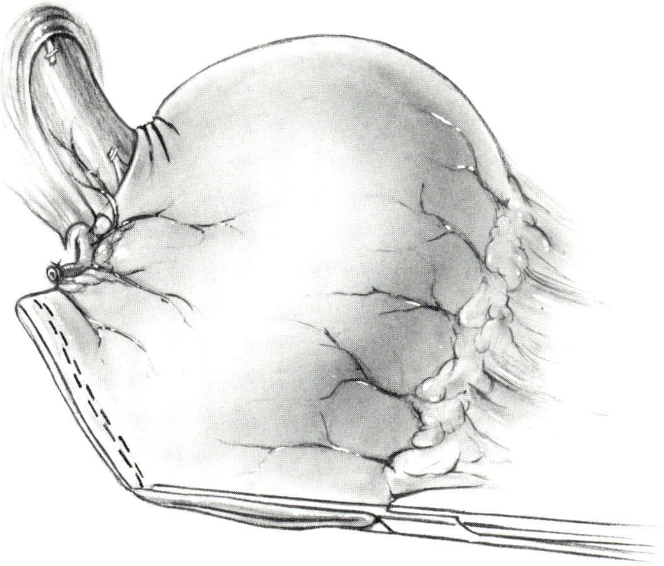

Fig. 15–9a

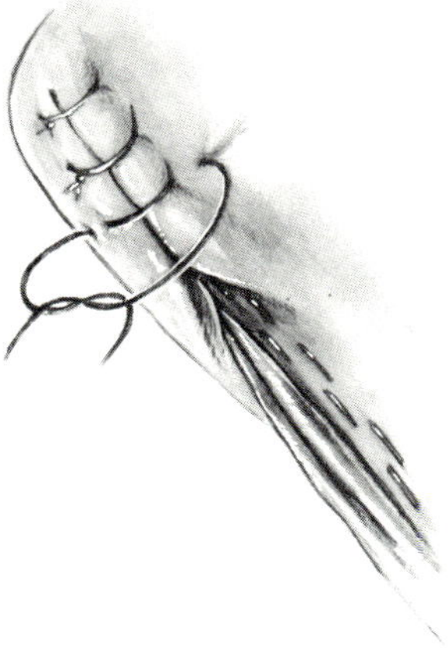

Fig. 15–9b

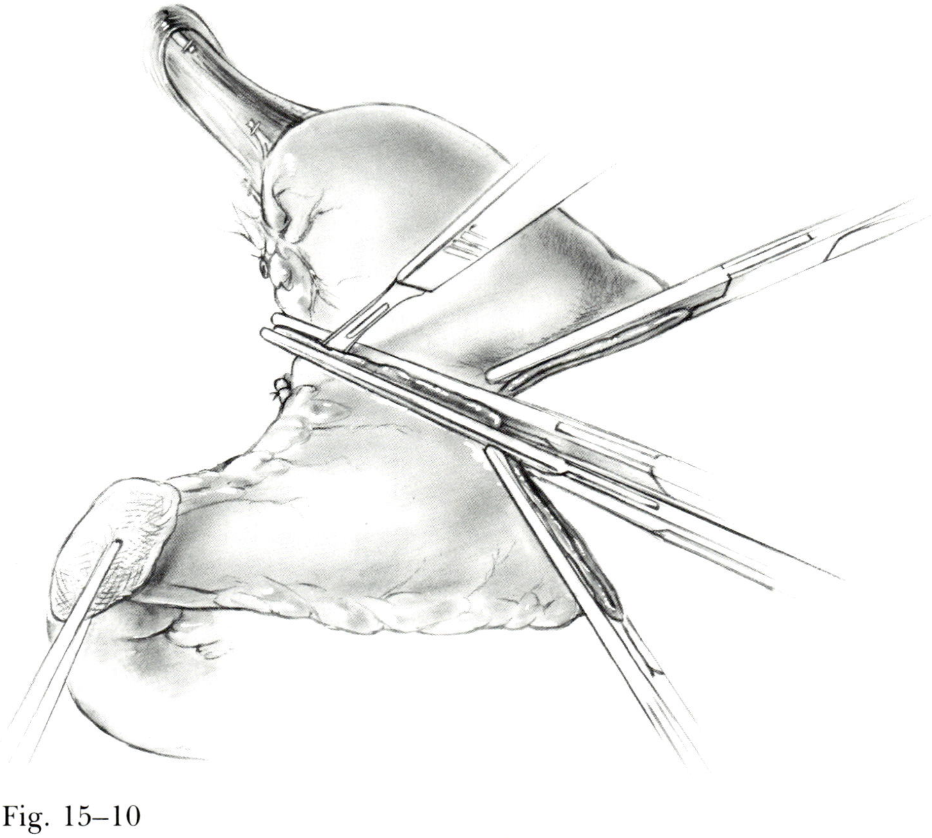

Fig. 15–10

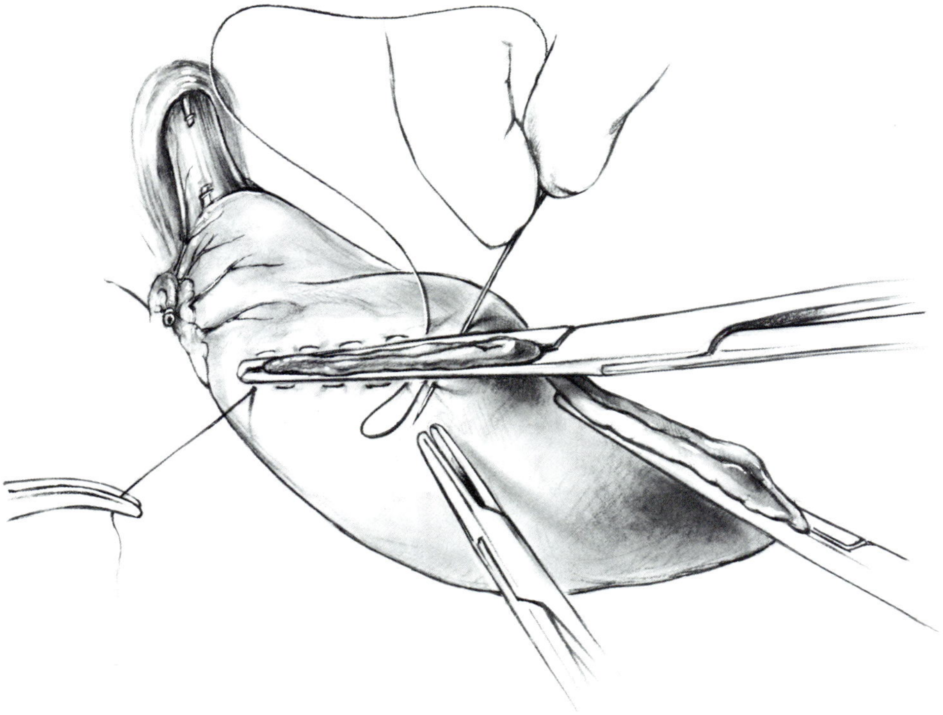

Fig. 15–11

Place another Allen clamp opposite the stapler and divide the gastric tissue flush with the stapler. Lightly electrocoagulate the gastric mucosa before removing the stapling device (**Fig. 15–9a**). Invert the stapled portion of gastric pouch, using a layer of interrupted 4–0 cotton Lembert sutures (**Fig. 15–9b**). Apply a gauze pad over the exposed mucosa on the specimen side and fix it in place with umbilical-tape ligatures, leaving the Allen clamps in position.

When a stapling device is not used, the lesser curvature should be divided between Allen clamps (**Fig. 15–10**) and then closed in several layers. For the first layer use 3–0 PG on a straight intestinal needle. Initiate this suture on the lesser curvature of the gastric pouch just beneath the Allen clamp. Then pass the straight needle back and forth beneath the Allen clamp to make a basting stitch, terminating it at the base of the Allen clamp (**Fig. 15–11**). After

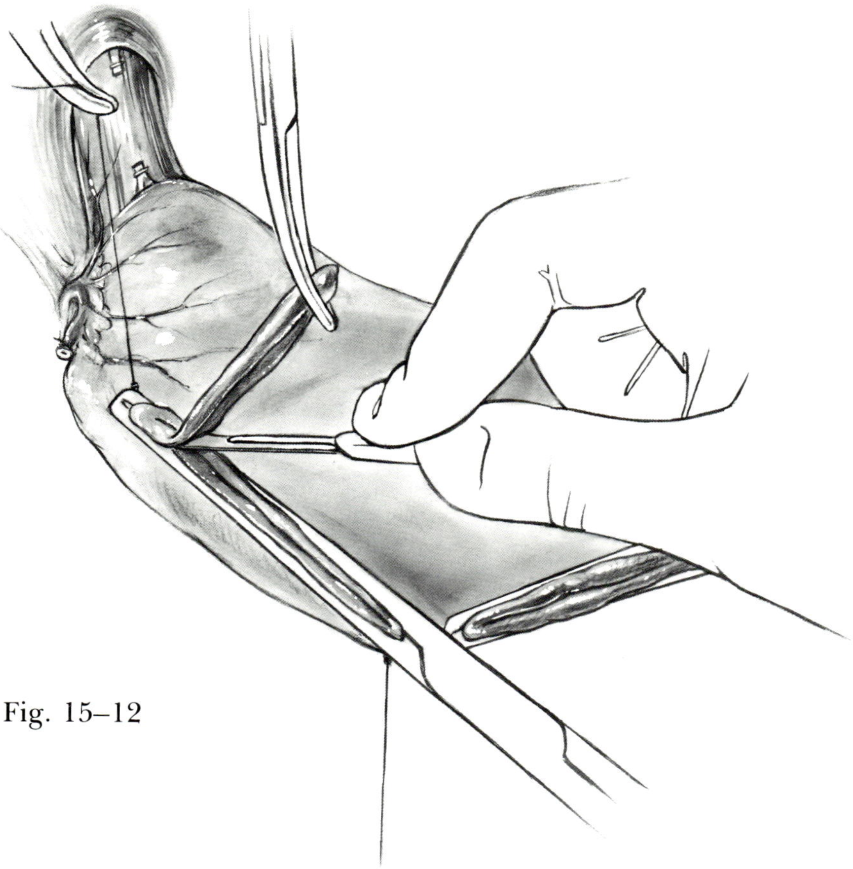

Fig. 15–12

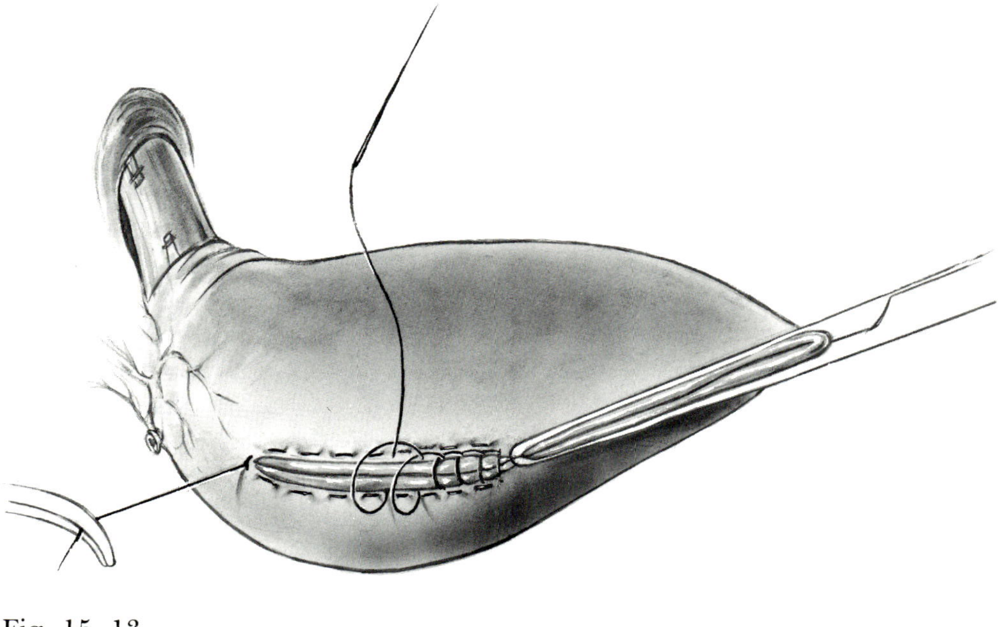

Fig. 15–13

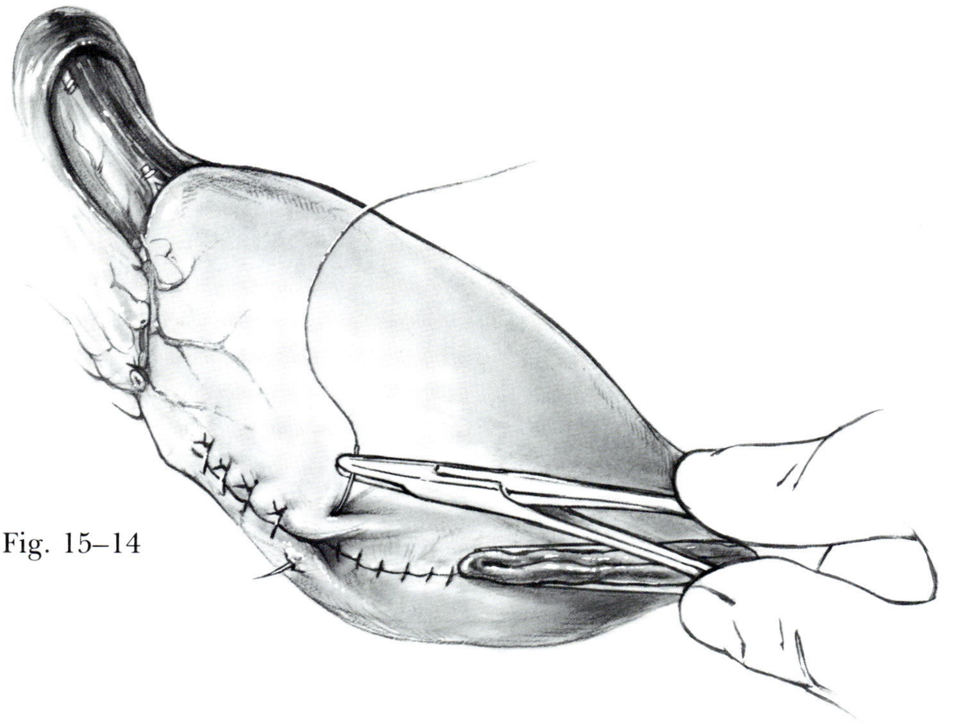

Fig. 15–14

trimming off excess gastric tissue (**Fig. 15–12**) remove the Allen clamp, return the same suture to its point of origin as a continuous locked suture (**Fig. 15–13**), and tie it to its point of origin. This will complete hemostasis of this suture line. Then invert the mucosa, using one layer of interrupted 4–0 cotton Lembert sutures (**Fig. 15–14**).

Duodenal Dissection in Absence of Advanced Pathology

Identify, ligate, and divide the right gastric artery (**Fig. 15–15**).

Apply traction to the specimen in an anterior direction to expose the posterior wall of the duodenum and the anterior surface of the pancreas. Five or six blood vessels of small size can usually be identified going from the pancreas to the back wall of the duodenum. Divide each between Crile hemostats and ligate each with 3–0 or 4–0 cotton. If there has been some scarring in this area, the stump of a small

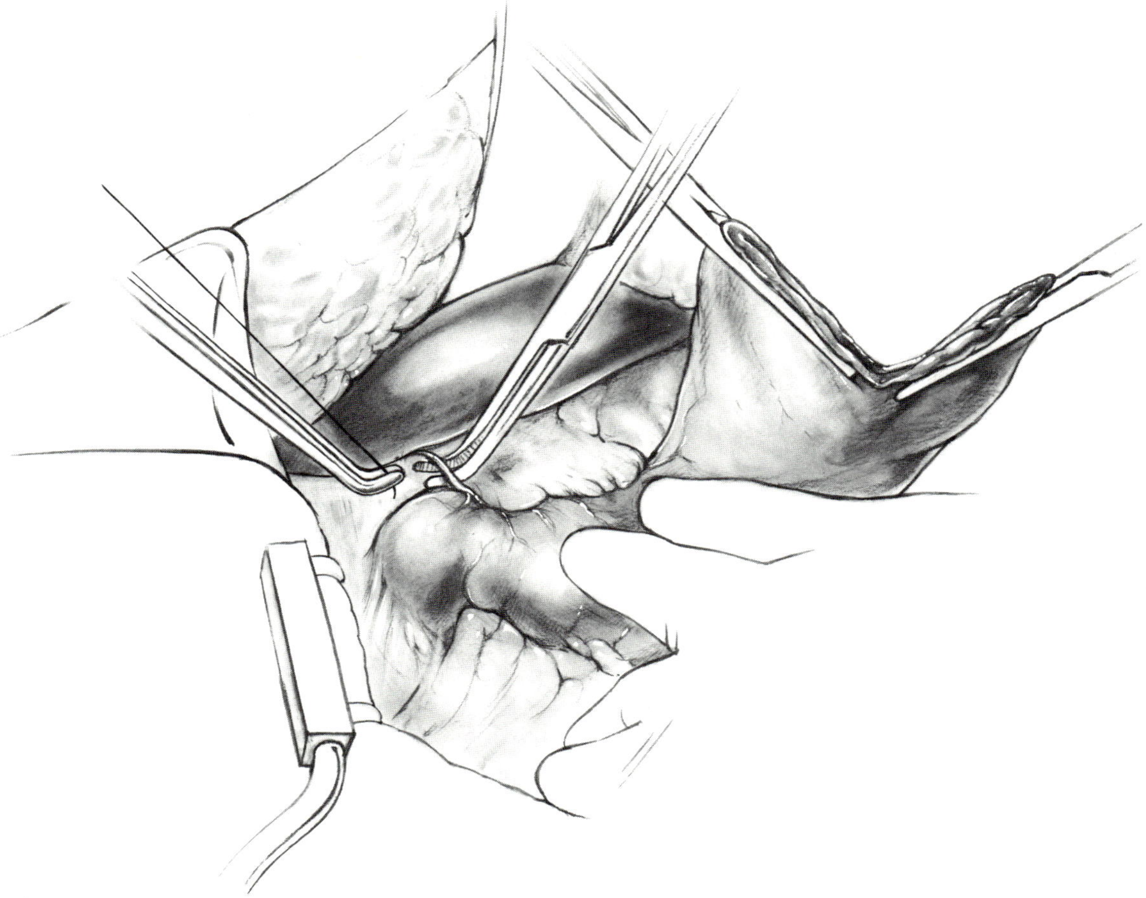

Fig. 15–15

artery may retract into the substance of the pancreas. In such a case it is prudent to control the bleeding with a mattress suture of 4–0 cotton. After 1.5 cm of the posterior duodenal wall has been freed from the underlying pancreas, dissection may be discontinued, as this is adequate either for turning in the duodenal stump or for gastroduodenal end-to-end anastomosis. In any case, the dissection should always be in a plane very close to the posterior wall of the duodenum.

Division of Duodenum

Apply an Allen clamp immediately distal to the pylorus and transect the duodenum flush with the clamp, which should be left on the specimen (**Fig. 15–16**). Before discarding the specimen, remove the clamp and inspect the distal end of the specimen to ascertain that a rim of duodenal mucosa has been removed. This will help assure that there is no remaining antral mucosa left behind in the duodenal stump. If there is still a question, the presence or absence of the antrum should be confirmed by frozen section examination of the distal end of the specimen.

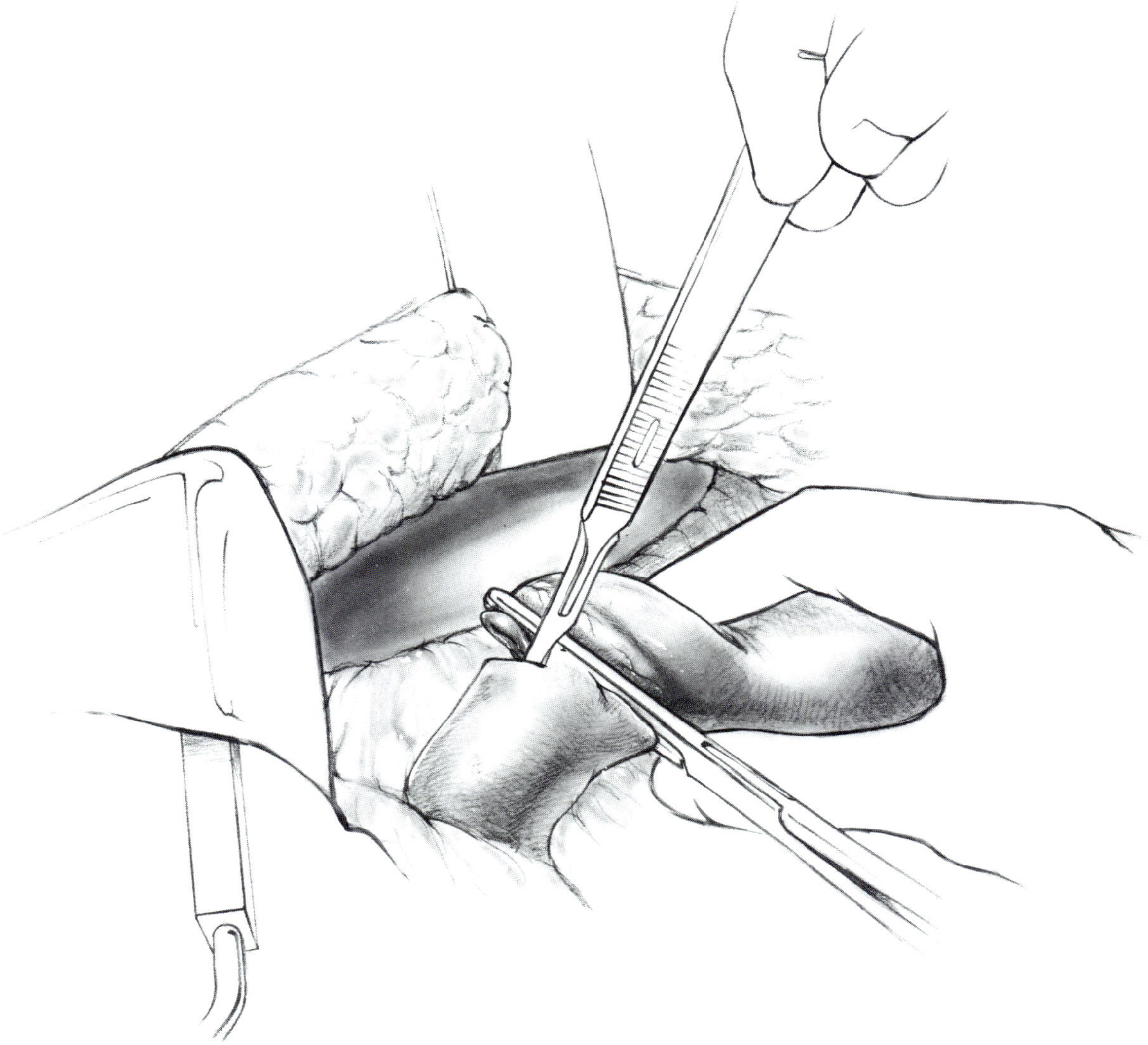

Fig. 15–16

Insert an index finger into the duodenal stump in order to check the location of the ampulla of Vater. The ampulla is situated on the posteromedial aspect of the descending duodenum at a point approximately 7 cm beyond the pylorus. Occasionally the orifice of the duct of Santorini can also be palpated along the back wall of the duodenum. If the duodenal dissection has not continued beyond the gastroduodenal artery, there need be no concern about damage to either the duct of Santorini or the main pancreatic duct. When the dissection continues beyond this point, special attention must be paid to these structures. When the duct of Santorini is divided, the open duct must be closed with a nonabsorbable suture-ligature. If the ampulla has been divided inadvertently and is separated from the duodenum, it should be reimplanted into the duodenal stump or into a Roux-Y segment of the jejunum.

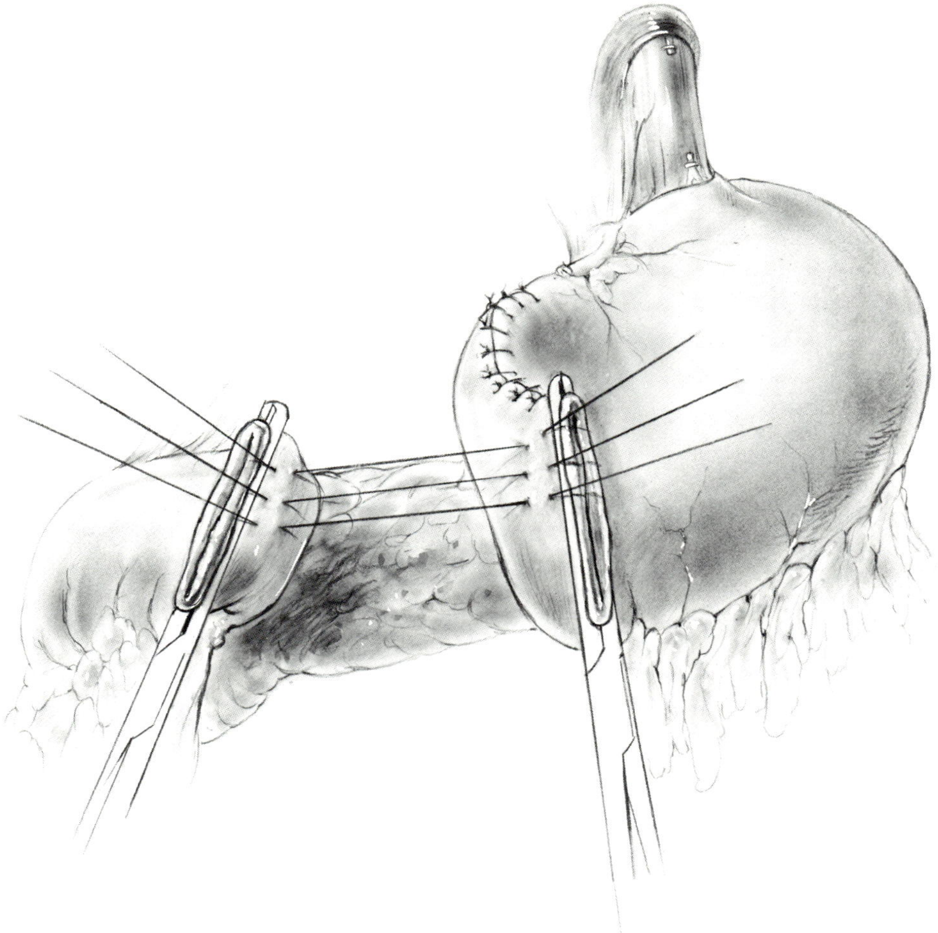

Fig. 15–17

Billroth I Gastroduodenal Anastomosis

When at least 1 cm of healthy posterior duodenal wall is available, a routine type of gastroduodenal anastomosis should be constructed. The Allen clamp previously applied to the unsutured portion of the gastric pouch should contain a length of stomach approximately equal to the diameter of the duodenal stump. Insert the corner sutures by the Cushing technique. Complete the remainder of the posterior layer with interrupted 4–0 cotton seromuscular Lembert sutures (**Fig. 15–17**). To prevent postoperative obstruction, care should be taken that an excessive amount of tissue is not inverted.

Remove the Allen clamp and approximate the mucosal layer by using a double-armed 4–0 PG suture, initiating it at the midpoint of the posterior layer where the knot is tied (**Fig. 15–18**). We prefer to use straight needles for this procedure. Take small bites, as a continuous locked suture is inserted (**Fig. 15–19**). Approximate the anterior mucosal layer with a continuous Connell or Cushing suture, which should be terminated at the middle point of the anterior layer (**Fig. 15–20**). This layer of sutures should be reinforced by a seromuscular layer of interrupted 4–0 cotton Lembert sutures (**Fig. 15–21**). At the "angle of sorrow," where the Hoffmeister shelf of the gastric pouch meets the duodenal suture line at its lateral margin, insert a crown stitch by taking seromuscular bites of the anterior wall of the gastric pouch, then of the posterior wall of the

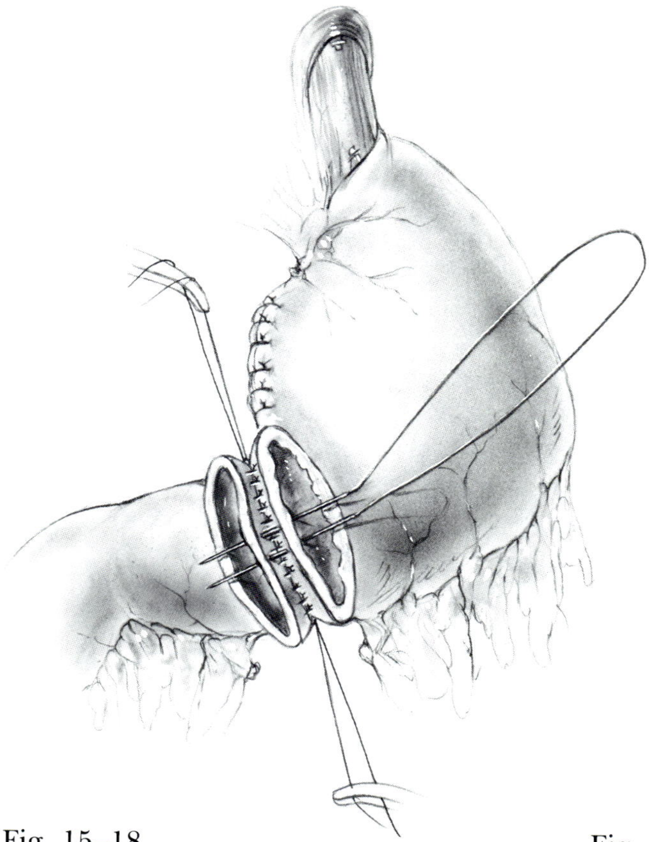

Fig. 15–18

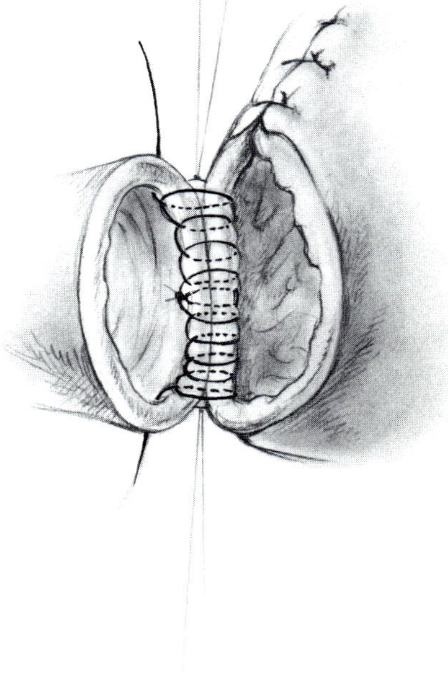

Fig. 15–19

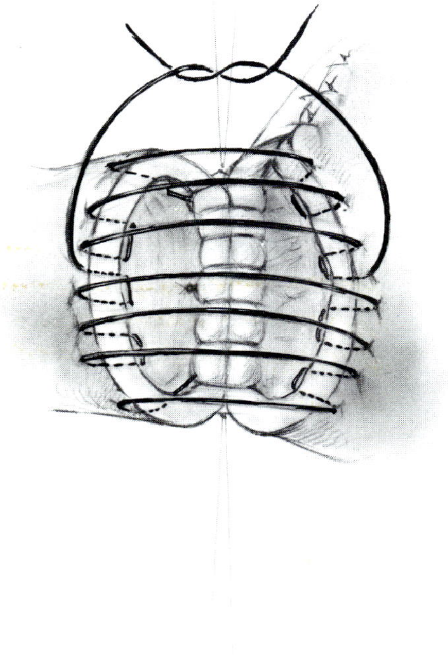

Fig. 15–20

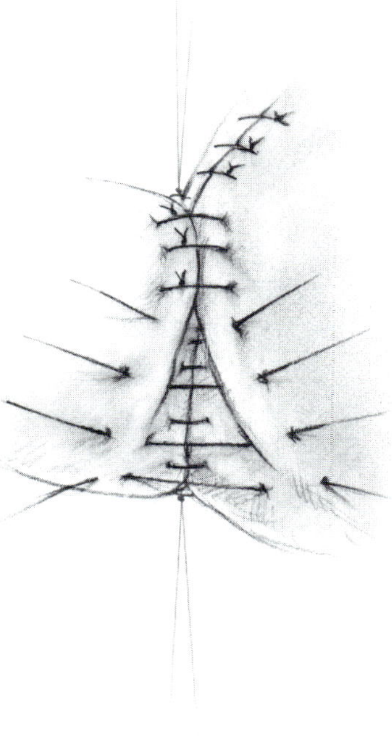

Fig. 15–21

Connell outside inside outside → outside inside outside

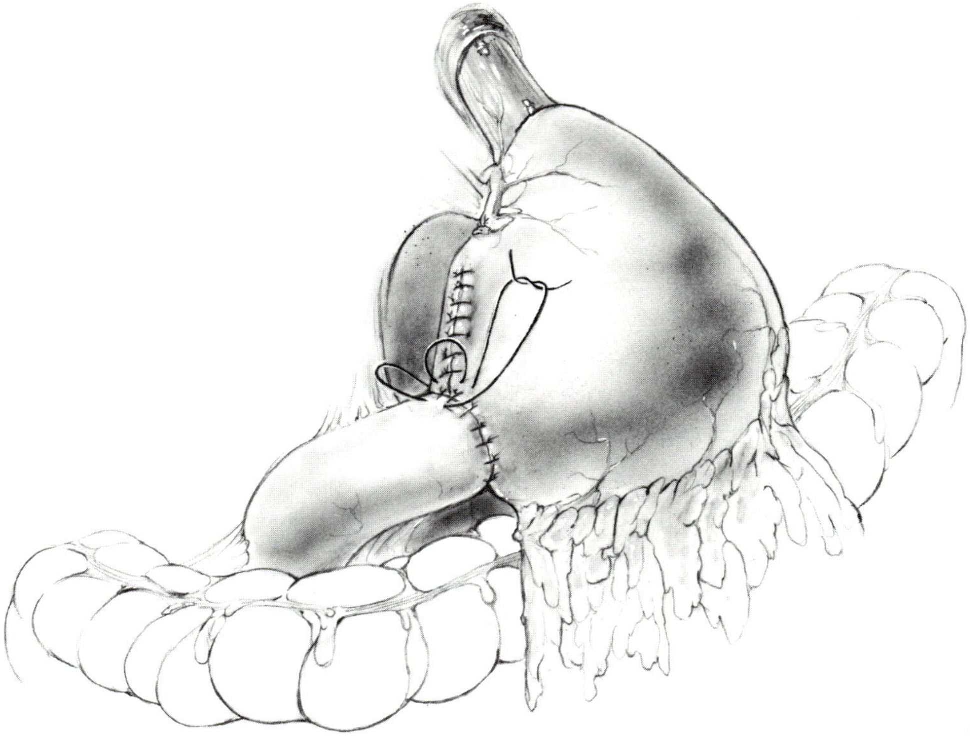

Fig. 15–22

gastric pouch, and then returning to catch the wall on the duodenal side (**Fig. 15–22**). If the sutures have been properly inserted, the lumen should admit the tip of the surgeon's thumb. Loosely suture omentum over the anastomosis.

Any bleeding points encountered in the cut edge of the stomach or duodenum during the above procedure should be occluded either by catgut suture-ligature or electrocoagulation.

Closure of Duodenal Stump

Closure of the healthy duodenal stump is generally accomplished by one layer of an inverting Connell suture of 4–0 PG supplemented by a layer of interrupted 4–0 cotton Lembert sutures. Initiate the Connell suture by placing a half purse-string stitch at the right lateral margin of the duodenum. Continue this strand to the middle of the duodenal stump, and initiate a second strand of 4–0 PG at the left margin of the duodenal stump. Continue this also to the middle of the stump, where it should be terminated by tying it to the first strand (**Fig. 15–23**).

Though it is simple to insert a layer of interrupted Lembert seromuscular sutures as a second layer when the tissues are not thickened (**Figs. 15–24 and 15–25**), suturing the fibrotic duodenum requires judgment and skill. If the stitch is placed deep, through the mucosa, and then tied with strangulating force, a fistula may result. Once a small leak occurs, the powerful duodenal digestive juices may erode the adjacent tissue—with disastrous results.

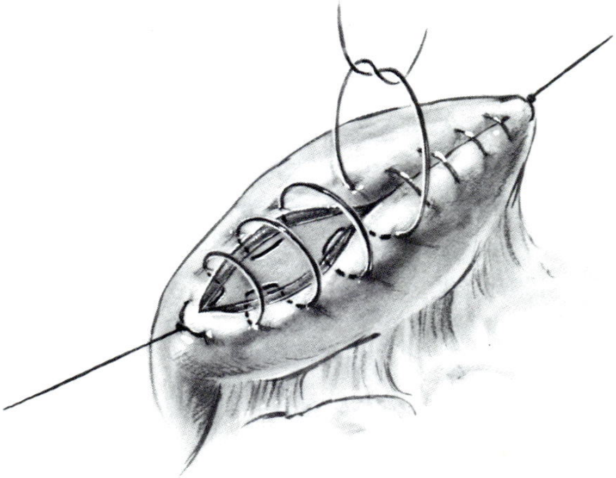

Fig. 15–23

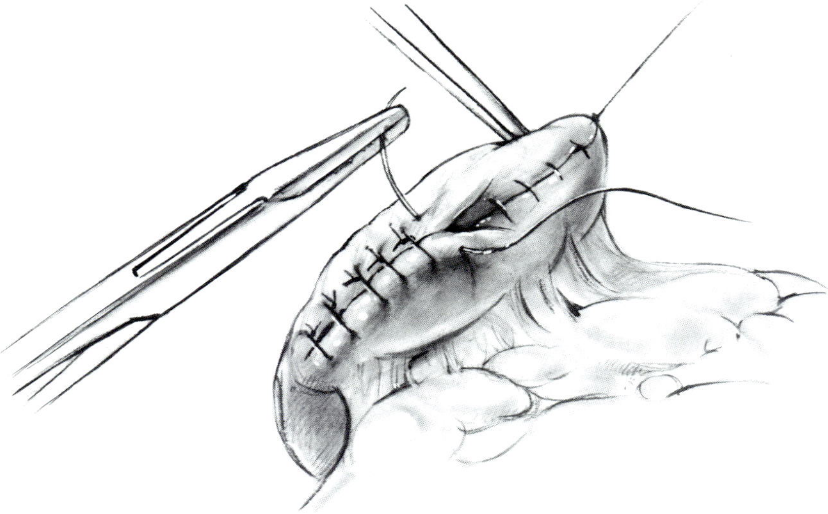

Fig. 15–24

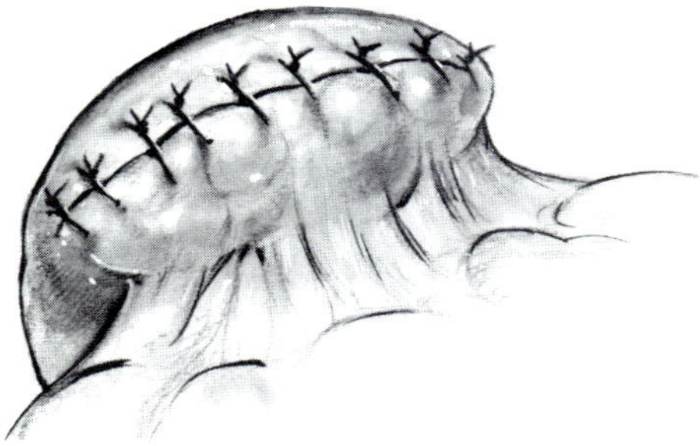

Fig. 15–25

After the Connell suture has been completed, take a forceps and test the flexibility of the tissue by pushing down tentatively on the suture line. Manipulating the tissue in this manner increases the accuracy of one's judgment about the best place for the Lembert sutures. A common error is to insert the seromuscular Lembert stitch too close to the Connell suture line. If this is done with a pliable duodenum of normal thickness, no harm will result. However, sewing thick, fibrotic tissue into apposition without first sufficiently inverting the Connell suture line creates a lateral shearing force that will

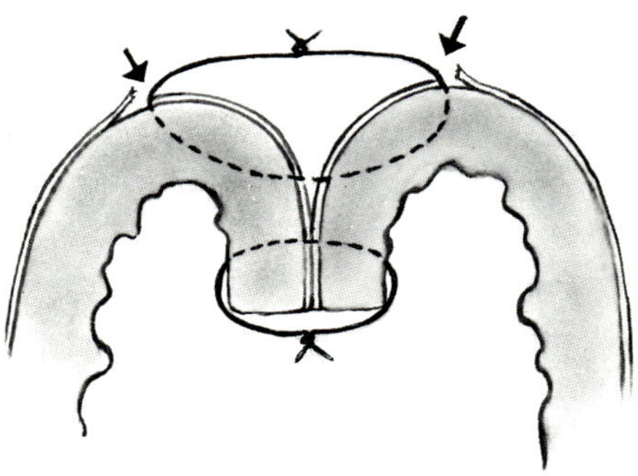

Fig. 15–26a

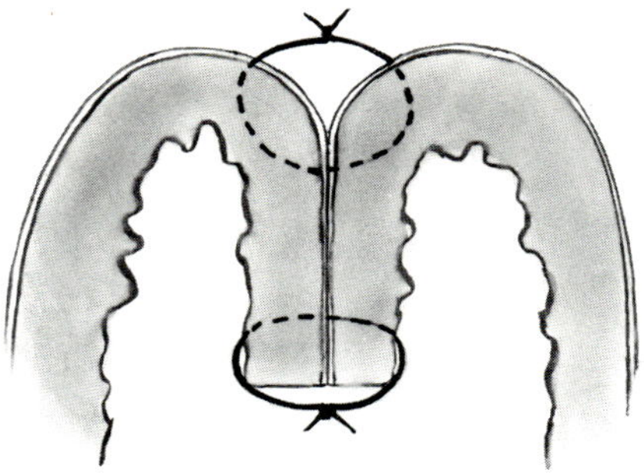

Fig. 15–26b

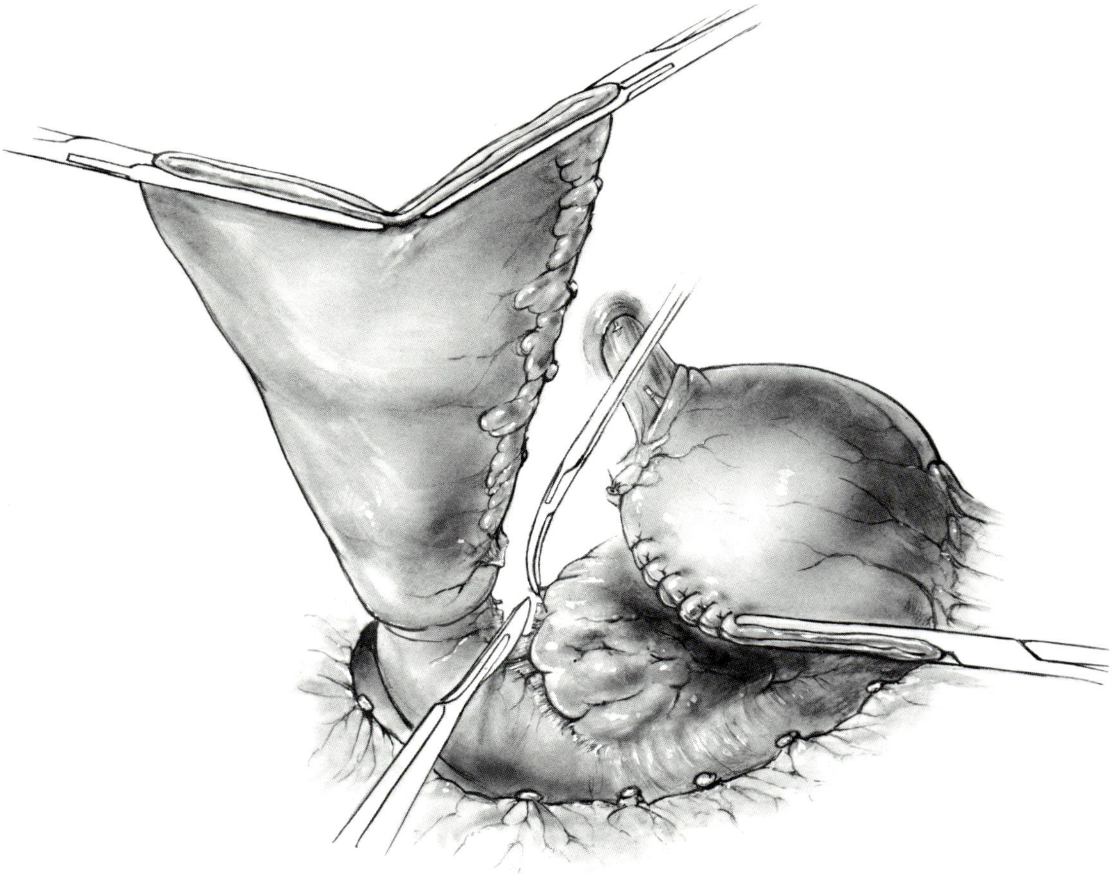

Fig. 15–27

cause a small tear when the suture is tied (**Fig. 15–26a**). If the suture also penetrates the mucosa of the duodenum, this mishap, combined with excessive shearing force, may produce a duodenal fistula. The fistula can be prevented if the surgeon inverts the Connell suture line for a distance of 2–3 mm before placing the Lembert suture (**Fig. 15–26b**). If the duodenal serosa has a small tear after the Lembert suture is tied, either the above error (Fig. 15–26a) was committed or the suture was tied too tightly.

Dissection of Difficult Duodenum

If the posterior duodenal wall and adjacent pancreas are replaced by fibrosis, scalpel, rather than scissors, dissection should be used (**Fig. 15–27**). It is not necessary to apply hemostats when incising dense scar tissue, but it is important to keep the plane of dissection close to the posterior wall of the duodenum, thus avoiding trauma to the pancreas. When the dissection enters the posterior duodenum at the site of the penetrating ulcer, this "window" in the duodenum should be enlarged by an incision extending proximally from the ulcer toward the pylorus. The incision permits the surgeon's index finger to be inserted into the duodenal lumen. With the finger as a guide, dissection around the borders of the ulcer may be resumed.

It is obviously not necessary to remove the *base* of the ulcer during this dissection. The base of the ulcer is really the anterior surface of the pancreas, which should not be disturbed. When the duodenum is dissected off the pancreas beyond the dense scar tissue, small hemostats may again be applied to the vessels on the pancreatic side. The vessels are then divided; any bleeding from the duodenum, which is generally minimal in the presence of fibrosis, can be ignored. If the dissection is successful, the caudal lip of the ulcer will be dissected away from the duodenum and, after a few more millimeters of dissection, the posterior duodenal wall may assume a fairly normal appearance. If at any point it appears that liberating the caudal lip of the ulcer is becoming dangerous, dissection should be discontinued and closure of the stump by the Nissen-Cooper technique (see below) carried out. Otherwise, 1.5 cm of posterior duodenal wall is liberated.

Another contraindication to further dissection of the caudal lip of the ulcer is contiguity of the ampulla of Vater. This should be checked by frequent palpation with the index finger in the duodenal lumen. After an adequate segment of posterior duodenum has been liberated, closure may be performed as described above (Figs. 15–23, 15–24, and 15–25).

When a posterior duodenal or pyloroduodenal penetrating ulcer involves the hepatoduodenal ligament, it may be necessary to identify the course of the common bile duct. Make an incision in the proximal common bile duct, for the insertion of a 16F catheter or a No. 4 Bakes dilator, either of which should be passed down to the ulcer. By noting the location of the guide, one can avoid damaging the duct.

Closure of Difficult Stump by Nissen-Cooper Technique

When it is deemed hazardous to free the posterior duodenum beyond a callous ulcer, closure can be accomplished by inserting interrupted 4–0 cotton Lembert sutures to attach the free anterior and anterolateral walls of the duodenum to the distal lip of the ulcer (**Fig. 15–28**). Use a

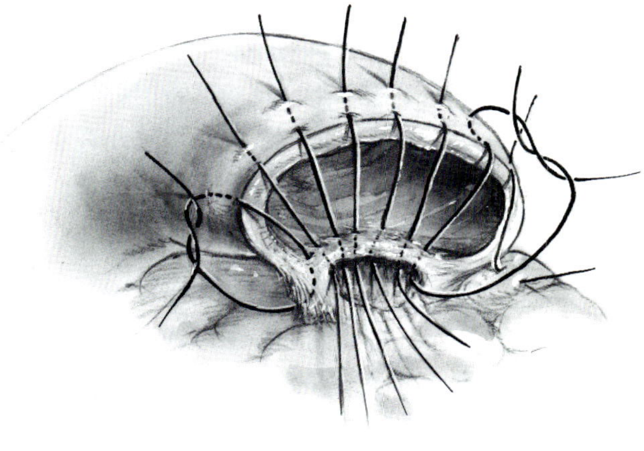

Fig. 15–28

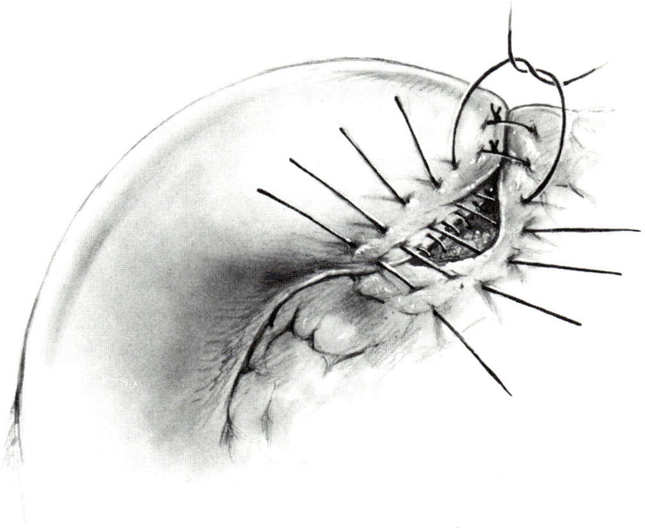

Fig. 15–29

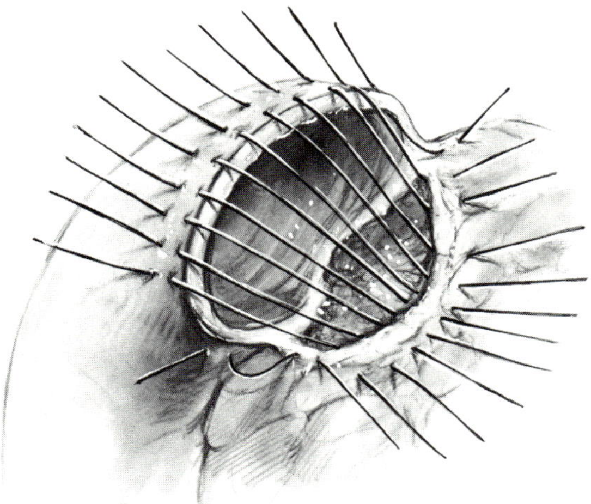

Fig. 15–30

second layer of Lembert sutures to invert the first suture line by suturing the pliable anterior wall to the proximal lip of the ulcer and to the adjacent pancreatic capsule (**Fig. 15–29**). Devised by Nissen and by Cooper, this technique was used extensively by Harrower. A variation of it (**Fig. 15–30**) involves inserting the first layer of sutures so as to attach the free anterior wall of the duodenum to the proximal lip of a large ulcer crater. This may be reinforced by a layer of Lembert sutures between the duodenum and adjacent pancreatic capsule. It is *essential* that the anterior wall of the duodenum be soft, pliable, and long enough for use in the Nissen-Cooper maneuver without causing tension on the suture line. A Kocher maneuver must be performed to liberate the duodenum for this type of closure.

Closure of Difficult Duodenal Stump—Duodenal Stenosis

Occasionally, chronic duodenal ulcer disease produces an annular stenosis at some point in the proximal 3–4 cm of the duodenum. If there is no active bleeding, it is safe to close a healthy duodenum proximal to an ulcer. On the other hand, it is unwise to attempt an inversion of the duodenal stump proximal to an area of marked stenosis. There simply is not enough room to invert the normal diameter of proximal duodenum into a stenotic segment. In such cases, the duodenum should be dissected down to the point of stenosis and perhaps 1 cm beyond (**Fig. 15–31**). It is then a simple matter to turn in the stenosed area. Usually only 3–4 interrupted Lembert sutures of 4–0 cotton are required for each of the two layers because of their narrow diameter (**Fig. 15–32**).

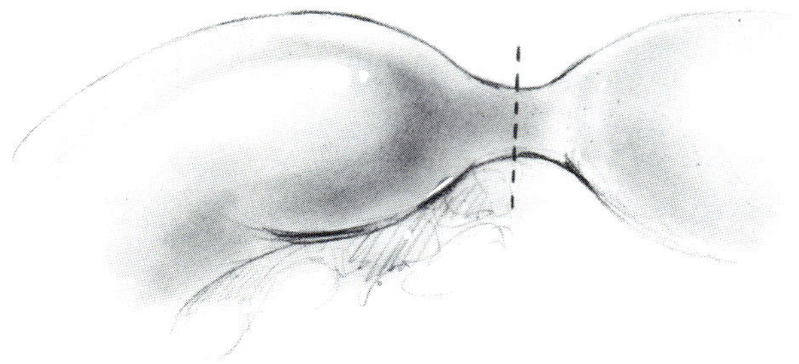

Fig. 15–31

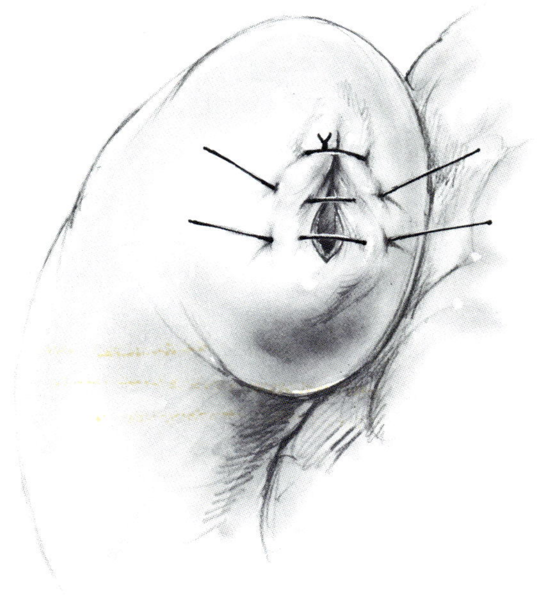

Fig. 15–32

Closure of Difficult Duodenal Stump—Catheter Duodenostomy

Surgeons at the Massachusetts General Hospital (as noted by Austen and Baue) and Parkland Hospital (as observed by Jones et al.) have reported their experience with catheter duodenostomy, which is designed to protect the integrity of a difficult duodenal stump closure. Properly performed, this technique, which prevents the buildup of intralumenal pressure against the newly sutured stump, has been surprisingly safe. If there is doubt about the integrity of the duodenal stump suture line, place a No. 14F whistle-tip or Foley catheter through a tiny incision in the lateral wall of the descending duodenum. This maneuver is easier to perform before the duodenal stump is closed. Pass a right-angled (Mixter) clamp into the open duodenum, press the tip of the clamp laterally against the duodenal wall, and make a 3 mm stab wound to allow the tip of the clamp to pass through the duodenal wall.

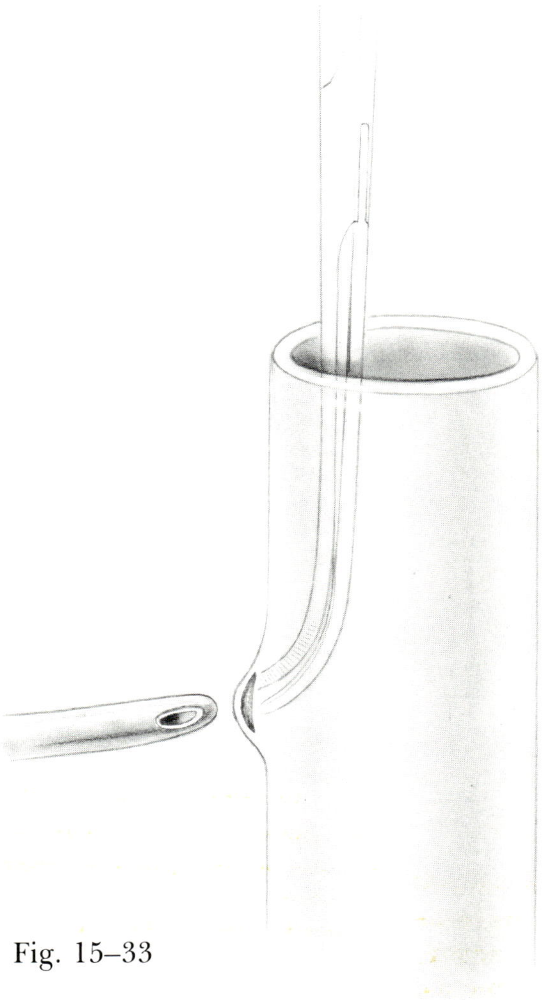

Fig. 15–33

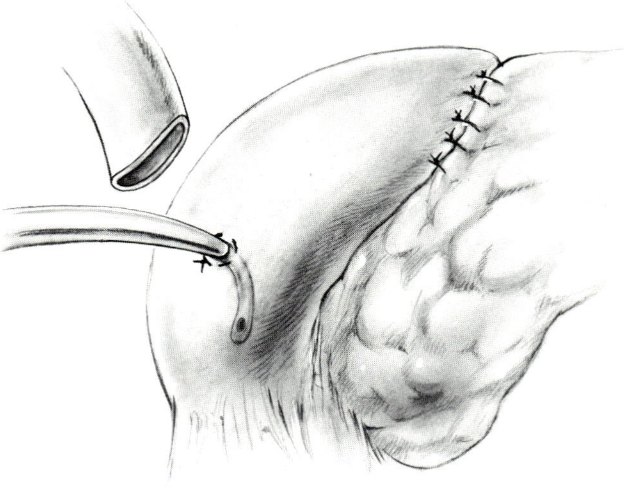

Fig. 15–34

Use the Mixter clamp to grasp the tip of the catheter and draw it into the duodenal lumen (**Fig. 15–33**). Close the incision around the catheter with a 4–0 cotton purse-string suture. Wrap the catheter with omentum and bring it out through a stab wound in the abdominal wall, *leaving some slack* to allow for postoperative abdominal distention. Suture the catheter to the skin with heavy silk. In addition, bring a latex Penrose drain from the area of the duodenotomy out through a separate stab wound in the lateral abdominal wall (**Fig. 15–34**).

There may be some occasions when the surgeon may find it impossible to invert the duodenal stump, even with the techniques described earlier. This should happen rarely, but if it does occur, the catheter may be placed directly in the stump of duodenum, which should be closed as well as possible around the catheter. The lateral duodenostomy is much to be preferred, however.

Following the operation, place the catheter on low suction until the patient passes flatus, after which it is attached to a tube leading to a plastic bag for gravity drainage. The catheter should be irrigated twice each day with 5 ml of sterile saline. If the patient does well, the Penrose drain can be removed by the eighth postoperative day. Three days later partly withdraw the catheter so its tip lies just outside the duodenum. Low suction should be applied. If the volume of suction drainage does not exceed 100 ml per day, the catheter can be gradually withdrawn over the next day or two.

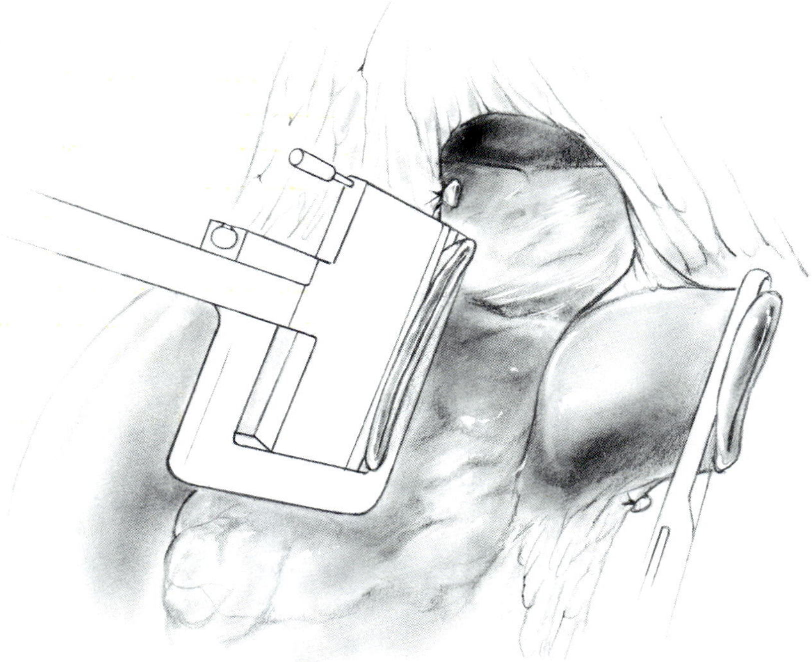

Fig. 15–35

Duodenal Closure with Surgical Staples

If the duodenal wall is not thickened markedly with fibrosis or edema, and if an 8–10 mm width of duodenum is available, the stump may safely be closed by the use of the Auto Suture TA–55 stapling device. Apply the stapler to the duodenal stump before dividing the specimen. After the stapler has been fired, apply an Allen clamp on the specimen side and with a scalpel transect the stump flush with the stapling device (**Fig. 15–35**). Lightly electrocoagulate the everted mucosa of the duodenal stump before removing the stapling device. Ravitch et al. (see Chap. 4) see no need to invert this closure with a layer of sutures. Their experimental and clinical evidence shows that despite the eversion of duodenal mucosa in this type of closure, healing is essentially equal to that of the sutured duodenal stump. Generally, we cover the stapled stump with omentum or the pancreatic capsule with a few sutures, but do not invert the mucosa.

When the duodenal wall is at all thickened, the larger size (4.8 mm) staples should be used, as this reduces somewhat the degree of compression applied to the tissues by the stapling device. There should be blood circulation to the narrow rim of tissue that lies distal to the staple line. This is generally manifested by a slight oozing from the tissues despite the staples. It must be emphasized again: If the duodenal wall is so diseased that it probably would not heal if closed by sutures, stapling it will fail too.

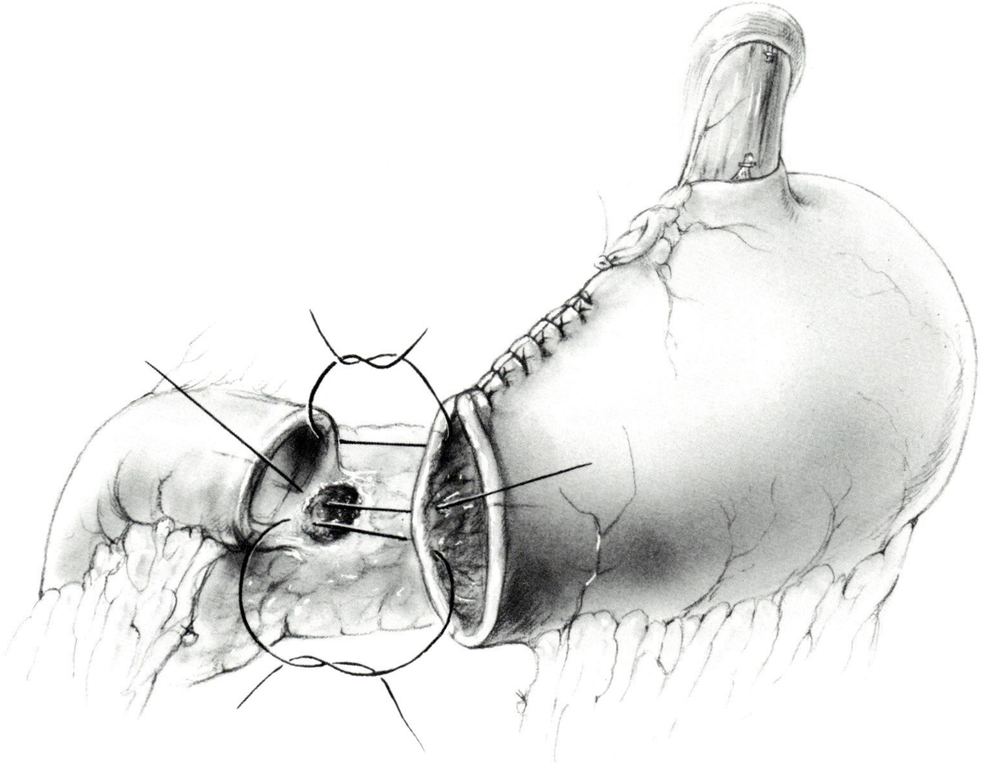

Fig. 15–36

Closure of Difficult Duodenal Stump by Billroth I Gastroduodenostomy

In the hands of an expert such as Nyhus, "If one can close the duodenum, one can anastomose to it." While it is not always necessary to liberate the *distal* lip of the ulcer crater, the duodenum should be dissected away from the pancreas at least to this point. The usual technique of gastroduodenal anastomosis, as described in Figs. 15–17 though 15–22, must be modified. In the region of the ulcer crater only one posterior layer of interrupted 4–0 cotton sutures should be inserted, taking a bite of stomach, of underlying fibrosed pancreas, and of the distal lip of the ulcer crater and duodenum, with the knot tied inside the lumen (**Fig. 15–36**). If the ulcer crater is so deep that the posterior anastomotic suture line will not be buttressed by the underlying pancreatic bed of the ulcer, the use of this technique may be hazardous. Because surgery for duodenal ulcer has declined in the past decade, fewer surgeons have had the opportunity to develop experience and judgment in managing the difficult duodenum. It is not wise for the inexperienced surgeon to perform a Billroth I anastomosis unless the above precautions are followed.

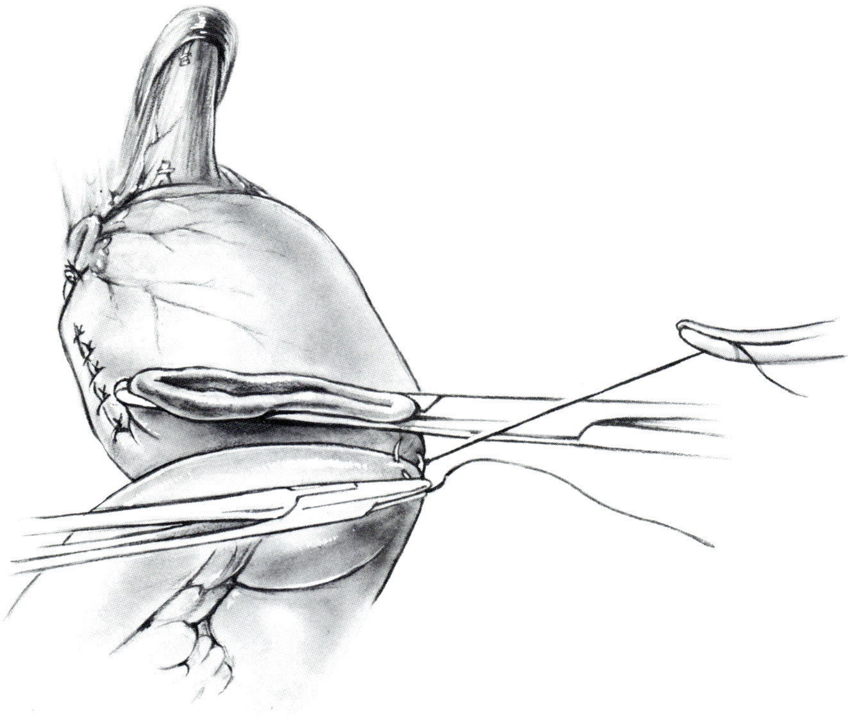

Fig. 15–37

Billroth II Gastrojejunal Anastomosis

Although there are many variations in the technique of constructing Billroth II anastomoses, we have preferred a short loop antecolonic anastomosis of the Schoemaker-Hoffmeister type. It does not seem to matter whether the afferent segment of the jejunum is attached to the greater curvature of the gastric pouch or to the lesser curvature. In most cases a shorter loop can be used when the afferent loop goes to the greater curvature of the pouch. The distance from the ligament of Treitz to the gastric pouch should be no greater than 12–15 cm. The major portions of the transverse colon and omentum should be brought to the patient's right for the antecolonic anastomosis.

The antimesenteric aspect of the jejunum should be scored by making a scratch line with a scalpel blade. Place the first posterior suture line posterior to but parallel with the scratch line. This assures that the stoma is accurately placed and may help prevent postoperative obstruction of the gastric outlet. Attach the jejunum to the gastric pouch with interrupted 4–0 cotton seromuscular Lembert sutures placed about 5 mm apart (**Fig. 15–37**). Attach hemostats to the first and last stitches which should be left long while all the remaining cotton tails are cut.

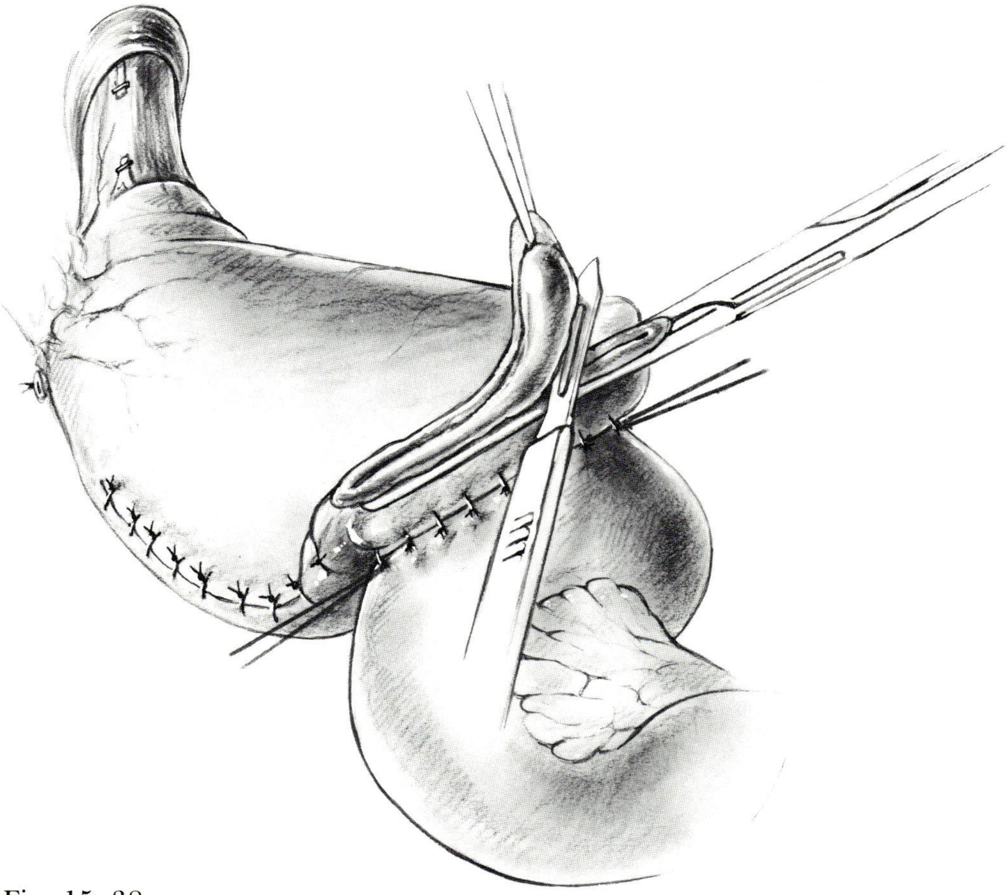

Fig. 15–38

If any gastric wall protrudes from the Allen clamp, remove the excess with a scalpel incision flush with the clamp (**Fig. 15–38**). Then make an incision along the antimesenteric scratch line in the jejunum. Open the mucosa of the jejunum (**Fig. 15–39**). Bleeding points may be controlled by electrocoagulation. The incision in the jejunum should be a few millimeters shorter than the diameter of the opening in the gastric pouch.

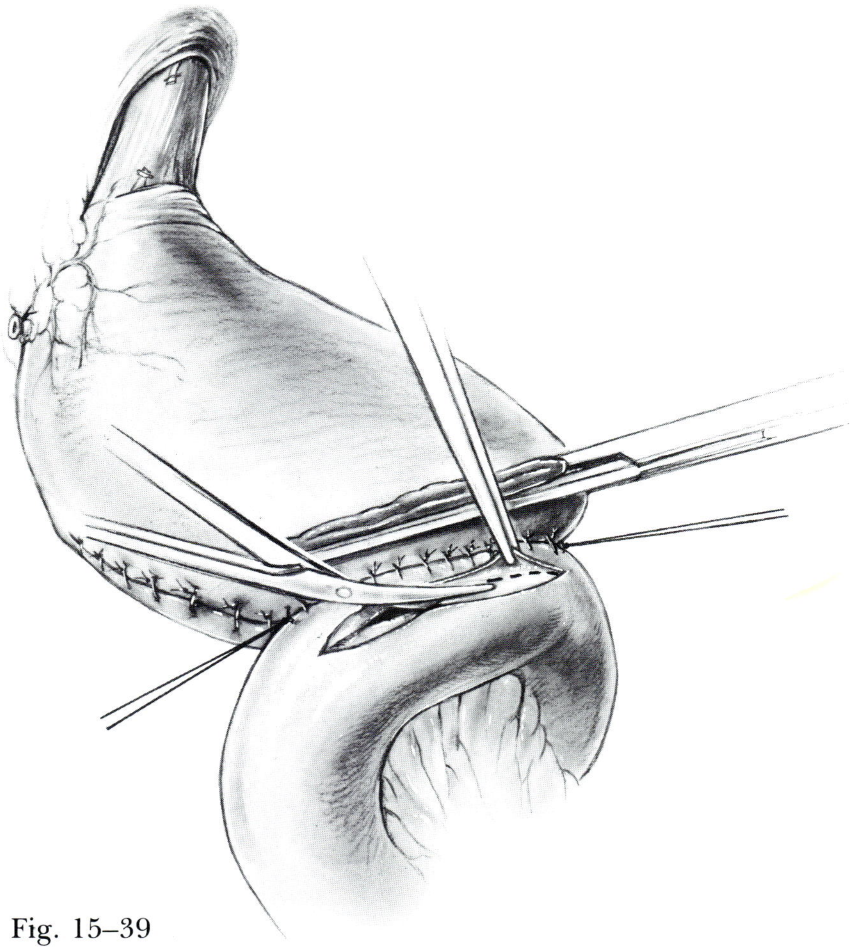

Fig. 15–39

The Allen clamp then should be removed and the gastric pouch opened. Bleeding points on the anterior aspect of the gastric pouch must be carefully controlled by means of 4–0 chromic suture-ligatures. The posterior wall will be controlled by the mucosal locked suture. Initiate this suture at the middle point of the posterior layer with a double-armed 3–0 chromic catgut or PG suture, which should be inserted through the full thickness of the gastric and jejunal walls and tied (**Figs. 15–40a, 15–40b, and 15–40c**). Straight intestinal needles are preferred for this procedure. Start a continuous locked suture

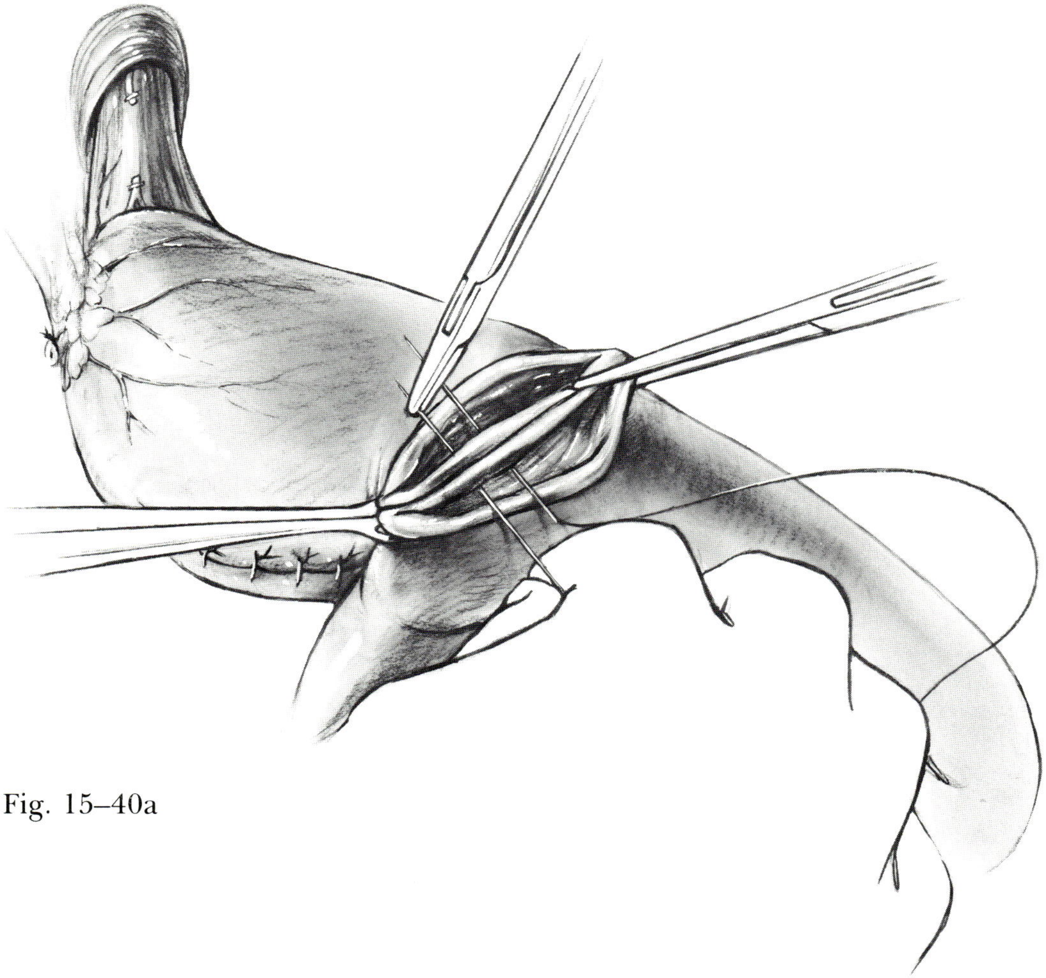

Fig. 15–40a

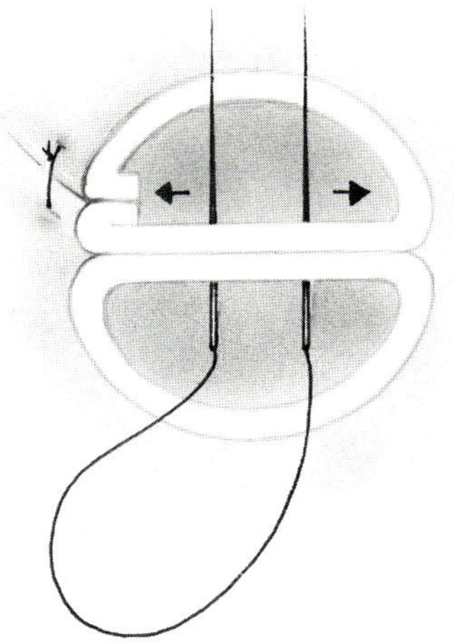

Fig. 15–40b

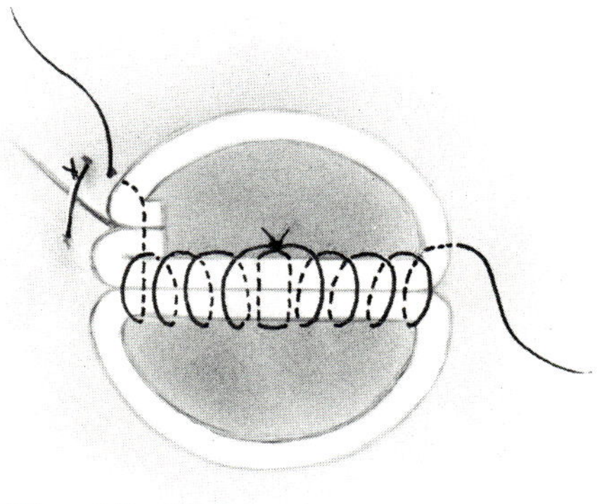

Fig. 15–40c

from the middle point and go first to the right and then to the left. Suturing is expedited if the first assistant grasps the straight needle with a straight hemostat, pulls it through the tissue and then hands it back to the surgeon. Accomplish the anterior mucosal layer with the same straight

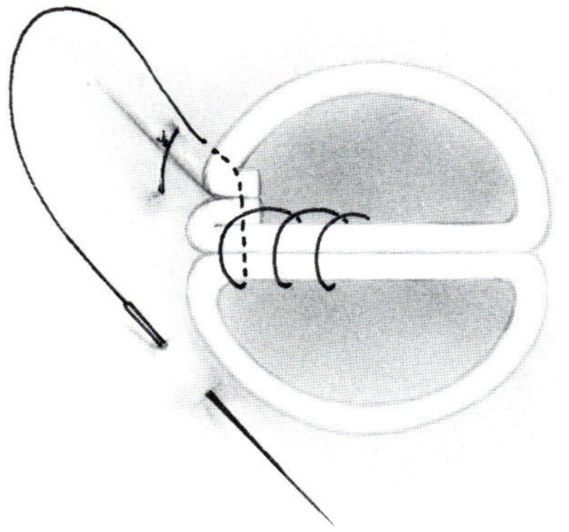

Fig. 15–41a

needle by means of a continuous Connell or continuous Cushing suture. Initiate the suture line first at the right-hand margin of the anastomosis (**Fig. 15–41a**) and then on the left (**Fig. 15–41b**), working both needles towards the middle point, where the two strands should be tied to each other (**Fig. 15–41c**). Complete the anterior layer with a row of interrupted 4–0 cotton seromuscular Lembert sutures (**Figs. 15–41d and 15–42**) on curved needles. At

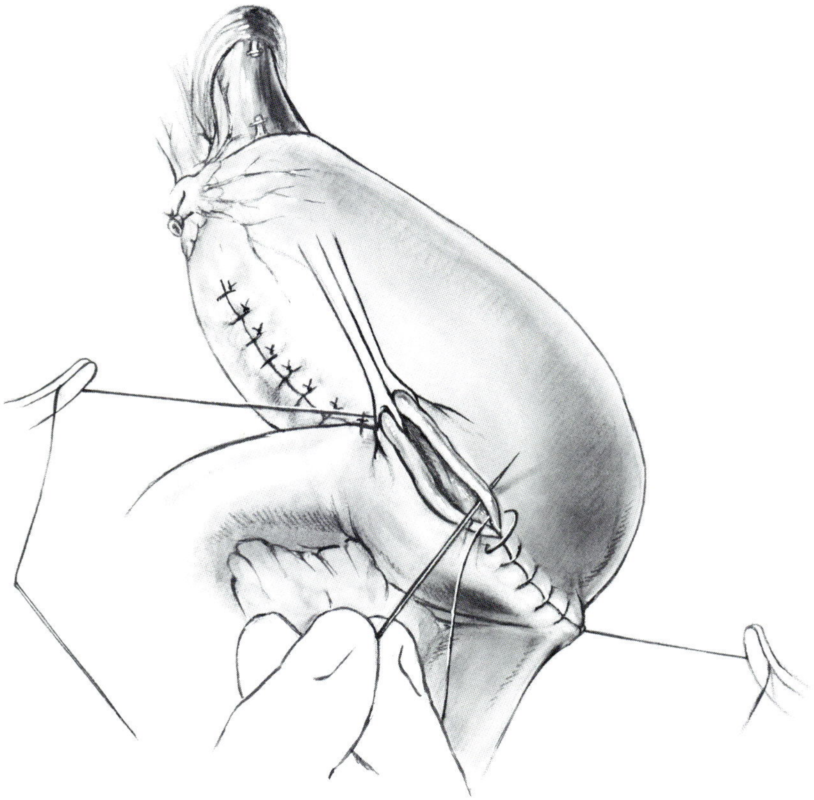

Fig. 15–41b

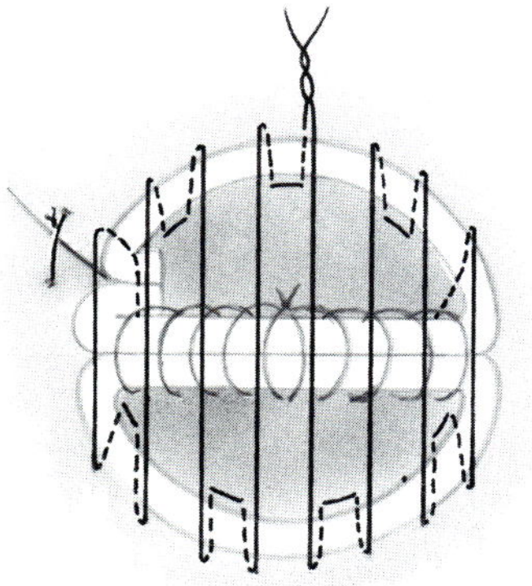

Fig. 15–41c

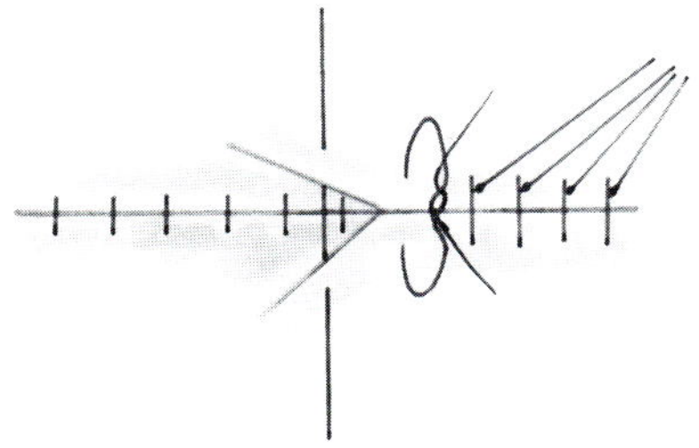

Fig. 15–41d

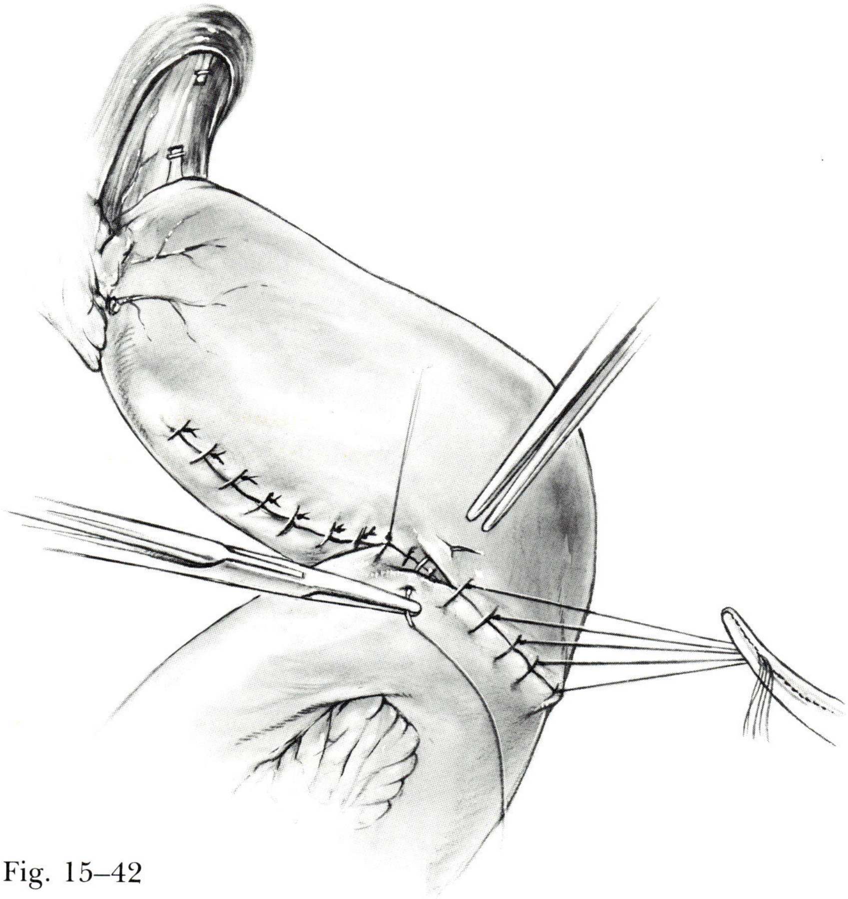

Fig. 15–42

the medial margin of the anastomosis, the "angle of sorrow," insert a crown stitch. (**Fig. 15–43**). Occasionally, two crown sutures are inserted for added security.

In the poor-risk patient, to minimize anesthesia time the seromuscular suture layer should be inserted in over-and-over continuous Lembert fashion using 3–0 PG instead of interrupted cotton or silk. The mucosal layer may be closed by the same technique as described above. When this anastomosis is performed with care, there seems to be no disadvantage to the use of a continuous PG seromuscular suture.

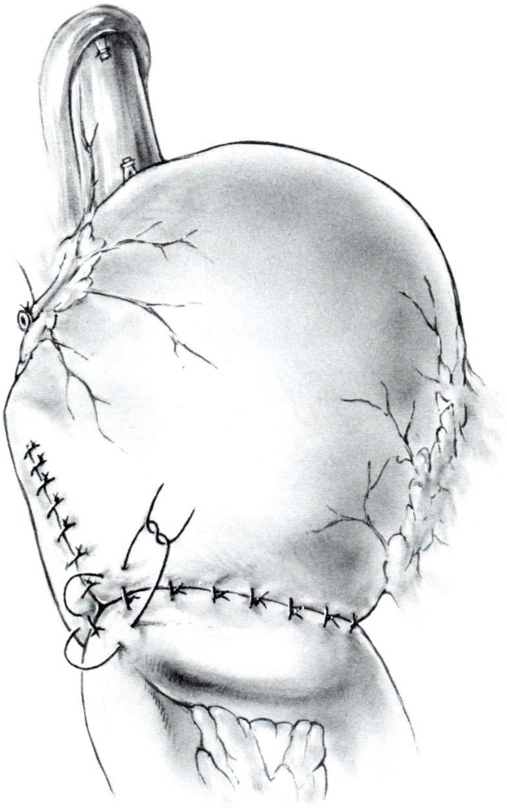

Fig. 15–43

Billroth II Gastrojejunal Anastomosis by Stapling Technique

Isolate the vasa breviae along the greater curvature individually by passing a Kelly hemostat behind the vessels. Then use the LDS instrument to divide the vessels and to apply stainless steel clips to both cut ends simultaneously (**Fig. 15–44**). When stapling is used, it is not necessary to close the lesser curvature as a separate step. Instead, apply a TA–90 stapler across the entire stomach, tighten it and fire. (**Fig. 15–45**). Generally, the 4.8 mm staples are used for this purpose. A large Payr clamp should be applied to the specimen side of the stomach, and the stomach divided flush with the TA–90 by a scalpel. Lightly electrocoagulate the everted mucosa and remove the TA–90 device. Close the duodenal stump by stapling with the TA–55 device, and remove the specimen. (**Fig. 15–46**).

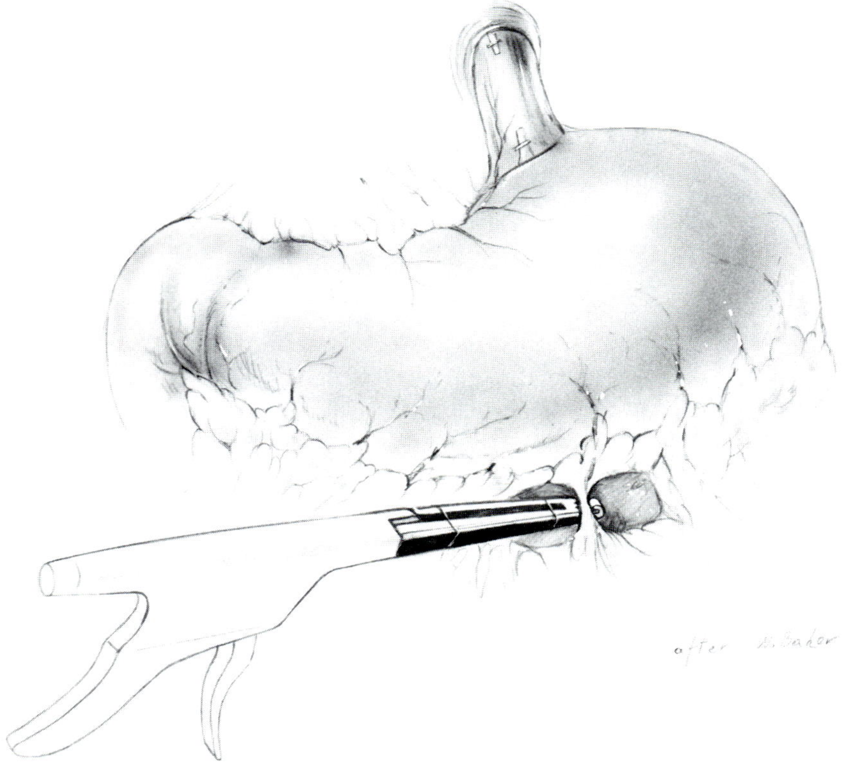

Fig. 15–44

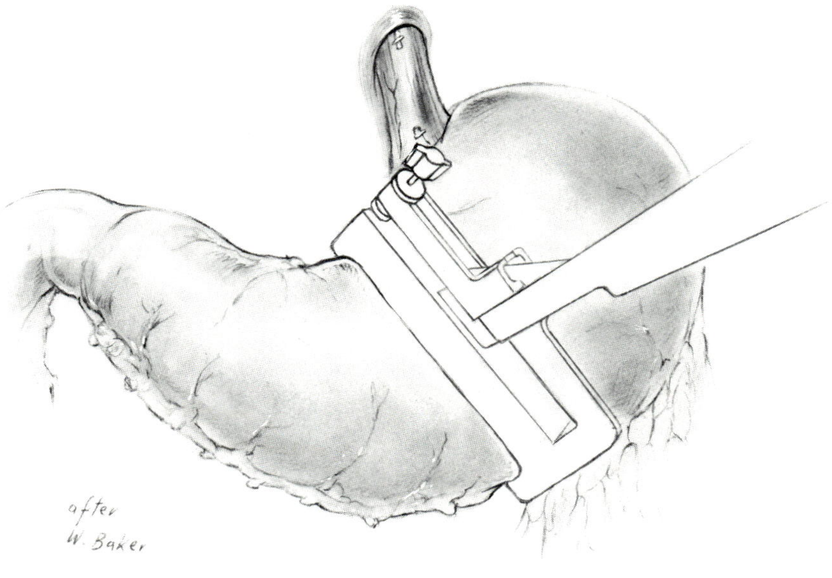

Fig. 15–45

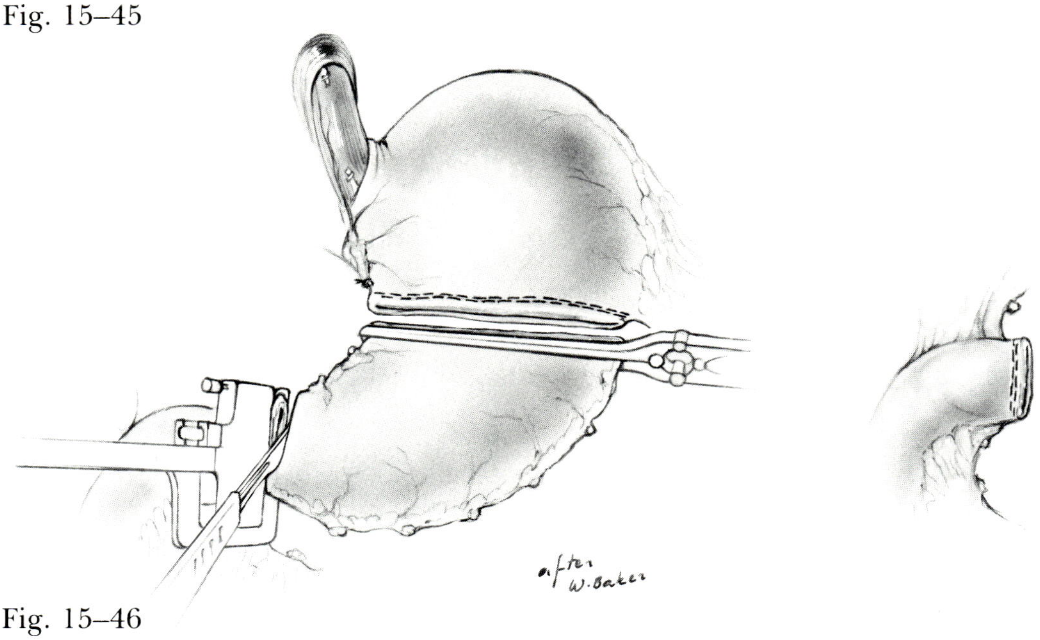

Fig. 15–46

It is imperative that the nasogastric tube not be permitted to lie anywhere in the vicinity of the staple line during this step. If the nasogastric tube gets trapped in the gastric staple line, it will not be possible to remove the tube postoperatively without another laparotomy.

Next identify the ligament of Treitz and bring a segment of proximal jejunum in antecolonic fashion to the greater curvature side of the gastric pouch. Approximate the antimesenteric border of the jejunum with a 4–0 cotton suture to a point on the greater curvature of the stomach about 2 cm proximal to the TA–90 staple line. Make small stab wounds in the gastric pouch and the jejunum adjacent to this suture and just deep to it. Then insert the GIA stapling device so that one fork enters the gastric pouch parallel to the TA–90

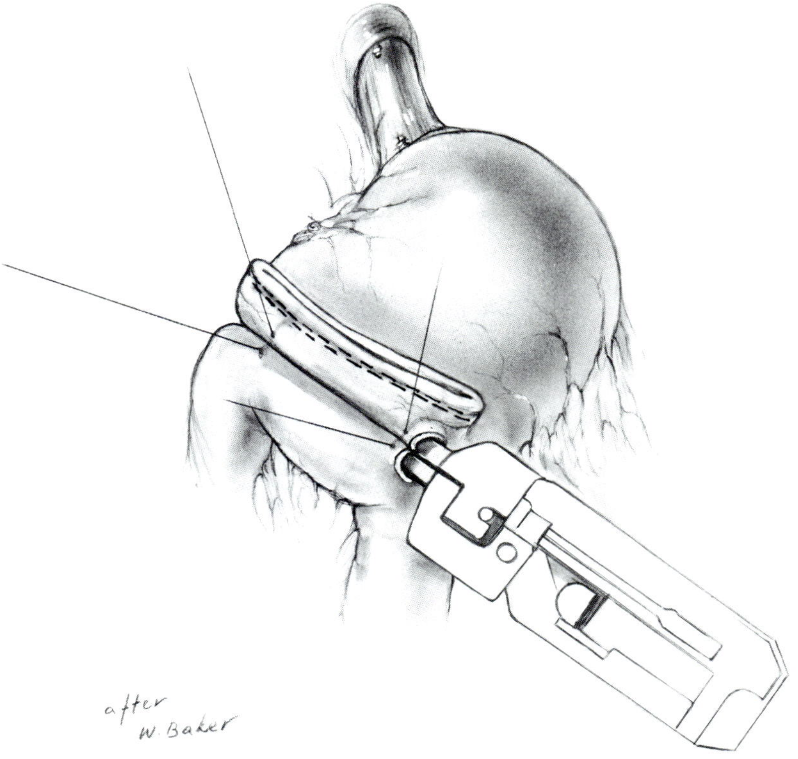

Fig. 15–47

staple line and the other fork enters the jejunum and is placed exactly along the antimesenteric border (**Fig. 15–47**). Care should be taken that no other organ or tissue is permitted to intrude between the stomach and jejunum being grasped by the GIA device. When the GIA stapler has been inserted to the 4 cm or 5 cm mark, close and lock the device (**Fig. 15–47**). Then reinspect the area. There should be a width of 2 cm of posterior gastric wall between the TA–90 staple line and the GIA staple line. Also, the gastric and jejunal tissues should be exactly apposed to each other in the hub of the GIA device. At this point fire and remove the GIA.

Apply an Allis clamp to the anterior termination of the GIA staple line and another to the posterior termination of the same staple line. Carefully inspect the mucosal surface of the GIA anastomosis for bleeding, as arterial spurting from the gastric wall may occur occasionally. If this should happen, transfix the vessel with a fine chromic or PG suture-ligature. Lesser bleeding may be controlled by cautious electrocoagulation. On rare occasions there may be multiple bleeding points: The entire mucosal suture line should then be oversewn with a locked continuous suture of 4–0 PG. The needle must be inserted deep to the staples in performing this maneuver. This should be necessary in no more than 1% or 2% of all cases, and generally indicates a defective, misaligned GIA device.

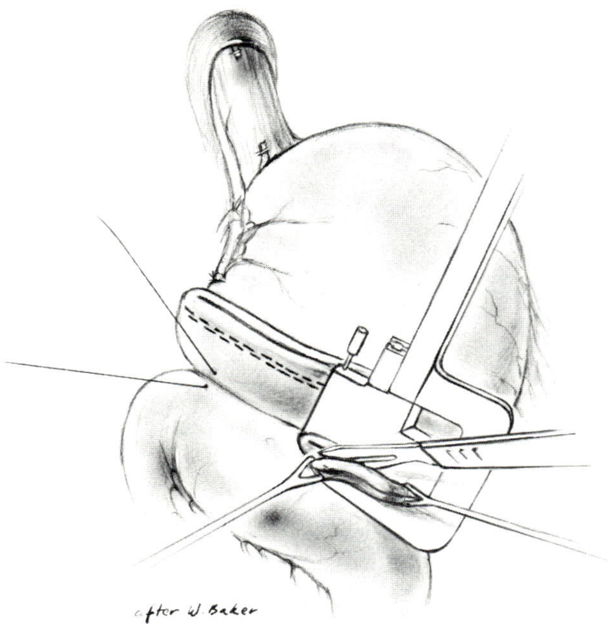

Fig. 15–48

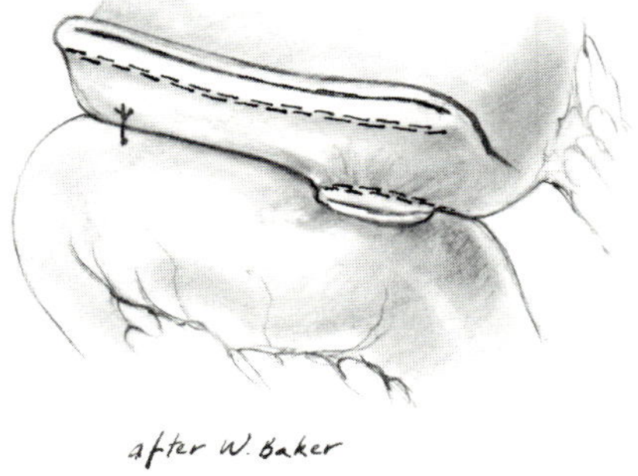

Fig. 15–49

After hemostasis is assured, approximate the gastric and jejunal layers of the open stab wounds in an everting fashion with several Allis or Babcock clamps. Close the defect with one application of a TA–55 stapler deep to the line of Allis clamps (**Fig. 15–48**). *This staple line must include the anterior and posterior terminations of the GIA staple line,* guaranteeing that there will be no defect between the two lines of staples. Excise the redundant tissue, lightly electrocoagulate the everted mucosa, and remove the TA–55 device. Alternatively, the stab-wound defect may be closed in an inverting fashion by various suturing techniques. Then place a single 4–0 cotton seromuscular suture at the right termination of the gastrojejunal GIA anastomosis (**Fig. 15–49**). Palpation of the gastrojejunal stoma should admit two fingers. A three-dimensional diagram of the anastomosis is shown in **Fig. 15–50**.

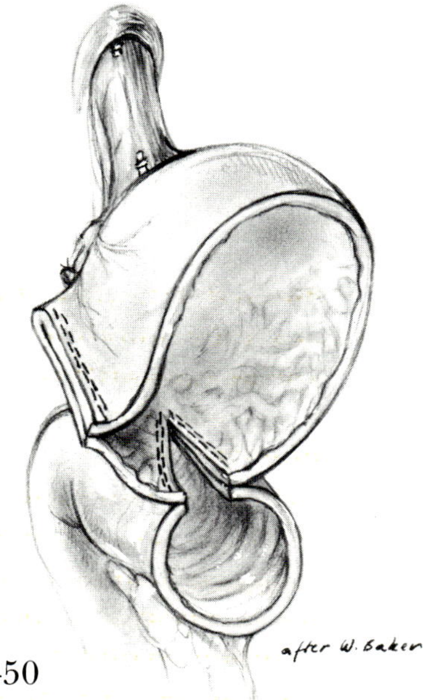

Fig. 15–50

Drainage, Irrigation, and Closure

To reduce the incidence of postoperative wound infection, especially when gastrectomy has been undertaken in the presence of active hemorrhage or to correct a long-standing gastric outlet obstruction, the abdominal cavity as well as the subcutaneous tissues should be irrigated thoroughly with an antibiotic solution.

In Billroth II operations, whenever the surgeon thinks that a duodenal closure is less than perfect, a closed-suction drain should be brought out from the vicinity of the duodenal stump through a stab wound in the right upper quadrant. The drain should be separated from the actual duodenal suture line by a layer of omentum. Accomplished this way, drainage does no harm to the patient. Close the abdominal wall in the usual fashion, after taking pains to assure that the efferent limb of the jejunum descends freely and without any kinks.

Postoperative Care

Nasogastric suction should be continued for several days.

Oral intake can be resumed when there is evidence of bowel function. For the first 4–6 weeks following gastric resection the composition of the diet should be low in carbohydrates and fluids and high in protein and fat, so as to reduce the osmolarity of the meals. Liquids should largely be eliminated from meals and be consumed beginning one hour after meals. Very sweet drinks should be avoided. If this course is followed, the transitory dumping symptoms, which many patients have in the early postgastrectomy period, will be eliminated. Generally, after 4–6 weeks most patients can take an unlimited diet.

Complications

Duodenal Fistula

In the presence of an adequate drain, the appearance of duodenal content in the drainage fluid without any other symptoms may not require vigorous therapy. On the other hand, if there are signs of spreading peritoneal irritation, prompt relaparotomy is indicated. If no drain was placed during the initial operation, immediate relaparotomy should be undertaken whenever there is reason to suspect duodenal leakage. On *rare* occasions, relaparotomy can be performed before the intense inflammatory reaction of the duodenal tissues occurs, and the defect may be closed by suture. This is very seldom possible, however. If suturing of the virgin duodenum at the first operation was not successful, an attempt at secondary suturing will fail unless considerable additional duodenum can be freed from the pancreas for a more adequate closure. In most cases the operation is done to provide excellent drainage. A small sump-suction drain should be inserted into the fistula, and additional latex and sumps placed in the area. If a controlled duodenocutaneous fistula can be achieved, this will generally close after a few weeks of intravenous hyperalimentation.

Leaks from Billroth I gastroduodenal anastomoses, while rare, are even more serious than from duodenal stump (Billroth II) procedures. Generally, they should be treated by the Graham technique of closing a perforated duodenal ulcer with a segment of viable omentum (see Figs. 16–2 and 16–3). Multiple sump drains should also be inserted.

Acute Pancreatitis

This serious complication can best be avoided by preventing trauma to the pancreas during the initial operation. Therapy here is identical with that for acute pancreatitis in the patient who has not undergone an operation.

Gastric Outlet Obstruction

In the gastroduodenal anastomosis, obstruction is generally due to the inversion of too much tissue, which produces a mechanical block. If this condition does not respond after a period of conservative treatment, reoperation to convert to a Billroth II anastomosis will probably be necessary.

Be aware that Billroth II gastrojejunal anastomosis occasionally develops an outlet obstruction, which appears to be due to a malfunction of the efferent loop of the jejunum. This diagnosis can be confirmed by postoperative gastroscopy, which demonstrates the absence of any mechanical stomal obstruction. Relaparotomy in these cases is of no value. Generally, a period of several weeks of conservative treatment with hyperalimentation intravenously will be successful. We managed one patient by inserting a 3 mm plastic nasogastric tube weighted with a small rubber finger cot containing 1 ml mercury. We passed this tube into the efferent jejunal loop for a distance of 10–12 cm. Continuous infusion of a blenderized diet was well tolerated by the patient for a period of 8 weeks, at the end of which time she had achieved complete recovery of function.

Hiatt advocates the use of the hormone coherin in similar cases.

Bilious Vomiting Syndrome

Toye and Williams have described an unusual syndrome following Billroth II gastrectomy: Patients are able to eat a satisfactory diet but are afflicted by episodes in which they vomit clear bile not accompanied by ingested food. Sometimes these episodes do not occur until several years after the operation. The patients tend tc remain well nourished. They do not experience pain after meals, as seen in alkaline gastritis. The syndrome appears to result from the gastric pouch's intolerance of the bile that enters from the afferent loop. This bile is promptly ejected by the stomach while ingested food remains undisturbed. There is no obstruction or malfunction of the afferent loop in these cases. This condition can be corrected surgically by using the technique illustrated in **Figs. 15–51 and 15–52.**

Transect the afferent limb of jejunum just at its point of entry into the gastric pouch. Use a TA–55 stapler to close the gastric side of the jejunum. Then anastomose the open end of the afferent segment to the side of the efferent segment of the jejunum. This anastomosis should take place at a point 50 cm distal to the gastrojejunostomy. It converts the efferent limb of the jejunum into a Roux-Y configuration. Vagotomy is necessary to prevent marginal ulceration following this type of Roux-Y anastomosis.

Alkaline Gastritis

The entrance of bile and other duodenal secretions into the gastric pouch sometimes results in severe gastritis accompanied by superficial ulcerations, metaplasia of the gastric mucosa, weight loss, and severe pain that is accentuated by eating. Alkaline gastritis may occur after the pylorus has been bypassed, removed, or rendered ineffective by pyloroplasty. Occasionally it is seen in a patient who has not been operated on but has a patulous pyloric sphincter.

After the diagnosis has been confirmed by endoscopy and biopsy, surgical relief can be obtained by total diversion of the bile and duodenal contents from the gastric pouch, as described above in the discussion of bilious vomiting.

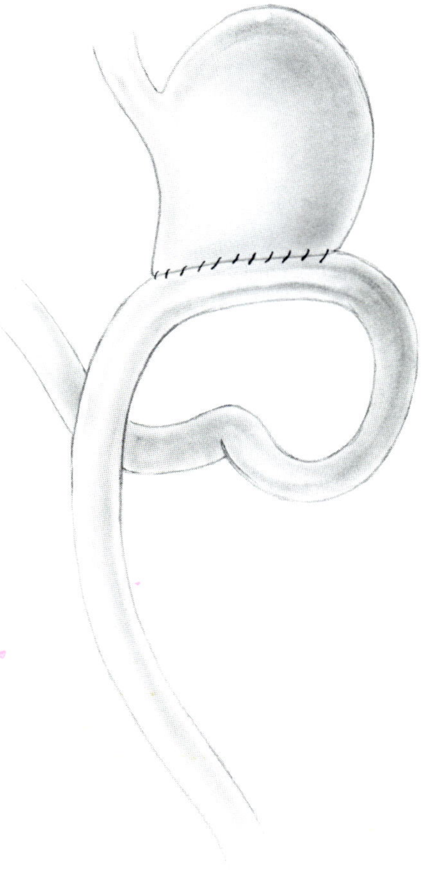

Fig. 15–51

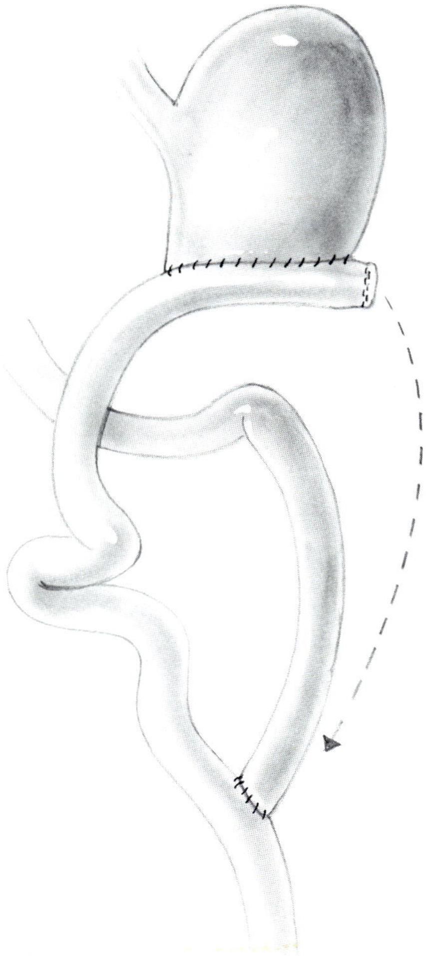

Fig. 15–52

Afferent Loop Syndrome

For many years the symptoms discussed under bilious vomiting and alkaline gastritis were attributed to intermittent afferent loop obstruction. It was hypothesized that a partial obstruction at the entrance of the afferent jejunum into the gastric pouch resulted in the accumulation of bile and duodenal contents under pressure in the afferent jejunum. Suddenly, it was alleged, the jejunum expelled its contents forcefully into the gastric pouch, which resulted in vomiting. This mechanism must be extremely rare, however. Patients who experience bilious vomiting syndrome and alkaline gastritis do not exhibit a dilated afferent loop; nor is there evidence of an obstructed afferent stoma in these cases.

On the other hand, complete mechanical blockage of the afferent stoma does result in an acute closed-loop obstruction, manifested by excruciating upper abdominal pain and retching. Gastrointestinal X rays at this moment will show a complete block at the afferent stoma, which can be confirmed by endoscopy. This situation is a surgical emergency, for if the distended afferent loop bursts lethal peritonitis will result. Obviously, emergency surgery for the correction of the obstruction is essential. When X rays reveal no dilatation of the afferent loop, and no other evidence of organic stomal obstruction can be discovered, afferent loop malfunction is probably not the cause of the patient's symptoms.

One cause of acute afferent stomal obstruction is jejunogastric intussusception, another condition that may require emergency surgical correction. This diagnosis can be confirmed by endoscopy.

Most afferent loop symptomatology can be prevented by assuring that the distance between the ligament of Treitz and the gastric pouch is never more than 12–15 cm. Enthusiasts of the Billroth I gastrectomy are quick to point out that gastroduodenostomy averts this group of complications.

Internal Hernia

Herniation of the small bowel into the antecolonic jejunal loop has been reported following antecolonic Billroth II gastrojejunal anastomoses. This complication is quite rare and has never been observed by us, but it does make another argument in favor of gastroduodenostomy.

Dumping Syndrome

Much has been written about the "dumping syndrome," which may occur in any patient whose pylorus has been rendered nonfunctional. It is more common in the patient who has an asthenic habitus and who has never achieved normal body weight, even before surgery. These patients should probably be subjected to a proximal gastric vagotomy rather than gastrectomy, even if the recurrence rate of duodenal ulcer is higher after this operation than after vagotomy–antrectomy. When dumping does occur, the best therapy is a low-carbohydrate, high-protein, high-fat diet, in which fluid is not permitted during mealtime. As Sawyers and Herrington have pointed out, *rarely* is a patient so disabled by dumping as to require the interposition of an antiperistaltic jejunal segment between the gastric pouch and the remainder of the alimentary canal.

Postvagotomy Diarrhea

Postvagotomy diarrhea appears to be rare in this region of the world, even after a truncal vagotomy. When diarrhea occurs, a complete investigative study to rule out other causes of this condition, such as nontropical sprue, should be carried out. Sawyers has reported some success in the control of intractable diarrhea by placing a reversed segment of the jejunum about 100 cm down from the ligament of Treitz.

Recurrent Ulcer

Recurrent peptic ulcer following a gastrectomy is often the result of the surgeon's having overlooked the right vagus trunk during a vagotomy or having failed to perform a vagotomy in a case of duodenal ulcer. Another cause of recurrent ulcer is the surgeon's having left behind gastrin-secreting antral mucosa on the duodenal stump following a Billroth II gastrectomy. Rarely will an ulcer recur because some residual antral mucosa was left behind in the gastric pouch. Here the secretion of gastric acid, even though subnormal following a vagotomy, is sufficent to suppress the secretion of gastrin. Yet another important cause of recurrent ulcer is the Zollinger-Ellison syndrome, which the surgeon may have overlooked during the diagnostic study of the peptic ulcer before the operation.

Malabsorption

Smith and Jeffries have made the following observations about malabsorption:

> Anemia may be caused by inadequate iron absorption. Folic acid and vitamin B_{12} deficiencies also may develop on rare occasions following gastrectomy.

Another late complication is osteomalacia or osteoporosis caused by poor calcium or vitamin D absorption.

Steatorrhea and diarrhea develop in some cases and may contribute to malnutrition. These cases should be studied for the presence of gluten enteropathy, which may be unmasked by the gastrectomy.

Although almost all the early complications are manageable, the occurrence of malabsorption and malnutrition many years after a gastrectomy is quite difficult to treat. Following a 40%–50% gastrectomy, these complications seem to be very rare, however. It is not certain that vagotomy and pyloroplasty are completely devoid of these late complications.

References

Austen WG, Baue AE (1964) Catheter duodenostomy for the difficult duodenum. Ann Surg 160:781

Berne CJ, Rosoff L (1969) Peptic ulcer perforation of the gastroduodenal artery complex. Ann Surg 169:141

Chassin JL (1978) Pros and cons. Surg Gynecol Obstet 146:619

Harrower HW (1966) Closure of the duodenal stump after gastrectomy for posterior ulcer. Am J Surg 111:488

Hiatt RB, Goodman I (1979) Physiological properties and therapeutic potential of coherin. Am J Surg 137:82

Jones RC et al. (1967) Difficult closures of the duodenal stump. Arch Surg 94:696

Nyhus LM, Wastell C (1977) Surgery of the stomach and duodenum. Little Brown, Boston, p 368

Sawyers JL, Herrington JL Jr (1973) Superiority of antiperistaltic jejunal segments in management of severe dumping symptoms. Ann Surg 178:311

Smith FW, Jeffries GH (1973) in Sleisinger MH, Fordtran JS Gastrointestinal disease. Saunders, Philadelphia, p. 826

Toye DKM, Williams JA (1965) Post-gastrectomy bile vomiting. Lancet 2:524

16 Perforated Peptic Ulcer

Concept

Perforated Gastric Ulcer

Not all free perforations of gastric ulcers are susceptible to simple plication techniques. Often the ulcer is quite large and surrounded by edema. When the perforation occurs on the posterior surface of the antrum, adequate repair by plication techniques is generally not possible. Also, gastric ulcers have a high rate of recurrence. For these reasons, in a good-risk patient, in whom the diagnosis of perforation has been made reasonably early, gastric resection is *preferred* to simple plication. If for technical reasons, a sound plication cannot be constructed, then gastric resection is *mandatory*, regardless of the risk, as a recurrent gastric leak into the peritoneal cavity is almost always fatal.

Perforated Duodenal Ulcer

If a perforated duodenal ulcer is treated with a simple closure, about one-third of the patients will remain nonsymptomatic. Perhaps two-thirds will develop recurrent ulcer symptoms, and one-half of these will require definitive surgery at a later date.

In the good-risk patient who comes to the operating room within 8 hours of the first sign of perforation, vagotomy and antrectomy or pyloroplasty has proved to be a safe operation, according to Jordan and associates. Consequently, in middle-aged patients, especially males, who have a history of chronic *duodenal ulcer symptoms*, a definitive operation including vagotomy and antrectomy or pyloroplasty or proximal gastric vagotomy is indicated unless the peritoneal insult is severe.

Another category of patients, in whom vagotomy and antrectomy should be done if possible, are those whose perforation is accompanied by acute bleeding. These patients have a posterior penetrating ulcer as well as the anterior perforation. They experience a high mortality rate unless a definitive operation is accomplished early.

Whether to do a plication or a definitive operation on young good-risk patients whose duodenal ulcer perforations are fresh and who have had *no prior ulcer symptoms* is a controversial matter, because over 60% of these patients will never need further definitive surgery if simple plication is done. The long-term ill effects of pyloroplasty or antrectomy are avoided if plication is combined with a proximal gastric vagotomy. Plication with proximal gastric vagotomy may well be the ideal treatment for these patients, but pending the accumulation of more data, it should be regarded as a procedure still under study.

Simple plication of the ulcer is indicated for patients in poor general health, the aged, and patients who have waited many hours between the onset of perforation and surgical therapy.

Preoperative Preparation

Fluid and electrolyte resuscitation, primarily with a balanced salt solution

Nasogastric suction

Systemic antibiotics

Monitoring of hourly urine output, central venous pressure, or pulmonary artery wedge pressure, as indicated

Pitfalls and Danger Points

Inadequate fluid and electrolyte resuscitation

Inadequate closure of perforation

Operative Strategy

The most important initial step in the operative strategy is to determine, on the basis of the principles discussed above, whether the patient should be treated by plication or by vagotomy and excisional therapy. On technical grounds alone, very large defects in the stomach or duodenum are better handled by resection than by attempted plication. Also, if it appears that plication will produce duodenal obstruction, a definitive procedure is indicated.

In most perforated duodenal ulcers, an attempt to close the defect by sutures alone will often result in the stitch tearing through the edematous tissue. It is preferable simply to place a plug of viable omentum over the defect and use through-and-through sutures to hold the omentum in contact with the wall of the duodenum. This avoids tension on the sutures.

It is important to irrigate the abdominal cavity thoroughly with large quantities of saline and then with a dilute antibiotic solution to remove the contamination from the peritoneal cavity.

Operative Technique of Plication

Incision

A midline incision from the xiphoid to the umbilicus provides good exposure and can be made rapidly.

Identification of Perforation

By following the lesser curvature aspect of the stomach down to the pylorus, the perforation along the anterior wall of the duodenum generally becomes quickly evident (**Fig. 16–1**). In some cases it is sealed off either by omentum or by the undersurface of the liver. If this area is not the site of the perforation, then the entire stomach must be carefully searched, up to the esophagus and including the entire posterior surface of the stomach in the lesser sac. On rare occasions an unusual type of perforation may be found somewhere in the small intestine or colon, as, for instance, that secondary to a sharp fish bone.

Plication of Perforation

Generally, insert 3–0 silk (or PG) on an atraumatic intestinal needle beginning at a point about 5 mm above the perforation. Bring the stitch out at a point 5 mm distal to the perforation and leave it untied. Two additional sutures of the same type are needed for the average perforation. Next, isolate a viable segment of omentum and place it over the perforation. Tie the three sutures over the plug of omentum in order to fasten it in place (**Figs. 16–2 and 16–3**).

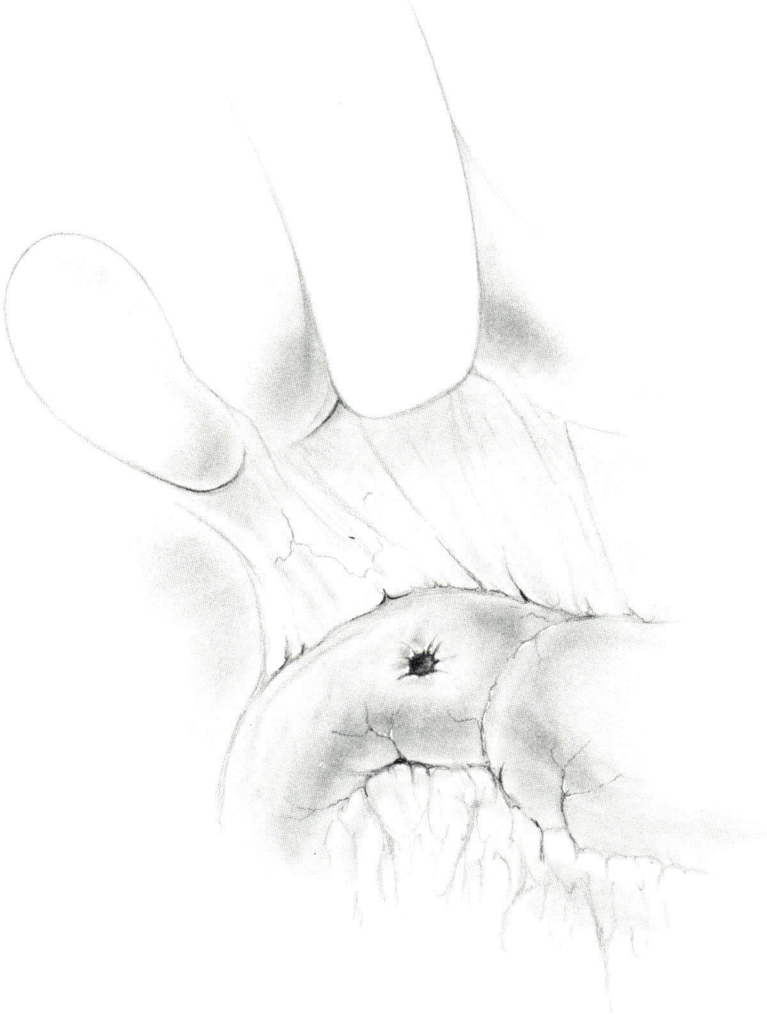

Fig. 16–1

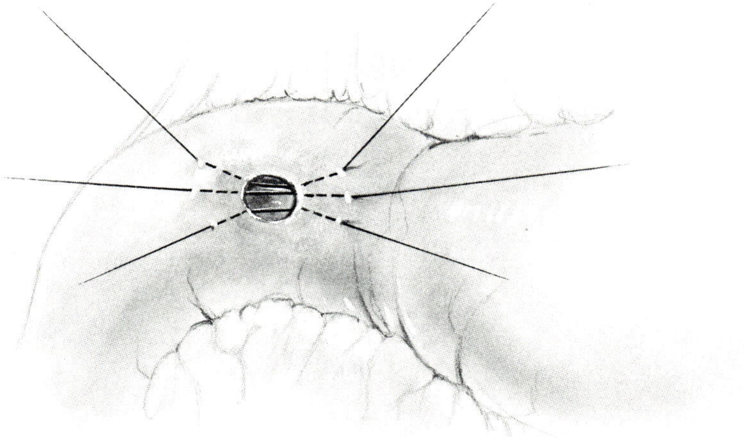

Fig. 16–2

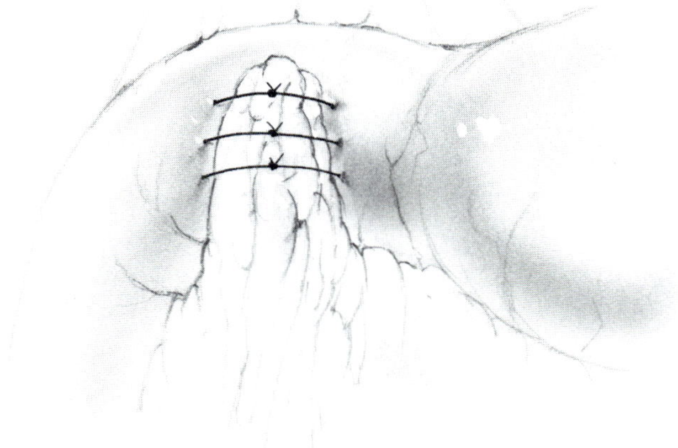

Fig. 16–3

Peritoneal Lavage

Using large volumes of warm saline, thoroughly lavage the peritoneal cavity with multiple aliquots until the gastric contents and fibrin are removed from the surfaces of the bowel and peritoneum. The final liter of lavage fluid should be a dilute antibiotic solution, all of which should then be aspirated.

Abdominal Closure

Close the midline incision without drainage by the modified Smead-Jones technique, using 2–0 monofilament stainless steel wire, as described in Chap. 5. Unless the patient has advanced peritonitis, the skin may be closed in routine fashion after inserting a closed-suction drain, as described in Chap. 2.

Postoperative Care

Nasogastric suction

Intravenous fluids; parenteral hyperalimentation for malnourished patients or those suffering advanced peritonitis

Systemic antibiotics, the selection of which is governed by the results of bacteriological cultures, aerobic and anaerobic, obtained during the operation

Complications

Subphrenic and subhepatic abscesses occur mainly in patients whose operations have been delayed for more than 8–12 hours after the perforation.

Duodenal obstruction, caused by the plication, should be suspected if gastric emptying has not returned to normal by the eighth or ninth postoperative day. This may be confirmed by a gastrointestinal X-ray series.

Reperforation of the same duodenal ulcer may occur in rare cases, and the surgeon must be alert to detect this complication. When it does occur, gastric resection is mandatory if there is to be any hope of stopping the duodenal leak.

Reference

Jordan GL Jr et al. (1966) Acute gastroduodenal perforation: comparative study of treatment with simple closure, subtotal gastrectomy and hemigastrectomy and vagotomy. Arch Surg 92:449

17 Gastrostomy

Indications

When gastric suction is to be achieved without traversing the esophagogastric junction or the nasopharynx

For gastric tube feeding

Concept

Patients who have a history of reflux esophagitis often tolerate nasogastric tubes poorly. Occasionally a patient who has unrecognized reflux esophagitis develops a virulent esophagitis after a period of 2 weeks with an indwelling nasogastric tube. This may progress rapidly to an extensive stricture. Although this complication is uncommon, when it does occur, management is extremely difficult.

Some surgeons believe that nasogastric intubation increases the incidence of bronchopneumonia in patients who have pulmonary problems or an inadequate gag reflex. Improved nursing care and good nasotracheal suction can successfully prevent postoperative pulmonary complications. Consequently, the need for gastrostomy is no longer as great as it was a decade ago.

For those rare patients who require long-term gastric tube feeding, the Janeway gastrostomy is more convenient than the usual Stamm gastrostomy, as the Janeway does not require an indwelling tube.

Pitfalls and Danger Points

Gastric leak into the peritoneal cavity

Operative Strategy

When constructing a tube gastrostomy, the gastrostomy opening must be carefully sutured to the anterior abdominal wall around the stab wound made for the exit of the tube. Otherwise, gastric contents may leak out around the tube and escape into the abdominal cavity.

Operative Technique

Stamm Gastrostomy

Tube gastrostomy is generally done as part of some other operation on the gastrointestinal tract, so the abdominal incision will already have been made. If necessary, it can be extended upward into the epigastrium to expose the stomach. Using 2–0 atraumatic PG, insert a circular purse-string suture with a 1.5 cm diameter. Do this in the midportion of the stomach, closer to the greater than to the lesser curvature (**Fig. 17–1**).

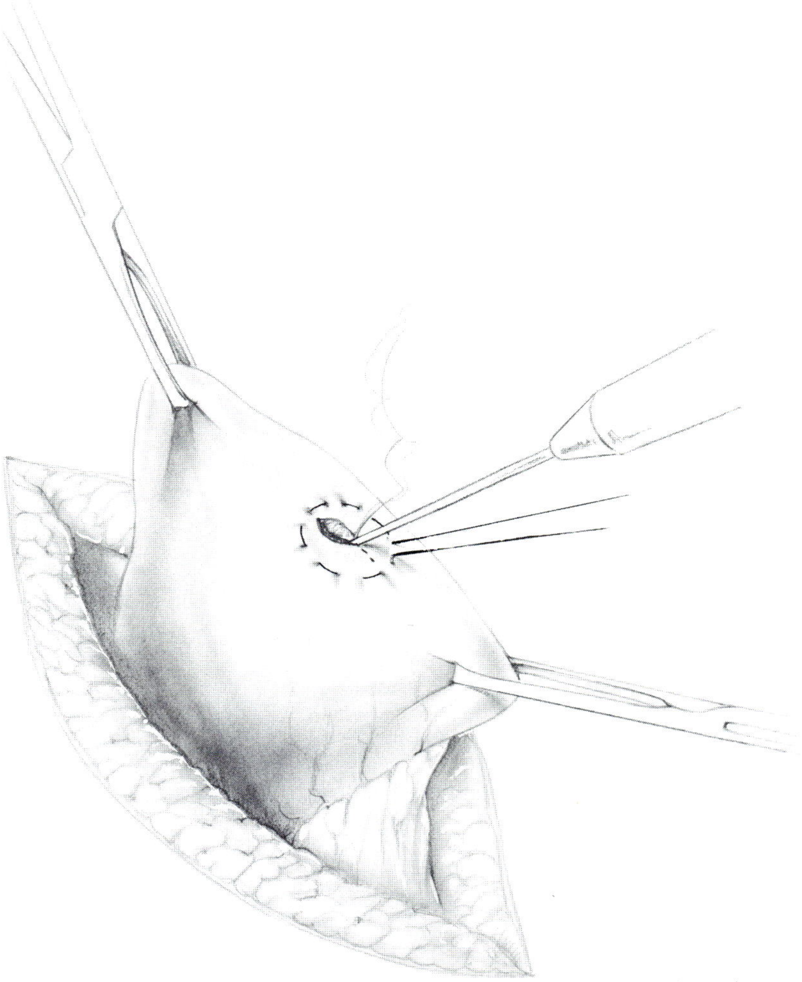

Fig. 17–1

Grasp the left side of the incised linea alba with a Kocher clamp and elevate it. Then make a stab wound through the middle third of the left rectus muscle at the level of the purse-string suture. Pass a Kelly hemostat through the stab wound from the peritoneum outward. The Kelly should grasp the tip of an 18F Foley catheter, which has a 5 ml bag. Draw the catheter into the abdominal cavity with the hemostat. With the electrocoagulator make a stab wound into the anterior gastric wall in the middle of the previously placed purse-string suture (**Fig. 17–1**). Insert the Foley catheter into the stomach, tighten

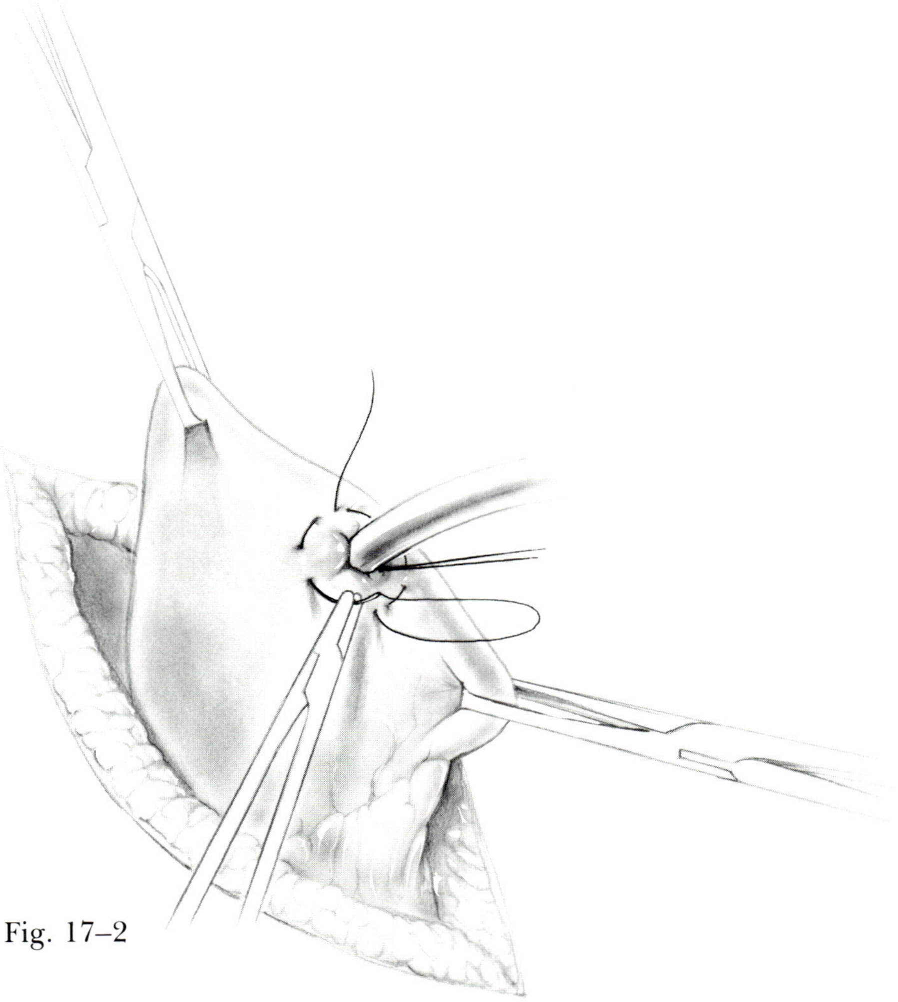

Fig. 17–2

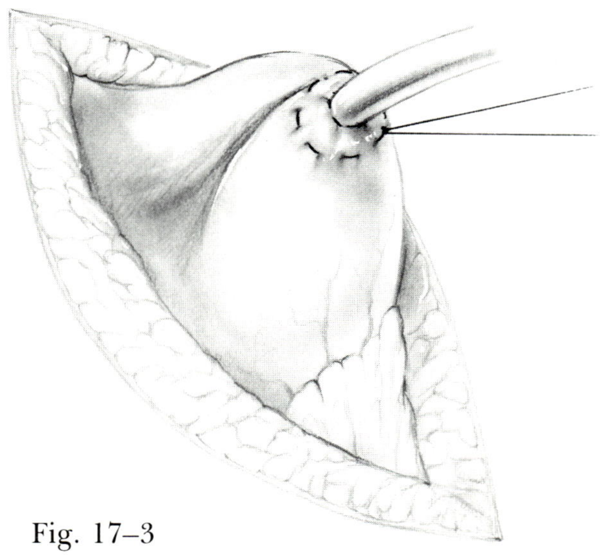

Fig. 17–3

the purse-string suture, and tie it so as to invert the gastric serosa (**Fig. 17–2**). Invert this purse-string suture in turn with a second concentric 2–0 PG purse-string suture (**Fig. 17–3**). Inflate the Foley catheter balloon and draw the stomach toward the anterior abdominal wall. Insert Lembert sutures of PG in four quadrants around the Foley catheter to sew the stomach to the anterior abdominal wall around the stab wound (**Fig. 17–4**). When these four Lembert sutures are tied, the anterior gastric wall will be firmly anchored to the abdominal wall (**Fig. 17–5**).

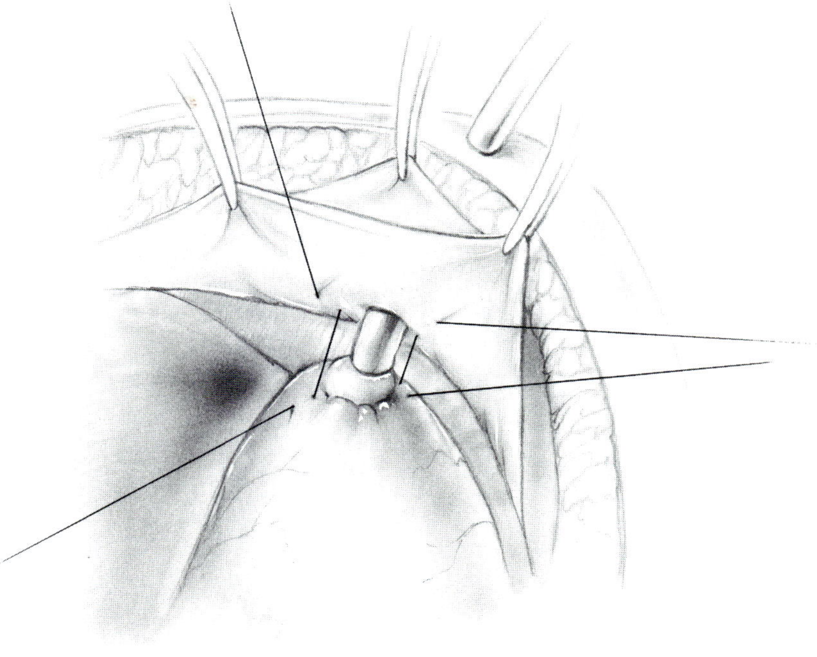

Fig. 17–4

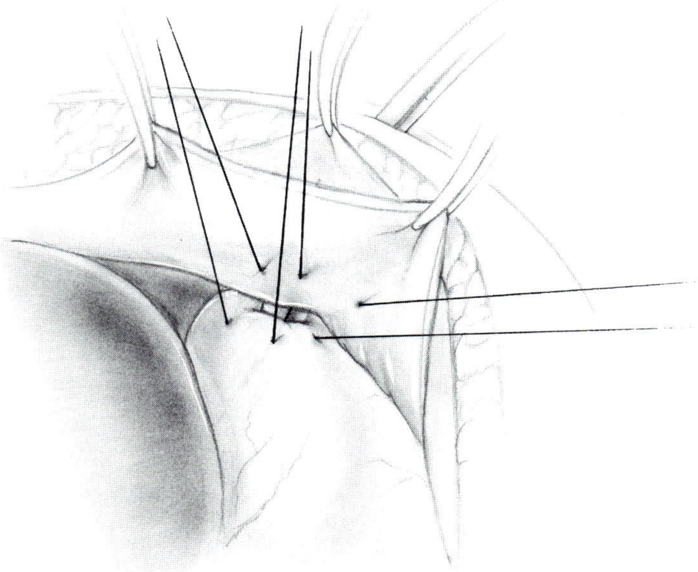

Fig. 17–5

Janeway Gastrostomy, Stapled

Make a midline incision in the mid-epigastrium for a distance of 10–12 cm. This may be performed under local anesthesia in the poor-risk patient. Apply Babcock clamps to the anterior gastric wall near the lesser curvature. Then apply the GIA stapling device (**Fig 17–6**). Fire the device, laying down four rows of staples, and incising for a distance of about 4 cm between the staples (**Fig. 17–7**). This pro-

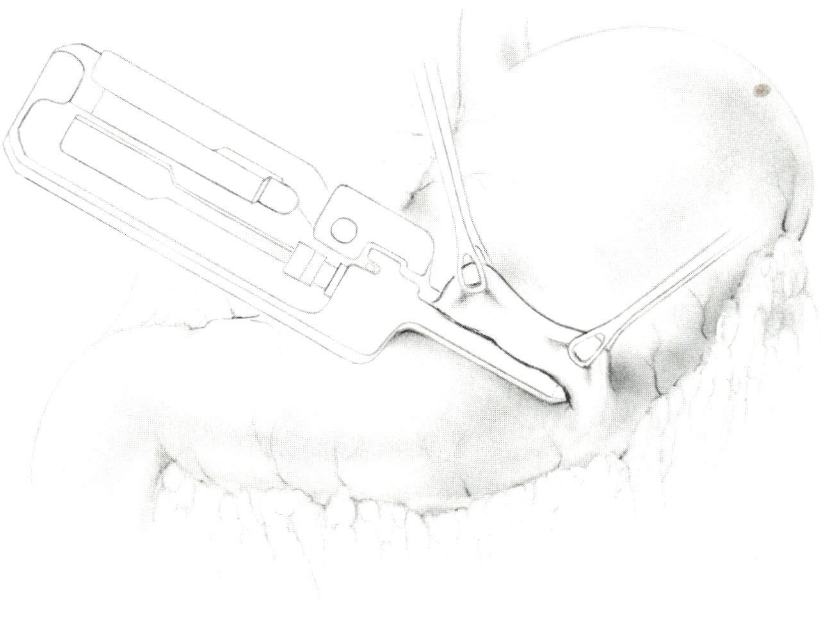

Fig. 17–6

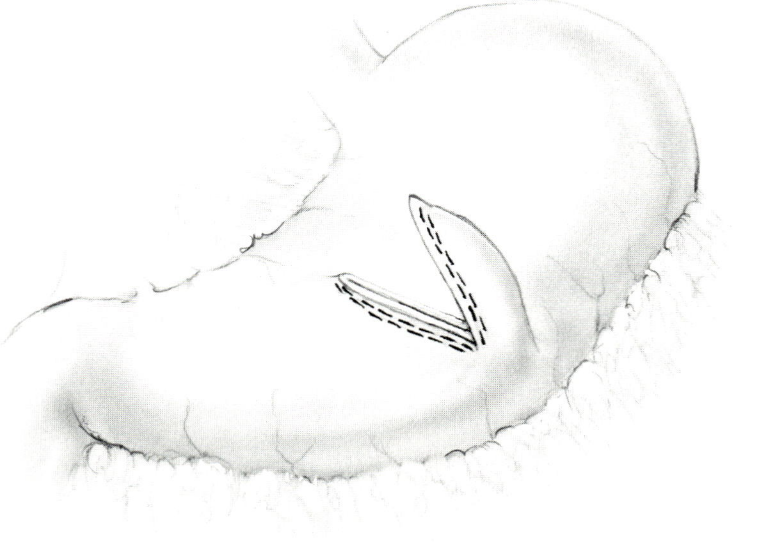

Fig. 17–7

vides a tunnel of gastric mucosa about 4 cm in length, which is sufficient to pass through the abdominal wall. Reinforce the line of staples with a layer of continuous 3–0 atraumatic PG seromuscular Lembert sutures, so as to invert the staples (**Fig. 17–8**).

Make a vertical incision, about 1.5 cm in length, in the skin overlying the middle third of the left rectus muscle. Deepen the incision through the rectus muscle with the aid of the electrocautery, then dilate it by inserting the index finger.

Grasp the gastric nipple and draw it to the outside by passing a Babcock clamp into the incision in the rectus muscle. This brings the gastric wall into contact with the

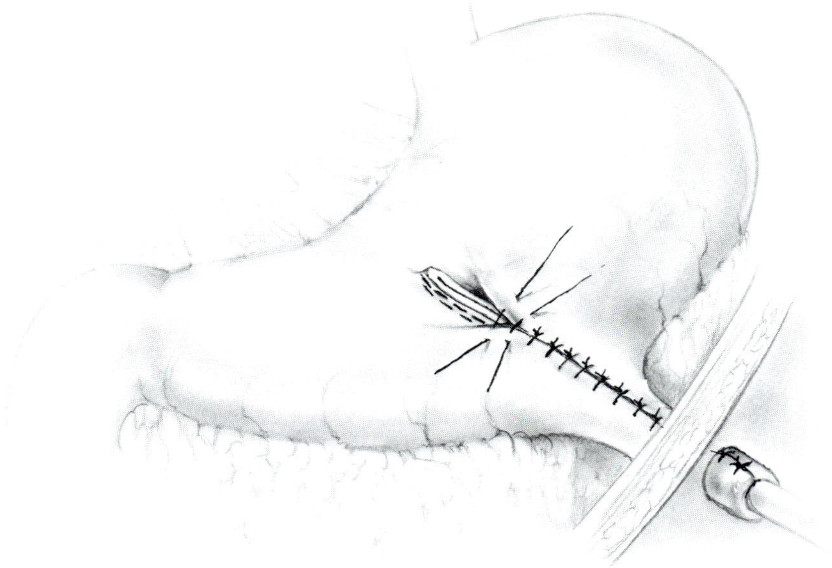

Fig. 17–8

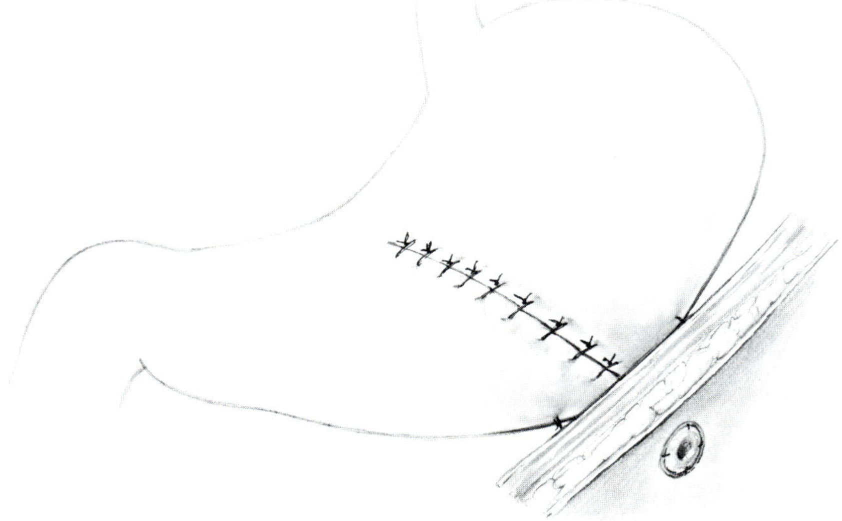

Fig. 17–9

anterior abdominal wall, to which it should be fixed with two Lembert sutures of 3–0 PG. Then transect the tip of the gastric nipple with a Mayo scissors, leaving enough gastric tissue to reach the skin level. Insert an 18F catheter into the stomach to test the channel.

Accomplish immediate maturation of the gastrostomy by interrupted mucocutaneous sutures of 3–0 PG, which should pass through the entire thickness of the gastric wall and catch the subcuticular layer of the skin.

Close the abdominal incision in the usual fashion and apply a sterile dressing (**Fig. 17–9**). Leave the catheter in place until the wound heals.

After healing has taken place, gastric feeding can be given by inserting a catheter into the stomach while the feeding is being administered. The catheter should be removed between meals.

18 Gastrectomy for Cancer

Concept: How Radical an Operation for Gastric Cancer?

Points of Controversy

For the past 30 years there has been great confusion over the choice of operations for gastric malignancies. The pendulum has swung from partial gastrectomy to total gastrectomy and back again. Lacking adequate data that correlates survival statistics with various lesions, surgeons have based their choice of operations on anatomical study of the distribution of lymphatic metastases. The *routine* use of total gastrectomy for all gastric malignancies has been shown not to improve survival of patients. Several major controversies still remain:

1) Proximal gastric lesions are treated by total gastrectomy by some surgeons and by resection of the lower esophagus and proximal stomach by others (see Chaps. 6 and 8).

2) According to Hoerr and to Nyhus, antral malignancy requires only a distal two-thirds gastrectomy, including adjacent lymph nodes, duodenum, and omentectomy. On the other hand, Menguy recommends an 80%–90% gastrectomy, with division of the left gastric artery at its origin, omentectomy, and splenectomy, followed by gastroduodenostomy or gastrojejunostomy.

Anatomical Zones of Spread

Direct Extension

Spread by direct invasion of gastric malignancy can involve a number of organs. Posteriorly, the tumor can invade the body or tail of the pancreas, the middle colic artery, or the transverse colon, all of which can be included in the specimen. Invasion of the aorta contraindicates resection. Extension into the left lobe of the liver is amenable to resection, as is extension into the crura of the diaphragm.

Lymphatic Metastasis

A malignancy of the cardia or fundus drains into the paracardial, left gastric, and pancreaticolienal lymph nodes. A tumor of the body or antrum drains into the left gastric and accompanying lymph nodes on the lesser curvature of the stomach, and into the greater curvature nodes. Cancer involving the prepyloric area drains into the hepatic artery and subpyloric node groups. In general, the more advanced tumors tend to metastasize to nodes at greater distances from the primary site than listed above.

Operation for Lesions of Cardia and Fundus

As described in Chaps. 6 and 8, small to medium-sized lesions of the proximal stomach and esophagogastric junction are best handled by resecting the lower esophagus and proximal stomach, including transection of the left gastric artery at the celiac axis to include these nodes in the specimen. The paracardial lymph nodes around the diaphragmatic crura should also be included. The spleen and lymph nodes around the tail and superior border of the pancreas should be removed. If the tail of the pancreas has been invaded by tumor, this too should be included in the specimen.

After the dissection has been completed, the surgeon can decide whether to perform an esophagogastric resection with end-to-side esophagogastric anastomosis or a total gastrectomy with Roux-Y esophagojejunostomy. The esophagogastric end-to-side reconstruction offers most patients the possibility of a normal diet and normal nutrition because the end-to-side technique generally prevents reflux esophagitis. If more than half the stomach has to be resected to provide an adequate margin beyond a proximal gastric carcinoma, and if the left gastric vessels and celiac lymph nodes are removed, what remains after the resection is a small tubular segment of gastric antrum. In this case an end-to-end esophagogastric anastomosis is doomed to failure because there is no way of preventing the reflux of bile and gastric juice. Also, as Chassin has reported, the rate of anastomotic leakage following the end-to-end anastomosis is much higher than after the end-to-side. Soga et al. advocated not only total gastrectomy but also hemipancreatectomy, splenectomy, and extensive lymphadenectomy for advanced lesions of the proximal one-third of the stomach.

On the other hand, a number of proximal lesions are localized in the area of the esophagogastric junction. These can be resected with an adequate margin, while sufficient stomach is preserved for the construction of an end-to-side anastomosis at a point 6–7 cm beyond the proximal cut edge of the remaining gastric segment. Sometimes the proximal portion of the residual gastric pouch can be shaped into a partial fundoplication. Even when this has not been done, we have rarely encountered a serious degree of gastroesophageal reflux in our end-to-side reconstructions.

In summary, if enough stomach can be spared for an end-to-side anastomosis, esophagogastrectomy is the procedure of choice. Otherwise, total gastrectomy followed by some type of esophagojejunal reconstruction on the Roux-Y principle is indicated. Whether the addition of a jejunal substitute pouch is of value in these cases has yet to be determined, although some experienced surgeons believe that the Hunt-Lawrence pouch is helpful.

Operation for Lesions of Body

A malignancy in the body of the stomach involving most of the lesser curvature requires total gastrectomy. Circumscribed lesions of the body may be treated by subtotal gastrectomy, as described below for lesions of the antrum.

Operation for Lesions of Antrum

Studies by Paulino and Roselli of the lymphatic distribution of metastases have demonstrated that when a lesion is confined to the antrum and is not so large as to extend into the body of the stomach, involvement of the splenic and pancreatic lymph nodes is rare. Consequently, it appears unnecessary to perform a routine splenectomy for lesions of the distal stomach. A major drawback of including the spleen in a resection, which also involves the ligation of the left gastric artery *at its origin*, is that ischemia or gangrene of the residual gastric pouch may develop. After a left gastric ligation and the division of the left gastroepiploic artery, the blood supply of the residual gastric pouch is limited. There is often a posterior gastric branch that arises from the splenic artery proximal to the origin of the left gastroepiploic. It is possible to preserve this artery if care is taken during the operation, but it is a small vessel and is easily traumatized. In addition, there are collateral branches from the inferior phrenic vessels and intramural circulation from the esophagus. Gangrene of the residual stomach following the combined gastrectomy and splenectomy has been reported by Spencer and by Thompson. If a rim of only a few centimeters of gastric tissue is left attached to the esophagus, intramural circulation will suffice. However, anastomosis of this tissue to the side of the jejunum or to the duodenum results in a high incidence of reflux alkaline esophagitis. The reconstruction here should be to a Roux-Y segment of the jejunum as in total gastrectomy. As to postoperative nutrition, this operation seems to offer no advantage over total gastrectomy.

Since there is insufficient data to demonstrate that this radical subtotal resection improves a patient's chances of survival, most surgeons agree with the conservative philosophy of Hoerr, who is supported by Nyhus, Cady, and Paulino and Roselli. The more conservative approach to treating malignancy of the distal stomach is to do a small operation for the small tumor and a large operation for the large tumor. If the tumor is localized to the antrum and is small, a two-thirds gastric resection that includes the accompanying omentum and adjacent lymph nodes plus 3–5 cm of the duodenum constitutes an adequate operation.

For larger carcinomas of the distal stomach, the left gastric artery may be ligated at its origin and included in the specimen, together with the nodes along the lesser curvature of the stomach and the lesser omentum. A hepatic artery node dissection down to the pylorus should be included, together with any visible subpyloric and right gastric nodes, the lymph glands around the origin of the right gastroepiploic artery and the upper border of the pancreas. The spleen should not be removed. The spleen provides a good blood supply to the gastric pouch through the short gastric vessels, which is important if the left gastric artery is divided at its origin. Adjacent organs should be included when there is evidence of direct invasion. Total gastrectomy should be done if most of the lesser curve of the stomach is invaded.

Unless a large margin (8–10 cm) of normal appearing gastric wall has been included in the specimen, frozen section histological examination of both ends of the specimen should be carried out as significant submucosal spread of cancer may occur.

Preoperative Preparation

The patient should receive nutritional rehabilitation by tube feeding when feasible or by intravenous hyperalimentation.

Antibiotic preparation of the stomach is necessary because necrotic tumor often harbors virulent bacteria similar to those in the colon. The same intestinal antibiotics are used here as are employed for colon preparation.

Perioperative systemic antibiotics also should be administered.

Operative Strategy

Blood Supply to Residual Gastric Pouch

As mentioned above, whenever the left gastric artery is divided at its origin and splenectomy is performed, the blood supply to the gastric pouch may be inadequate. Thus one should avoid a splenectomy in these cases unless so little gastric pouch is left behind that it may receive adequate nourishment through the intramural channels from the esophagus if the posterior gastric and inferior phrenic collaterals prove inadequate. If there is any doubt about the adequacy of the blood supply, perform a total gastrectomy.

Duct of Santorini

When carcinoma approaches the pyloric region, microscopic spread into the proximal 4–5 cm of the duodenum is possible. When as much as 5 cm of the duodenum is mobilized, the dissection will have progressed beyond the gastroduodenal artery. In this area there is a risk that the duct of Santorini will be transected. Since the duodenal wall is free of inflammation in cases of this type, this structure may well be identifiable in which case it should be divided and ligated. If the duct of Santorini communicates with the duct of Wirsung, the pancreatic juice will then drain freely into the larger duct, and there should be no postoperative difficulty. In some cases, the duct of Santorini does not communicate with the main duct. In this event, despite the ligature, a pancreatic fistula may well develop. This will probably require a secondary operation to anastomose a Roux-Y segment of the jejunum to the transected duct for internal drainage. Fortunately, in most cases the two ducts do communicate.

Operative Technique

The technique for removing lesions of the cardia and fundus is described in Chap. 8. Distal gastrectomy in the usual case of antral carcinoma is performed by the same technique described for peptic ulcer (Chap. 15), except that additional duodenum may have to be resected. Frozen section examination should be performed on the distal margin of the duodenum in such cases. Omentectomy should be carried out, and the left gastric artery may be divided at its origin, as described in Chap. 19. Remove the lymph nodes along the left gastric, the gastroduodenal, the right gastric, and the right gastroepiploic arteries together with the gastrohepatic omentum along the lesser curve.

Lavage of the operative site with a dilute antibiotic solution helps to counteract bacterial contamination.

Postoperative Care

Postoperative care is identical to that following gastrectomy for peptic ulcer (Chap. 15), with the addition of intravenous hyperalimentation when indicated.

Complications

Complications are similar to those following gastrectomy for peptic ulcer (Chap. 15), but subphrenic and subhepatic sepsis is more common because of the increased bacterial contamination in carcinoma cases.

References

Cady B et al. (1977) Gastric cancer, contemporary aspects. Am J Surg 133:423

Chassin JL (1978) Esophagogastrectomy: data favoring end-to-side anastomosis. Ann Surg 188:22

Hoerr S (1973) Prognosis for carcinoma of the stomach. Surg Gynecol Obstet 137:205

Menguy R (1974) Surgical treatment of gastric adenocarcinoma. JAMA 228:1286

Nyhus LM, Wastell C (1977) Surgery of the stomach and duodenum, Little, Brown, Boston, p. 672

Paulino F, Roselli A (1973) Carcinoma of the stomach. Curr Probl Surg

Soga J et al. (1979) The role of lymphadenectomy in curvative surgery for gastric cancer. World J Surg 3:701

Spencer FC (1956) Ischemic necrosis of the remaining stomach following subtotal gastrectomy. Arch Surg 73:844

Thompson, NW (1963) Ischemic necrosis of proximal gastric remnant following subtotal gastrectomy. Surgery 54:434

19 Total Gastrectomy

Indications

Zollinger-Ellison syndrome

Malignant tumors arising from midportion of stomach and occupying more than two-thirds of the lesser curvature

Malignant tumors arising in proximal stomach, if more than 50% of stomach must be resected

Palliation in patients who have obstructing or bleeding tumor, provided that degree of metastasis is not massive and that primary tumor is not technically difficult to resect

On rare occasions, life-threatening hemorrhage from extensive erosive gastritis

Preoperative Preparation

Preoperative gastroscopic biopsy or lavage cytology should be positive for malignancy before a total gastrectomy is elected. Otherwise, the diagnosis should be confirmed by frozen section at surgery.

For malnourished patients, administer preoperative intravenous hyperalimentation.

Administer perioperative systemic antibiotics.

Carry out mechanical and antibiotic preparation of the colon if there is a possibility that the tumor has invaded the middle colic artery or the transverse colon.

Insert a nasogastric tube.

Pitfalls and Danger Points

1) Improper reconstruction of alimentary tract, which can lead to postoperative reflux alkaline esophagitis.

2) Erroneous diagnosis of malignancy: Patients have undergone total gastrectomy when surgeons have misdiagnosed a large posterior penetrating ulcer as a malignant tumor. Because benign gastric ulcer can be cured by relatively simple surgery, this error may have serious consequences for the patient. If preoperative gastroscopic biopsy has been negative, perform a gastrotomy and with a scalpel or a biopsy punch obtain a direct biopsy of edge of ulcer in four quadrants.

3) Inadequate anastomotic technique, resulting in leak or stricture.

4) Sepsis, either in wound or subhepatic and subphrenic spaces, due to contamination by gastric contents.

5) Failure to identify submucosal infiltration of carcinoma in esophagus or duodenum beyond the line of resection.

Operative Strategy

Exposure

If the primary lesion is a malignancy of the body of the stomach that does not invade the lower esophagus, a midline incision from the xiphocostal junction to a point 6–8 cm below the umbilicus may prove adequate for total gastrectomy if the Upper Hand or "chain" retractor is used to elevate the lower sternum. If the tumor is approaching the esophagogastric junction, it may be necessary to include 6–10 cm of lower esophagus in the specimen to circumvent submucosal infiltration by the tumor. In this case a left thoracoabdominal incision is indicated, as described in Chap. 8. No esophageal anastomosis should ever be performed unless there is excellent exposure.

Esophageal Anastomosis

We prefer an end-to-side esophagojejunal anastomosis because it permits invagination of the esophagus into the jejunum. This results in a lower incidence of leakage. With end-to-end esophagojejunostomy, invagination would result in constriction of the lumen.

The lumen of the anastomosis can be increased also if the anterior wall of the esophagus is left 1 cm longer than the posterior wall. This converts the anastomosis from a circular shape to an elliptical one, adding to its circumference.

The anastomotic technique requires close attention, for, according to Schrock and Way, two-thirds of the fatalities that followed total gastrectomies they did were caused by leakage, and one-fifth of all resections for cancer resulted in anastomotic disruption.

Prevention of Reflux Alkaline Esophagitis

An anastomosis between the end of the esophagus and the side of the jejunum combined with a side-to-side jejunojejunostomy (**Fig. 19–1**), results in a high incidence of *disabling* postoperative alkaline esophagitis, according to Scott et al. (1965), Schrock and Way, and Paulino and Roselli. This must be prevented by utilizing the Roux-Y principle in all cases. The distance between the esophagojejunal anastomosis and the jejunojejunal anastomosis must be 50 cm to prevent reflux of the duodenal contents into the esophagus. This is a far more important consideration than is the construction of a jejunal pouch for a reservoir. Although we have used the Hunt-Lawrence [as described by Scott et al. (1965)] and the Paulino pouches in good-risk patients, metabolic studies done by Scott et al. (1968) have not produced sufficient data to demonstrate their superiority over a single-limb esophagojejunostomy done by the Roux-Y principle. When a jejunal pouch is employed, we prefer to use a stapling technique for its construction in order to save time in an already lengthy operation. The technique described below was free of complications in nine cases studied.

Extent of the Operation

When performing a total gastrectomy for adenocarcinoma of the stomach, the surgeon must be aware that microscopic submucosal infiltration may occur in the esophagus as far as 10 cm proximal to a grossly visible tumor and occasionally well down into the duodenum. Frozen section microscopic examination of both the esophageal and duodenal ends of the specimen should be obtained in order to avoid leaving behind residual submucosal carcinoma. In Schrock's series, microscopic tumor was found at the esophageal or duodenal margin or both in 33% of patients.

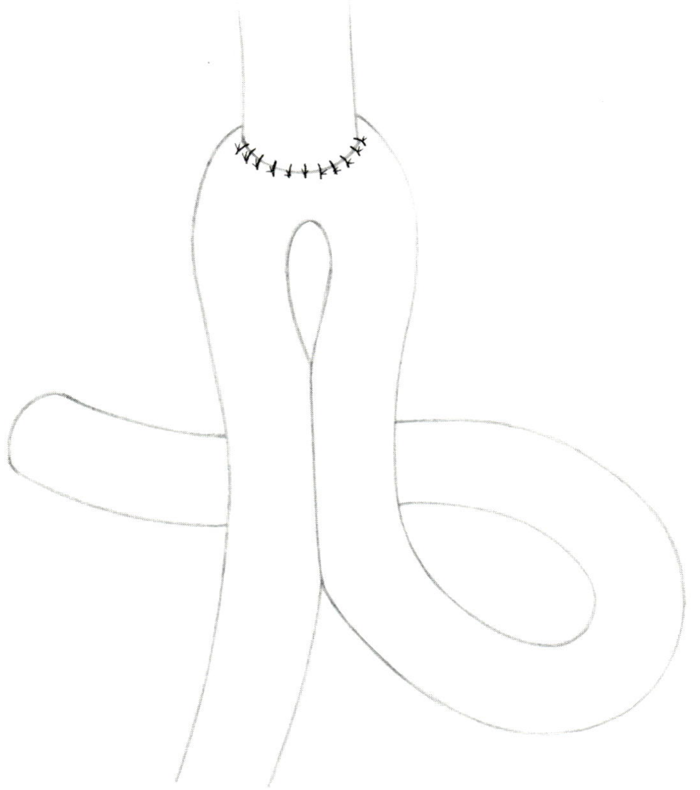

Fig. 19–1

The lymph nodes along the celiac axis should be swept up with the specimen when the left gastric artery is divided at its origin. The lymphatics along the hepatic artery also should be removed, along with those at the origin of the right gastroepiploic artery. Whether it is beneficial to skeletonize the hepatic artery and portal vein all the way to the hilus of the liver is not clear.

Routine resection of the body and tail of the pancreas increases the mortality rate from this operation because pancreatic complications can occur; at the same time it has not been proved that this additional step improves a patient's long-term survival. However, if the tail of the pancreas shows evidence of tumor invasion, then this portion of the pancreas should be included in the resection.

The anatomy of the structures involved in this operation can be seen in **Fig. 19–2**.

Ulcerated and necrotic gastric tumors may harbor virulent bacteria, so patients with these maladies should be prepared by being given preoperative intestinal antisepsis as well as prophylactic systemic antibiotics. This appears to be especially applicable to malignant lymphoma. The abdominal cavity should be irrigated with an antibiotic solution at intervals during the operation in order to minimize the effect of local contamination.

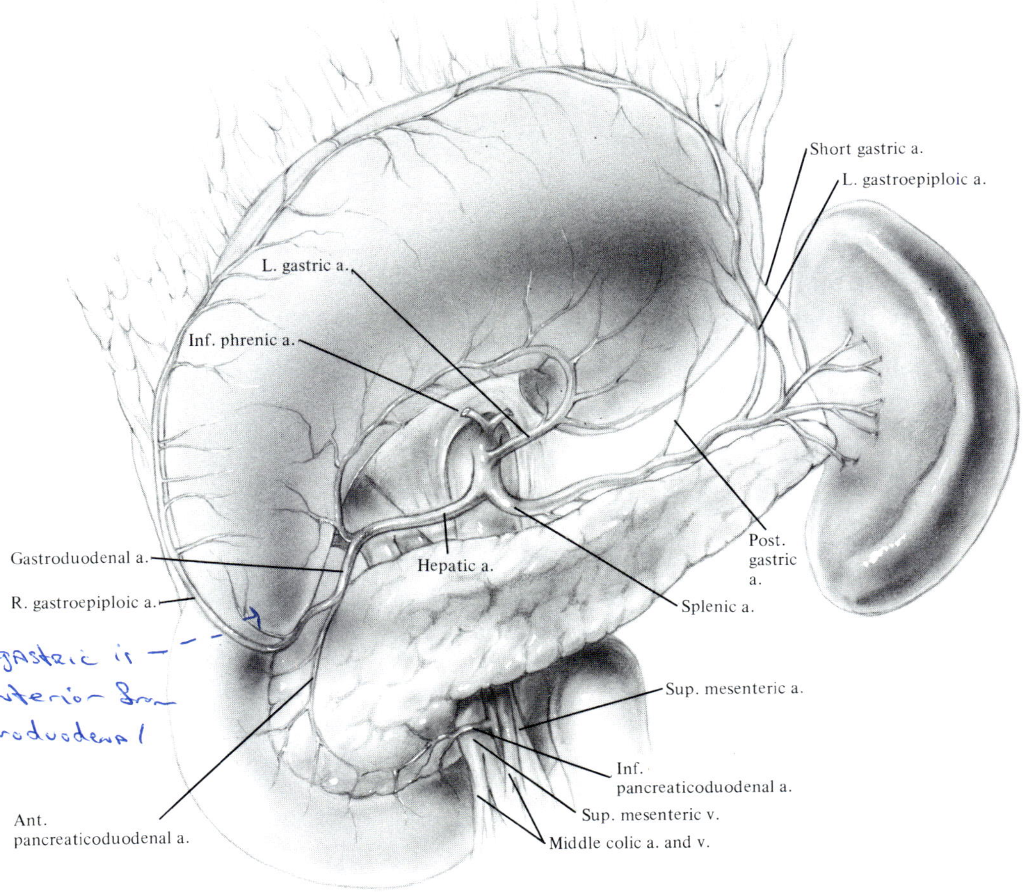

Fig. 19–2

Operative Technique

Incision and Exposure

In many cases adequate exposure is obtained by a midline incision from the xiphocostal junction to a point 6 cm below the umbilicus, along with the use of an Upper Hand or "chain" retractor. When the carcinoma approaches the esophagogastric junction, a left thoracoabdominal approach should be used.

Exploration and Determination of Operability

Tumors are considered nonresectable when there is posterior invasion of the aorta, the vena cava, or the celiac axis. Invasion of the body or tail of the pancreas is not a contraindication to operation; nor is invasion of the left lobe of the liver, as these structures can be included in the specimen if necessary.

When there is only a moderate degree of distant metastasis in the presence of marked symptomatology (obstruction or hemorrhage), a palliative resection may be indicated if it can be done safely.

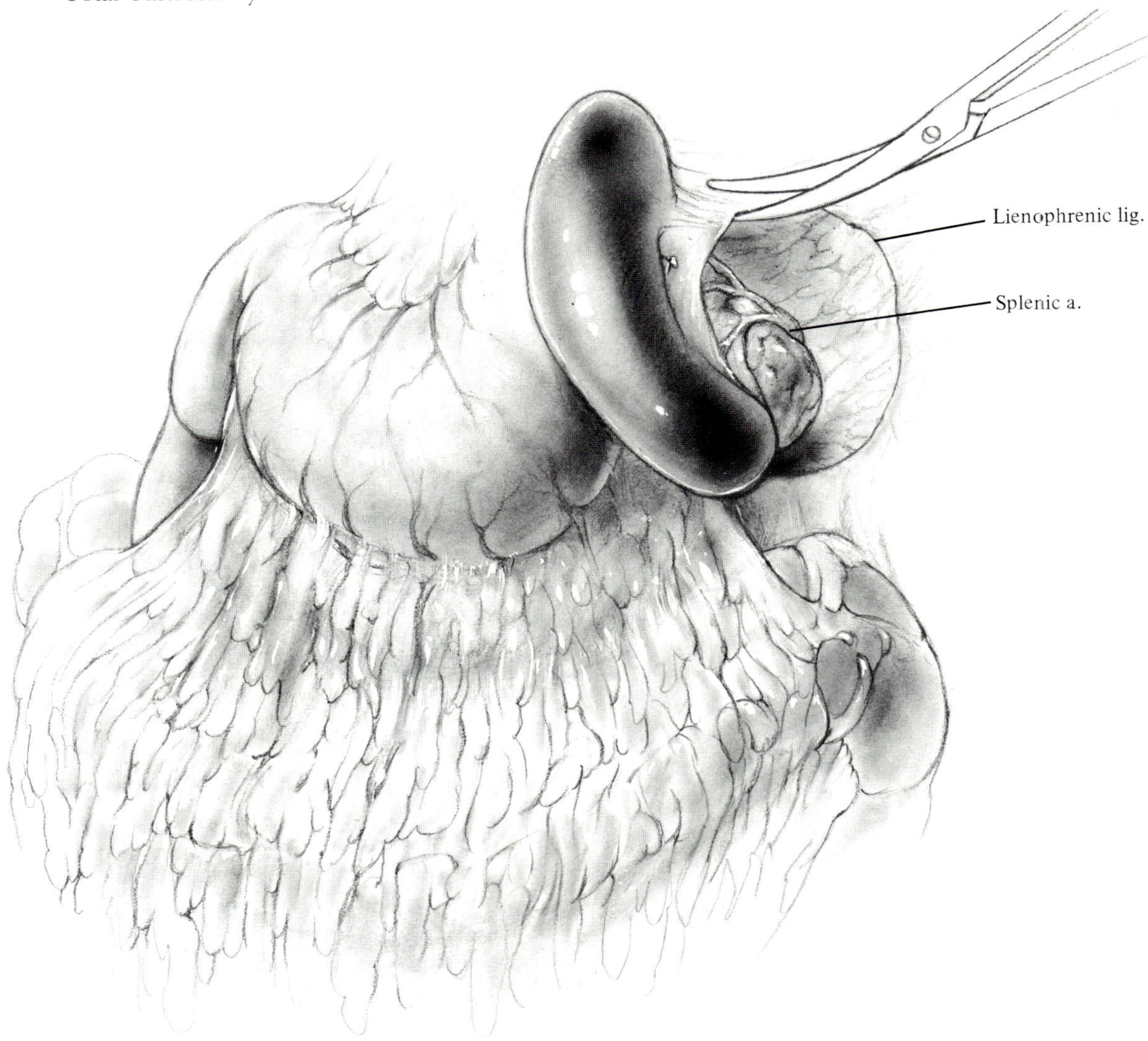

Fig. 19–3

Invasion of the root of the mesocolon, including the middle colic artery, does not contraindicate resection if leaving these structures attached to the specimen removes the tumor. This often requires the concomitant resection of a segment of the transverse colon. It is surprising that, in some patients, removing a short segment of the main middle colic artery does not impair the viability of the transverse colon, as long as there is good collateral circulation.

Splenectomy

With a scalpel or Metzenbaum scissors incise the avascular lienophrenic ligament that attaches the lateral aspect of the spleen to the undersurface of the diaphragm (**Fig. 19–3**). As this incision reaches the inferior pole of the spleen, divide the lienocolic ligament; the posterior surface of the pancreatic tail then can be seen. This can be elevated gently from the retroperitoneal space. Palpate the splenic artery near the distal end of the pancreas, encircle it with 2–0 cotton, and ligate it and the splenic vein. Divide these vessels between ligatures, releasing the tip of the pancreas from the hilus of the spleen. In-

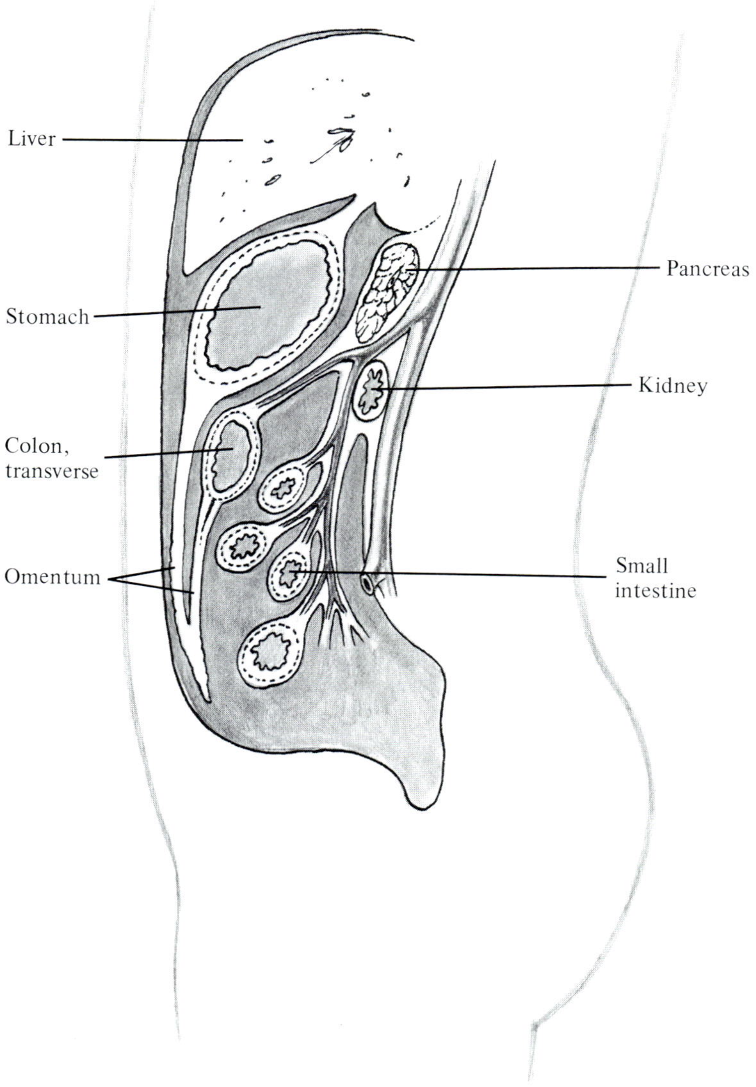

Fig. 19–4

cise a fold of posterior parietal peritoneum along the upper border of the body of the pancreas to separate the pancreas from the specimen. The spleen may be left attached to the greater curvature of the stomach, or it may be more convenient to divide and ligate the short gastric vessels and remove the spleen as a separate specimen. In the retroperitoneal dissection, expose the fascia of Gerota and the left adrenal gland. If there is evidence of tumor invasion, include these structures in the specimen.

Lift up omentum
Dissect posteriorly
to remove omentum from colon.

Omentectomy

Separate the entire gastrocolic omentum from the transverse colon by scalpel and scissors dissection through the avascular embryonic fusion plane, as seen in the coronal section of the abdomen in **Fig. 19–4**. Be alert to the difference in texture and color of the fat in the epiploic appendices of the colon and that of the omentum. Considerable bleeding will be

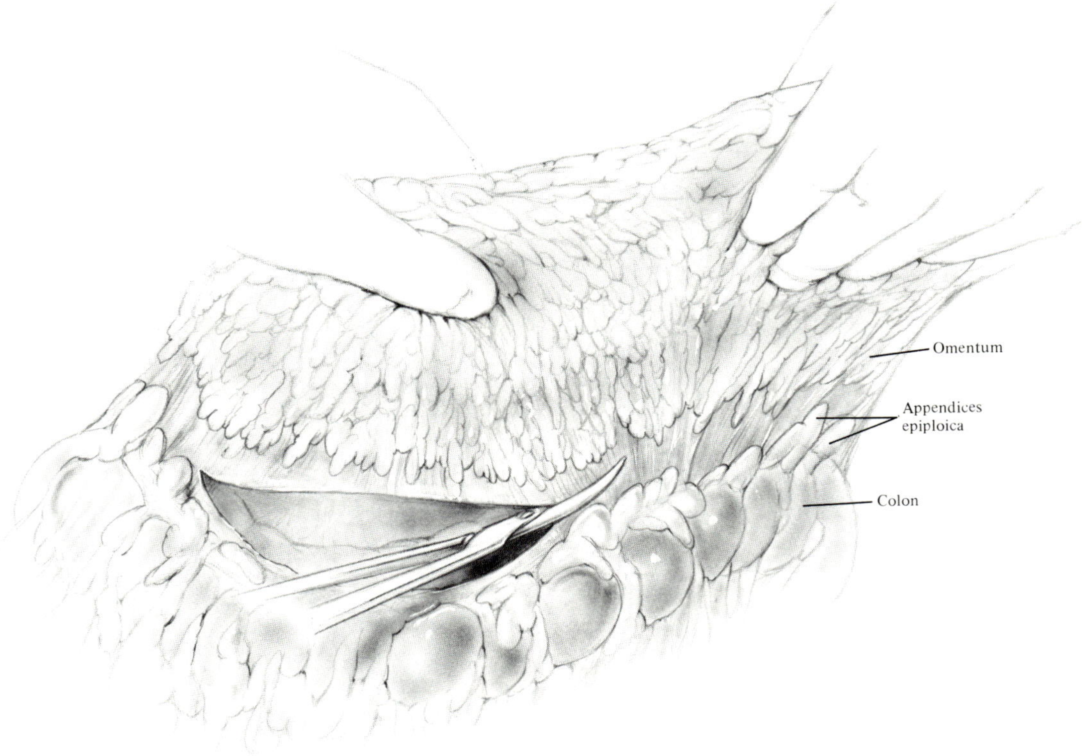

Fig. 19–5

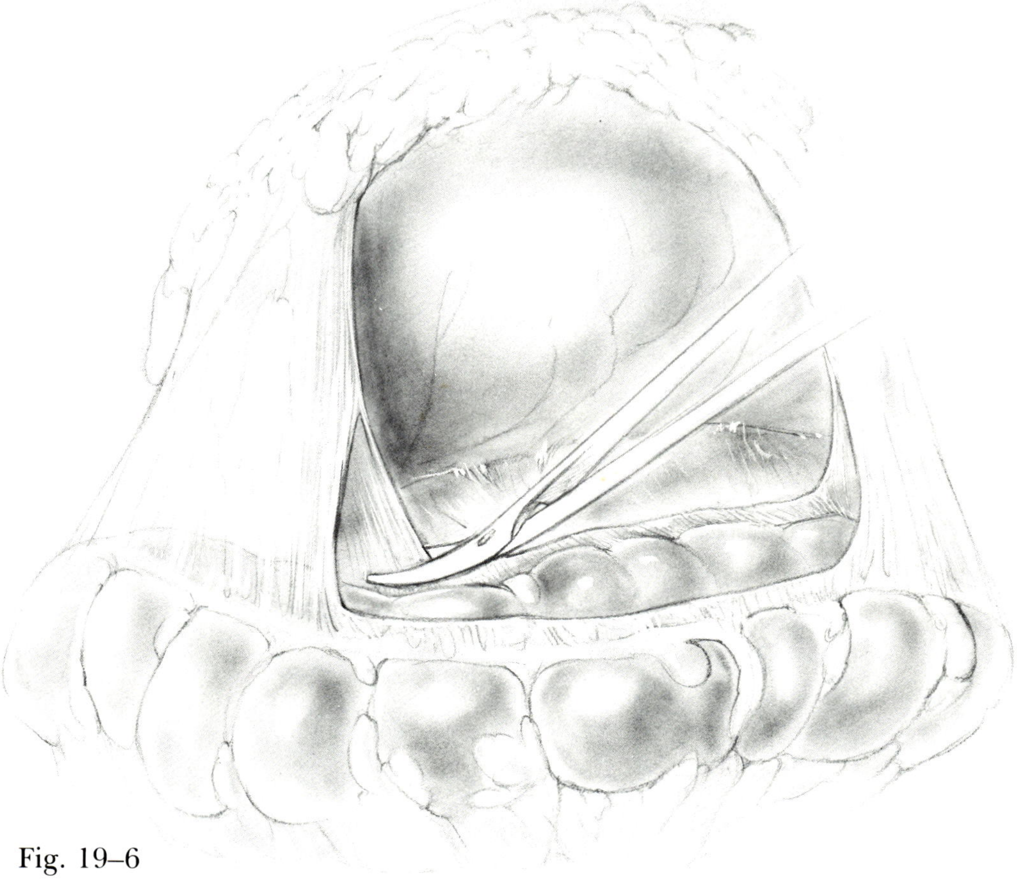

Fig. 19–6

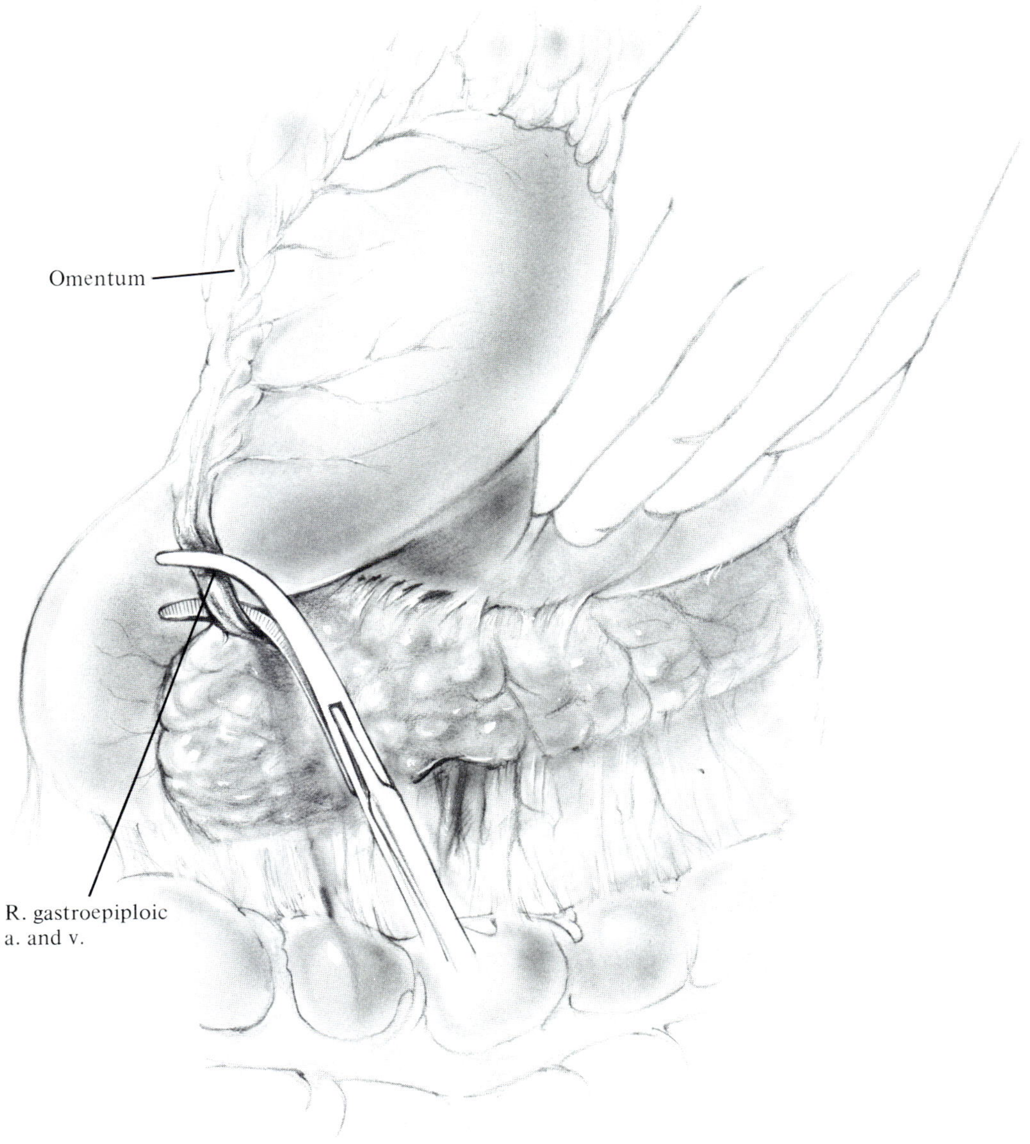

Fig. 19–7

avoided by keeping the plane of dissection between the appendices and omentum (**Fig. 19–5**). Next elevate the omentum from the transverse mesocolon (**Fig. 19–6**). Expose the anterior surfaces of the pancreas and duodenum, along with the origin of the right gastroepiploic vessels. Ligate the latter at their origin with 2–0 cotton and divide them, sweeping all adjacent lymph nodes toward the specimen (**Fig. 19–7**).

Pancreatic Resection

If the body and tail of the pancreas are to be resected, incise the peritoneum along the lower border of the pancreas. Ligate the splenic artery near its origin from the celiac axis and divide it. Trace the splenic vein to its junction with the portal vein, and ligate and divide it there. The inferior mesenteric vein enters the splenic near its termination. Divide and ligate this vessel also. If the pancreas is of average thickness, apply a TA–55 stapler

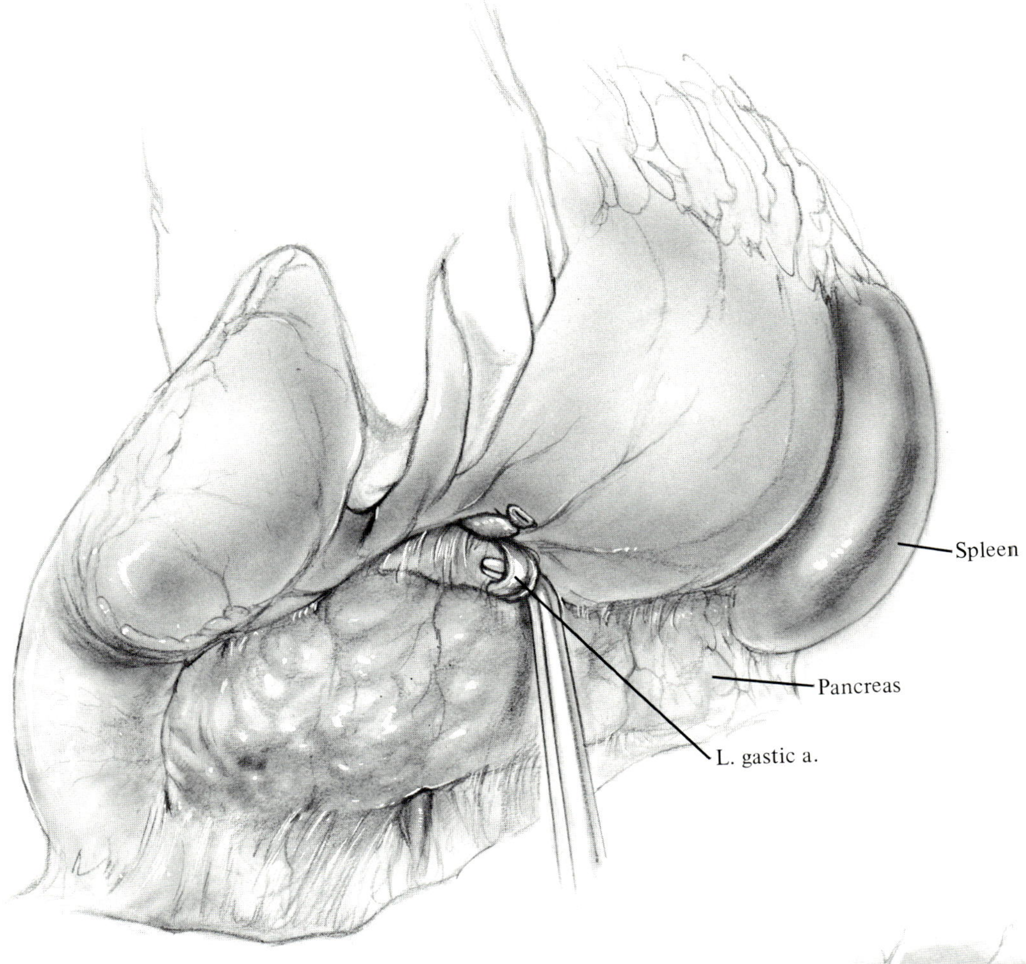

Fig. 19–8a

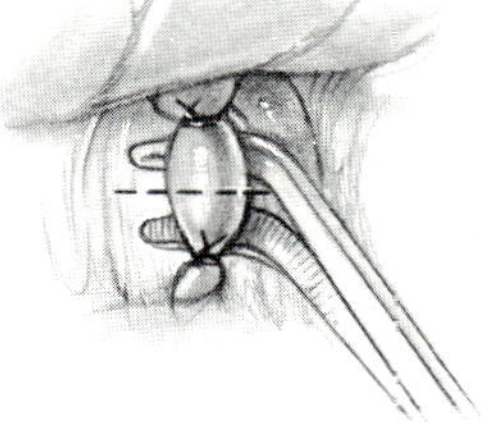

Fig. 19–8b

with 3.5 mm staples across the neck of pancreas and fire it, in the manner of Pachter et al. Incise the pancreas along the stapler and leave the tail of the pancreas attached to the specimen. If the body of pancreas is too thick to undergo stapling, even with 4.8 mm staples, divide the organ with a scalpel and close the cut end by overlapping interrupted mattress sutures of 3–0 Prolene. Occlude the pancreatic duct by an individual suture-ligature.

The pancreas should be resected only when invaded by tumor.

Celiac Axis Dissection and Division of Left Gastric Vessels

With the greater curvature of the stomach elevated and retracted toward the patient's right, it is a simple matter to palpate the left gastric artery as it travels from the region of the aorta, anteriorly, to meet the lesser curvature of the stomach. When there is tumor in this area, either the splenic or hepatic artery may be followed in a proximal direction. This will lead to the celiac axis and to the origin of the left gastric. By dissecting the areolar and lymphatic tissue away, the artery may

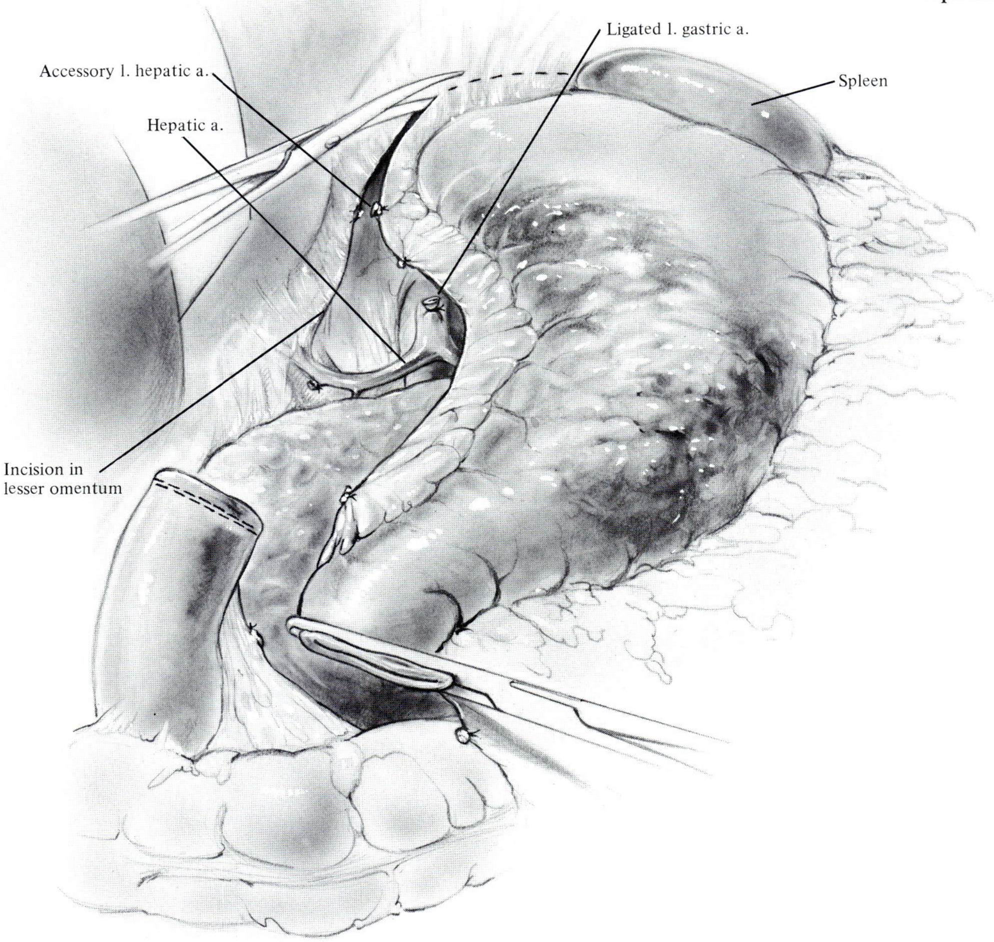

Fig. 19–9

be skeletonized (**Fig. 19–8**). A blunt-tipped Mixter right-angle clamp is very helpful in delineating the circumference of the artery. Use the clamp to pass 2–0 cotton ligatures around the vessel. After it has been doubly ligated, divide it. The coronary vein, which is situated just caudal to the artery, often is identified first in the course of the dissection. This, too, should be divided and ligated, and the lymphatic tissue swept toward the specimen. At the conclusion of this step, the superior border of the adjacent pancreas and the anterior surface of the celiac axis and the aorta should be free of lymphatic tissue.

Hepatic Artery Node Dissection

Make an incision in the peritoneum overlying the common hepatic artery as it leaves the celiac axis. Carry this incision down to the origin of the gastroduodenal artery. There are lymph nodes overlying the hepatic artery; dissect them toward the lesser curve of the gastric specimen, leaving the artery skeletonized (**Fig. 19–9**). If desirable, the lymph node dissection may be pursued to the hilus of the liver by skeletonizing the hepatic artery, portal vein, and common bile duct. Adequate data are not yet available to indicate how extensive a lymph node dissection should be done. Consequently, we do not routinely extend the hepatic artery dissection beyond the origin of the gastroduodenal.

Suspicious nodes in the subpyloric region and the superior margin of pancreas should be excised and the splenic artery should be skeletonized up to the distal end of the pancreas.

Division of Duodenum

Divide and ligate the right gastric artery. Perform a Kocher maneuver, and if the malignancy involves the distal stomach dissect the duodenum from the anterior surface of the pancreas for a distance of 5 cm. Extensive duodenal dissection is not necessary when the distal antrum is free of tumor.

If a stapled closure of the duodenum is elected, apply the TA–55 Auto Suture stapler to the duodenal stump. Generally, 4.8 mm staples are used. Fire the stapler and apply an Allen clamp to the specimen side of the duodenum. Divide the duodenum flush with the stapling device, as in Fig. 15–45. Ligate the distal end of the specimen with umbilical tape behind the Allen clamp and remove the clamp. Cover the distal end of the specimen with a sterile rubber glove, which should be fixed in place with an additional umbilical tape ligature.

When it is elected to suture the duodenal stump, the technique illustrated in Figs. 15–23, 15–24, and 15–25 should be followed.

Dissection of the Esophagocardiac Junction: Vagotomy

After the triangular ligament has been divided, retract the left lobe of the liver to the patient's right and incise the peritoneum overlying the abdominal esophagus. Using a peanut dissector, dissect away the esophagus from the right and left branches of the diaphragmatic crux. Then encircle the esophagus with the index finger and perform a bilateral truncal vagotomy, as described in Chap. 10. Incise the peritoneum overlying the right crux (Fig. 19–9). Identify the cephalad edge of the gastrohepatic ligament, which contains an accessory left hepatic branch of the left gastric artery. Divide this structure between clamps at a point close to the liver, thus completing the division of the gastrohepatic ligament.

Pass the left hand behind the esophagocardiac junction, a maneuver that will delineate the avascular gastrophrenic and any remaining esophagophrenic ligaments, all of which should be divided (**Fig. 19–10**). This frees the posterior wall of the stomach. In order to minimize further spill of neoplastic cells into the esophageal lumen, occlude the esophagogastric junction with umbilical tape or an application of staples with the TA–55.

Preparation of Roux-Y Jejunal Segment

After identifying the ligament of Treitz, elevate the proximal jejunum from the abdominal cavity and inspect the mesentery to determine how it will reach the apex of the abdominal cavity for the esophagojejunal anastomosis. In some patients who have lost considerable weight before the operation, the jejunum will reach the esophagus without the need to divide anything but the marginal artery. In patients whose jejunal mesentery is short, it may be necessary to divide several arcade vessels. Transillumination is a valuable aid in dissecting the mesentery without undue trauma.

Generally, the point of division of the jejunum is about 15 cm distal to the ligament of Treitz, between the second and third arcade vessels. Make an incision in the mesentery across the marginal vessels, and divide and ligate them with 2–0 cotton. Divide and ligate one to three additional arcade vessels to provide an ade-

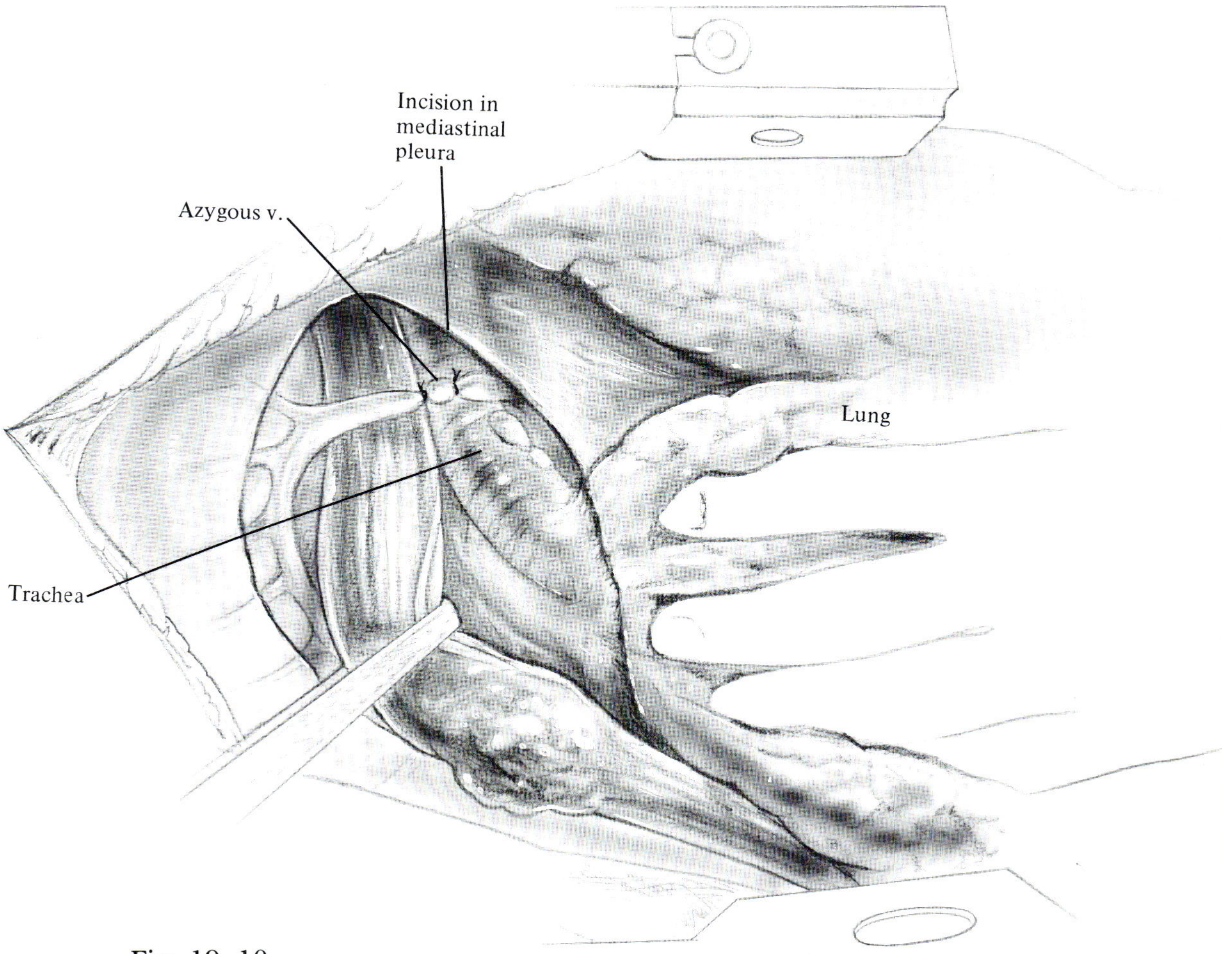

Fig. 19–10

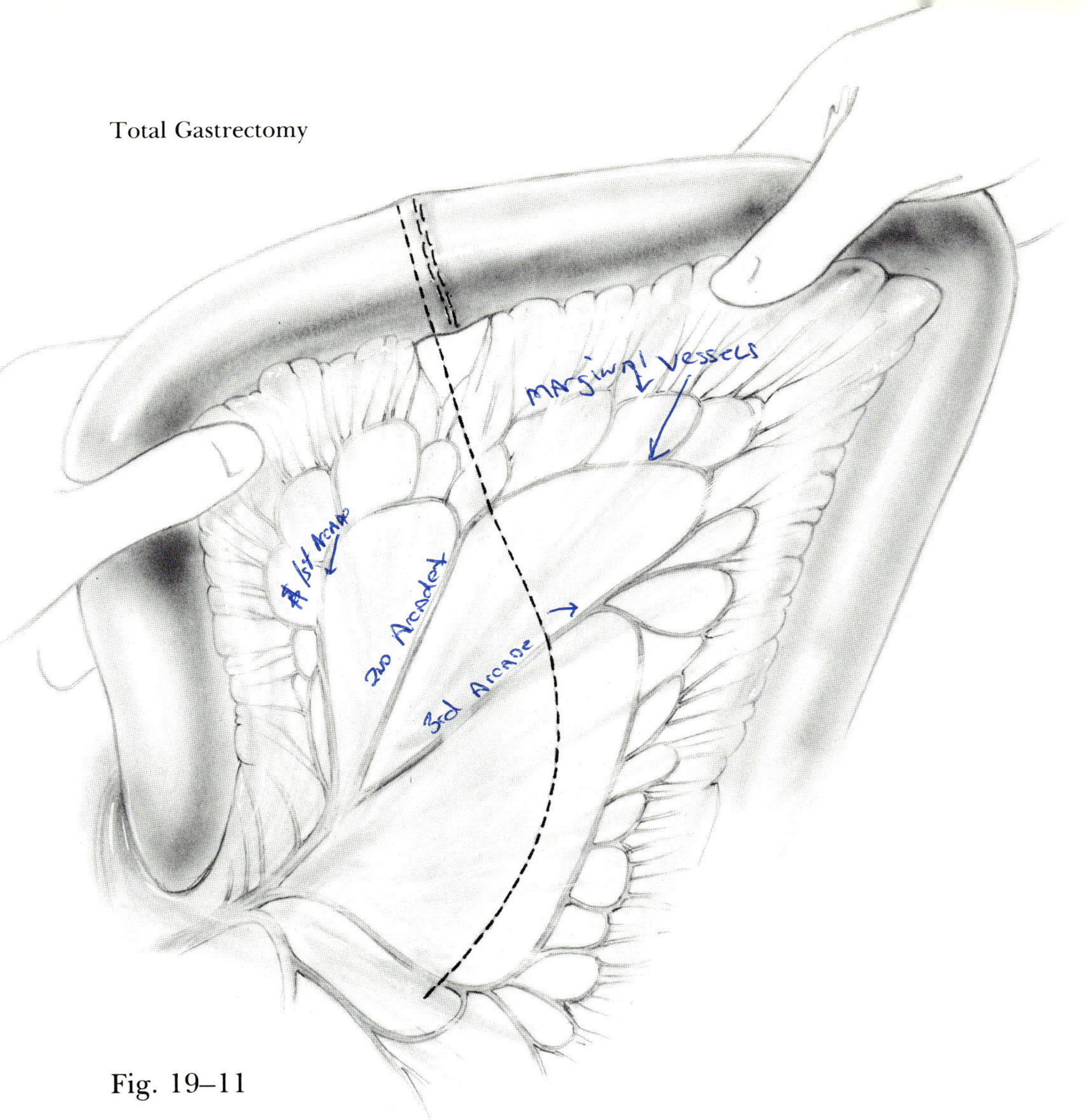

Fig. 19–11

quate length of the jejunum to reach the esophagus without tension (**Fig. 19–11**).

Apply a TA–55 stapler to the point on the jejunum previously selected for division. Fire the stapler. Apply an Allen clamp just *proximal* to the stapler and divide the jejunum flush with the stapler. Lightly electrocoagulate the everted edge and remove the stapler.

Next make a 3–4 cm incision in the avascular portion of the transverse mesocolon to the left of the middle colic artery. Deliver the stapled end of the jejunum through the incision in the mesocolon to the region of the esophagus. After the jejunal segment is properly positioned, suture the defect in the mesocolon to the wall of the jejunum in order to prevent herniation later.

Whenever the mesenteric dissection for the Roux-Y offers difficulty or threatens the blood supply of the jejunum, this step may be simplified by resecting a segment of the jejunum (**Fig. 19–12**). This technique avoids the division of any arcade blood vessels.

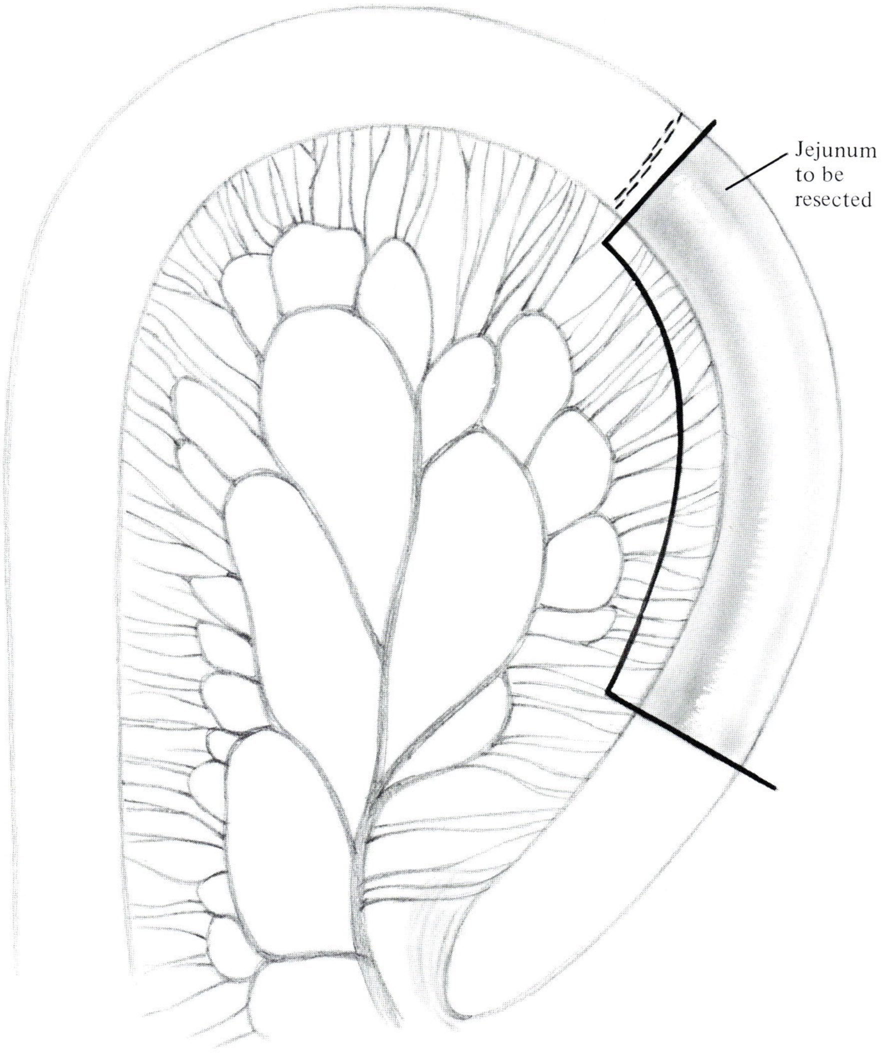

Fig. 19–12

End-to-Side Esophagojejunostomy

For reasons discussed in Chap. 8, we prefer an anastomosis of the end-to-side type. The anticipated site of the esophageal transection should be 6–10 cm above the proximal margin of the visible tumor. If the diaphragmatic hiatus is excessively large, narrow it with one or two 2–0 cotton sutures (**Fig. 19–13**). Then insert several interrupted 3–0 cotton sutures between the undersurface of the diaphragm and the posterior wall of the jejunum to prevent tension on the anastomosis caused by gravity. The sutures should be placed fairly close to the point at which the mesentery meets the jejunum, so as to preserve the antimesenteric border for anastomosis.

Before beginning to construct the anastomosis, mark the exact site of the anticipated jejunal incision by making a scratch with a scalpel along the antimesenteric border of the jejunum. This will serve as a guide for the insertion of the first layer of esophagojejunal sutures. Then place the specimen on the patient's chest. This will expose the posterior wall of the esophagus for the first layer of anasto-

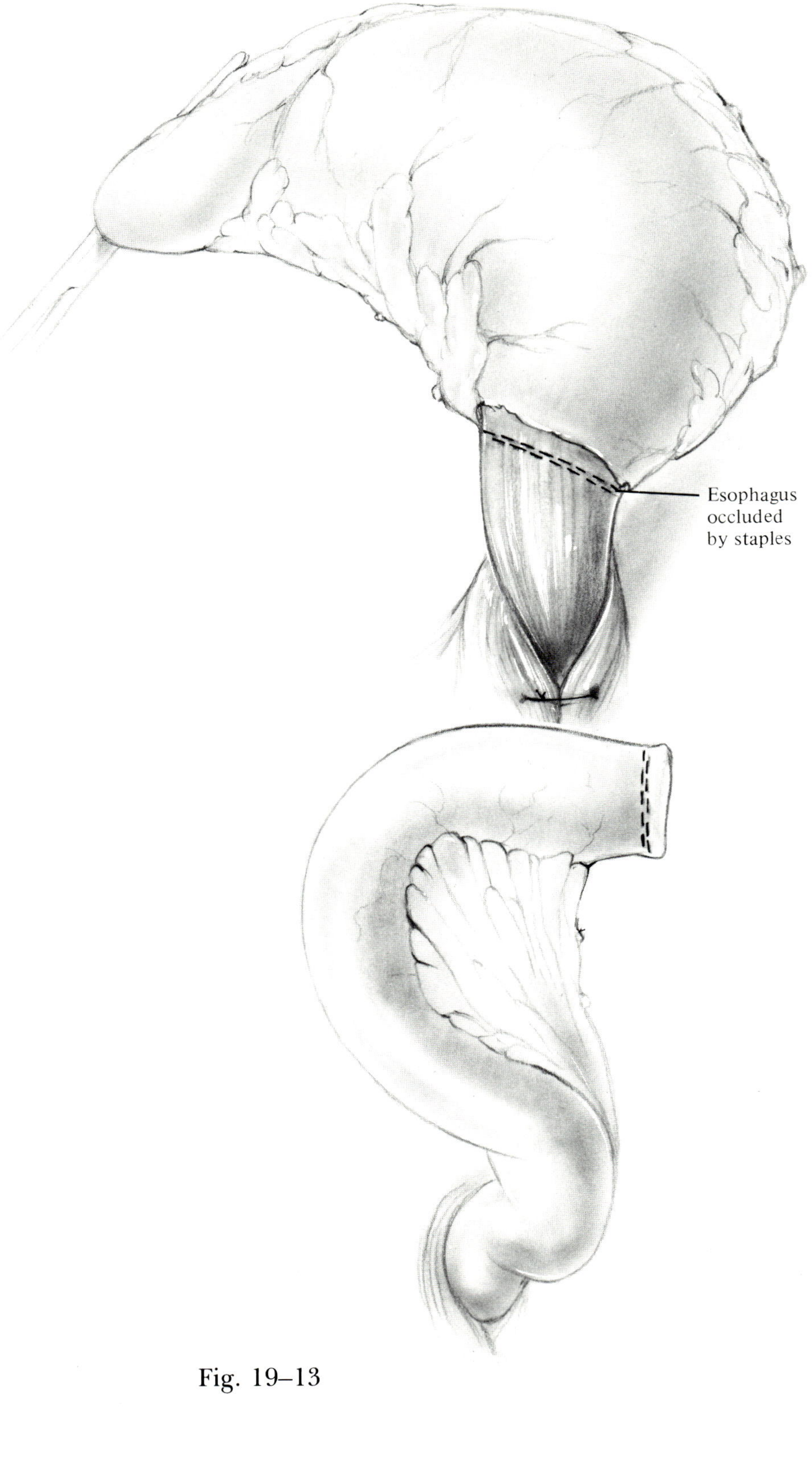

Fig. 19–13

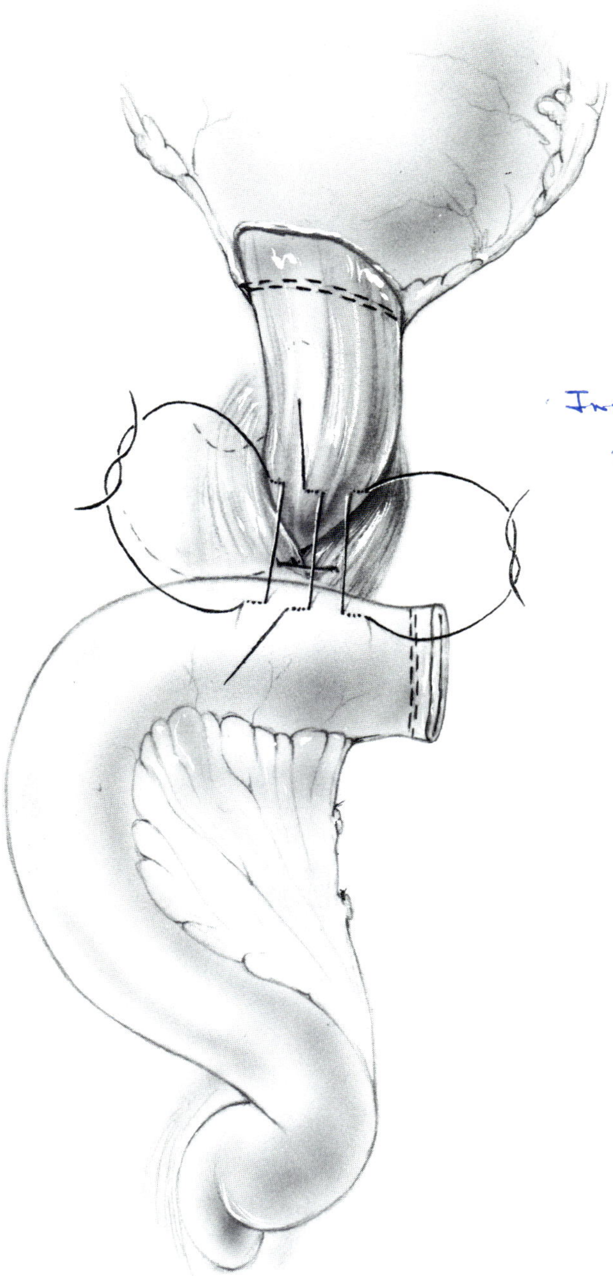

Insert Transverse suture into esophagus.

Fig. 19–14

motic sutures. Place a 4–0 atraumatic cotton Cushing suture beginning at the right lateral portion of the esophagus. With the same needle take a bite at the right lateral margin of the jejunal scratch mark. Place a similar suture at the left lateral margins of the esophagus and jejunum. Apply hemostats to each suture, as none will be tied until the suture line has been completed (**Fig. 19–14**). Note that the anticipated incision in the jejunum will be slightly longer than the diameter of the esophagus.

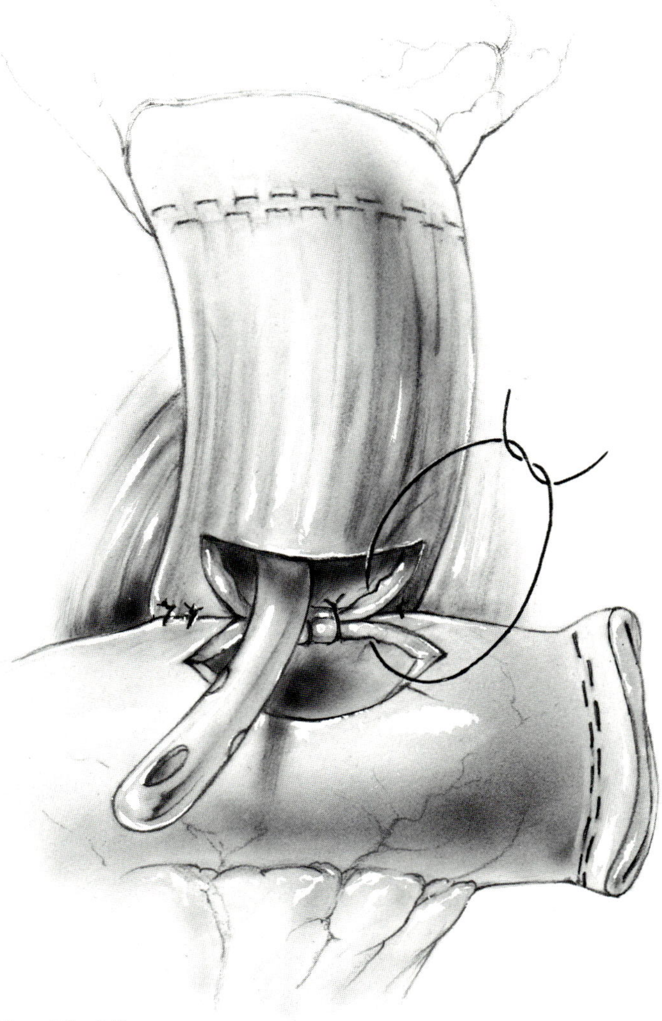

Fig. 19–15

With three or four additional Cushing sutures of 4–0 cotton, complete the posterior seromuscular layer of the anastomosis by successive bisection (see Figs. B–22 and B–23). After inserting the sutures, but before tying them, it is helpful to divide the posterior wall of the esophagus. Do this in a transverse manner, using a scalpel, until the mucosa has been transected. Complete the incision with a Metzenbaum scissors, leaving the anterior wall of esophagus intact. Now tie and cut the sutures, but leave the right and left lateralmost sutures long, with the identifying hemostats attached.

Make an incision in the antimesenteric border of the jejunum, as previously marked. If there appears to be considerable redundant mucosa, this may be excised with a Metzenbaum scissors. Control excessive bleeding with 4–0 PG suture-ligatures or careful electrocoagulation. Now approximate the posterior mucosal layers by interrupted sutures of atraumatic 4–0 PG, with the knots tied inside the lumen (**Fig. 19–15**). Instruct the anesthesiologist to pass the nasogastric tube farther down the esophagus. When the tube appears in the esophageal orifice, guide it down the jejunum.

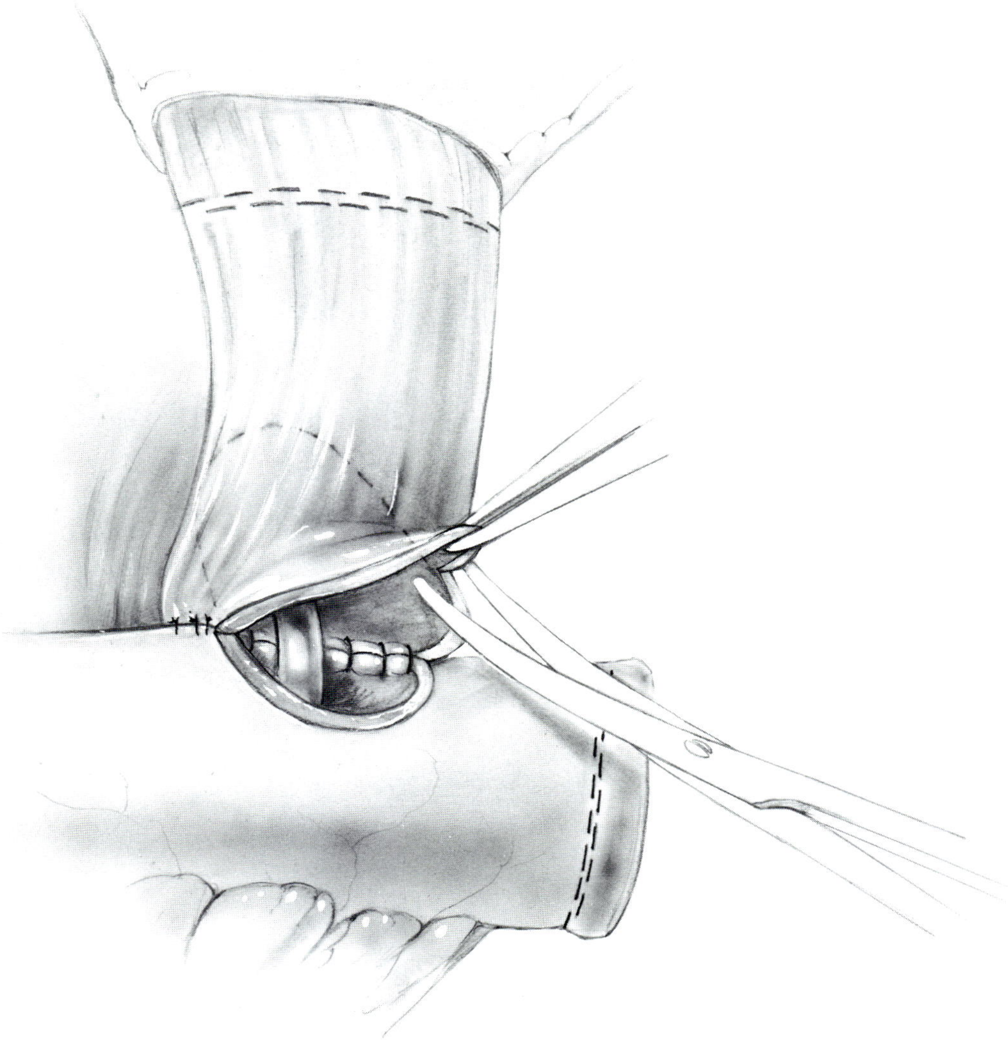

Fig. 19–16

Divide the remaining esophagus so that the anterior wall is 1 cm longer than the already anastomosed posterior wall (**Figs. 19–16, 19–17, 19–18, 19–19**). Remove the specimen and ask the pathologist to perform a frozen section examination of both the proximal and distal margins. If the frozen section examination is positive for malignancy, further excision is indicated.

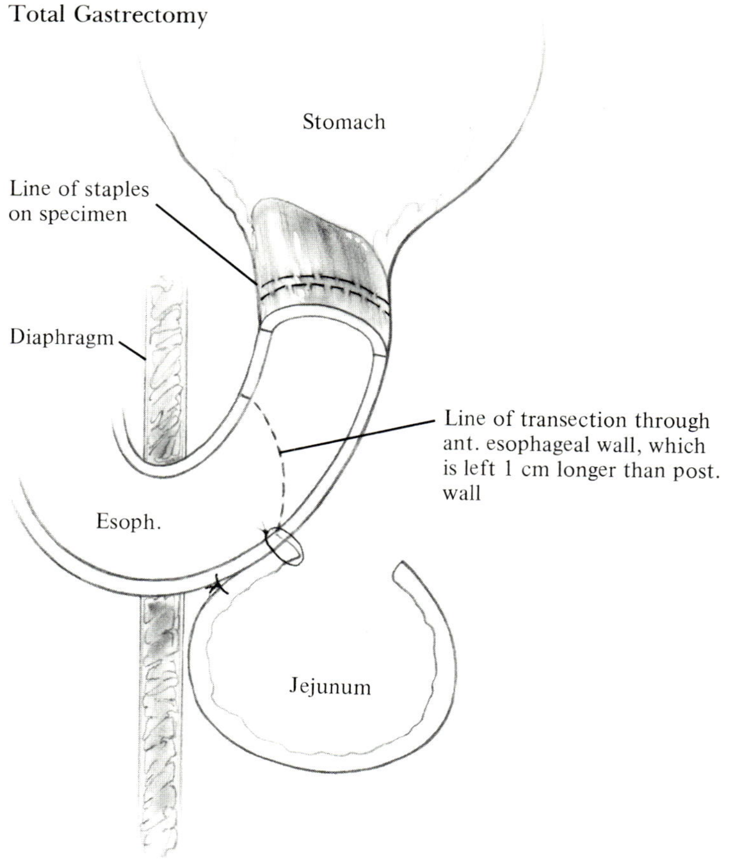

Fig. 19–17

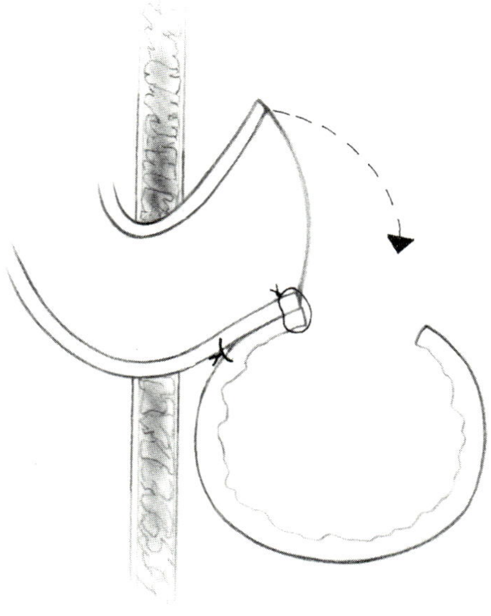

Fig. 19–18

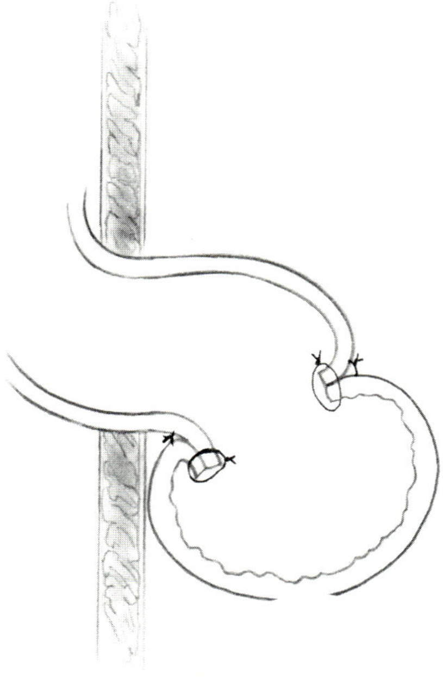

Fig. 19–19

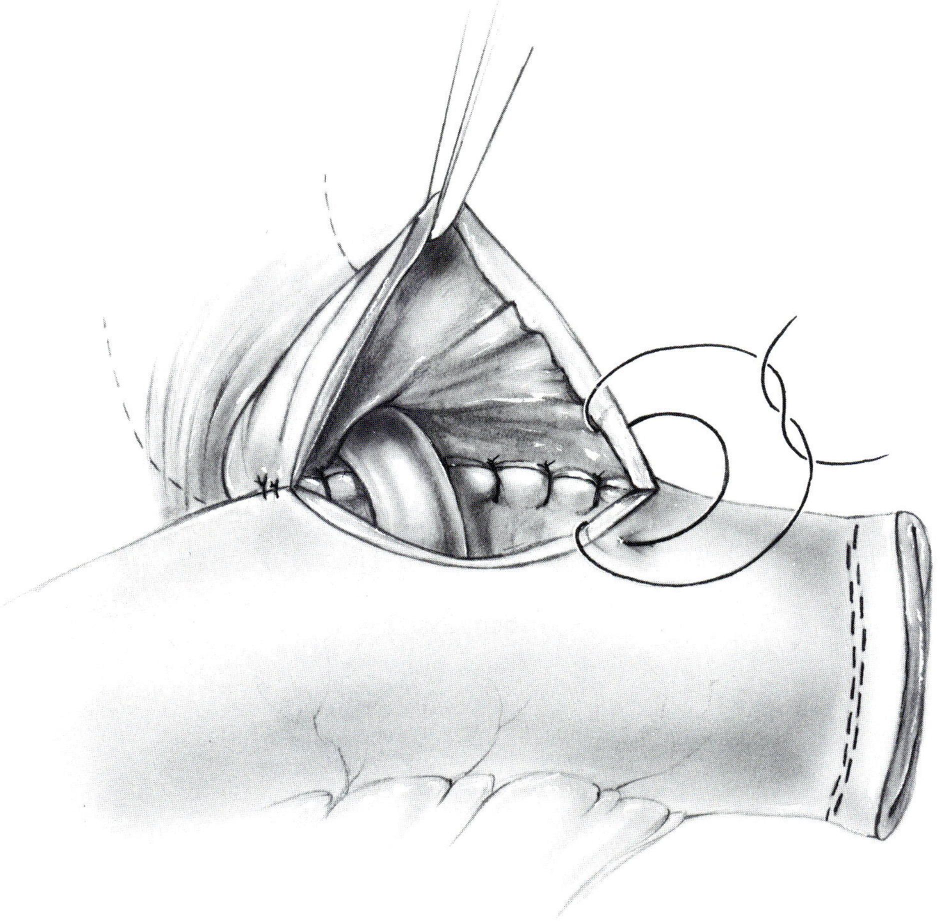

Fig. 19–20

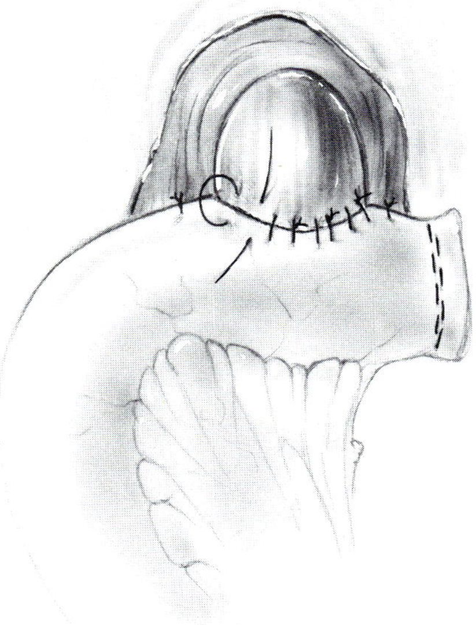

Fig. 19–21

Approximate and invert the anterior mucosal layer by 4–0 PG atraumatic sutures, interrupted, with the knots tied inside the lumen (**Fig. 19–20**). If it is difficult to invert the mucosa by this technique, the procedure may be accomplished with interrupted "seromucosal" sutures of 4–0 PG, 4–5 mm wide, inserted so as to include the cut end of the esophageal muscularis and mucosa (Fig. B–16).

Complete the final anastomotic layer by inserting interrupted 4–0 cotton Cushing sutures to approximate the outer layers of the esophagus and jejunum (**Fig. 19–21**). Each suture should encompass a bite of about 5 mm of esophagus and of jejunum. The peritoneum overlying the diaphragmatic hiatus can now be brought

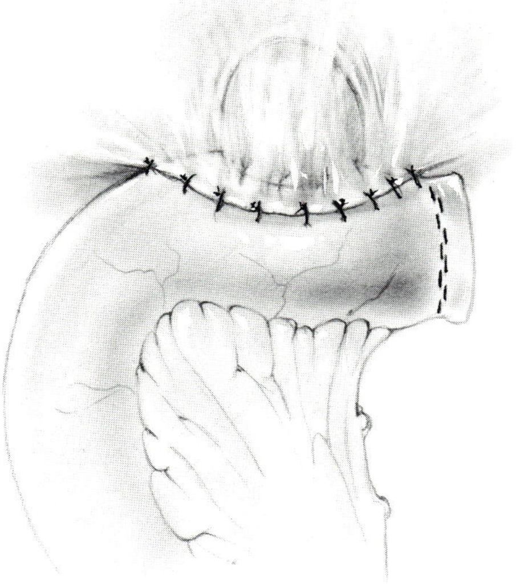

Fig. 19–22

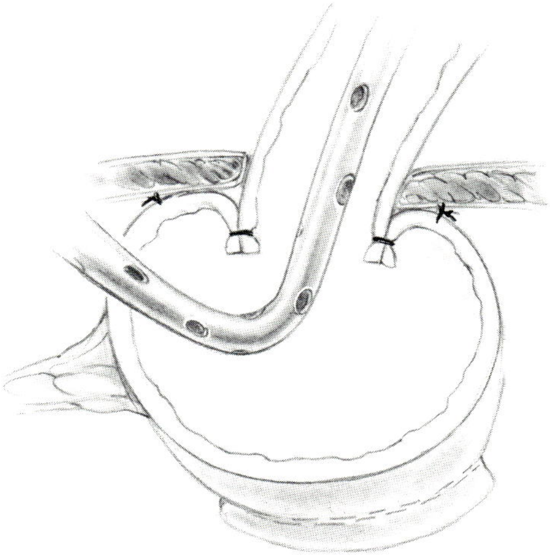

Fig. 19–23

down over the anastomosis. Attach it to the anterior wall of the jejunum by several interrupted 4–0 cotton stitches (**Fig. 19–22**). A sagittal section of the completed anastomosis can be seen in **Fig. 19–23**.

On occasion the esophagus will appear to be unusually narrow, secondary either to spasm or atrophy. In this case *gentle* digital dilatation by the surgeon before constructing the anastomosis may serve to accomplish a somewhat larger anastomotic lumen than would otherwise be the case. If desired, it is possible to perform the anastomosis over a 40F Hurst or Maloney esophageal bougie instead of the nasogastric tube.

The area should be irrigated intermittently with an antibiotic solution.

Construction of Stapled Substitute Gastric Pouch

Experienced surgeons such as Scott et al. (1965) and Paulino and Roselli believe that the Hunt-Lawrence type pouch may be advantageous, so we shall describe this technique. To save operating time we developed a staple technique for the construction of this pouch. The technique has proved to be rapid and safe.

Draw the transverse colon in a cephalad direction and inspect the proximal jejunum. Select a segment that will reach most easily to the esophagus and pass this segment through an incision in the transverse mesocolon. The afferent loop of the jejunum is generally placed to the patient's left and the efferent loop to the patient's right. Sufficient jejunum (about 50 cm) should be delivered into the supramesocolic space to provide for an end-to-side esophagojejunal anastomosis and then for a side-to-side jejunojejunostomy about 15 cm in length. When the proper amount of jejunum has been laid out in the upper abdomen, select a point for division on the afferent limb of the jejunum. Divide the mesentery of the jejunum for a short distance. Then apply a TA–55 stapler to the jejunum and fire it. Apply an Allen clamp to the jejunum proximal to the stapler and divide the jejunum flush with the stapler. Lightly electrocoagulate the everted mucosa on the stapler. Pass the segment of the jejunum grasped by the Allen clamp down through the incision in the mesocolon, to be used later for the end-to-side

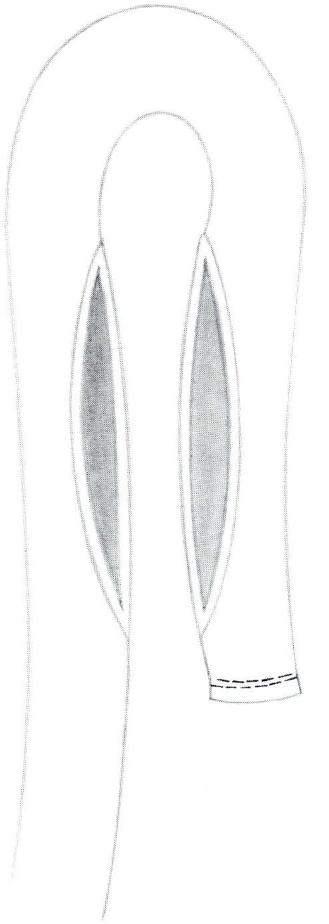

Fig. 19–24

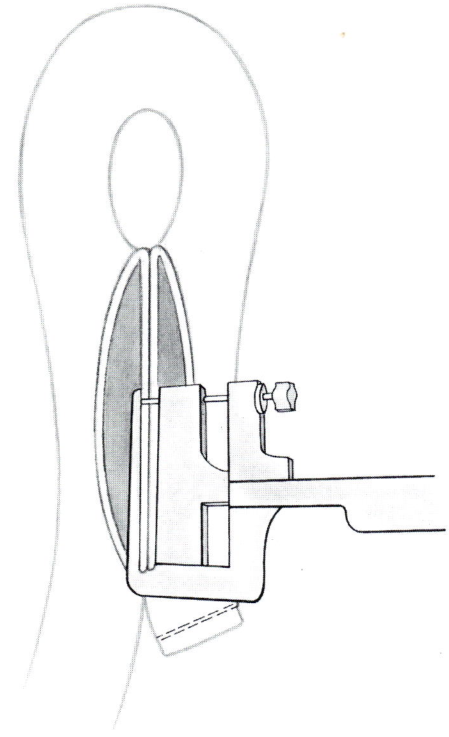

Fig. 19–25

jejunojejunostomy. Most of the time it will not be necessary to divide a single major arcade vessel in the mesentery to accomplish this step.

Now construct a side-to-side anastomosis between the antimesenteric margins of the afferent and efferent limbs of the jejunum. A distance of 8 cm should be left between the anticipated site of the esophagojejunostomy and the beginning of the side-to-side jejunojejunostomy. The first step in the latter procedure is to make a long incision—approximately 16 cm—through the antimesenteric wall of the ascending limb of the jejunum. Make an incision of the identical length through the antimesenteric wall of the descending limb of the jejunum (**Fig. 19–24**). Continue this incision within 1 cm of the closed, stapled end of the ascending jejunum. Apply multiple Allis clamps to the posterior cut edges of both limbs of the jejunum to approximate them. Apply a TA–90 stapling device, loaded with 3.5 mm staples, deep to the Allis clamps to accomplish approximately half of the posterior layer of the jejunojejunostomy. Rotate into place the thumb screw that aligns the TA–90 device. Tighten the TA–90 to the proper guidelines and fire it (**Fig. 19–25**). Excise the redundant mucosa superficial to the TA–90 and electrocoagulate the mucosa. Remove the TA–90 and apply additional Allis clamps to the remaining posterior walls of the jejunum. Make certain to apply one of the Allis clamps so that *the previously applied line of staples will be crossed by the second application of the TA–90.* Apply the TA–90 stapler, adjust it, and fire (**Fig. 19–26**); this completes the posterior anastomosis (**Fig. 19–27**). Again excise redundant mucosa.

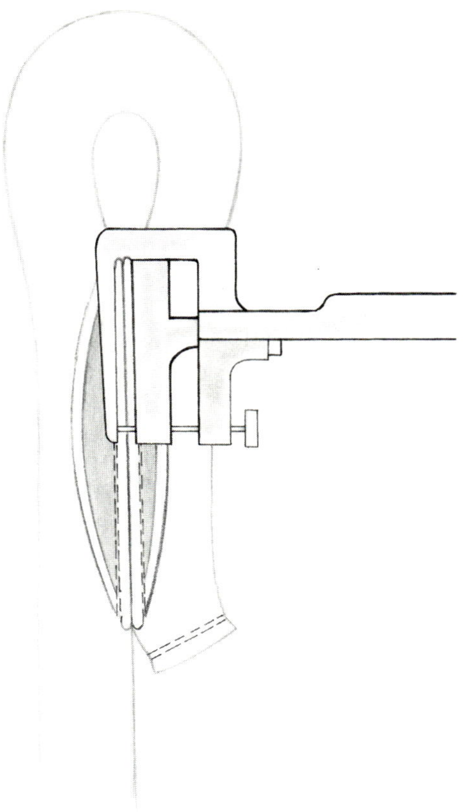

Fig. 19–26

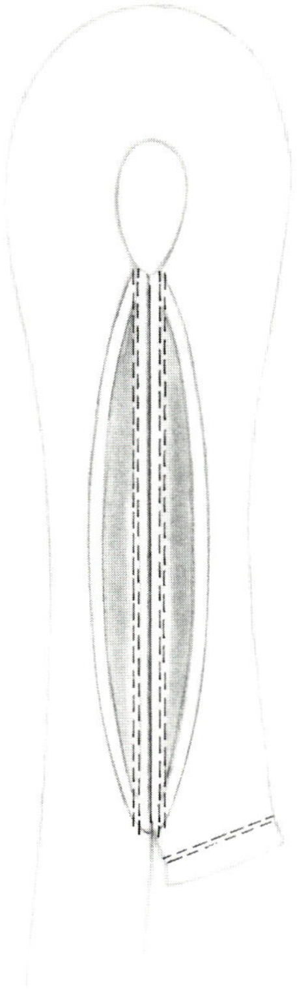

Fig. 19–27

Bleeding points may be controlled with electrocoagulation or suture-ligatures of 4–0 PG. On rare occasions the posterior line of staples may bleed enough to require a continuous locked 4–0 PG suture to the mucosa. Although the posterior anastomosis has been constructed in an inverting fashion, the anterior walls of the jejunum should be joined in an *everting* fashion by applying Allis clamps to approximate the anterior layers of the jejunum, mucosa to mucosa.

Be sure to apply an Allis clamp to the serosal surface of the proximal termination of the *posterior* TA–90 staple line, so that the staple line will be included in the next application of staples and will form the anterior anastomosis. Again apply the TA–90 deep to the Allis clamps, adjust, and fire (**Fig. 19–28**). Follow this by excising the redundant tissue.

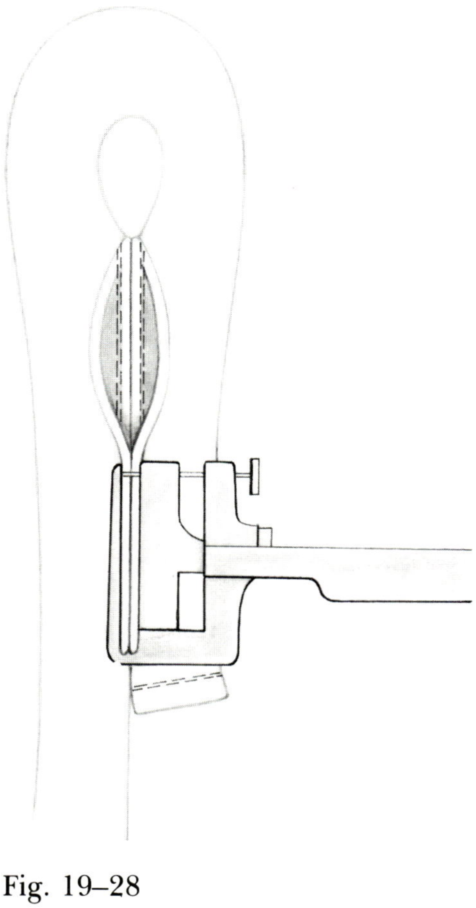

Fig. 19–28

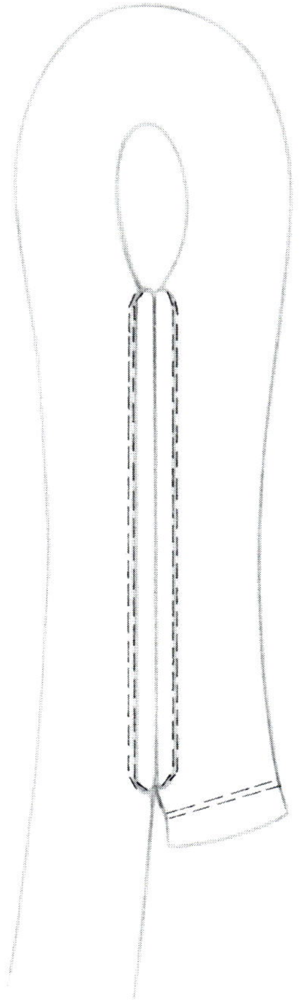

Fig. 19–29

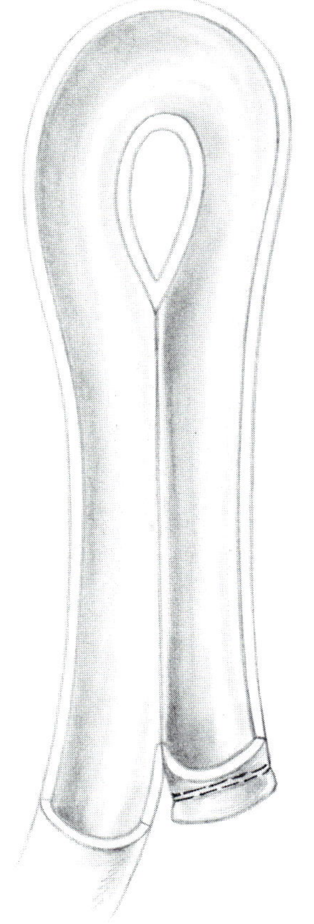

Fig. 19–30

The final step in the anastomosis begins with the application of an Allis clamp to the serosal surface of the distal margin of the *posterior* line of staples. Apply a second Allis clamp to the proximal margin of the remaining defect in the anastomosis so as to make the final TA–90 staple line include both terminations of the everted lines of staples. Apply the stapler deep to the Allis clamps, adjust, and fire.

Again, excise the redundant tissue flush with the stapling device and lightly electrocoagulate the mucosa (**Fig. 19–29**). After removing the TA–90 stapler, transfix or electrocoagulate any bleeding points. *Carefully inspect the entire staple line* to catch technical errors or mechanical failures in the closure of the staples. Then ask the anesthesiologist to inject 400–500 ml of a methylene blue solution into the newly fashioned gastric pouch so that any possible point of leakage may be detected. **Fig. 19–30** illustrates the pouch in coronal section.

Now construct an end-to-side esophagojejunal anastomosis by the suture method illustrated in Figs. 19–14 through 19–23.

Anastomose the divided proximal segment of the jejunum, which is being held by an Allen clamp, to the side of the descending limb of the jejunum at a point *50 cm from the distal end of the newly constructed pouch*. Complete this after removing the Allen clamp, by the Roux-Y stapling technique described below.

Any defects in the mesentery that might permit herniation of the small bowel should be closed by appropriate sutures of interrupted cotton or continuous PG.

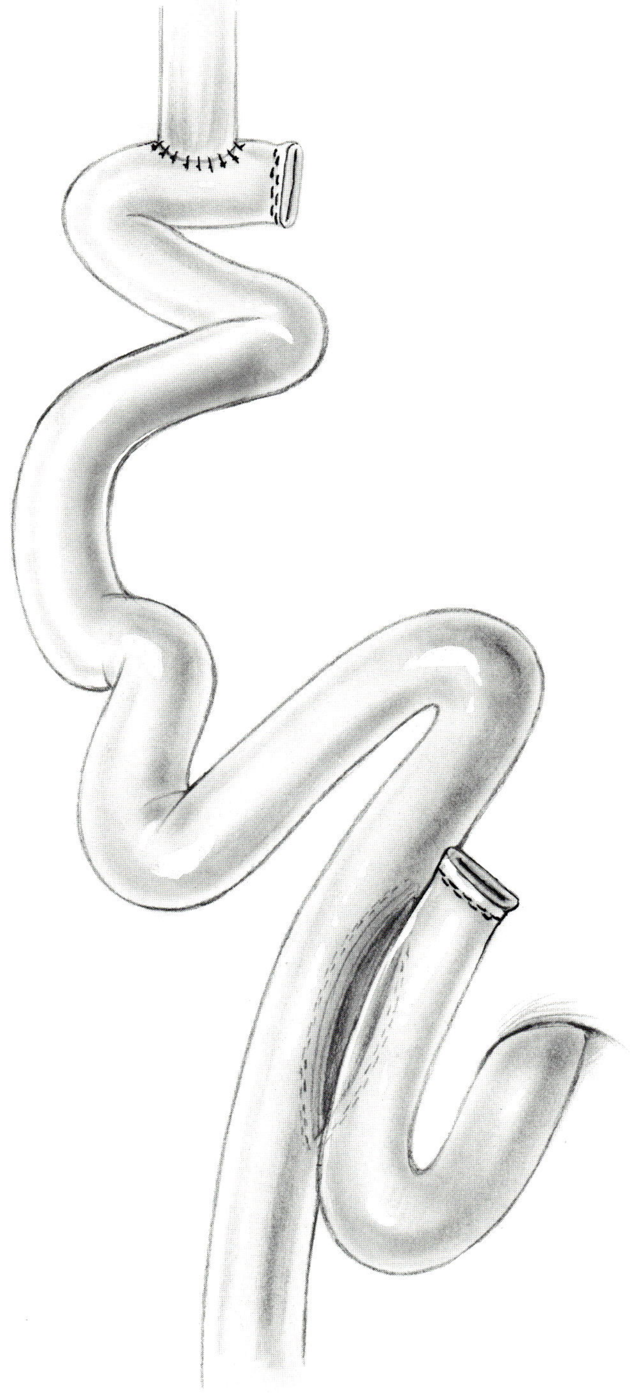

Fig. 19–31

Although no extensive experience with it has yet been reported, the distal pouch described by Paulino has many attractive features. It is illustrated in **Fig. 19–31**. There is one anastomosis less than in the Hunt-Lawrence method. It is easily performed by a stapling technique similar to that described for the Hunt-Lawrence pouch (Figs. 19–24 through 19–30). Although Paulino reported leaving 25 cm between the esophagojejunostomy and the pouch, we prefer a distance of 50 cm.

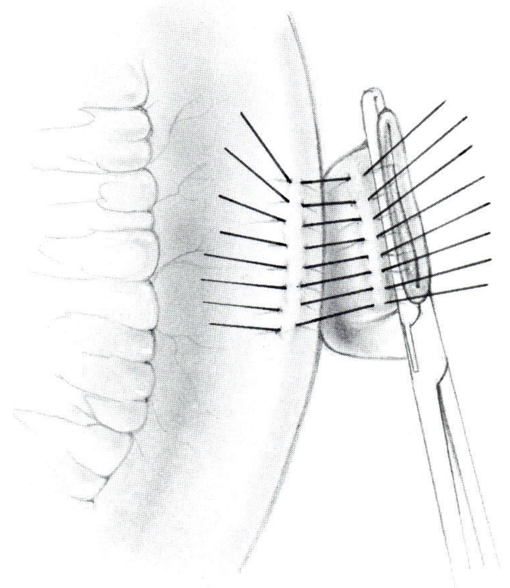

Fig. 19–32

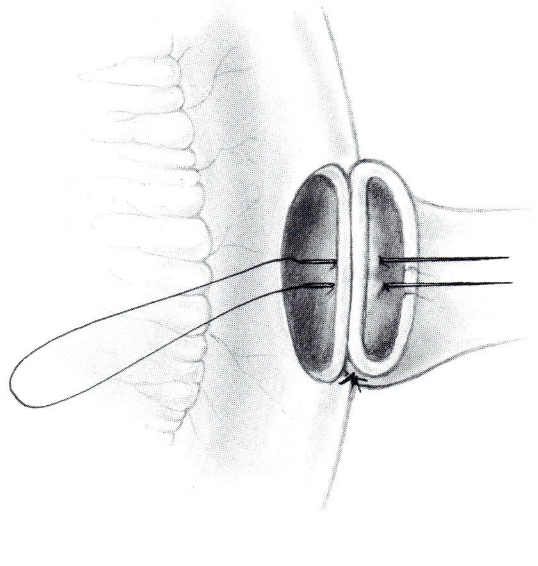

Fig. 19–33

Roux-Y Jejunojejunostomy, Sutured

Attention should now be directed to restoring the continuity of the small intestine by doing an end-to-side anastomosis between the cut end of the proximal jejunum and the side of the Roux-Y limb. This anastomosis should be made 50 cm from the esophagojejunal anastomosis in order to prevent bile reflux. After the proper site on the antimesenteric border of jejunum has been selected, make a longitudinal scratch mark with a scalpel. Use interrupted 4–0 cotton Lembert sutures for the posterior seromuscular layer of the end-to-side anastomosis (**Fig. 19–32**). When all these sutures have been placed, make an incision along the previously marked area of the jejunum and remove the Allen clamp from the proximal segment of the jejunum. Approximate the mucosal layers, using 4–0 chromic catgut doubly armed with straight needles (**Fig. 19–33**). Take the first stitch in the middle of the posterior layer and tie it. Close the remainder of the posterior mucosal layer with a continuous locked suture (**Fig. 19–34**). Approximate the anterior mucosal layer with a continuous suture of either the Connell or Cushing type. Then close the final anterior seromuscular layer with interrupted 4–0 cotton Lembert sutures (**Fig. 19–35**). Test the lumen by invaginating the jejunum with the index finger.

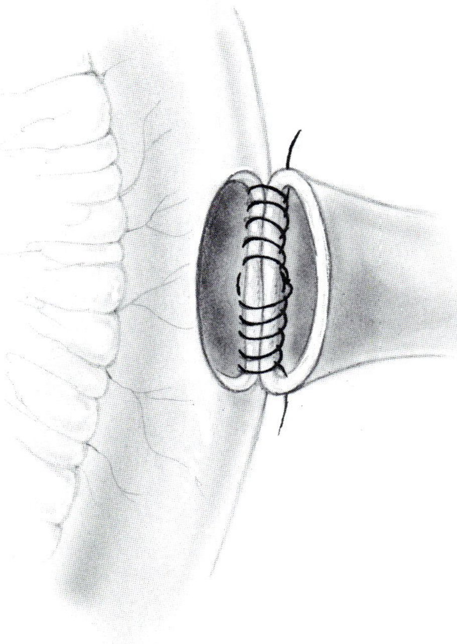

Fig. 19–34

Stapled Roux-Y Jejunojejunostomy

In most cases, especially those involving poor-risk patients, we prefer to perform the Roux-Y jejunojejunostomy with a stapling technique. To accomplish this,

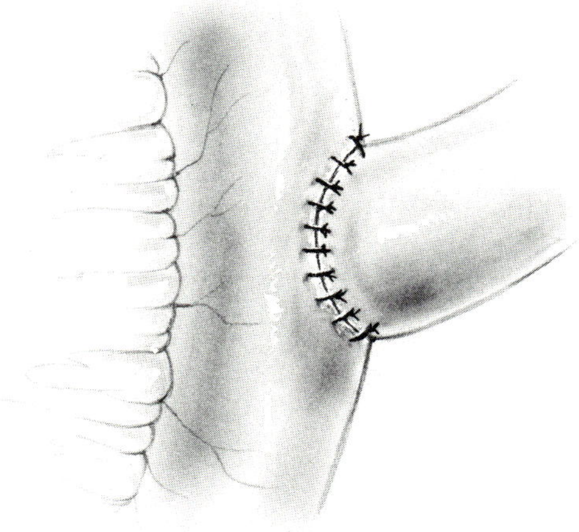

Fig. 19–35

the proximal segment of the jejunum is approximated to the Roux-Y limb. With the electrocautery make a 1.5 cm longitudinal incision on the antimesenteric border. Insert a GIA stapling device, one fork into the descending segment of the jejunum and the other fork into the open end of the proximal segment of the jejunum (**Fig. 19–36**). Be certain that the *open end of the proximal segment of jejunum is placed so that the opening faces in a cephalad*

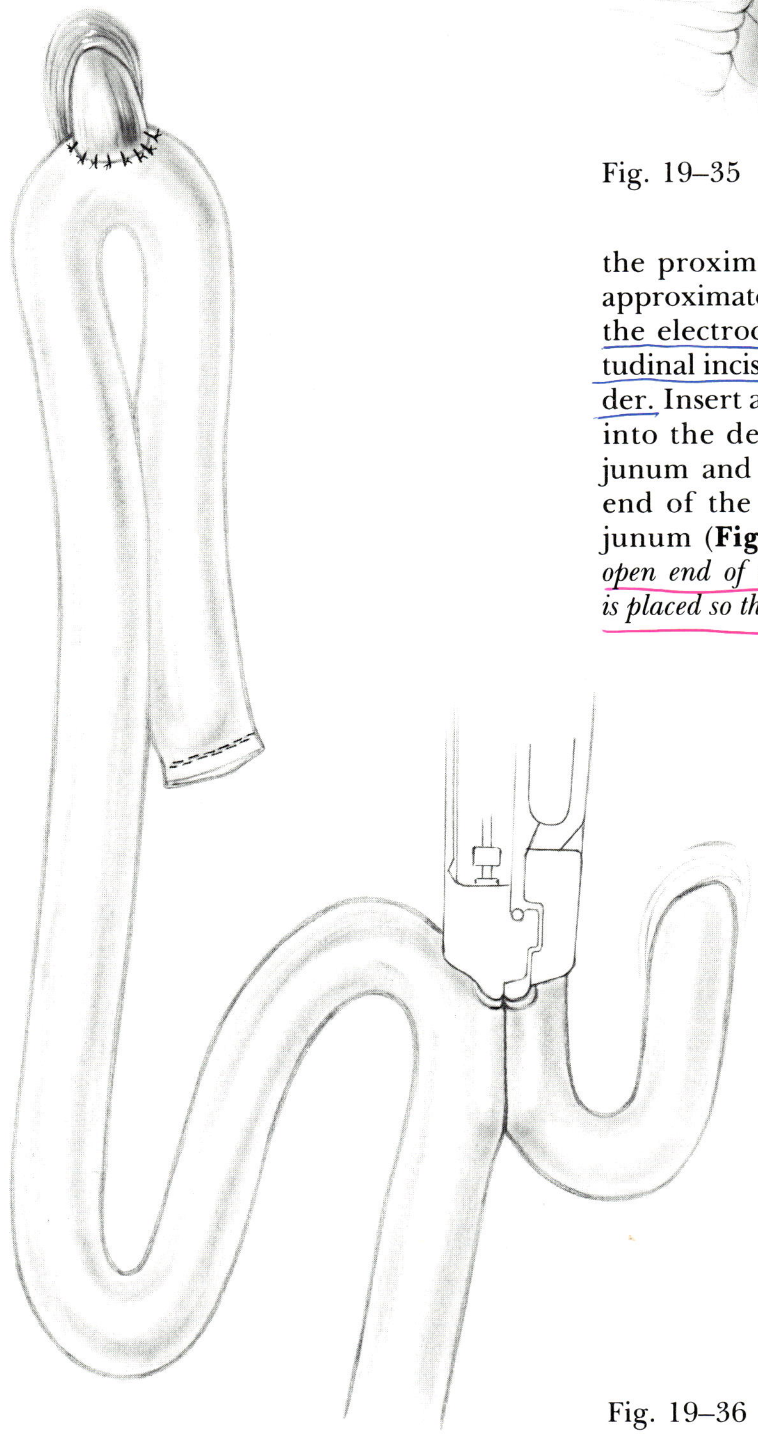

Fig. 19–36

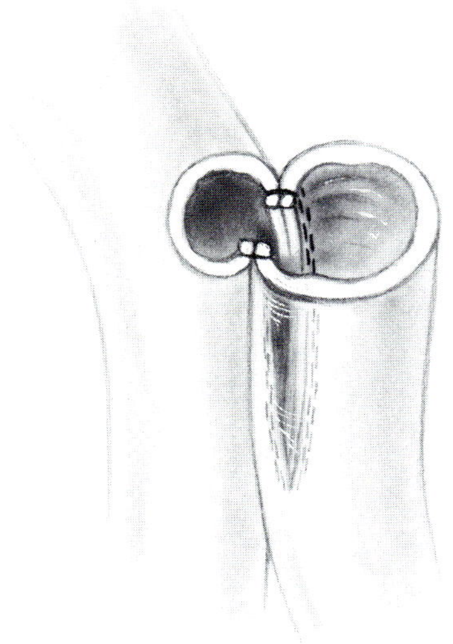

Fig. 19–37

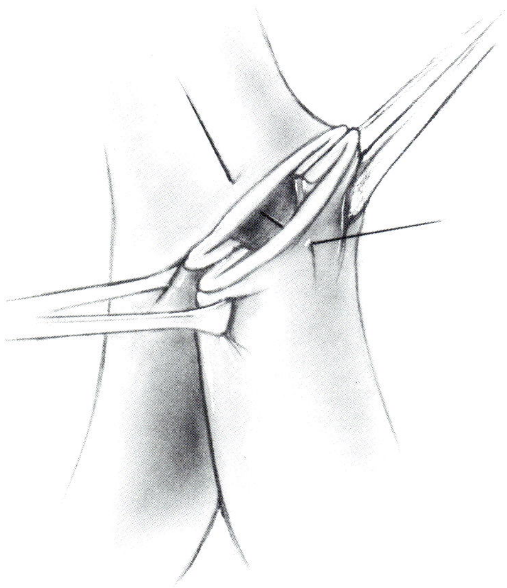

Fig. 19–38

direction. If the limbs of the jejunum are not joined in this manner, there is increased risk of narrowing the lumen of the jejunum. When the GIA device is in place, lock, and fire; it will be seen that the first layer of the anastomosis has been completed in a side-to-side fashion between the antimesenteric borders of both segments of the jejunum (**Fig. 19–37**).

To close the remaining defect in the anastomosis, apply an Allis clamp to the right-hand termination of the staple line and another Allis to the left-hand termination of the staple line. Insert a guy suture into the midpoint of the remaining defect on the proximal segment of the jejunum and pass it through the midpoint of the defect on the distal segment of the jejunum (**Fig. 19–38**). When the guy suture approximates these two points, apply Allis clamps to the right side of the defect to approximate the two segments of the jejunum in an everting fashion. Complete this part of the anastomosis by applying and firing the TA–55 stapling device deep to the Allis clamps and the guy suture (**Fig. 19–39**). Excise the redundant mucosa flush with the stapling device, but preserve the guy suture. Lightly electrocoagulate the everted mucosa.

Use Allis clamps again to close the remaining defect and apply the TA–55 stapler once more deep to the Allis clamps and the guy suture. When the stapler is fired and the redundant mucosa excised, the anastomosis is complete. It can be seen that the lumen is quite large (**Fig. 19–40**).

Close the remaining potential defects between the mesentery of the proximal and distal jejunum with interrupted sutures of 4–0 cotton to prevent herniation.

Modifications of Operative Technique for Patients with Zollinger-Ellison Syndrome or Benign Disease

When total gastrectomy is being performed for the Zollinger-Ellison syndrome or for benign disease, several modifications are indicated. First, it is not necessary to excise considerable lengths of the esophagus or duodenum. Both these structures are divided close to the margins of the stomach. Second, it is not necessary to remove the spleen or omentum, and the greater curvature dissection can be carried out by dividing each of the vasa breviae

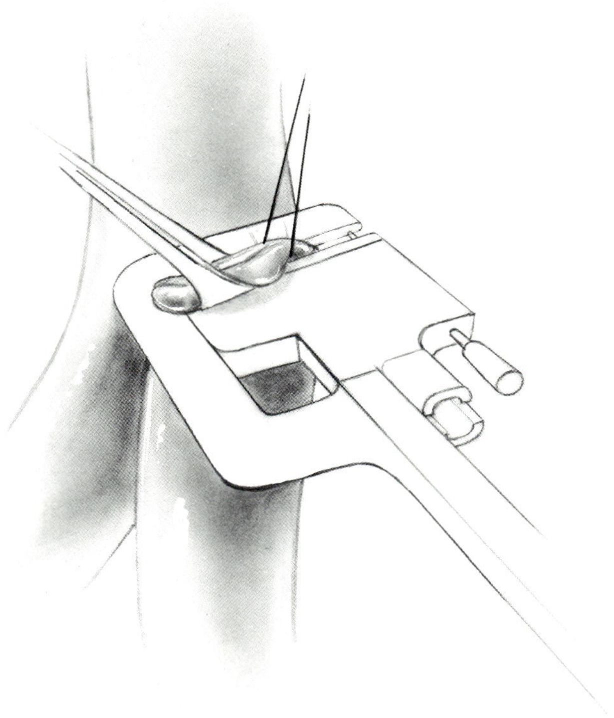

Fig. 19–39

between the greater curvature of the stomach and the greater omentum, leaving the omentum behind. Third, dissection of the lymph nodes in the region of the celiac axis, hepatic artery, and pancreas is not indicated. But for the foregoing modifications, the technique is essentially the same as for cancer operations; however, the incidence of postoperative complications is far lower in patients with the Zollinger-Ellison syndrome.

Wound Closure

Irrigate the abdominal cavity again with saline and antibiotic solution. If hemostasis is excellent and the anastomoses have been performed with accuracy, we do *not* insert drains into the abdominal cavity. Otherwise, one or two 6 mm Silastic Jackson-Pratt catheters may be brought out from the vicinity of the anastomosis through puncture wounds in the abdominal wall and attached to closed-suction drainage. Kanamycin in a dosage of 25 mg in 25 ml of sterile saline should be injected every 8 hours into each drainage catheter for a few days.

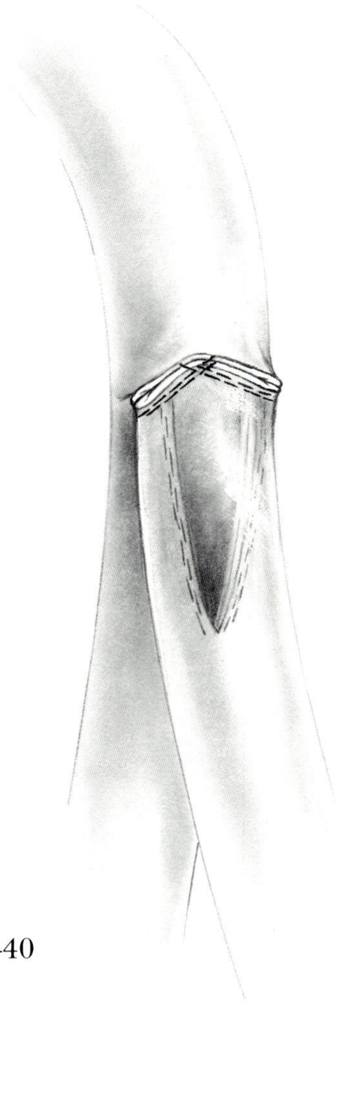

Fig. 19–40

Postoperative Care

Administer nasogastric suction for 4 days. If a pouch has been constructed, suction may be continued longer.

Administer perioperative antibiotics.

Patients who required intravenous hyperalimentation for nutritional rehabilitation before the operation should continue with this therapy.

As in other esophageal anastomoses, absolutely nothing should be permitted by mouth until the seventh postoperative day, at which time an esophagram should be performed in the X-ray department. If no leakage is identified, a liquid diet should be initiated. This may be increased rapidly according to the patient's tolerance.

Long-term postoperative management requires all patients to be on a dietary regimen that counteracts dumping. The diet should be high in protein and fat while low in carbohydrate and liquids. Frequent small feedings are indicated. Liquids should not be consumed during and 1 or 2 hours after meals in order to prevent hyperosmolarity in the lumen of the proximal jejunum. Some patients may require several months of repeated encouragement to establish adequate caloric intake following total gastrectomy. Others seem to do well with no dietary restrictions.

Dietary supplements of vitamins, iron, and calcium as well as continued injections of vitamin B_{12} are necessary in the long-term management of patients following total gastrectomy.

Complications

Sepsis of the abdominal wound or the subphrenic space is one complication that follows surgery for an ulcerated gastric malignancy. Early diagnosis and management are necessary.

Leakage from the esophagojejunal anastomosis is the most serious postoperative complication, but should occur *rarely* if proper technique has been used. A minor degree of leakage may be managed by prompt institution of adequate sump suction drainage in the region, supplemented every 8 hours by injection through the drainage catheter of 50 ml of saline with suitable antibiotics. A nasogastric tube of the sump type should be passed to a point just proximal to the esophagojejunal anastomosis for continuous suction. Nutritional support by parenteral hyperalimentation is essential, as are systemic antibiotics. In more serious cases, a diverting cervical esophagostomy may be required. Fortunately, a properly performed Roux-Y anastomosis will divert duodenal and pancreatic enzymes from the leak. If the Roux-Y technique has not been used, exteriorization of the jejunal segment, temporary occlusion of the distal esophagus, and cervical esophagostomy become necessary to control the septic process.

References

Pachter HL et al. (1979) Simplified distal pancreatectomy with the Auto Suture stapler: preliminary clinical observations. Surgery 85:166

Paulino F, Roselli A (1973) Carcinoma of the stomach. Curr Probl Surg

Schrock TR, Way LW (1978) Total gastrectomy. Am J Surg 135:348

Scott HW Jr et al. (1965) Clinical experience with a jejunal pouch (Hunt-Lawrence) as a substitute stomach after total gastrectomy. Surg Gynecol Obstet 121:1231

Scott HW Jr et al. (1968) Clinical and metabolic studies after total gastrectomy with a Hunt-Lawrence food pouch. Am J Surg 115:148

Small Intestine

20 Exposure of the Third and Fourth Portions of the Duodenum

Indications

Tumor

Bleeding

Concept

Because the third portion of the duodenum is located behind the superior mesenteric vessels and transverse mesocolon, a direct approach to it would be hazardous. Liberating the right colon and small bowel mesentery from their attachments to the posterior abdominal wall permits the surgeon to elevate the right colon and entire small bowel to a position over the patient's thorax. This changes the course of the superior mesenteric and middle colic vessels so that they travel directly cephalad, leaving the transverse portion of the duodenum completely exposed.

Preoperative Care

Nasogastric tube

Some lesions in the third and fourth portions of the duodenum may be biopsied by the endoscopist, which permits more accurate planning of the operation

Pitfalls and Danger Points

Trauma to superior mesenteric artery or vein

Trauma to pancreas

Operative Strategy

After liberating the right colon by incising the peritoneum of the right paracolic gutter, divide the renocolic attachments. Continuing in this plane, the surgeon will be able to free the entire mesentery of the small intestine in an entirely avascular dissection. It is important to devote special attention to the superior mesenteric vein as it emerges from the pancreas; rough traction in the area may avulse one of its branches, producing troublesome bleeding.

In planning a resection of the third and fourth portions of the duodenum, it should be noted that to the right of the superior mesenteric vessels the blood supply of the third portion of the duodenum arises from many small branches of the inferior pancreaticoduodenal arcade. These must be dissected, divided, and ligated delicately, one by one, to avoid pancreatic trauma and postoperative acute pancreatitis. The distal duodenum is not attached to the body of the pancreas to the left of the superior mesenteric vessels; its blood supply arises from branches of the superior mesenteric artery, as does that of the proximal jejunum. These are easy to identify and control.

If the pancreas has not been invaded, it is possible to resect the third and fourth portions of the duodenum for tumor and then to construct an anastomosis between the descending duodenum and the jejunum, so long as the ampulla is not involved. When working in this area, it is essential that the ampulla of Vater be identified early in the dissection.

Operative Technique

Incision

A long midline incision from the midepigastrium to the pubis gives excellent exposure for this operation.

Liberation of Right Colon

Make a Metzenbaum incision in the peritoneum of the right paracolic gutter. Insert the index finger to separate the peritoneum from underlying fat and areolar tissue; this will provide an avascular plane. When the hepatic flexure is encountered, the electrocoagulator can help control bleeding as the peritoneum is cut. It is not generally necessary to dissect the greater omentum off the transverse colon in this operation. It is important, however, to continue the division of the paracolic peritoneum around the inferior portion of the cecum and to move on medially to liberate the terminal ileum, all in the same plane (**Fig. 20–1**). Identify the renocolic ligament at the medial margin of Gerota's fascia. Division of this thin, ligamentous structure will completely free the right mesocolon.

Liberation of Small Bowel Mesentery

Insert the left index finger beneath the remaining avascular attachments between the mesentery of the small bowel

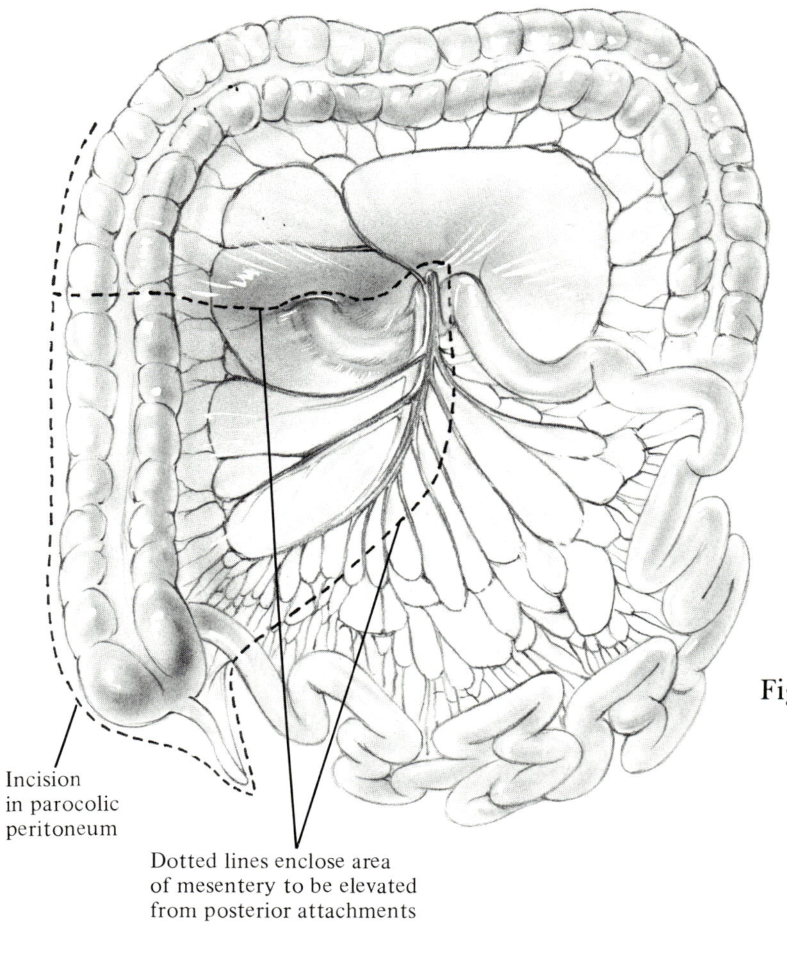

Fig. 20–1

and the posterior wall of the abdomen; incise these attachments until the entire small intestine up to the ligament of Treitz is free and can be positioned over the patient's thorax. This configuration resembles the anatomy of patients who have a congenital failure of rotation or malrotation of the bowel (**Fig. 20–2**).

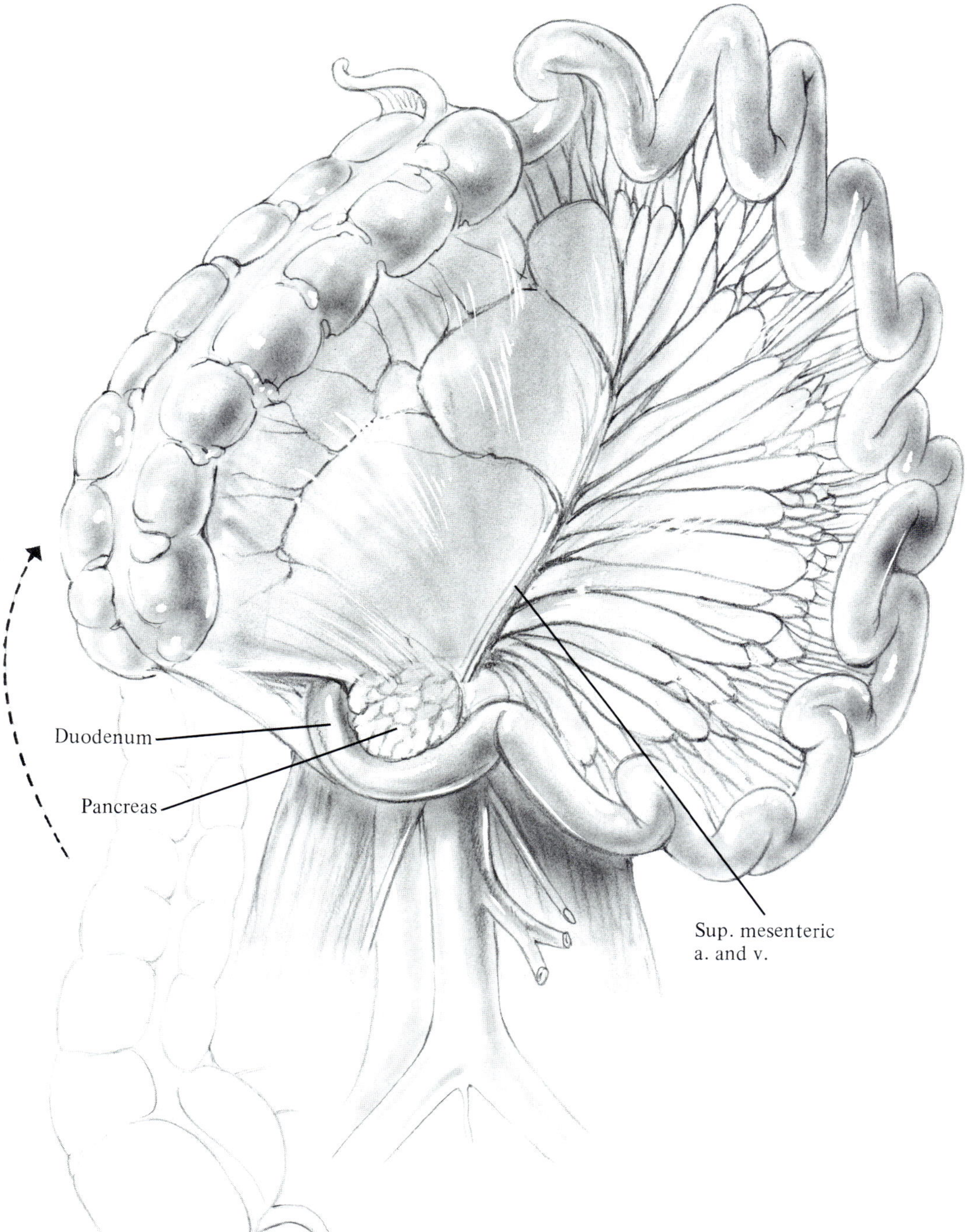

Fig. 20–2

Resection of Duodenum

There is no structure lying over the third and fourth portions of the duodenum or proximal jejunum at this time. If a tumor of the duodenum is to be resected, it is important to determine now if it is safe to do so. If some portion of the pancreas has been invaded, a decision will have to be made whether a partial or total pancreatectomy is indicated for the patient's pathology. If the duodenum is free, dissection is best begun by identifying the blood supply of the distal duodenum, dividing each vessel between clamps, and ligating. As the pancreatic head is approached, the dissection should be done with delicacy. It is possible to identify and divide each of the small vessels arising from the pancreas. This frees the duodenum and permits resection and anastomosis.

About 1 cm of the duodenum should be freed from the pancreas proximal to the point of transection. This permits an end-to-end anastomosis between the proximal duodenum and a segment of the jejunum that is brought over for this purpose. Mere closure of the distal duodenum plus a gastrojejunostomy is not a satisfactory operation, as the proximal duodenum will eventually dilate to huge proportions and form a blind loop. If for some reason the end of the duodenum is suitable for closure but not for anastomosis, a side-to-side anastomosis between the second portion of the duodenum and proximal jejunum is a second-best alternative.

Closure

After the anastomosis has been performed, return the right colon and small bowel to the abdomen. Make no attempt to reestablish the posterior attachments of the mesentery. Close the abdomen in routine fashion.

Postoperative Care

Aside from the administration of nasogastric suction until bowel function has resumed with the passage of flatus, postoperative care is routine. Be aware that acute pancreatitis is a possible complication of any dissection in the region of the pancreas. If the serum amylase remains elevated and the patient shows any signs of acute pancreatitis, nasogastric suction should be continued until no danger exists.

Postoperative Complications

Pancreatitis

Anastomotic leaks

21 Small Bowel Resection and Anastomosis

Indications

Tumor
Trauma
Strangulation
Crohn's enteritis with complications
Ischemic enteritis

Preoperative Preparation

Nasogastric intubation
Perioperative antibiotics

Pitfalls and Danger Points

The small bowel anastomosis is generally quite safe unless there is also some impairment of the blood supply or advanced peritoneal sepsis. When the small bowel anastomosis fails because of mechanical errors, the leak almost invariably occurs at the mesenteric border, where the serosa has not been adequately cleared of blood vessels and fat.

Operative Strategy

Requirements for Successful Bowel Anastomosis

1) A *good blood supply* is required for optimal healing. Determine this by noting the pulsatile flow after dividing a terminal arterial branch in the region where the bowel is to be transected. There should be no hematoma near the anastomosis, as this may impair circulation.

2) *Accurate apposition of the seromuscular coats* is essential. There should be no fat or other tissue between the two bowel walls being sutured. The seromuscular suture must catch the submucosa, where most of the tensile strength of the intestine is situated. Optimal healing of an anastomosis requires serosa-to-serosa approximation. Special attention must be devoted to the mesenteric border of any anastomosis. This is the point at which several terminal blood vessels and accompanying fat are dissected off the bowel wall to provide the surgeon with sufficient visibility to permit accurate insertion of the seromuscular suture. If fat and blood vessels are cleared away from a 1 cm width of serosa around the circumference of an anastomosis, there need be no worry about impairing the blood supply of the bowel. The increased accuracy with which the sutures are inserted will minimize anastomotic complications.

3) A *sufficient length of bowel must be freed* proximal and distal to each anastomosis to insure there will be no tension whatever on the healing suture line. Allowance should be made for some degree

of foreshortening of the length of the intestine in case postoperative distension occurs.

4) *Do not apply excessive force* in tying the anastomotic sutures as this will result in strangulation of tissue. If the suture should inadvertently have been placed through the full thickness of the bowel and into the lumen, strangulating the suture will cause the intestinal contents to leak. The suture should be tied with no more tension than is needed to approximate both intestinal walls.

5) *Avoid using the electrocoagulator for transecting the bowel.* According to Kott and Lurie, when the bowel is transected with the electrocautery device, especially if the device is set for coagulating current, the tissue trauma thus induced prolongs the lag period that precedes the development of tensile strength in the healing anastomosis.

6) *Do not apply excessive force to the forceps* when manipulating the ends of the bowel to be anastomosed. If the imprint of forceps teeth is visible on the serosa after the forceps has been removed, the surgeon obviously has compressed the tissue with too much force. When a curved needle is used, the needle must be passed through the tissue with a rotatory motion to minimize trauma. As discussed in detail in Appendix B, it does not matter whether an intestinal anastomosis is constructed with one or two layers or whether a stapling method is used, as long as proper technique is employed.

7) *Before constructing stapled intestinal anastomoses, learn the pitfalls,* both technical and conceptual, of the method. Study the strategy of avoiding the complications of surgical stapling (see Chap. 4). We have published a report demonstrating that when done by those who have learned the technique, stapled anastomoses are no more prone to complications than are sewn anastomoses. This is surprising, considering that many stapled anastomoses are, in part, of the *everting* type, which most surgeons believe is not conducive to optimal healing in the sutured anastomosis.

8) Some errors often are made by residents who are learning the art of anastomotic suturing. One is inserting the outer layer of seromuscular sutures with the collapsed bowel resting on a flat surface. An even worse error consists in putting the left index finger underneath the back of the anastomosis while inserting the anterior seromuscular sutures. Both errors make it possible to pass the seromuscular suture through the bowel lumen and then to catch a portion of the posterior wall. When the sutures are tied, an obstruction is created. While some of these sutures may later tear out of the back wall in response to peristalsis, others may remain permanently in place and produce a stenosis. In order to prevent this complication, simply have the assistant *grasp the tails of those anastomotic sutures that have already been tied.* Skyward traction on these sutures keeps the lumen of the anastomosis wide open while the surgeon inserts additional sutures.

9) Another error consists in inserting anastomotic sutures while the bowel is under linear tension. This stretches the bowel wall so that it becomes relatively thin, making it difficult to enclose a substantial bite of tissue in the suture. *A sufficient length of the intestine, proximal and distal, should be loosely placed in the operative field.* After the first seromuscular bite has been taken, the needle is then ready to be reinserted into the wall of the opposite segment of intestine. At this time it is often helpful to use forceps to elevate the distal bowel at a point 3–4 cm distal to the anastomosis. Elevation relaxes this segment of the bowel and permits the suture to catch a substantial bite of tissue, including the submucosa. Each bite should encompass about 5 mm of tissue. These stitches should be placed about 5 mm from each other.

Contraindications to Anastomosis

Because of the excellent blood supply and substantial submucosal strength of the small bowel, anastomoses are often successful even in the presence of such adverse circumstances as intestinal obstruction and gross contamination of the abdominal cavity. Consequently, the only major contraindications to a primary small bowel anastomosis are peritoneal sepsis, questionable blood supply, or a patient whose condition on the operating table is precarious. In these cases both ends of the divided small bowel may be brought to the skin as temporary enterostomies.

Operative Technique: Small Bowel Anastomosis by Suturing

Incision

For the best exposure of the small bowel, use a midline vertical incision.

Division of Mesentery

Expose the segment of intestine to be resected by laying it flat on a moist gauze pad on the abdominal wall. With a scalpel make a V-type incision in the mesentery to be removed, carrying it through the superficial peritoneal layer only, in order to expose the underlying blood vessels (**Fig. 21–1**). Apply medium-size hemostats in pairs to the intervening tissue. Divide the tissue between hemostats and ligate each with 2–0 cotton. After the wedge of mes-

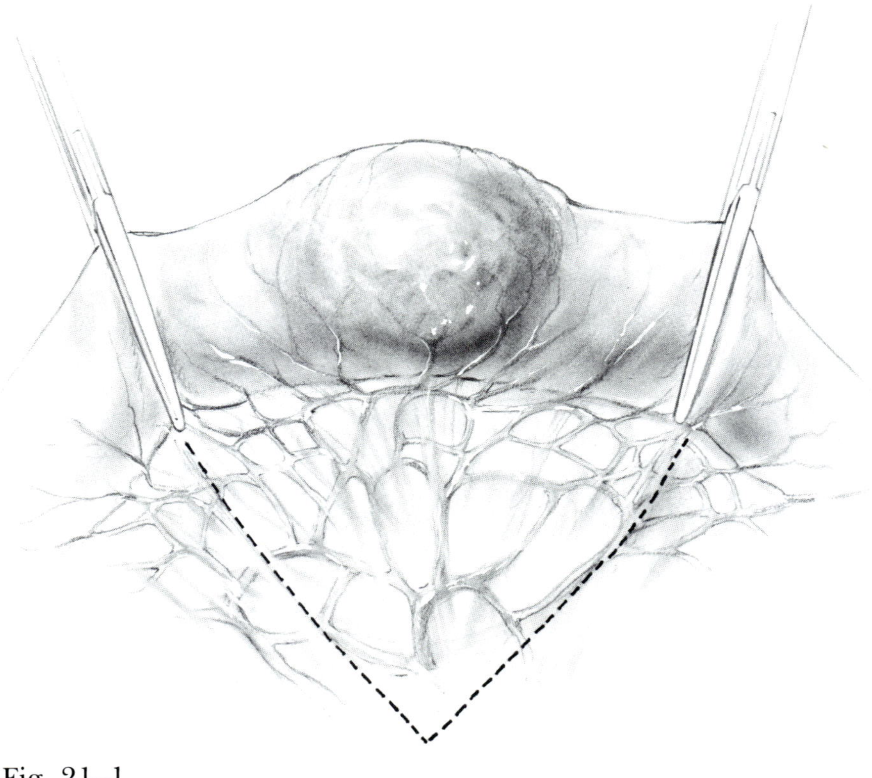

Fig. 21–1

entery has been completely freed, apply Allen clamps to the bowel on the specimen sides. Apply linen-shod Doyen noncrushing intestinal clamps proximal and distal to prevent spillage of intestinal contents. Remove the diseased segment of intestine by scalpel division.

Open Two-Layer Anastomosis

Considerable manipulative trauma to the bowel wall can be eliminated if the anterior seromuscular layer of sutures is the first layer to be inserted. This should be done by the technique of successive bisection (see Appendix B). First, insert a Lembert 4–0 cotton atraumatic seromuscular suture on the antimesenteric border. Then insert the second suture on the mesenteric border, (**Fig. 21–2**). Tie both sutures. Next, bisect the distance between these two sutures and insert and tie the third Lembert suture at this point. Follow this sequence until the anterior seromuscular layer has been completed (**Fig. 21–3a**). Retain the two end sutures as guys, but cut

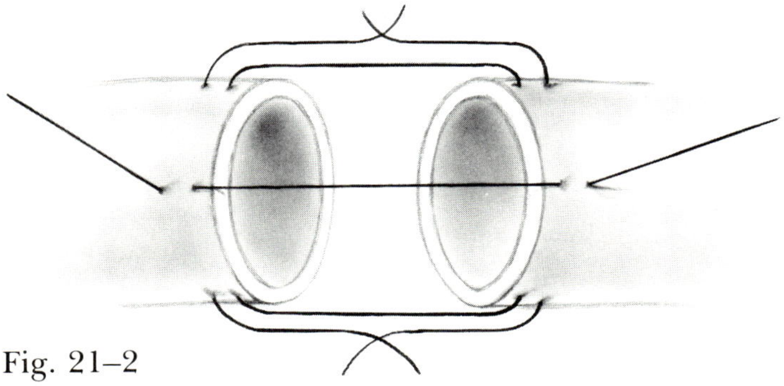

Fig. 21–2

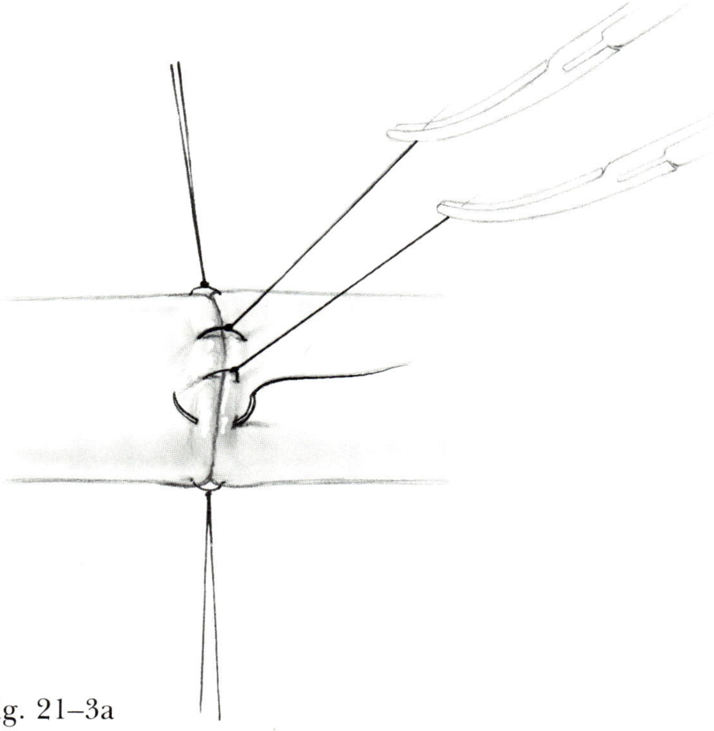

Fig. 21–3a

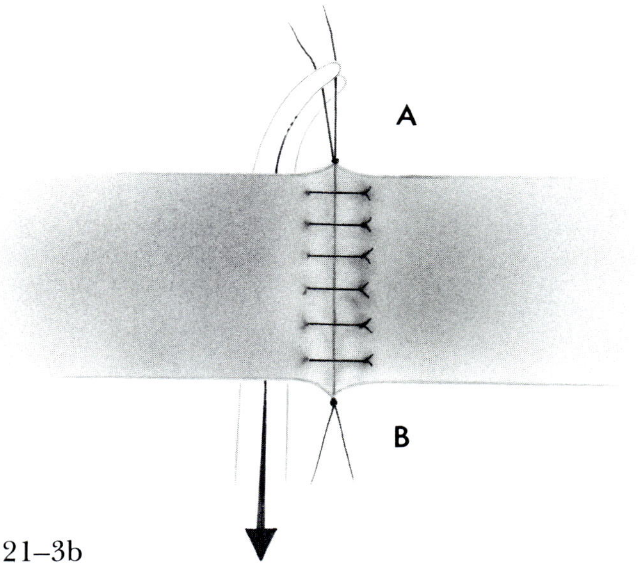

Fig. 21–3b

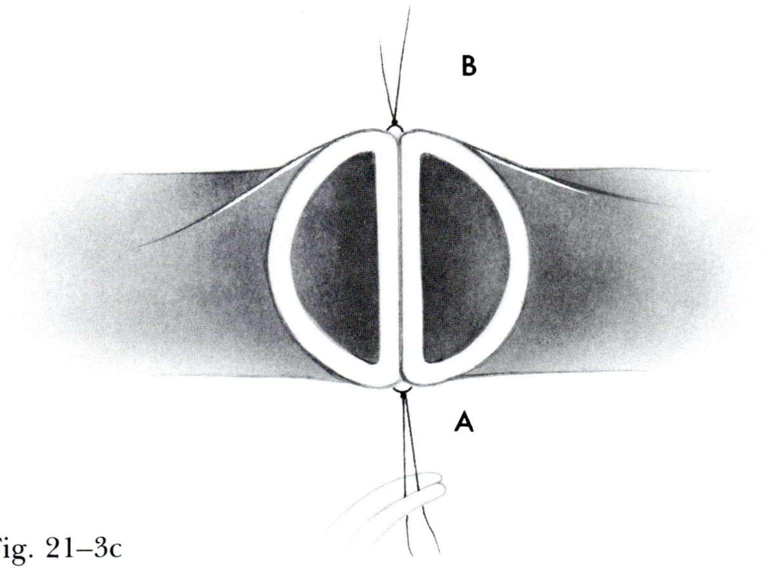

Fig. 21–3c

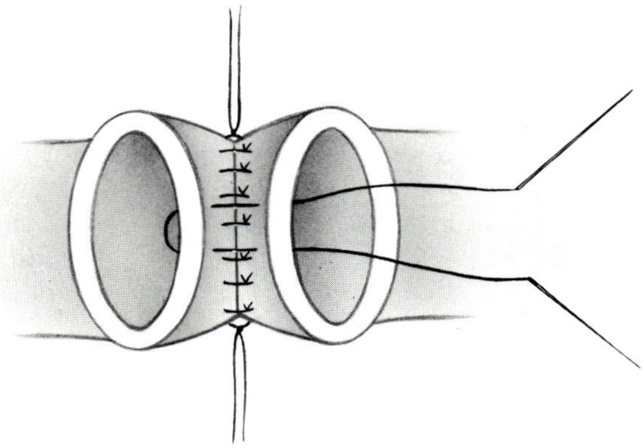

Fig. 21–4

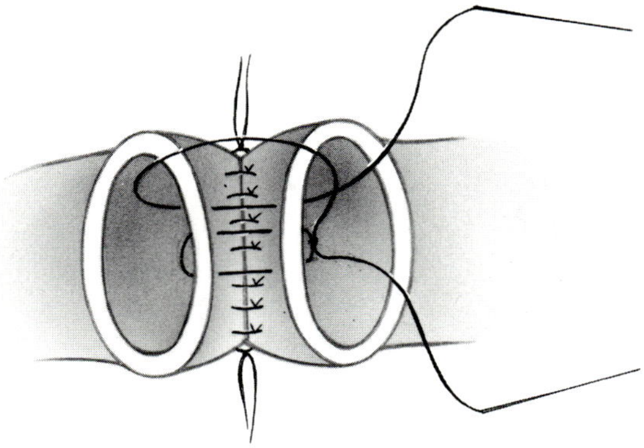

Fig. 21–5

the tails of all the remaining sutures. *The bowel should then be rotated by passing guy suture A behind the anastomosis* (**Fig. 21–3b**) so that the posterior layer is on top (**Fig. 21–3c**).

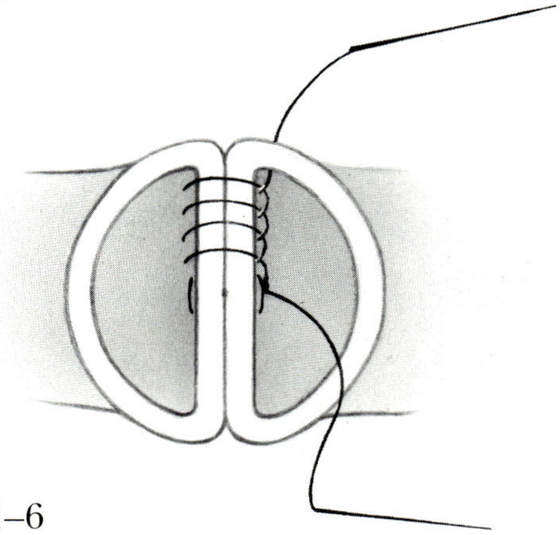

Fig. 21–6

Accomplish closure of the mucosal layer with 4–0 chromic catgut, preferably double-armed with straight needles. Insert the two needles at the midpoint of the deep layer (**Fig. 21–4**). Tie the suture and close the posterior layer, which should include both mucosa and a bit of seromuscular tissue, with a continuous locked suture (**Figs. 21–5, 21–6, and 21–7**). Turning in the corners with this technique is simple. Bring the needle from inside out through the outer wall of the intestine (**Fig. 21–8**). Then complete the final mucosal layer, using either the Connell technique or a continuous Cushing suture (**Fig. 21–9**). After this mucosal layer has

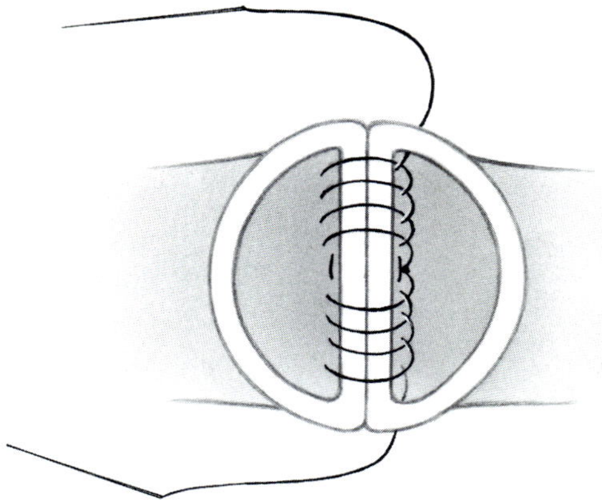

Fig. 21–7

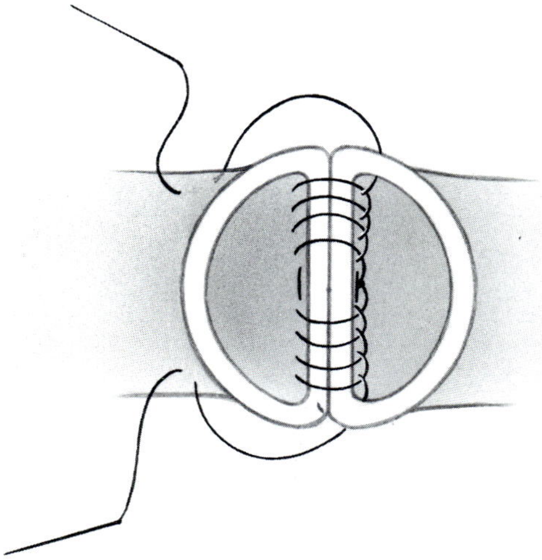

Fig. 21–8

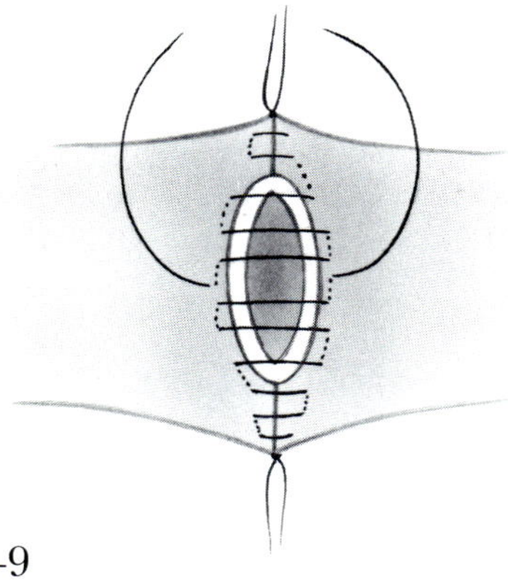

Fig. 21–9

been completed, insert the final seromuscular layer of interrupted 4–0 Lemberts (**Fig. 21–10**). The technique of successive bisection is not necessary in the final layer because the two segments of bowel are already in accurate apposition.

After all the suture tails have been cut, inspect carefully for imperfections in the suture line, especially at the mesenteric margin. Test the patency of the lumen by invaginating one wall of the intestine through the anastomosis with the tip of the index finger.

Open One-Layer Anastomosis

The first step in constructing an end-to-end anastomosis in one layer is identical with Figs. 21–2 and 21–3a. Insert interrupted Lemberts on the anterior seromuscular layer. Cut the tails of all the sutures except the two at the end, and rotate the bowel to expose the opposite, unsutured bowel (see Figs. 21–3b and 21–3c). Approximate this too with interrupted 4–0 cotton *seromuscular* Lembert sutures, paying special attention to the mesenteric border, where fat and blood vessels may hide the seromuscular tissue from view if the dissection has not been thorough.

After the anastomosis is completed, check it closely for defects. Test the size of the lumen by invaginating the wall with a fingertip.

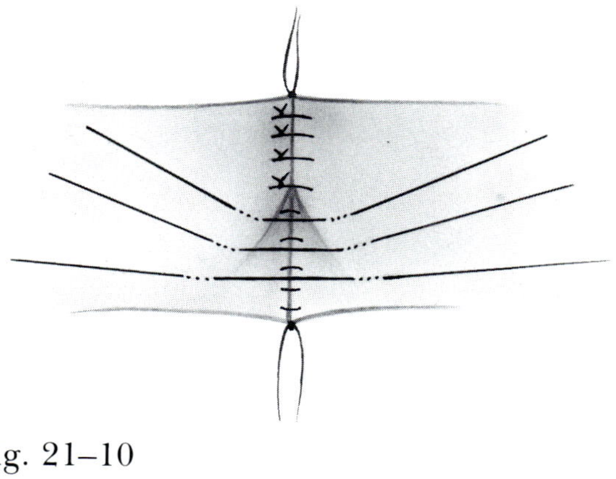

Fig. 21–10

Alternatively, instead of Lemberts, "seromucosal" stitches may be inserted (**Fig. 21–11**). This suture enters the seromuscular layer and like the Lembert penetrates the submucosa, but instead of emerging from the serosa the needle emerges just beyond the junction of the cut edge of the serosa and underlying mucosa. This stitch has the advantage of inverting a smaller cuff of tissue than does the Lembert or Cushing technique and may therefore be useful when the small bowel lumen is small. When inserted properly the seromucosal suture does invert the mucosa, but not to the extent that the Lembert stitch does.

Closure of Mesentery

Close the defect in the mesentery by a continuous suture of 2–0 PG on a large, intestinal-type needle. Take care not to pierce the blood vessels.

Operative Technique: Small Bowel Anastomosis Using Stapling Technique

In our experience, the most efficient method of stapling the small bowel is a two-step functional end-to-end technique which we have developed. This requires the two open-ended segments of the small bowel to be positioned so that their antimesenteric borders are in apposition. Insert a GIA stapling device, one fork into the proximal and the other fork into the distal segment of the intestine (**Fig. 21–12**). Fire the GIA instrument, which will form one layer of the anastomosis in an inverting fashion (**Fig. 21–13**). Apply one Allis to the left-handed termination of the staple line and the other Allis to the right-handed termination. Then draw the two Allises apart (**Figs. 21–14 and 21–15**). Close the remaining defect in the anastomosis in an everting fashion after applying 4–5 Allises to maintain apposition of the walls of the proximal and distal segments of bowel (**Fig. 21–16**).

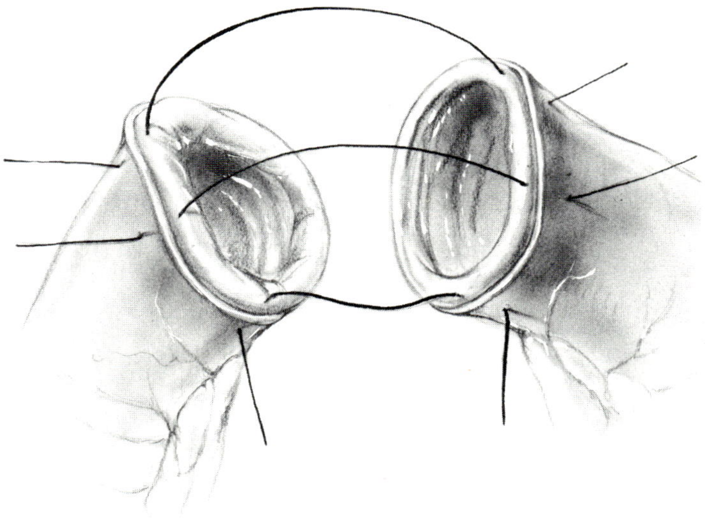

Fig. 21–11

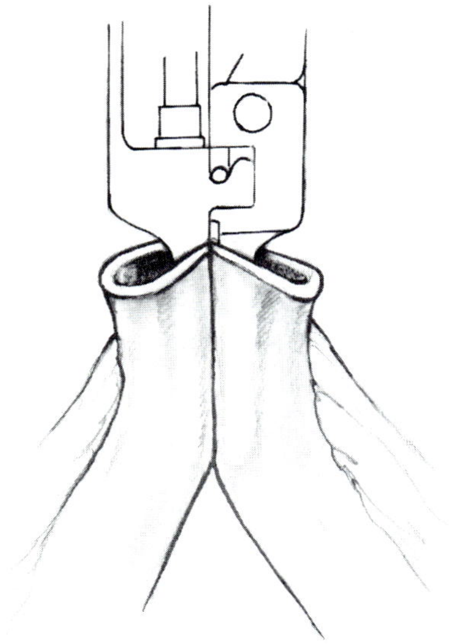

Fig. 21–12

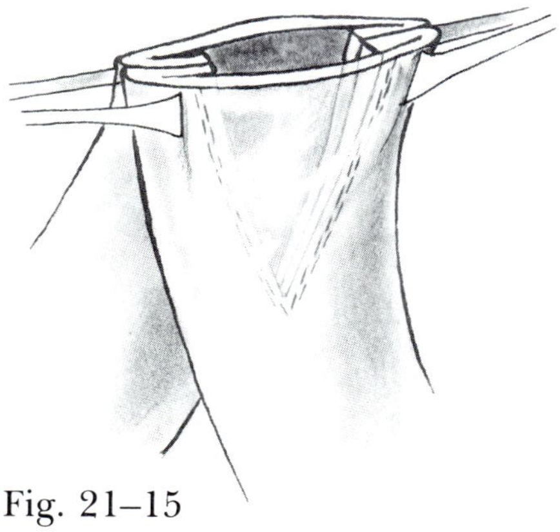

Fig. 21–15

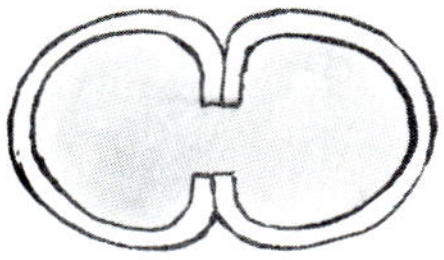

Fig. 21–13

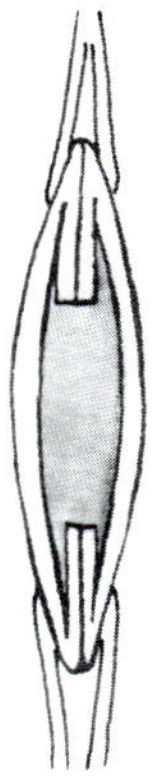

Fig. 21–14

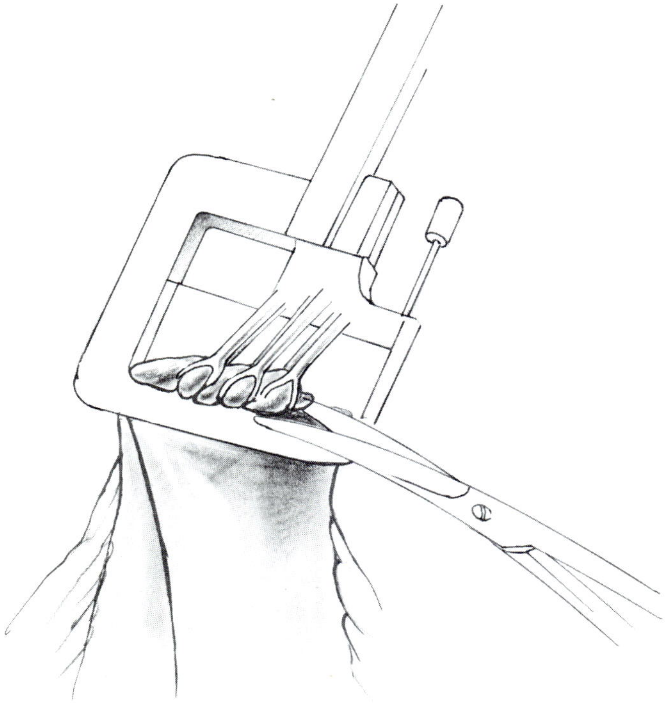

Fig. 21–16

After all the Allis clamps have been aligned, staple the bowel in eversion by applying a TA–90 device just deep to the Allis clamps. Insert and tighten the alignment pin, tighten the wing nut until the two black bands overlap, and fire the device (Fig. 21–16). To be sure there are no gaps in the closure it is essential that the line of staples cross both the right-handed and left-handed terminations of the GIA staple line. Generally, staples of 3.5 mm size should be used unless the bowel wall is very thick, in which case 4.8 mm staples are preferable. Excise the redundant bowel flush with the stapling device, using Mayo scissors. Lightly electrocoagulate the everted mucosa.

Carefully inspect the staple line to be sure each staple has formed a proper B. Bleeding may be controlled by conservative electrocoagulation or by using 4–0 atraumatic PG sutures.

Close the defect in the mesentery with a continuous 2–0 atraumatic PG suture. If feasible, cover the everted mucosa by the mesenteric suture line to minimize the possibility of it becoming a nidus of adhesion formation.

Whether the anastomosis is sutured or stapled, it is advisable to cover it with a layer of omentum, whenever possible, to prevent adhesions.

Postoperative Care

Administer nasogastric suction until bowel function resumes, as indicated by the passage of flatus.

Complications

Although it is quite uncommon for the patient to develop complications following a small bowel anastomosis, postoperative obstruction does occasionally occur. Anastomotic leaks accompanied by intraperitoneal sepsis or enterocutaneous fistula are rare except after resection in the face of sepsis or when mesenteric circulation is impaired.

References

Chassin JL et al. (1978) The stapled gastrointestinal tract anastomosis: incidence of postoperative complications compared with the sutured anastomosis. Ann Surg 188:689

Kott I, Lurie M (1973) The effects of electrosurgery and the surgical knife on the healing of intestinal anastomoses. Dis Colon Rectum 16:33

22 Enterolysis for Intestinal Obstruction

Indications

Enterolysis is indicated in acute cases of complete small bowel obstruction.

Concept: When to Operate?

Despite long years of experience, in cases of acute small bowel obstruction a surgeon *often* can not determine preoperatively whether strangulation has taken place. Numerous retrospective studies confirm this fact. There is more risk in overlooking strangulation of the intestine than there is in possibly performing an unnecessary operation on a patient who might have been salvaged by successful long-tube suction. Consequently, most surgeons feel that a patient suffering a recent onset of acute complete intestinal obstruction, confirmed by flat X rays of the abdomen, should be operated upon as soon as rehydration has taken place. When strangulation is suspected, rapid resuscitation may be accomplished within 1 hour and continued in the operating room with appropriate monitoring.

Many surgeons are willing to attempt conservative treatment for a longer period of time in the postoperative patient in the belief that the adhesions are fibrinous and may be disrupted by the passage of a long intestinal tube. Another common explanation of postoperative obstructions is to call them paralytic ileus. In most operations, after the seventh postoperative day the persistence of ileus, as manifested by intestinal distention and failure of the patient to pass stool or flatus, is probably the result of anastomotic obstruction or some intraperitoneal pathology such as hematoma or sepsis. An internal hernia of the small intestine through a pelvic suture line following abdominoperineal resection or abdominal hysterectomy is another common cause of this clinical complex. For these reasons, even in the postoperative patient conservative treatment should be limited to a fixed number of days. If no response is forthcoming, relaparotomy is safer than continued persistence in conservative management.

Preoperative Preparation

Nasogastric or long-tube suction should be instituted before the operation.

Pitfalls and Danger Points

Inadvertent laceration and spillage of the contents of the intestine is a hazard of this procedure.

Operative Strategy

Approach to Densely Adherent Abdomen

While the contents of the normal small intestine may be sterile, in intestinal obstruction the stagnation of bowel content often results in an accumulation of virulent bacteria and toxic products. When these are spilled in the peritoneal cavity, the likelihood of postoperative mortality and infection increases. To avoid this mishap, dissection should be done carefully and patiently.

The basic dissection strategy consists of entering the abdominal cavity through a scar-free area. Even though an old midline scar is frequently used to reenter an abdomen to relieve an obstruction, it is advantageous to make some part of the incision through an area of the abdomen above or below the old scar. Access to the peritoneal cavity through an unscarred area often gives the surgeon an opportunity to assess the location of adhesions in the vicinity of the anticipated incision. After the free abdominal cavity is entered and any adherent segments of intestine freed, the remainder of the incision should be carefully opened. If the earlier incision was closed with wire sutures, the electrocautery device, set on a mild cutting current, should be used to incise the linea alba until the wires are identified, cut, and removed. The electrocautery is more efficient than cold-steel scalpel blades, which become dull each time they strike a wire and must be changed frequently.

The next aspect of the strategy employed to free a densely adherent abdomen is to attach Kocher clamps to the peritoneum and linea alba on one side of the incision. After the clamps are elevated, a Metzenbaum scissors can generally be insinuated behind the various layers of avascular adhesions to incise them (see Fig. 22–1). If the left index finger can be passed around a loop of bowel adherent to the abdominal wall, this will help guide the dissection. The aim is to free all the intestine from the anterior and lateral abdominal wall, first on one side of the incision and then on the opposite, so the anterior and lateral layers of parietal peritoneum are completely free of intestinal attachments (see Fig. 22–2).

Once the intestine has been freed, trace a normal-looking segment to the nearest adhesion. If possible, insert an index finger into the leaves of mesentery separating the two adherent limbs of the intestine. By gently bringing the index finger up between the leaves of mesentery, often the adherent layer can be stretched into a fine, filmy membrane, which is easily divided with a scissors (see Fig. 22–3). In general, the strategy is to insinuate either the left index finger or the closed blunt-tipped curved Metzenbaum scissors beneath an adhesion to delineate the plane, then to withdraw the closed scissors and to cut the fibrous layer. A guiding principle should be to *perform the easy dissection first.* If this principle always is followed, the difficult portion of a dissection will become easy. Avoid tackling a dense adherent mass head on; if the loops of intestine going to and coming from the adherent mass are dissected on their way in and on their way out of the mass of adhesions, a sometimes confusing collection of intestine can be easily untangled.

In the case of an acute small bowel obstruction, frequently there are only one or two adhesions and a markedly distended proximal bowel. When this occurs, be careful not to permit the distended bowel to leap out of a small portion of the incision, as it may be torn inadvertently in the process. If possible, first deliver the collapsed bowel (distal to the point of obstruction) and then trace it retrograde up to the point of obstruction. The adhesion can then be divided under direct vision and the entire bowel freed.

Relaparotomy for Postoperative Obstruction

To reexplore the postoperative abdomen we most often reenter the same incision, usually in the midline. Since most relaparotomy operations are done after the eighth to tenth postoperative day, some sharp dissection may be necessary to enter the abdomen.

To divide adhesions in these cases, many of the loops of bowel can be separated by inserting the index finger between the leaves of adjoining mesentery. By elevating the finger, the adhesion can be stretched between the bowel segments. Often the adhesion may be disrupted by pinching it *gently* between the thumb and index finger without damaging the serosa of the bowel.

When multiple abscesses between the leaves of mesentery contribute to the bowel obstruction, it is best to excise each abscess by gently peeling off its fibrinous walls from the mesentery and serosa, aided by copious irrigation with warm saline, according to the technique described by Hudspeth. This is feasible, if the dissection is done patiently, in most cases in which the diagnosis has not been delayed so long that the abscess walls have become fibrotic.

Operative Intestinal Decompression

If the diameter of the small bowel appears to be so distended that closing the incision would be difficult, operative decompression of the bowel will make the abdominal closure simpler and may improve the patient's postoperative course. Decompression may also lessen the risk of inadvertent laceration of the tensely distended intestine.

For this procedure we prefer to use the Baker intestinal tube. This is essentially a plastic Foley catheter, 270 cm long, with a 5 ml balloon at its tip. It may be passed through the patient's nose by the anesthesiologist or introduced by the surgeon through a Stamm gastrostomy. It is then passed through the pylorus with the balloon deflated. The balloon is partially inflated and the tube milked around the duodenum to the ligament of Treitz and then down the small intestine. Meanwhile, intermittent suction should be applied for the aspiration of gas and intestinal content. Caution should be exercised in milking the tube through the intestine, as the distended bowel has impaired tensile strength and can easily be torn. In patients who have relatively few adhesions, the Baker tube may be removed at the conclusion of the decompression and a nasogastric tube substituted for postoperative suction. In patients who have extensive serosal damage due to universal adhesions, it may be desirable to perform a stitchless plication by leaving the Baker tube in place for 10–14 days.

Management of Serosal Damage

Small areas of intestine from which the serosa has been avulsed by dissection require no sutures for repair if the submucosa has remained intact. This is evident in areas where some remnants of muscle fibers remain. Otherwise, when only thin mucosa bulges out and the mucosa is so transparent that bubbles of fluid can be seen through it, the damage is extensive enough to require inversion of the area with several interrupted 4–0 cotton Lembert sutures.

Operative Technique

Incision and Bowel Mobilization

A long midline incision is preferable. If the site has an earlier incision, start the new incision 3–5 cm cephalad to the upper margin of the old incision so that the abdomen can be entered through virgin territory. Carry the skin incision through the middle of the old scar and down to the linea alba. After opening the upper portion of the incision, identify the peritoneal cavity, then carefully incise the remainder of the scar. At the same time dissect away any adherent segments of underlying intestine (**Fig. 22–1**).

Divide adhesions by the method described above in "Operative Strategy," until the entire anterior and lateral portion of the abdominal wall and parietal peritoneum are free of underlying adhesions (see **Fig. 22–2**). Thereupon, free the remainder of the bowel of adhesions, from the ligament of Treitz to the ileocaecal valve. Accomplish this by delicate Metzenbaum scissors dissection, alternately sliding the scissors underneath a layer of fibrous tissue to visualize its extent and then cutting the adhesion. This can be

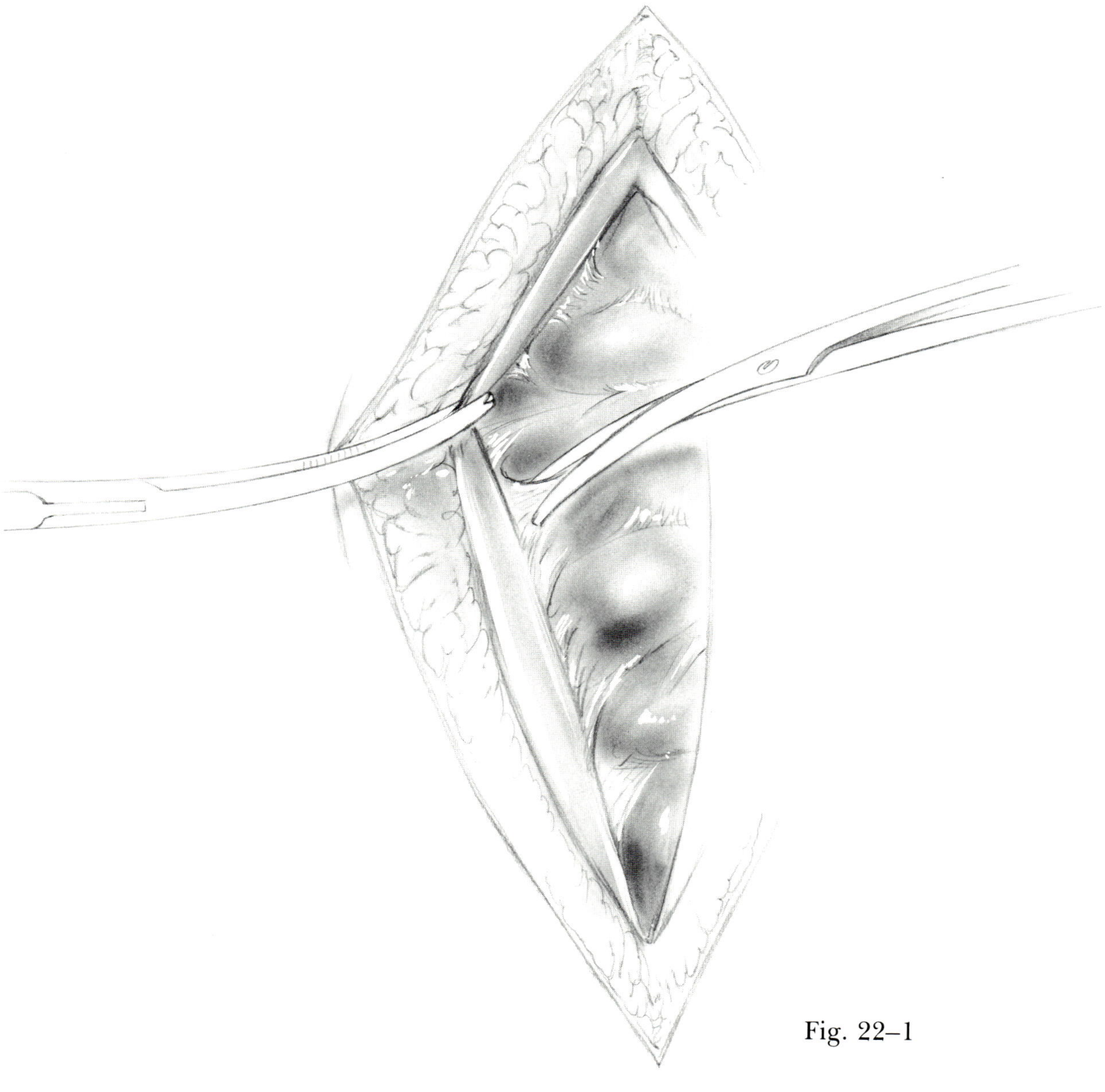

Fig. 22–1

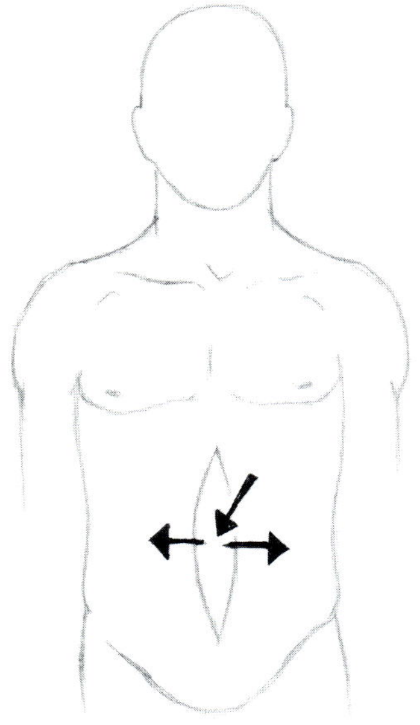

Fig. 22–2

done more efficiently if the left index finger can be insinuated in such a way as to circumscribe the adherent area, or if the index finger can be brought between the leaves of mesentery separating the adherent bowel, thereby placing the adhesion on stretch and making it visible (**Fig. 22–3**). In some cases there are adhesions of a cartilaginous nature, especially in patients whose obstruction is due to multiple malignant implants. Bold scalpel incisions should be made to divide adhesions of this type. Again, by doing the easy dissection first, the difficult parts will become easier.

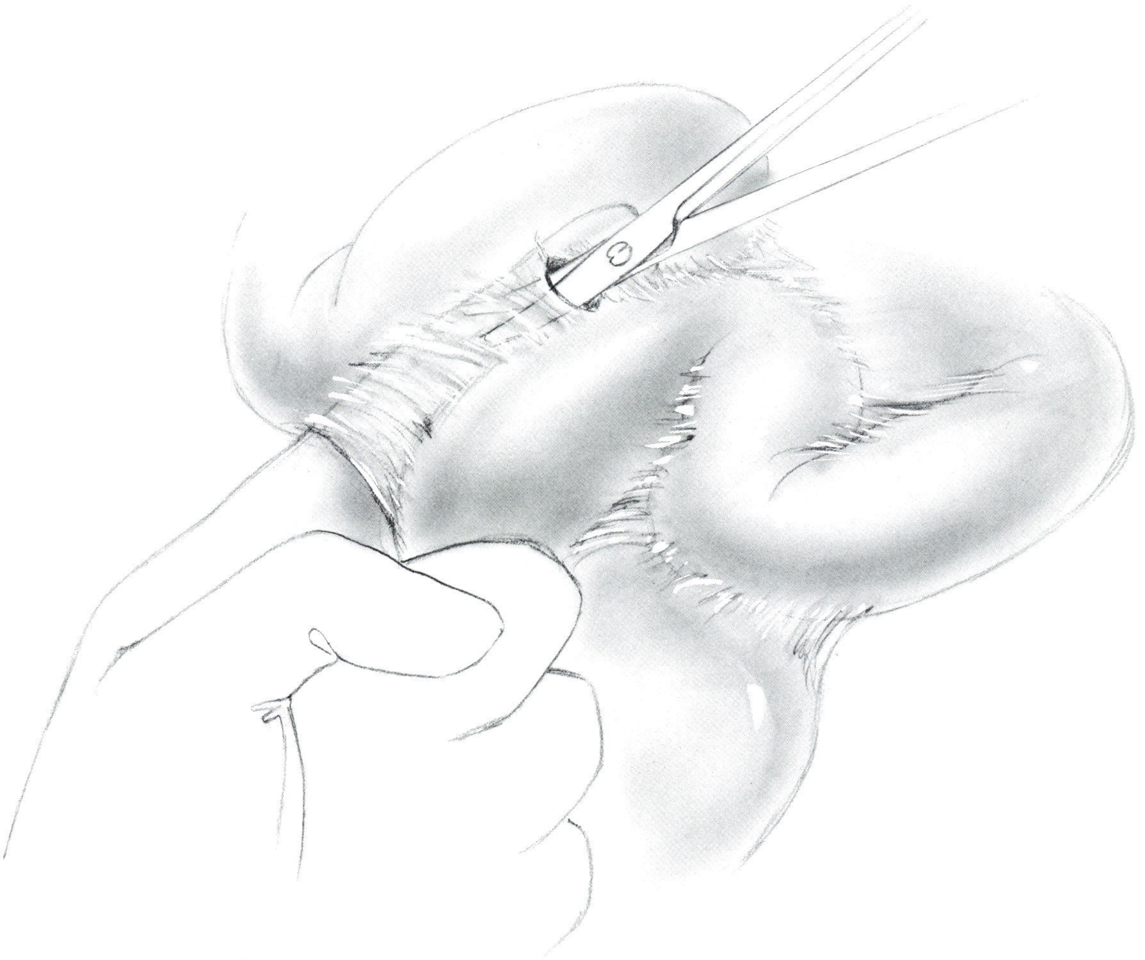

Fig. 22–3

Repair of Damage to Bowel Wall

Small areas of damage to the bowel wall, as evidenced by the protrusion of a thin transparent layer of mucosa, should be repaired by interrupted 4–0 cotton seromuscular Lembert sutures. If there are larger areas of damage, such as a longitudinal rent, they may be repaired by one or two layers of Lembert sutures in a transverse manner. Extensive damage requires a bowel resection with anastomosis either by sutures or stapling.

Closure

After decompressing the bowel, replace it in the abdominal cavity. If there has been any spillage, thoroughly irrigate the abdominal cavity with large volumes of warm saline solution followed by lavage with a dilute antibiotic solution. Close the abdominal wall in the usual fashion with a modified Smead-Jones technique (see Chap. 5).

Postoperative Care

Nasogastric or long intestinal tube suction will be required postoperatively until evidence of bowel function returns, as manifested by the passage of flatus or stool per rectum, or active bowel sounds.

Perioperative antibiotics

Complications

Recurrent intestinal obstruction

Intestinal fistula or peritonitis

Reference

Hudspeth AS (1975) Radical surgical debridement in the treatment of advanced generalized bacterial peritonitis. Arch Surg 110:1233

23 Baker Tube Stitchless Plication

Indications

Operations for intestinal obstruction due to extensive adhesions, when patient has already undergone numerous similar operations

Patients who suffer extensive serosal damage following division of many adhesions

Concept

After extensive adhesions involving most of the small intestine have been dissected, or the patient has undergone numerous similar operations, it can be anticipated that adhesions will reform after enterolysis. With the aim of causing these adhesions to form in an orderly fashion, Noble, and Childs and Phillips, performed a suture plication of the entire small intestine so that the bowel could not twist around localized adhesions.

Baker has developed a technique for accomplishing the same end by passing a 270 cm tube through a jejunostomy opening down to the cecum. This decompresses the small bowel after enterolysis. In addition, by leaving the tube in place for 10 days and by arranging the bowel in an orderly fashion (**Fig. 23–1**), any adhesions that develop presumably will form in a similar orderly fashion. In a series of 52 cases reported by Baker, 46 results were excellent and only one developed a postoperative obstruction, which responded to suction through a long intestinal tube.

Since Baker's is a simpler procedure, it has largely replaced the intestinal suture-plications of the Noble or Childs type for patients who have recurrent obstructions due to adhesions.

Preoperative Preparation

Nasogastric or long-tube suction should be administered to the patient before the operation.

Pitfalls and Danger Points

Trauma to the bowel while passing the Baker tube is a hazard of this procedure.

Operative Strategy

The 18F Baker tube, 270 cm long with a 5 ml bag at its tip, should be passed either through a jejunostomy or a gastrostomy. Of the two routes, the gastrostomy has far fewer postoperative complications than the jejunostomy and is the much preferred method. A gastrostomy of the Stamm type should be used (see Figs. 17–1 through 17–5). It is not advisable to pass the tube by the nasogastric route, as the tube must remain in place for at least 10 days. Also, in some cases a second nasogastric tube may be required to decompress the stomach postoperatively.

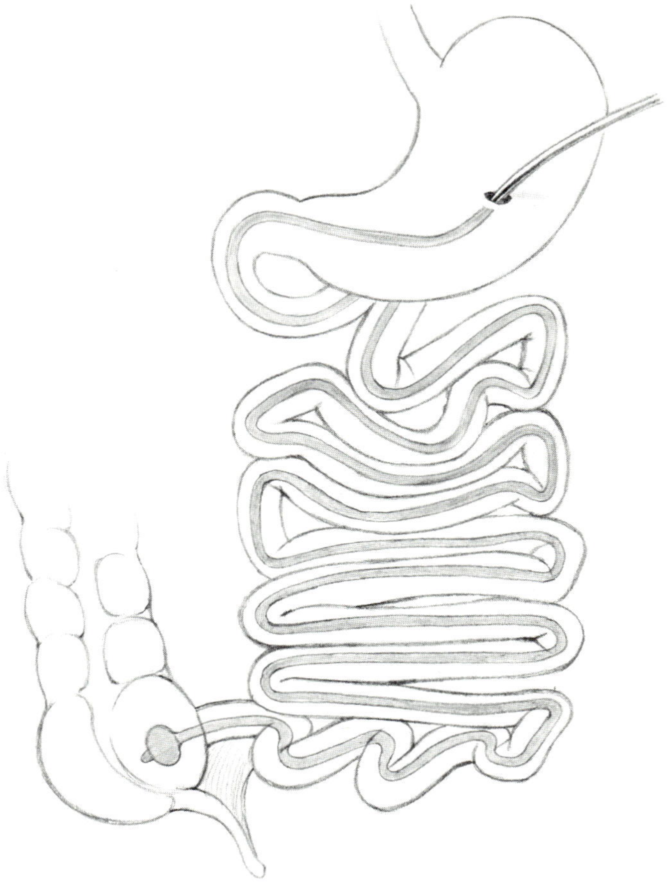

Fig. 23–1

If the stomach or the duodenum has been the site of a previous operation that would impede construction of a gastrostomy, then pass the Baker tube retrograde through a cecostomy up to the jejunum. This route too is safer than is the jejunostomy as the jejunostomy sometimes leaks or causes intestinal obstruction after the Baker tube is removed.

Operative Technique

Enterolysis of the entire small bowel should be performed as the first step of this operation. Pass the sterile tube through a puncture wound in the abdominal wall and then into a gastrostomy. Then pass it through the pylorus and partially inflate the balloon. By milking the balloon along the intestinal tract the tube may be drawn through the entire length of the intestine. Supply intermittent suction to the tube to evacuate gas and intestinal content. Pass the balloon through the ileocecal valve, where it should be inflated to 5 ml.

Distribute the length of the intestine evenly over the length of the tube. Then arrange the intestine in the shape of multiple S's. Complete the Stamm gastrostomy by suturing the stomach to the anterior abdominal wall in the vicinity of the stab wound. Irrigate the peritoneal cavity with a dilute antibiotic solution and close the abdomen in the usual fashion. If there has been any spillage of bowel content during the dissection, if gangrenous bowel has been resected, or if an enterotomy has been performed for intestinal decompression, the skin incision should not be closed primarily. Stewardson et al. have pointed out that over 50% of the patients they treated who had these conditions developed wound infections. An alternative way of preventing wound infections is McIlrath's method of inserting a closed suction subcutaneous catheter (see Fig. 2–3) and injecting antibiotics into the catheter postoperatively.

When local factors contraindicate a gastrostomy, pass the Baker tube through a stab wound near McBurney's point. Then construct a cecostomy by the Stamm technique. Insert a purse-string suture using 3–0 PG in a portion of the cecum that is near the stab wound. Make a puncture wound in the center of the purse-string, insert the Baker tube, and hold the purse-string taut. To pass the Baker tube through the ileocecal valve, make a 3–4 mm puncture wound in the distal ileum. Then insert a Kelly hemostat into the wound and pass the hemostat into the cecum. Grasp the Baker tube with the hemostat and draw the tube into the ileum. Close the puncture wound with sutures or staples.

Inflate the balloon of the Baker tube and milk the balloon in a cephalad direction until the tip of the Baker tube has reached a location proximal to the point of obstruction and to any area of bowel that has suffered serosal damage. Suction all the bowel contents through the Baker tube and deflate the balloon.

Insert a second 3–0 PG purse-string suture inverting the first purse-string. Then suture the cecostomy to the abdominal wall with one 3–0 PG suture in each quadrant surrounding the abdominal stab wound.

Postoperative Care

Deflate the balloon at the end of the Baker tube on the second postoperative day. However, leave the tube in place for at least 10 days if a stitchless plication is to be achieved. Some surgeons believe that the tube should be left in place from 14–21 days following the operation. An additional nasogastric tube for suction may be required for several days. The patient should be permitted to eat when evidence of bowel function returns, at which time the Baker tube suction can be discontinued.

Antibiotics should be given postoperatively to patients who have had intraoperative spill of intestinal contents.

Postoperative Complications

Wound infection

References

Baker JW (1968) Stitchless plication for recurring obstruction of the small bowel. Am J Surg 116:316

Childs WA, Phillips RB (1960) Experience with intestinal plication and a proposed modification. Ann Surg 152:258

Noble TB (1937) Plication of small intestine as prophylaxis against adhesions. Am J Surg 35:41

Stewardson RH et al. (1978) Critical operative management of small bowel obstruction. Ann Surg 187:189

Colon and Rectum

24 Appendectomy

Indications

Acute appendicitis

Interval appendectomy following conservative treatment of appendiceal abscess

Mucocoele of appendix

Adenocarcinoma and carcinoid of appendix may require right colon resection in addition to appendectomy, especially if there is suspicion of metastases in lymph nodes

Concept

Probably 85% of the time acute appendicitis is the result of a closed-loop obstruction generally secondary to an appendiceal fecalith. The base of the appendix, which is proximal to the obstructing fecalith, usually is fairly healthy even in the presence of advanced inflammation or even if the remainder of the organ is gangrenous. This makes ligature or inversion of the appendiceal stump a safe procedure.

There has been a decline in the incidence of acute appendicitis in the United States during the past two decades, while the accuracy of the diagnosis has increased. In good hospitals less than 15% of all appendectomies done are cases in which histological finding is of a normal appendix. Accuracy of diagnosis can be increased if in all doubtful cases the surgeon rechecks the physical findings every 4–8 hours. Frequently, by the end of 24 hours the presence or absence of acute appendicitis is clarified, at minimal risk to the patient. The most difficult diagnosis is of young women, in whom disease of the pelvic organs can be a source of confusion.

Whether an immediate operation is indicated in a patient who first presents with an appendiceal abscess in the right lower quadrant remains a matter of controversy. If the signs are well localized and the patient shows improvement with antibiotic therapy, conservative management will probably prove successful. In this case an interval appendectomy should be done in 6 weeks. If there is any progression in the abdominal findings or in the patient's toxicity, prompt laparotomy should be done to drain the abscess.

In cases of spreading peritonitis secondary to a feeding focus at the appendix, it may be necessary to perform an emergency ileocecal resection.

Preoperative Preparation

Intravenous fluids

Perioperative antibiotics

Nasogastric tube if ileus is present

Pitfalls and Danger Points

Inadvertent laceration of inflamed cecum during blunt dissection

Inadequate control of blood vessels in edematous mesoappendix

Operative Strategy

Incision

When classic signs of acute appendicitis present themselves, the McBurney incision is an appropriate one. Because this procedure splits the muscles along the lines of their fibers, each in a somewhat different direction, the healed scar is usually quite strong and the cosmetic result good. For most cases the incision proves to be centered over the base of the appendix. If the exposure is inadequate, the incision may be carried in a medial direction by dividing the rectus sheath. If necessary the right rectus muscle itself may be transected for the exposure of the pelvic organs.

If it is obvious that even with an extension the exposure will be inadequate, a new vertical incision should be made, suitable to the pathology, and the McBurney incision closed.

The McBurney incision is contraindicated for young women in whom the diagnosis is not clear-cut. Either a midline or paramedian incision should be made.

Management of Appendiceal Stump

After the appendix has been removed, the stump may be managed either by simple ligation or by inversion with a purse-string suture around its base. There does not appear to be any proof of the superiority of either method, although one would suspect that a purse-string inversion might produce fewer adhesions than a simple ligation, which permits eversion of a bit of the mucosa. Inversion is preferable in simple cases, but if the area is quite edematous, making inversion difficult, simple ligation is preferable.

Indication for Drainage

The presence of inflammation or even of free pus due to a perforated appendix is not an indication for external drainage. The abdominal wall should be closed without drainage after thorough irrigation of the abdominal cavity and pelvis. In cases of perforated appendix, to avoid wound sepsis the surgeon should leave the skin wound open for secondary closure at a later date. If an abscess with rigid walls is encountered, then it may be indicated to insert a drain through a stab wound in the abdominal wall.

Operative Technique

Incision

Draw an imaginary line from the right anterior superior iliac spine to the umbilicus. At a point 3–4 cm medial to the anterior spine, draw a perpendicular to this line (**Fig. 24–1**). This is the general direction of the McBurney skin incision. About one-third of the incision should be above the imaginary line between the iliac spine and umbilicus and two-thirds below this line. The average length of this incision is 6 cm.

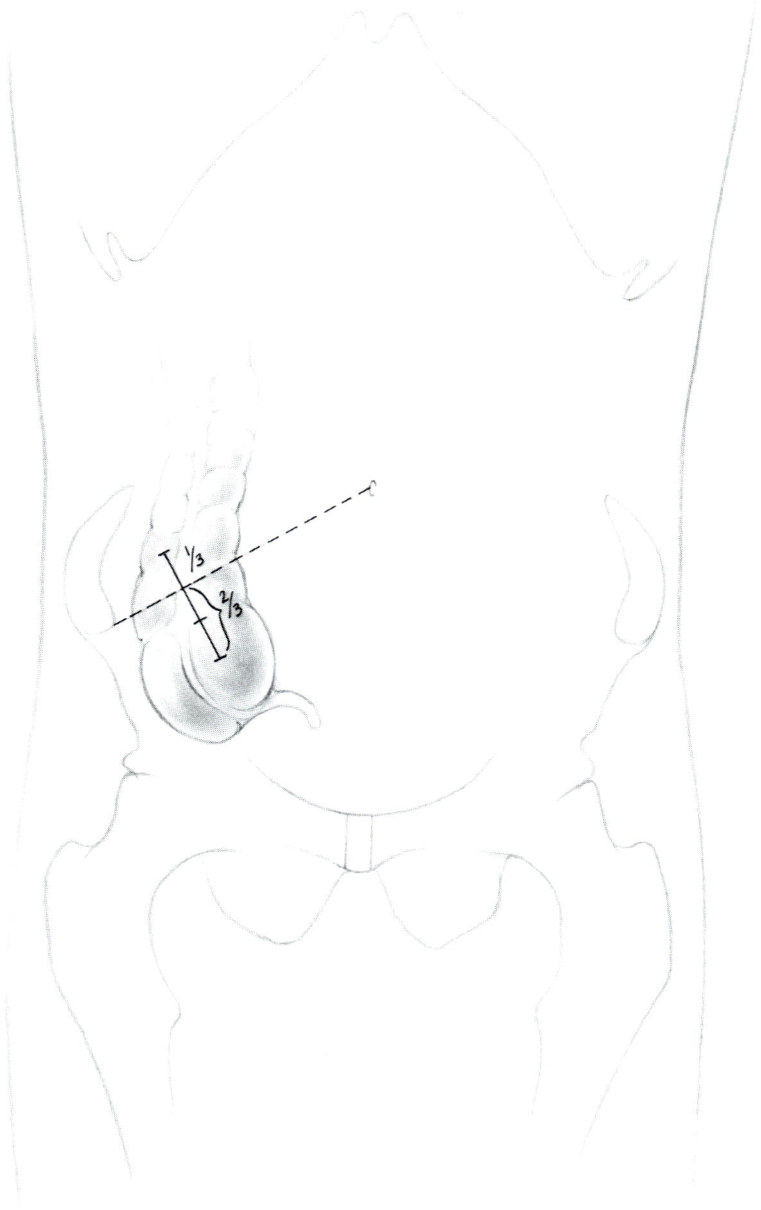

Fig. 24–1

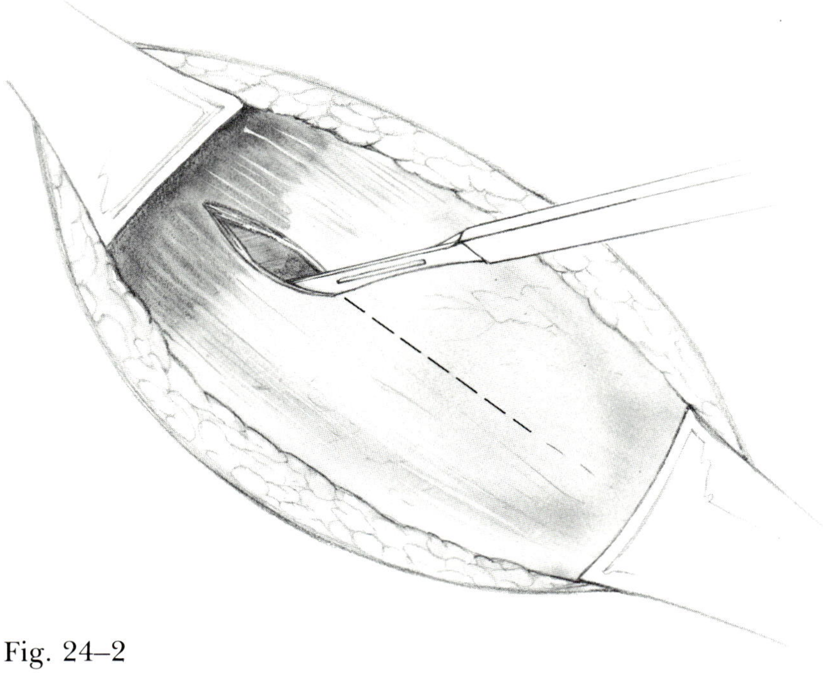

Fig. 24–2

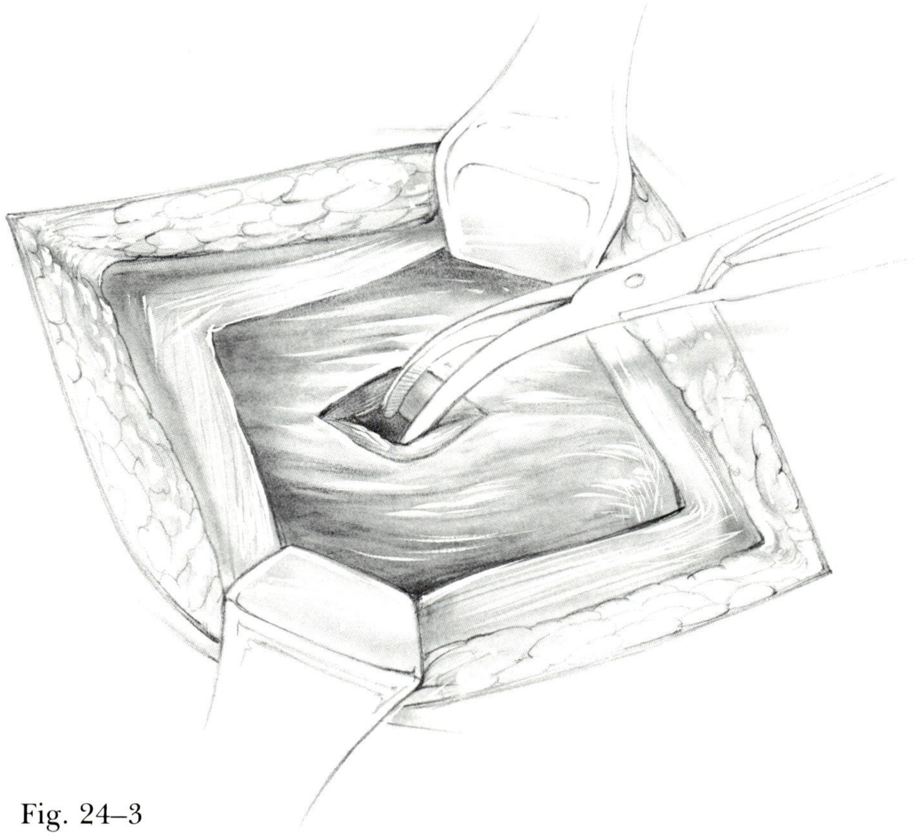

Fig. 24–3

Make an incision identical to that in the skin in the external oblique aponeurosis, along the line of its fibers (**Fig. 24–2**). After this incision has been initiated with a scalpel and extended with a Metzenbaum scissors, elevate the medial and lateral leaves of the external oblique from the underlying muscle, and separate them between retractors (**Fig. 24–3**).

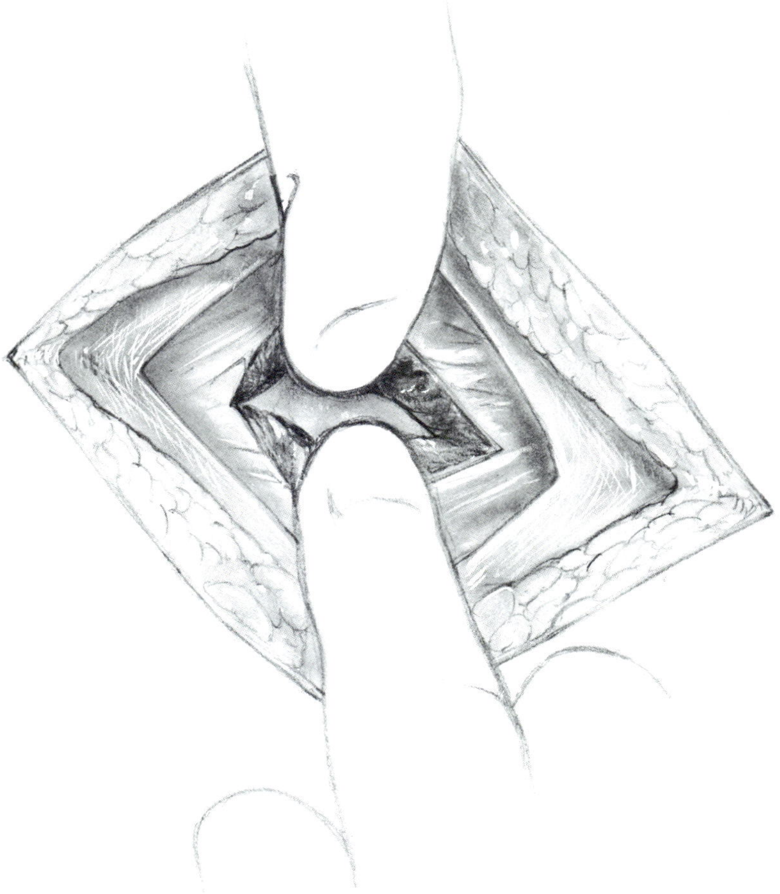

Fig. 24–4

Note now that the internal oblique muscle, which is fairly thick, and the transversus muscle, which is deep to the internal oblique, run in a transverse direction. Make an incision just below the level of the anterior superior iliac spine into the thin fascia of the internal oblique muscle. Then insert a Kelly hemostat to separate the muscle fibers of the internal oblique and underlying transversus muscle (Fig. 24–3). Using either two Kelly hemostats or both index fingers, enlarge this incision sufficiently to insert small Richardson retractors (**Fig. 24–4**).

By electrocoagulation, obtain adequate hemostasis of one or two vessels in the internal oblique. Then note the layer of fat that adjoins the peritoneum. By teasing the fat off the peritoneum lateral to the rectus muscle, a clear area of peritoneum can be identified. Elevate this between two hemostats and make an incision into the peritoneal cavity (**Fig. 24–5**). Enlarge this sufficiently to insert Richardson retractors. Then explore the region.

For additional exposure in a medial direction when, for example, it is necessary to identify a woman's pelvic organs, a medial extension of about 2 cm can be made across the anterior rectus sheath. Following this, a similar division of the posterior sheath can be carried out and the rectus muscle retracted medially.

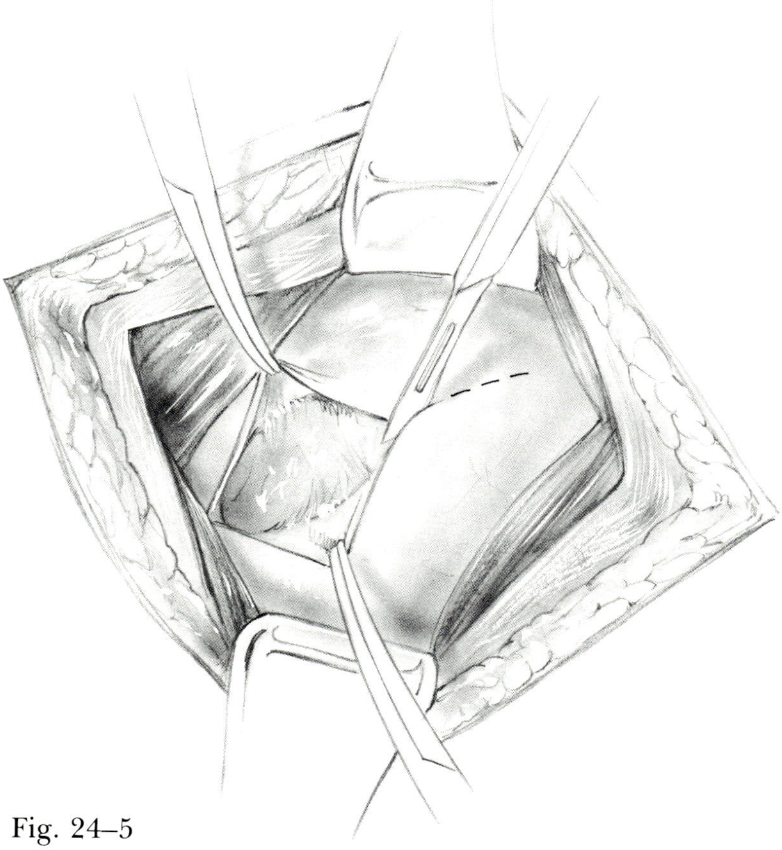

Fig. 24–5

When the lateral extremity of the McBurney incision must be extended, the surgeon has two choices: 1) Close the McBurney incision and make a separate vertical incision of adequate length for exposure. 2) If only a few centimeters of additional exposure are needed, the oblique and transverse muscles may be deliberately divided with the electrocautery in a cephalad direction along the lateral portion of the abdominal wall. Be aware that if this vertical extension along the lateral abdominal wall is continued for *more* than 4–5 cm, two or more intercostal nerves are likely to be divided, resulting in muscular weakness of the lower abdomen. If a 4–5 cm extension of the incision is closed carefully, generally no serious problems of weakness or herniation will develop.

Delivery of Appendix

Insert small Richardson retractors into the peritoneal cavity and grasp the anterior wall of the cecum with a moist gauze pad (**Fig. 24–6**). With the cecum partially exteriorized, identify the appendix. If the appendix cannot be seen, exploration with the index finger may reveal an inflammatory mass consisting of inflamed appendix and mesoappendix. By gentle digital manipulation around the borders of this mass, it can usually be delivered into the incision.

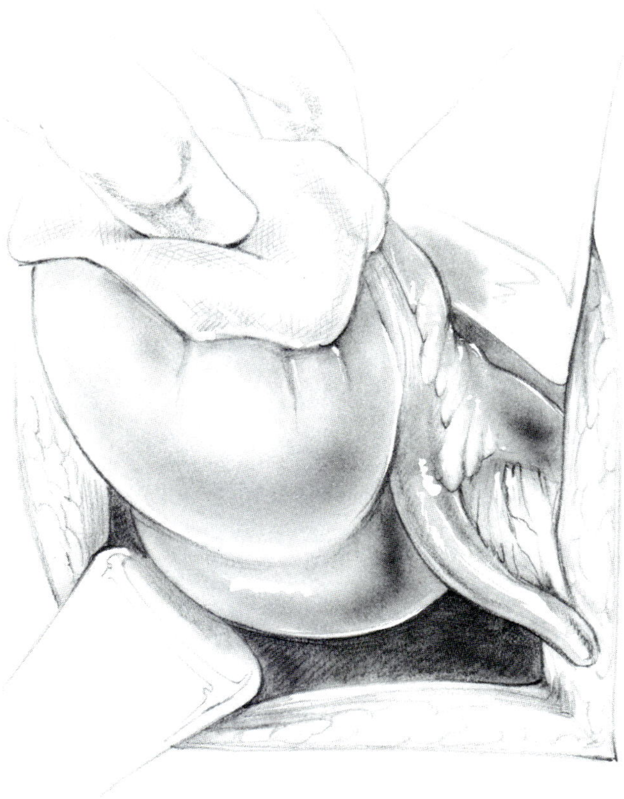

Fig. 24–6

If this palpatory maneuver is not successful in locating the appendix, follow the taenia on the anterior wall of the cecum in a caudal direction. This leads to the base of the appendix, which can then be grasped in a Babcock clamp. Apply a second Babcock clamp to the tip of the appendix and deliver it into the incision.

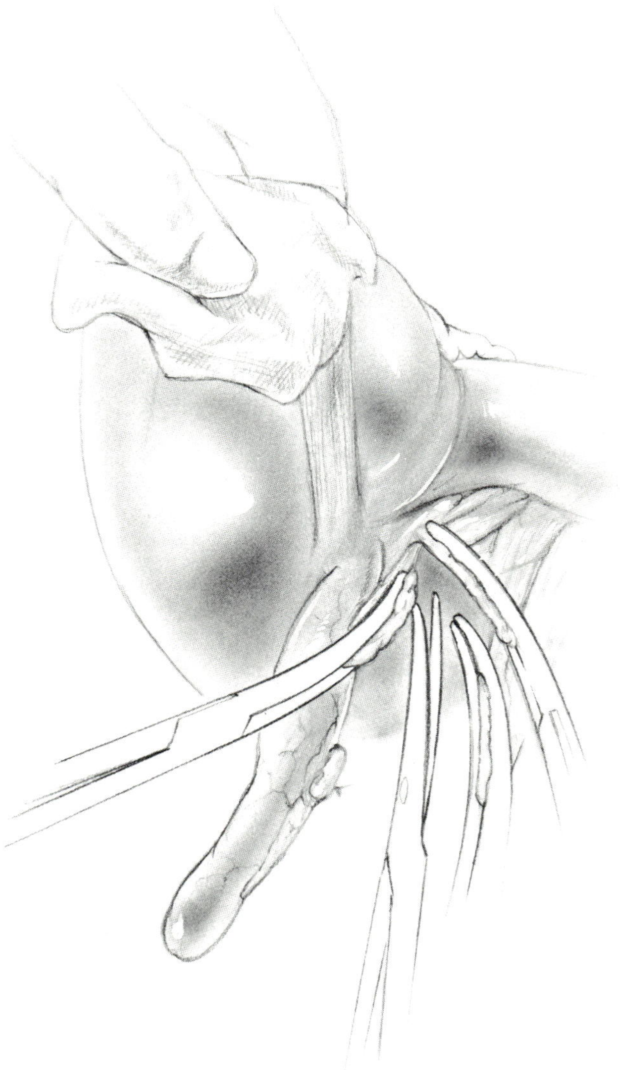

Fig. 24–7

Division of Mesoappendix

If the base of the mesoappendix is not thick it may be encompassed by a single ligature of 2–0 PG. Otherwise, divide the mesoappendix between serially applied hemostats, and ligate each with 2–0 or 3–0 PG until the base of the appendix has been dissected free (**Fig. 24–7**).

Ligation of Appendiceal Stump

Hold the tip of the appendix in a Babcock clamp and doubly ligate the base with 2–0 PG or chromic catgut at a point 4–6 mm from the cecum. Apply a straight hemostat to the appendix 1 cm distal to the ligature. Then transect the appendix with a scalpel 5–6 mm distal to the ligature (**Fig. 24–8**) and remove the specimen. The appendiceal stump may be cleansed with phenol and alcohol, if desired, or the mucosa of the stump may be lightly electrocoagulated. Or nothing at all need be done to the stump except to return it to the abdominal cavity (**Fig. 24–9**).

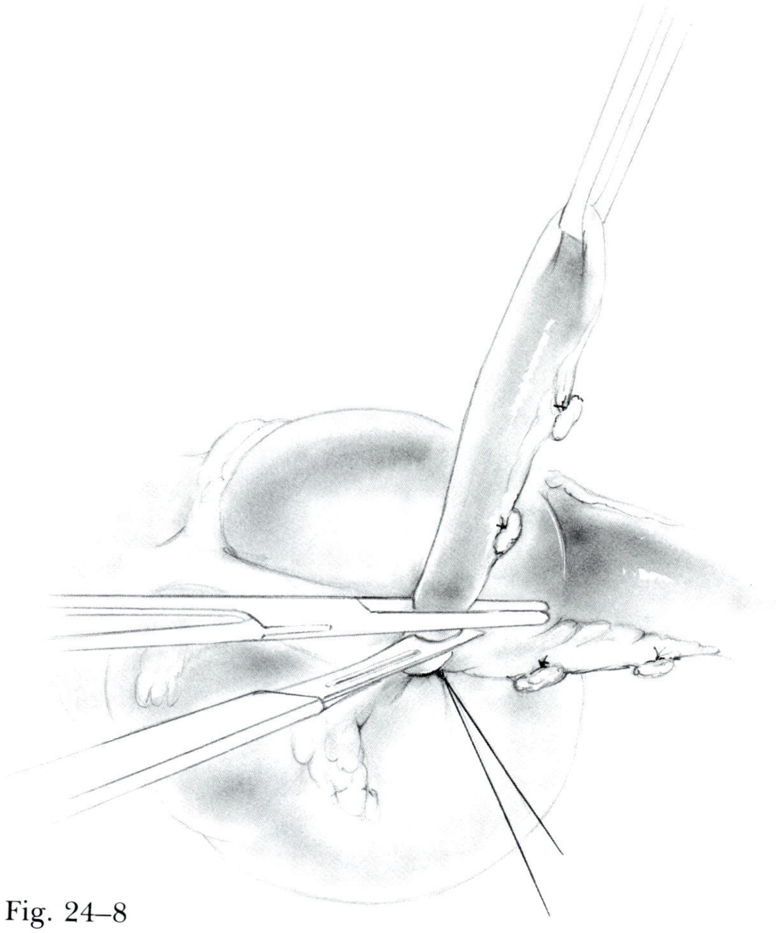

Fig. 24–8

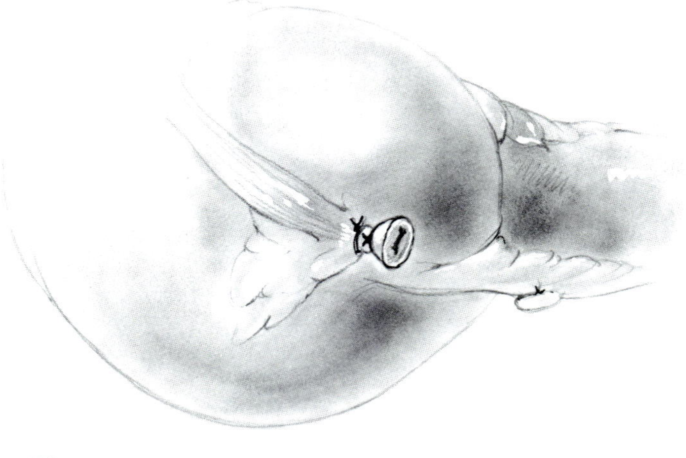

Fig. 24–9

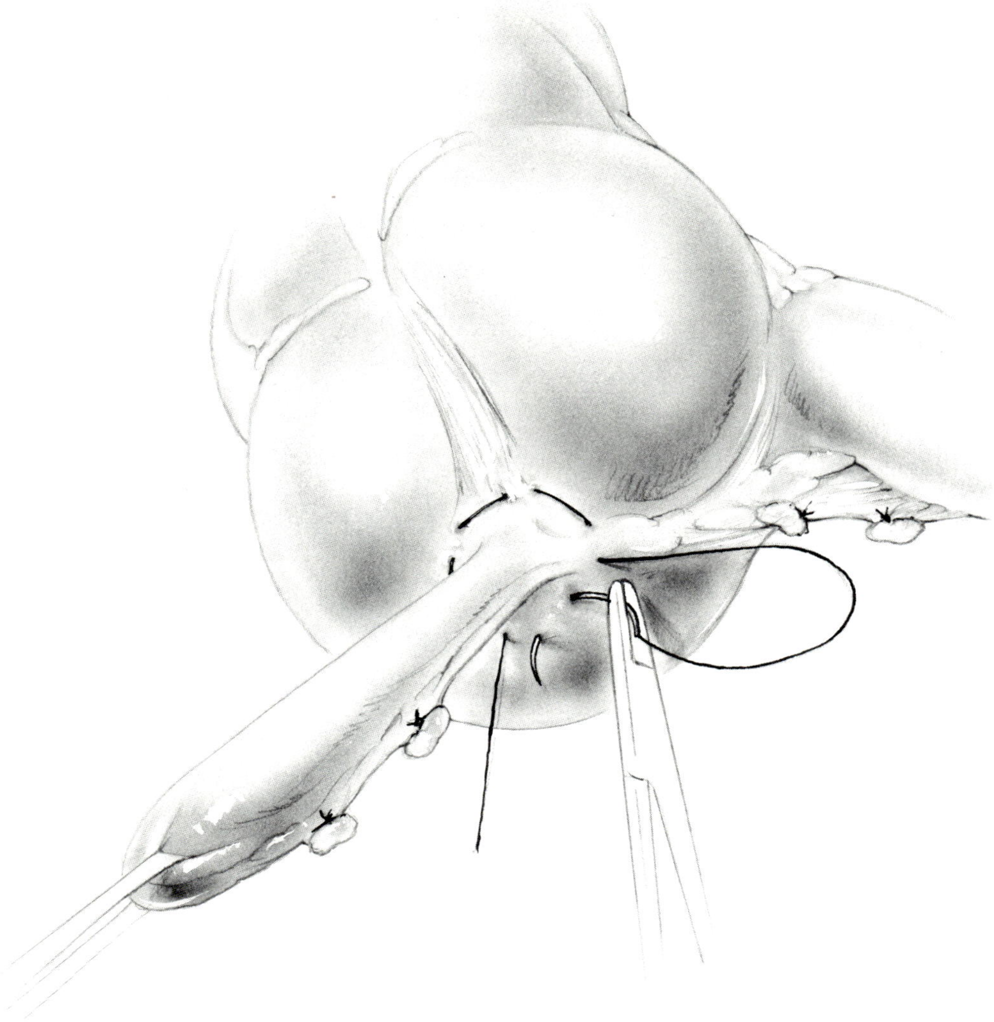

Fig. 24–10

Inversion of Appendiceal Stump

To invert the stump, insert a purse-string suture around the base of the appendix, using 3–0 PG or silk on an atraumatic needle. The radius of this purse-string should exceed the anticipated length of the appendiceal stump (**Fig. 24–10**). Apply a small straight hemostat to the base of the appendix at a point 5–6 mm from the cecum. Apply a second hemostat 1 cm distal to the first. Using a scalpel, transect the appendix just distal to the first hemostat (**Fig. 24–11**), which should now be used to invert the sump into the previously placed purse-string suture (**Fig. 24–12**). As the first knot is being tied, gradually withdraw the hemostat, thus completing the purse-string tie. The single suture should be sufficient; if there is some doubt of its adequacy, it may be reinforced with a figure-of-eight suture of the same material.

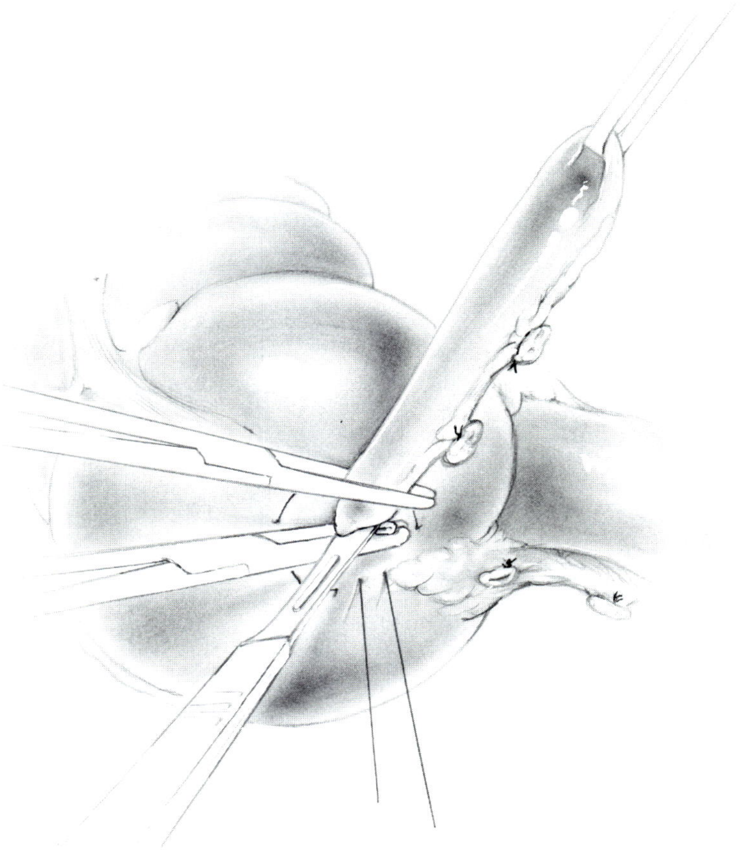

Fig. 24–11

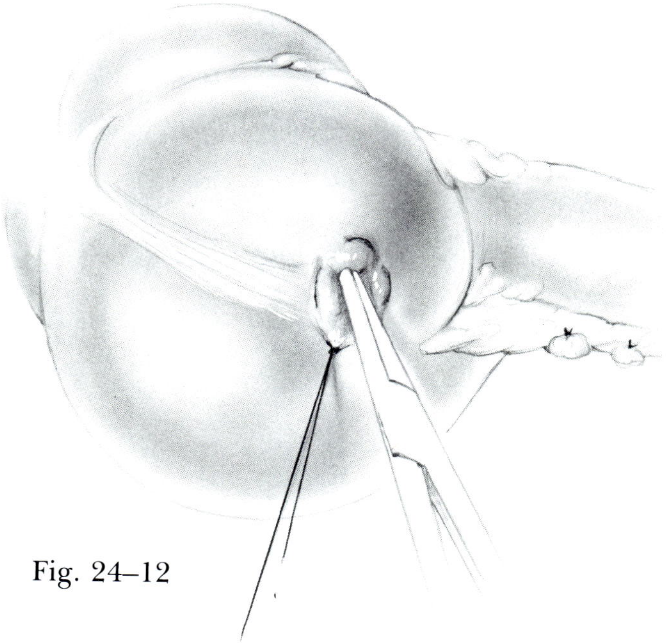

Fig. 24–12

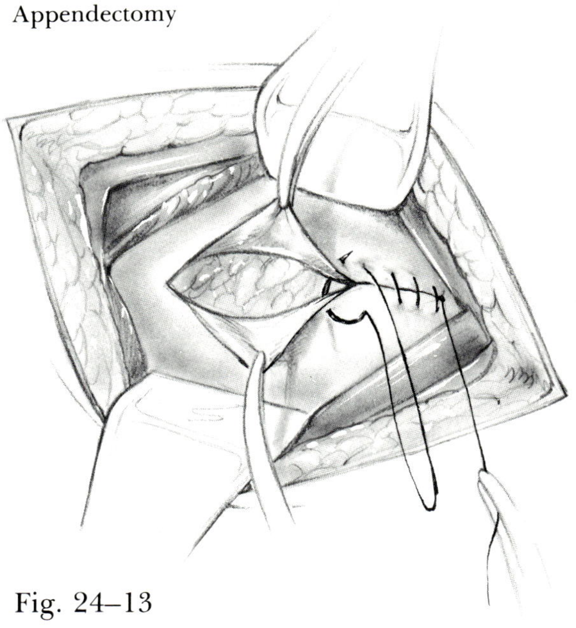

Fig. 24–13

Closure of Incision

Irrigate the right lower quadrant and pelvis with a dilute antibiotic solution. Then apply four hemostats to the cut ends of the peritoneum. Close the peritoneum with continuous 3–0 atraumatic PG suture (**Fig. 24–13**). Close the internal oblique and transversus muscles as a single layer with interrupted sutures of 2–0 PG tied loosely (**Fig. 24–14**). Close the external oblique aponeurosis with either continuous or interrupted sutures of 2–0 PG (**Fig. 24–15**).

If intraperitoneal pus or a gangrenous appendix is present, no attempt should be made at primary closure of the skin incision. Rather, a few vertical mattress sutures of 4–0 nylon may be inserted but not tied. Insert just enough gauze into the incision to keep the skin edges separated.

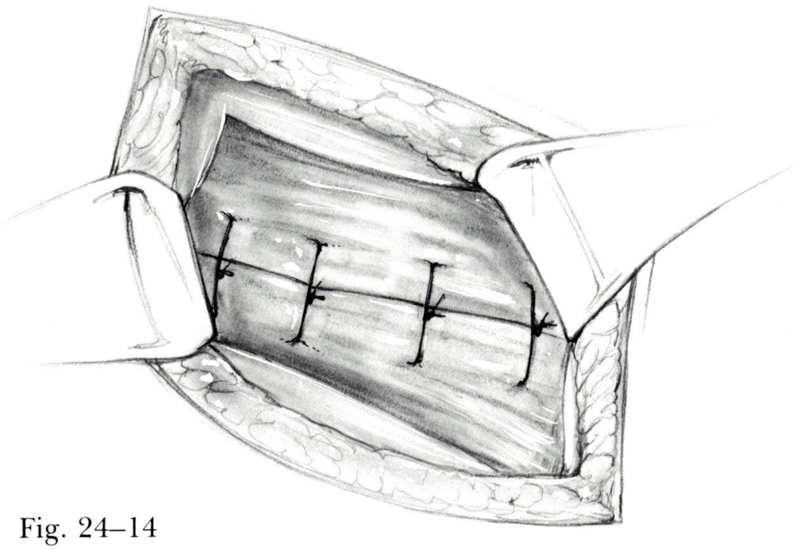

Fig. 24–14

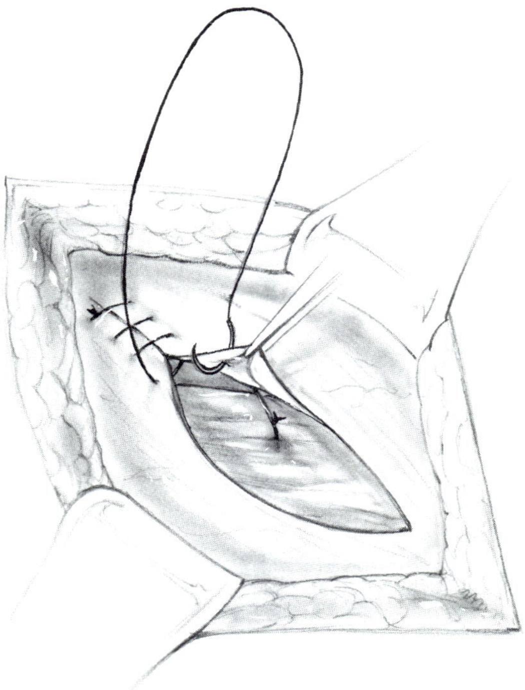

Fig. 24–15

Postoperative Care

In the absence of pus or perforation, postoperative antibiotics need not be administered beyond the perioperative period (24 hours). Otherwise, appropriate systemic antibiotics are indicated.

Most patients recover rapidly following an appendectomy. They usually do not require nasogastric suction or intravenous fluid for more than 1 day.

If the skin wound has been packed open, the packing should be changed daily. If the area is clean, the previously placed skin sutures may be tied after the fourth postoperative day.

Complications

Postoperative sepsis, either in the form of peritonitis or a pelvic abscess, is the most serious postoperative complication of an appendectomy. If the patient's temperature is elevated after the fourth or fifth postoperative day, a rectal or pelvic examination should be performed daily to try to detect a pelvic abscess. Often this can be discovered when the tip of the examining finger feels a fluctuant and tender mass pressing on the anterior wall of the rectum. If the abscess has progressed on antibiotic therapy, incision and drainage should be performed with general anesthesia. To do so, dilate the anus; then pass a needle into the palpable mass. Aspiration should reveal pus just deep to the rectal wall. If pus is found, insert a hemostat along the needle tract to make a 1–2 cm drainage opening.

Wound infection following an appendectomy for a perforated appendicitis is another cause of fever. This may be prevented by delaying closure of the skin. Otherwise, when a wound abscess is detected, the overlying skin must be opened for drainage.

Intestinal obstruction due to adhesions occasionally occurs in the postoperative period, especially when there is some degree of peritonitis. Early relaparotomy is indicated for a complete obstruction.

25 Colon Resection

Resection of the colon is performed in such conditions as carcinoma, diverticulitis, inflammatory bowel disease, ischemic colitis, volvulus, polyposis, arteriovenous malformation, and trauma. The nature of the dissection and the extent of the colectomy will vary with the pathology. The principles of performing an anastomosis of the colon remain constant.

Concept: Principles of Successful Colon Anastomosis

According to Schrock et al., if during an elective operation two segments of well-prepared, healthy colon are properly anastomosed, and infection and other adverse factors are not present, 98% of all cases can be expected to heal without clinical leakage. A number of technical requirements must be met, however, before this level of excellence can be reached.

Blood Supply

The end of each segment of colon should have demonstrable pulsatile arterial blood flow in the mesentery at the cut edge of the bowel. It is a valuable routine to make an incision in one of the small end-arteries near the point at which the colon is transected to determine if this is indeed so. An intramural hematoma at the anastomosis or a hematoma in the adjacent mesentery may impair blood flow. Generally, this impairment requires re-resection of the involved bowel or mesentery.

Suturing

Although it probably does not matter whether the anastomosis is constructed with one or two layers of sutures, it is essential that seromuscular apposition be accurate. There should be no blood clot or interposition of globs of fat between these two layers. This requires that a 1 cm cuff of serosa be completely cleared of fat, mesentery, and epoploic appendices. *Most leaks in anastomoses occur on the mesenteric side of the bowel,* where there is greater difficulty in clearing off fat and blood vessels. Special attention should be devoted to accomplishing an accurate inversion of the bowel at this place. Submucosa must be included in each suture. Seromuscular sutures should not be tied with excessive force, as this may bring on strangulation necrosis.

Tension

Enough colon should be liberated from the surrounding ligaments and omentum to guarantee that there will be no linear tension on the anastomosis during the healing process. Remember: In the postoperative period the colon will distend and thus become shorter. Consequently, any tension on the anastomosis at the time of the operation will be increased during the next 5–7 days and may produce disruption.

Perianastomotic Hematoma

The accumulation of blood or serum in the vicinity of an anastomosis, especially in the pelvis, is an invitation to localized sepsis, for absolute sterility of the colon's lumen is not possible. Many leaks from anastomoses in the pelvis occur when an abscess from an infected hematoma erodes into the lumen of the rectum. Prevention requires good hemostasis as well as postoperative suction-drainage of the presacral space.

Dead Space

If the surgeon closes the pelvic peritoneum proximal to a colorectal anastomosis in the pelvis, considerable dead space may be left in the vicinity of the colorectal anastomosis. This dead space is conducive to anastomotic leakage. Anastomoses are more certain to heal when they are surrounded by adjacent viable tissue, such as *small bowel* or omentum. Consequently, it is wise to leave the pelvic peritoneum unsutured after performing colorectal anastomosis. This allows the small bowel to help eliminate the dead space. Another way to eliminate dead space is to liberate omentum and bring it into the pelvis. In addition, enough proximal colon should be liberated to permit the hollow of the sacrum to be occupied by redundant descending colon, thereby helping to eliminate dead space.

Drainage

There appears to be no advantage in draining an anastomosis in the intraperitoneal space. On the other hand, it is very important to use closed-suction drains in the presacral space to evacuate serum and blood from the pelvic cavity. Leakage from low colorectal anastomoses is often caused by an infected presacral hematoma. Suction catheters can be kept open for an indefinite period if 50 ml of an antibiotic solution are instilled every 6 hours.

Omental Wrap

Some authorities believe that wrapping an anastomosis with omentum is important to prevent leakage. While we use this technique when the omentum is easily available, we do not perform elaborate omentum-lengthening maneuvers to accomplish an omental wrap. A properly constructed anastomosis does not require the contiguity of the omentum to heal without leaking.

Conditions Conducive to Anastomotic Leakage

(The figures given in this section are taken from the extensive statistical study by Schrock et al. of clinical leakage following anastomoses of the colon.)

Sepsis

The presence of infection in the vicinity of colon anastomoses had long been believed to increase the incidence of leakage. Schrock et al. found that "Peritonitis, abscess, or fistula strongly favored leakage regardless of the segment anastomosed." The *clinical* leak rate in 909 intraperitoneal ileocolonic or colocolonic anastomoses, performed in the absence of intra-abdominal infection, was 2.4%–3.1%. When infection was present, 6.9% of 87 ileocolonic anastomoses leaked and 12.1% of 58 colocolonic anastomoses disrupted. The figures are equally striking for extraperitoneal coloproctostomy: In the absence of infection 7.9% of 329 anastomoses leaked, and 20.5% of 39 anastomoses disrupted if infection was encountered during the operation. In summary, *when infection was encountered during the operation, there was an increase of 150%–500% in the incidence of postoperative leakage of anastomoses.*

Although this result is less marked in ileocolonic anastomoses, even here the surgeon should be cautious about electing to perform a primary ileocolostomy in the presence of serious abdominal sepsis.

Shock, Major Hemorrhage

Diminution of systolic blood pressure by more than 50 mm Hg below the base line for 15 minutes or longer during the operation resulted in a 150% increase in the rate of leakage. If four or more units of blood replacement were required during the 24-hour period following the induction of anesthesia, there was a 400% increase in the rate.

Carcinoma at the Anastomotic Margin

Carcinoma at the margin of anastomoses was associated with a 20% leakage rate compared with 4.2% for cancer operations in which the margins were free of tumor.

Preoperative Radiation Therapy

Anastomoses failed three times as frequently in a group of 35 irradiated patients as in the remaining cases.

Segment Anastomosed

Ileocolonic and colocolonic anastomoses showed no significant difference in the incidence of leakage as long as extraperitoneal colorectal anastomoses were excluded from the comparison. Intraperitoneal anastomoses of all types leaked 3.4% of the time; extraperitoneal anastomoses disrupted in 10.4% of the cases.

Emergency Operations

When primary anastomoses were performed in emergency operations on the left colon, the rate of leakage increased from 3.0% to 10.8%. For coloproctostomies the rate went from 8.4% to 21.7%. On the other hand, in the ileocolonic anastomoses the increase from 3.3% to 5.4% was not statistically significant. It is not clear exactly what it is about an emergency operation that produces these adverse results. It might logically be assumed that lack of opportunity for preoperative cleansing of the colon plays an important role.

In summary, it is obvious that abdominal sepsis, massive hemorrhage, emergency operations, and preoperative radiation therapy all mitigate against primary healing. In many cases, colon resection should be followed by exteriorization of the proximal segment as an end colostomy or ileostomy and conversion of the distal segment into a mucous fistula. This is especially valid for the left colon. Ileocolonic anastomoses seem to tolerate some of these adverse factors better than do the colocolonic anastomoses. Performing a complementary colostomy proximal to an anastomosis did not reduce the incidence of leakage in the anastomoses Schrock et al. studied. However, proximal colostomy did indeed sharply reduce the rate of fatalities from leakage. Details of technique, such as open or closed, one or two layers, or end-to-end, did not make a significant difference in the rate of leakage in anastomoses. Tube cecostomy did *not* significantly reduce the mortality rate from leakage in anastomoses following coloproctostomy.

If a good-risk patient is found to have sepsis from a *localized* cecal perforation, it is permissible to perform an ileocolonic anastomosis following a right colectomy, provided the two intestinal segments to be anastomosed are free of inflammation. Also, the anastomosis should be placed in the upper abdomen, away from the abscess. The same principle can be applied to a resection of the sigmoid colon if there is an intramural diverticular abscess—but only if the pelvis, where the anastomosis will be constructed, is clean, and if the colon is not packed with feces. Where contamination and inflammation are not well localized, primary anastomoses are hazardous.

Preoperative Preparation

Barium colon enema

Sigmoidoscopy or colonoscopy

Intravenous pyelogram

Blood transfusions to correct anemia

Nutritional rehabilitation if necessary

Nasogastric tube on morning of operation

Insert a Foley catheter in the bladder

Perioperative systemic antibiotics

Bowel Preparation

Preoperative Day No. 3
Minimum residue diet

Bisacodyl, 1 capsule p.o. at 6:00 P.M.

Preoperative Day No. 2
Clear liquid diet

Magnesium sulfate, 30 ml 50% solution at 10:00 A.M., 2:00 P.M., and 6:00 P.M.

Enema at 7:00 P.M. and 8:00 P.M. Repeated if necessary until no return of solid feces

Preoperative Day No. 1
Clear liquid diet

Magnesium sulfate, 30 ml 50% solution at 10:00 A.M. and 2:00 P.M.

Neomycin and erythromycin base, 1 g each at 1:00 P.M., 2:00 P.M., and 11:00 P.M.

Initiate intravenous fluids 24 hours before surgery to correct the dehydrating effect of bowel cleansing.

Operative Strategy: The Colon Anastomosis

Type of Anastomosis

No one technique of colon anastomosis has been demonstrated to have any inherent superiority over the others. What is most important is the skill with which the surgeon constructs the union between the two bowel segments. The most commonly employed method is the two-layer end-to-end anastomosis with interrupted Lembert seromuscular sutures and a continuous mucosal suture. If one segment of bowel has a diameter which is considerably less than that of the other segment, this may be corrected by making a so-called Cheatle slit, which is a longitudinal incision along the antimesenteric border of the smaller limb. This enlarges the circumference and thereby equalizes the diameter of the two segments. One pitfall in constructing the two-layer anastomosis is that too much bowel may be turned in, thereby producing stenosis. The diameter of the colon should be large enough to prevent this problem.

A second method of anastomosis is the closed technique using one layer of sutures. This is often done by applying narrow-blade straight Dennis clamps to each of the two cut ends of colon, or by using the Furniss technique. One advantage of the closed technique is that it reduces fecal contamination. It is also more rapid to execute than the two-layer method and minimizes narrowing of the lumen. The closed technique requires greater skill and experience of the surgeon, as each stitch must be placed with perfection when a second reinforcing layer of sutures is omitted. The closed technique also introduces the danger that the opposite wall may be included in one or more of the sutures, producing an obstructed anastomosis. The closed technique does not allow visualization of the lumen when the sutures are inserted. For these reasons, the technique is not suitable for those surgeons who have not been trained in its use. The closed one-layer technique is not used for anastomosis in the pelvis because there is inadequate space to permit the placement of straight clamps or the Furniss clamp.

A third technique is the open method of doing the one-layer anastomosis with interrupted seromuscular sutures.

A fourth method of anastomosis is based on the use of *surgical staples.* In a study we completed, patients who underwent stapled anastomoses did not develop a greater number of complications than did patients on whom sutures were used. There are, however, just as many pitfalls in the use of stapling techniques as in suturing. In order to achieve equal results, the surgeon must learn the details of stapling techniques, just as the surgeon learned how to sew. Stapling is by far the most rapid method of completing an anastomosis. Stenosis is easily prevented by using stapling techniques. The bowel should not be stapled when there is gross infection, the blood supply is poor, or there is tension on the anastomosis. Any segment of bowel that is not fit to be sewn should not be stapled. Stapling is especially valuable in operating upon the poor-risk or critically ill patient, when reducing operating time may be important.

Lembert, Cushing, or Halstead Suture Technique

There are no solid data demonstrating an intrinsic superiority of any of these suture techniques over the others, so the choice depends upon personal preference, familiarity, and the efficiency with which the suture may be inserted. For instance, in colorectal and esophagogastric anastomoses, the exposure is sometimes such that a Cushing type stitch can be inserted more efficiently than the Lembert or Halstead types.

Of more importance than the suture technique is the judgment exercised as to the exact point at which the needle should penetrate the bowel wall, as well as the exact point of exit. In general, the needle containing the seromuscular suture should *emerge* from the serosa at a point 1–2 mm behind the cut edge of the muscular coat. A width of approximately 4–5 mm should be included in each bite, and the sutures should be about 4–5 mm apart. The muscularis and submucosa must be included in each stitch, for the latter layer has been demonstrated to have the greatest holding power. The sutures should not be tied with such force that the enclosed bowel will be strangulated. When a suture incorrectly is passed deep through the mucosa and tied with excessive force, strangulation may lead to leakage of the anastomosis. When the sutures are tied, apply only the force needed to accomplish apposition.

Closing the Mucosal Layer: The Connell Suture

When Connell in 1892 first reported the technique that bears his name, he was describing a one-layer bowel anastomosis. In a two-layer anastomosis, it is the seromuscular suture layer that constitutes the major source of strength. Far too much time and effort has been expended on the undeviating perpetuation of the Connell technique for approximating the mucosal layer. It does not matter whether this layer is accomplished by the method of Connell or by continuous or interrupted sutures of the Cushing, Lembert, or seromucosal (see Fig. B–16) type.

If a continuous suture is used, care must be taken not to apply excessive force when drawing up the suture after each bite, as this exerts a purse-string constricting effect and narrows the lumen. A loose suture should be employed. If the lumen of the bowel being approximated is already narrow, then *interrupted* sutures should be used exclusively. Another aid in avoiding the purse-string effect is the use of absorbable 4–0 catgut for the mucosal layer, as catgut sutures may be absorbed by the seventh or eighth postoperative day. This permits enlargement of the lumen as stool begins to pass through.

Selection of Suture Material

While absorbable suture material has been the invariable choice for mucosal approximation, most surgeons prefer nonabsorbable material for the seromuscular sutures. The size of the suture material should not exceed 4–0, as this is adequate in strength to maintain approximation accompanied by minimum foreign-body reaction. We prefer cotton, but silk, polyester, and Tevdek have their proponents, as do the monofilament sutures like Prolene and 5–0 wire. Although the latter two have the advantage of inciting the least amount of inflammatory reaction and granuloma formation, it is more difficult to tie knots with monofilament material.

The polyglycolic synthetics (Dexon or Vicryl) are unique in that they maintain adequate tensile strength for 12–14 days before being absorbed. Another favorable aspect of the polyglycolic sutures is that they are *not* digested by proteolytic enzymes. Consequently, local sepsis does not accelerate the rate of absorption as it does with catgut. These two features seem to indicate that the polyglycolics are suitable for seromuscular suturing as well as for approximating the mucosa, especially in those cases in which *large* anastomoses (e.g., gastrojejunostomy) lend themselves to continuous sutures in the seromuscular as well as mucosal layers. At present, there are insufficient data to support the routine adoption of this technique for the small or large bowel.

Side-to-End Coloproctostomy (Baker)

Several difficulties present themselves after a low anterior resection with anastomosis to the extraperitoneal rectum. The diameter of the rectal ampulla is frequently much larger than that of the proximal segment of colon to which it is being anastomosed. Correction of this disproportion with a Cheatle slit followed by end-to-end anastomosis, requires a surgeon to be highly skilled in suture technique. On the other hand, the lumen of a side-to-end anastomosis can easily be made quite large, while the end of the rectum can be invaginated into the side of the colon for additional protection against leakage, without the risk of creating stenosis. There need be no fear that a blind-loop syndrome will result from the closed end of the colon, because the anastomosis will extend to within 1 cm of this closed end. In agreement with Zollinger and Sheppard, and Baker, we are convinced that this suture technique is a more efficient method of reconstruction following low anterior resection than is end-to-end anastomosis. It has been followed by a lower incidence of leakage and of stenosis of the anastomosis in this location than has been the experience with end-to-end anastomoses.

The side-to-end principle may also be applied to the ileocolonic anastomosis in order to correct a large disparity between the diameter of the ileum and transverse colon. However, in this location the use of the Cheatle slit in the ileum, followed by end-to-end anastomosis, is generally not difficult and is faster than side-to-end.

Strategy of Postoperative Care

How Long Nasogastric Suction?

Surgeons vary widely in their prescriptions for the duration of nasogastric suction following colon resection. In the absence of food, gas will not be produced in the gastrointestinal tract, and nasogastric suction should eliminate air that has been swallowed. While on intravenous fluids, patients secrete more gastric juice than the intestinal tract, in a state of postoperative ileus, can propel forward. Nasogastric suction prevents these patients from aspirating gastric juice, which can bring on serious complications, especially in elderly patients whose gag reflex is inadequate. Nasogastric suction should be continued until there is evidence of effective bowel activity. If the patient is passing flatus, this is conclusive evidence. It is reasonable to discontinue nasogastric suction in patients whose bowel sounds are vigorous and who do not have any abdominal distention. In most cases these events occur between the fourth and seventh postoperative days.

When to Feed the Patient

Studies of wound healing in animals show that before the seventh postoperative day intrinsic tensile strength is inadequate to withstand the application of a disruptive force. From the 3rd to the 7th days there is a rapid increase in the tensile strength of the healing wound. Thereafter, the rate of increase levels off sharply.

In humans it makes sense to rest an anastomosis of the colon for 7 days following the operation. If the bowel has been properly prepared, the intestinal tract should be empty of anything save intestinal secretions. If the patient does not receive any oral feeding at all for this period, it is likely that any minor imperfections the surgeon has produced in the anastomosis will have an opportunity to heal spontaneously without resulting in leakage. In malnourished patients, for whom 7 days of caloric starvation would constitute an added insult, intravenous hyperalimentation is indicated, rather than the early institution of oral feeding. Because there is a 2% incidence of clinical leakage following colon anastomoses, and since modern means of intravenous nutrition can safeguard the patient against caloric deficiency, it seems the caution of postponing oral intake until the seventh postoperative day can enhance the surgeon's efforts to reduce the 1%–2% surgical mortality rate that follows elective colectomy. This is especially applicable to low colorectal anastomoses below the peritoneal reflection, which have the highest rate of postoperative leakage and sepsis.

References

Baker JW (1950) Low end to side anastomosis. Arch Surg 61:143

Chassin JL et al. (1978) The stapled gastrointestinal tract anastomosis: incidence of postoperative complications compared with the sutured anastomosis. Ann Surg 188:689

Clarke JS et al. (1977) Preoperative oral antibiotics reduce septic complications of colon operations. Ann Surg 186:251

Connell ME (1892) An experimental contribution looking to an improved technique in enterorrhapy whereby the number of knots is reduced to two or even one. Med Record 42:335

Schrock TR et al. (1973) Factors contributing to leakage of colonic anastomoses. Ann Surg 177:513

Zollinger RM, Sheppard MH (1971) Carcinoma of the rectum and the rectosigmoid. Arch Surg 102:335

26 Colon Resection for Cancer

Concept: Extent of Colon Resection

Considerable data have been reported by Turnbull et al. and by Stearns and Schottenfeld suggesting that wide resection of colon neoplasms results in a higher percentage of 5-year survivals than does conservative excision. This is especially true of Duke's stage C lesions, those that have histologically positive lymph nodes. It is not that the length of colon removed results in increased survival, but that wide resection permits higher dissection of the mesentery and its lymphovascular complex. Because the lymphatic network tends to follow the course of the veins, a more extensive dissection of the lymph nodes requires a concomitant extensive resection of the blood vessels. Thus an additional length of colon must be removed.

Tumors of the cecum drain along the ileocolic vein. Here the apex of the lymph-node dissection is at the junction of the ileocolic and the superior mesenteric veins. The middle colic lymph nodes are not likely to harbor metastases unless the ileocolic lymph nodes are saturated with tumor. This is uncommon in any case in which there is some hope of cure. **Fig. 26–1** illustrates the extent of the resection in cases of cecal cancer.

When the tumor is situated near the hepatic flexure, lymphatic drainage both to the ileocolic and middle colic lymph nodes may be anticipated. Consequently, the apex of the dissection in this instance should be situated at the upper reaches of both the ileocolic and the middle colic veins (**Fig. 26–2**). For lesions of the mid-transverse colon, the apex of the lymph-node dissection should be located at the origin of the middle colic vessels (**Fig. 26–3**). Tumors of the splenic flexure require that the left colic vessels be resected (**Fig. 26–4**).

Neoplasms situated in the descending and sigmoid colon drain into lymphatics along the left colic and the inferior mesenteric vessels. The inferior mesenteric artery should be divided at the aorta and the inferior mesenteric vein removed if one wishes to extend the lymphovascular dissection to the farthest practical limit (**Fig. 26–5**).

Although in advanced stages of splenic flexure carcinoma metastatic lymph nodes may sometimes be observed in the area between the pancreatic tail and the splenic hilum, there is no data to show that *routine* splenectomy improves the survival of patients who have lesions in this location.

There is some controversy, in treating carcinoma of the rectum, over the optimal point for dividing the lymphovascular bundle: Is it the origin of the inferior mesenteric artery at the aorta, or is it a point on the inferior mesenteric artery just distal to the take-off of the left colic artery? Unless there is clear evidence to indicate otherwise, we generally select the latter point (**Fig. 26–6**) as the apex of the dissection for carcinoma of the rectum

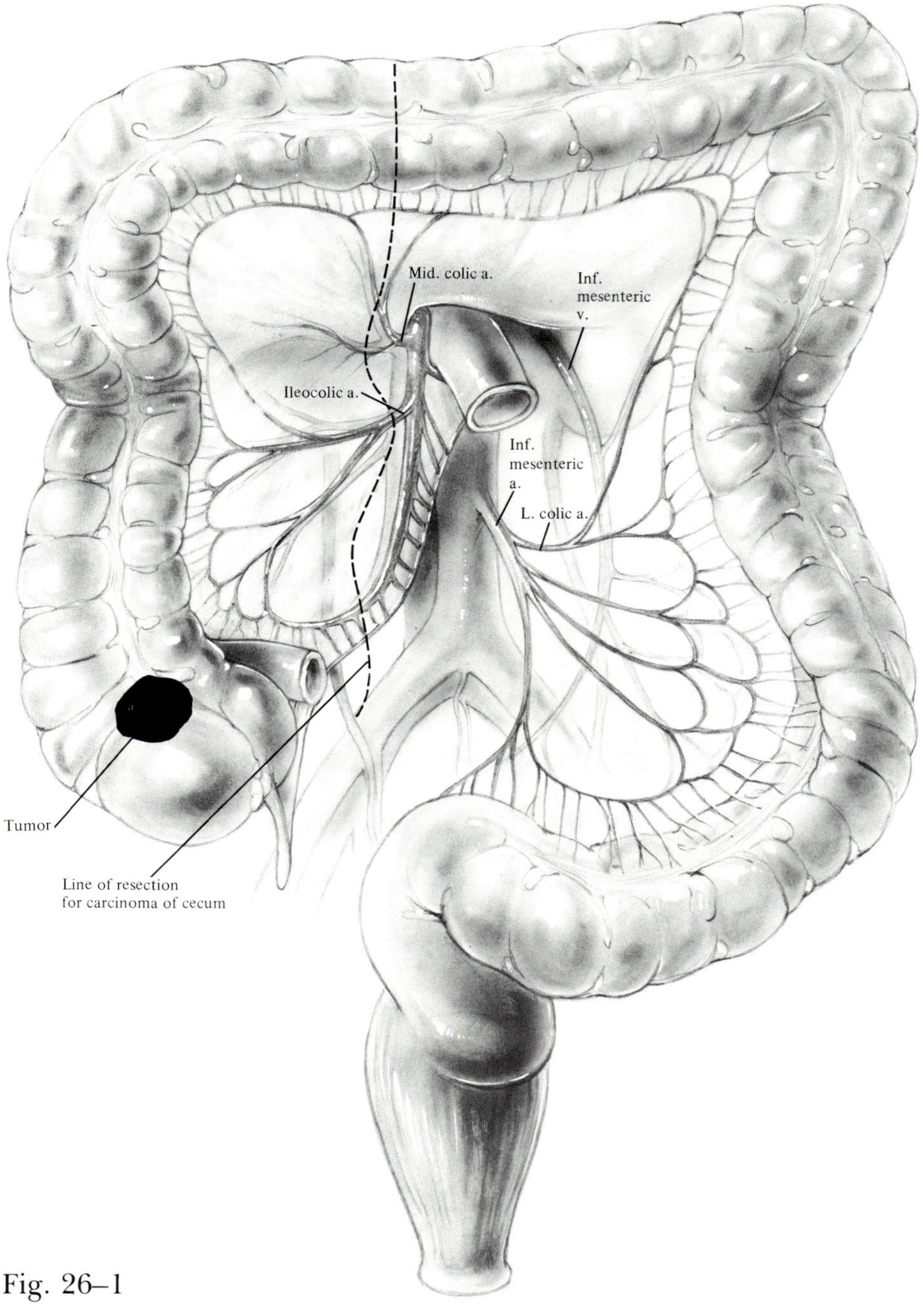

Fig. 26–1

and rectosigmoid junction. Goligher, and Stearns and Schottenfeld, prefer to transect the inferior mesenteric artery at the aorta (**Fig. 26–7**) and to rely upon the middle colic artery to supply adequate circulation to the descending colon.

Concept: The No-Touch Technique

A "no-touch" technique of right colon resection for carcinoma was first described in 1952 by Barnes. Serious attention was paid to this concept only 15 years later, when Turnbull et al. of the Cleveland Clinic demonstrated an improved 5-year survival rate in their patients who had

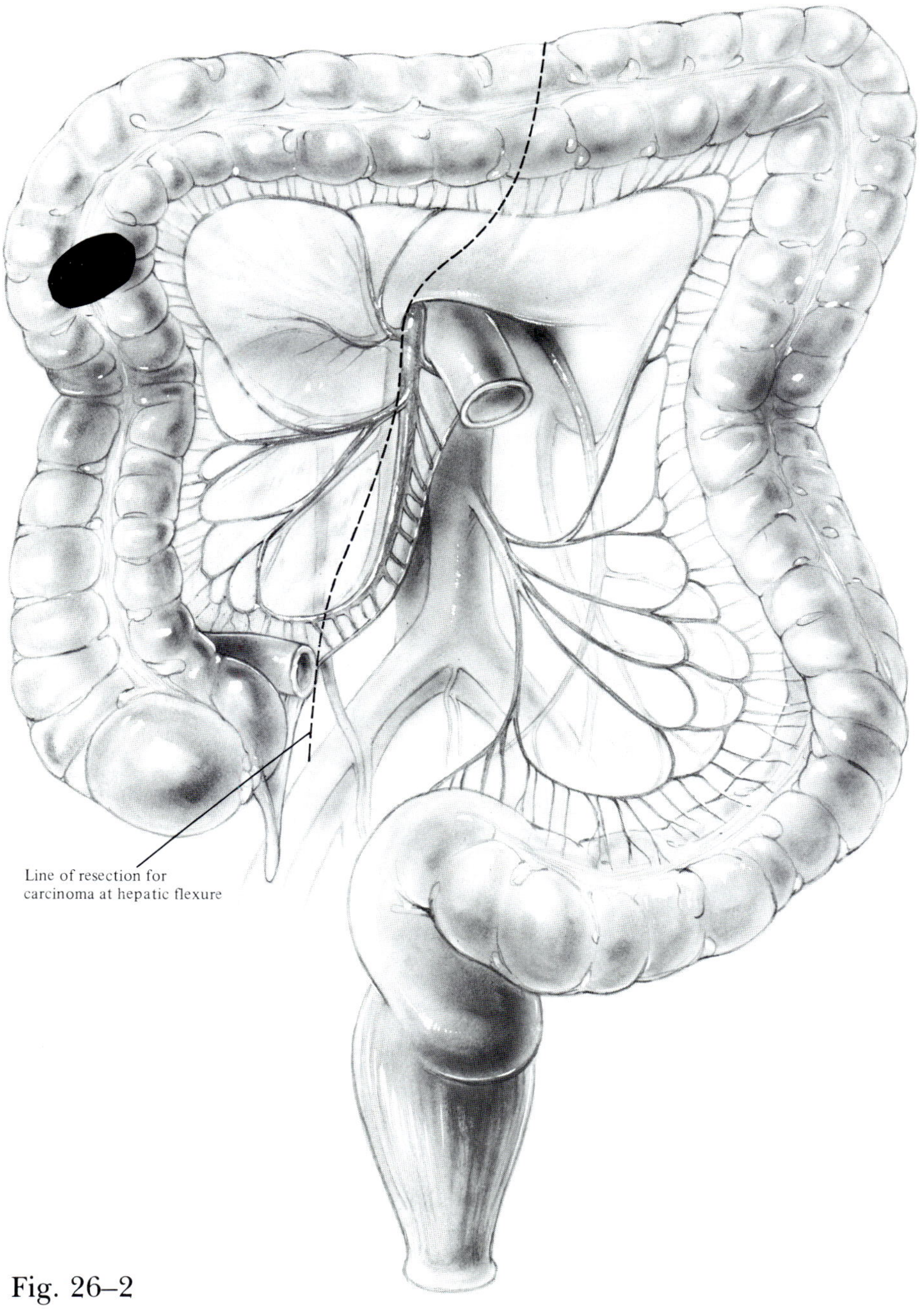

Fig. 26–2

been resected by this technique as compared with patients who had been operated upon by other surgeons at the same hospital. It is not clear whether this improved survival rate was a result of the no-touch isolation technique or simply because this technique also entailed a considerably wider resection of colon and mesentery than was routinely practiced by the other surgeons. Stearns and Schottenfeld achieved almost the same survival rate in patients whose operations had not been performed by the no-touch technique, but in whom equally extensive resections had been carried out.

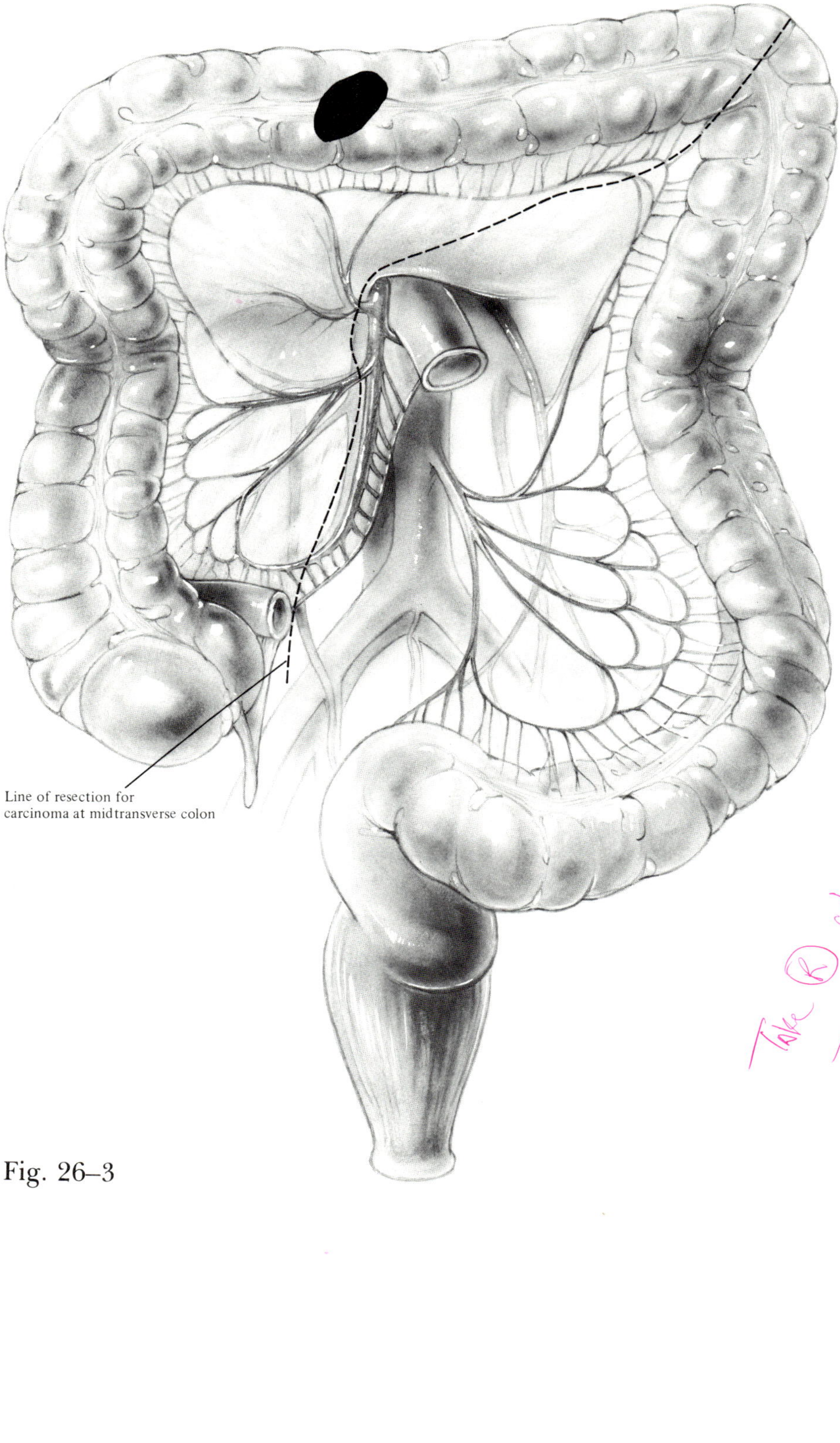

Fig. 26–3

Take (R) colon for mid Transverse lesion of colon

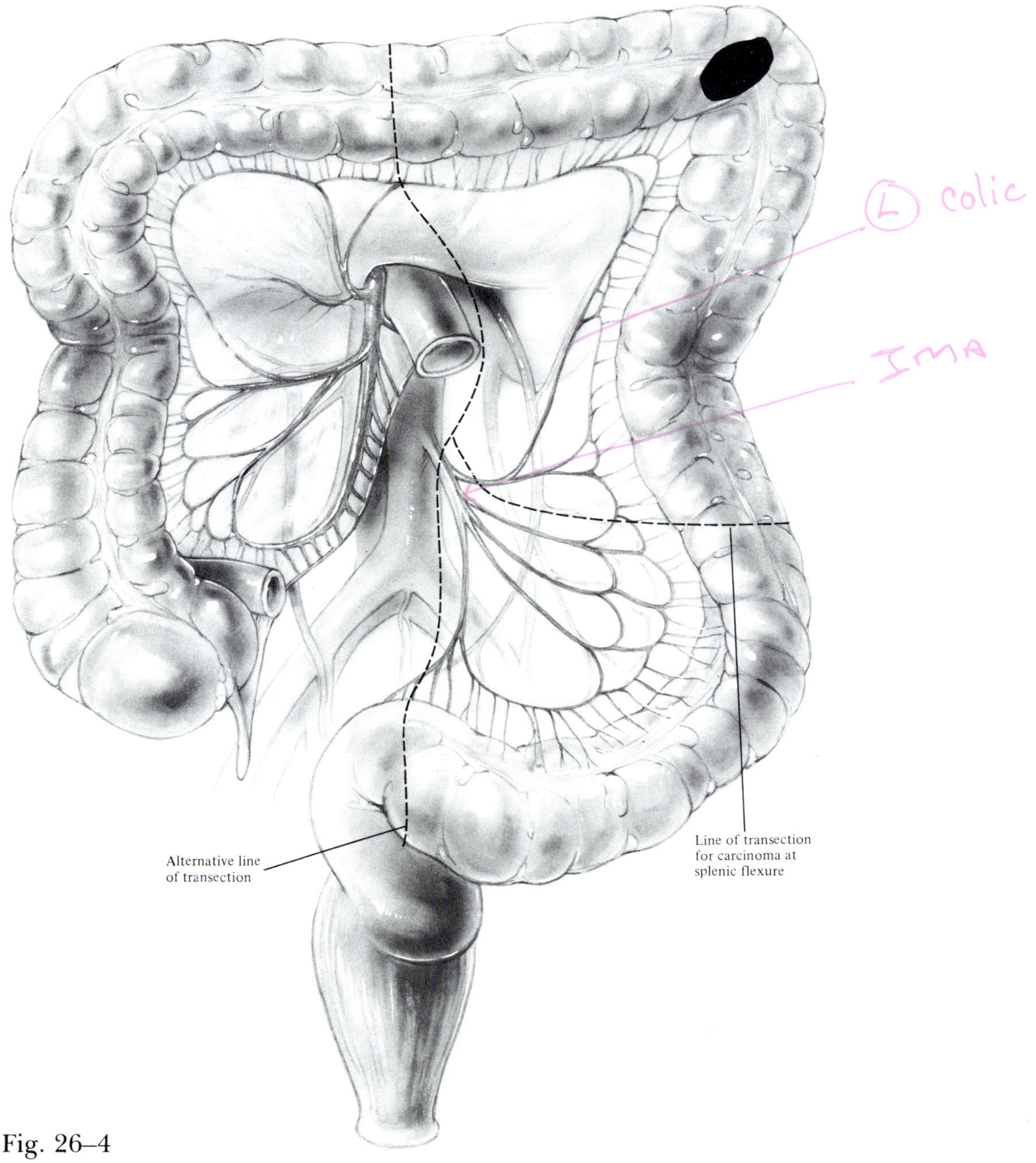

Fig. 26–4

The no-touch technique requires that the primary tumor not be manipulated until the section of colon in which it is located has been completely isolated from all lymphovascular connections to the patient. In other words, the tumor is not to be dissected until the blood supply has been divided and ligated and the lumen of the colon has been occluded.

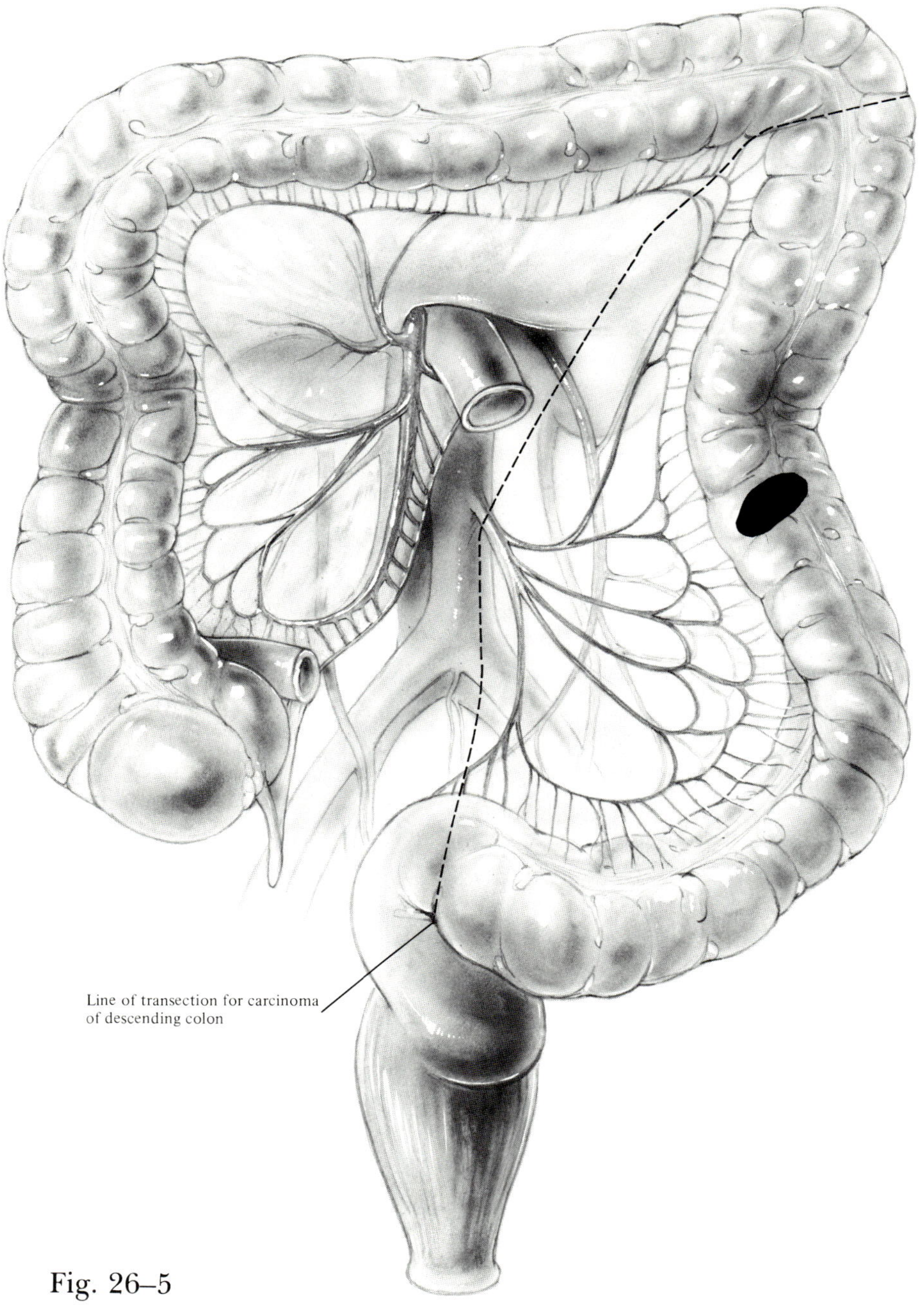

Fig. 26–5

It seems to us that in many cases it is not particularly difficult to add the no-touch isolation technique to an extensive resection of colon and mesentery. Consequently, when an operation is done for a cure in good-risk patients, the no-touch technique is generally used for lesions proximal to the splenic flexure.

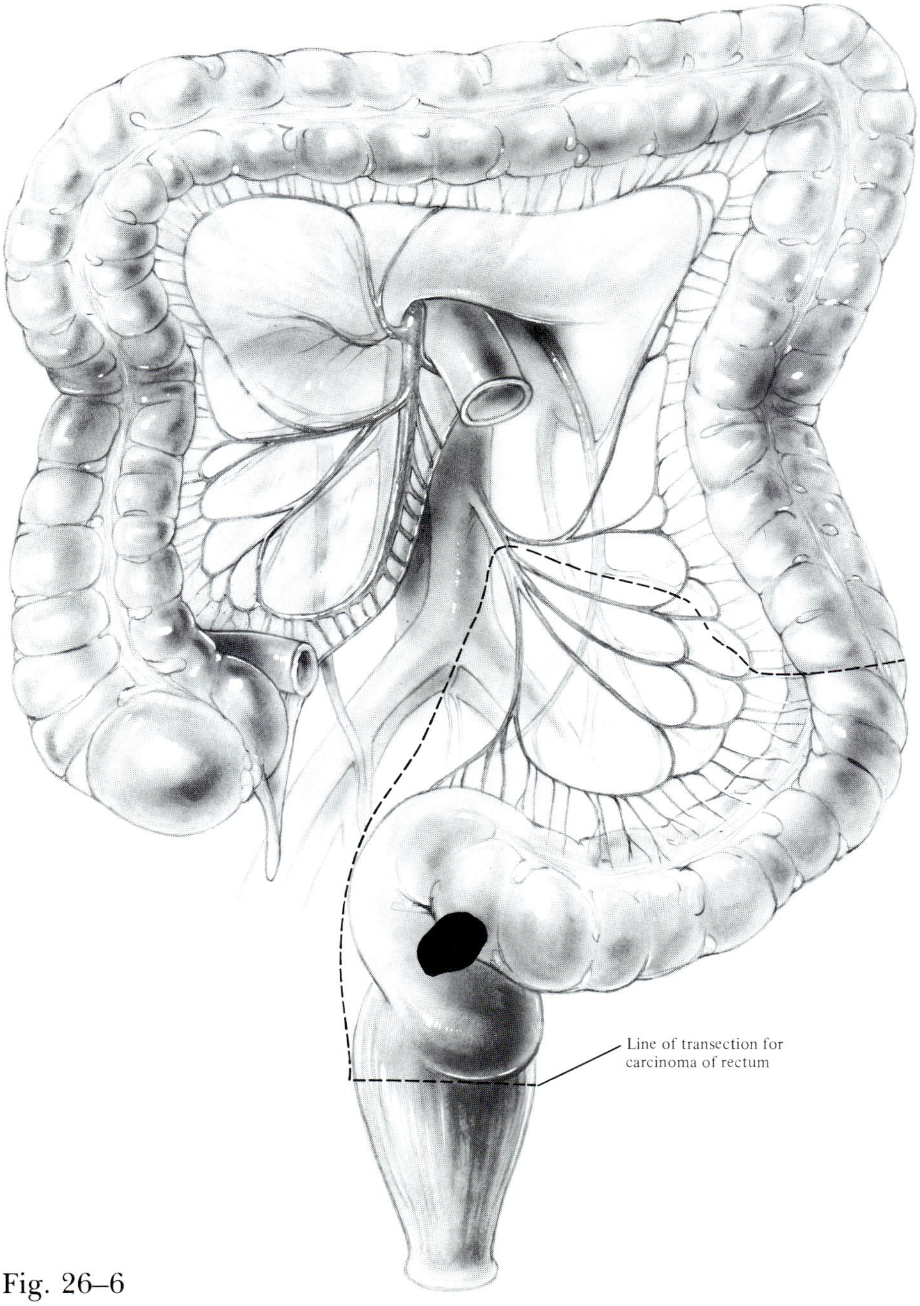

Fig. 26–6

Concept: Prevention of Suture-Line Recurrence

Cole et al. stated emphatically that most suture-line recurrences were preventable. They hypothesized that cancer cells got implanted into the suture line because the needle and suture material carried the cells through the wall of the colon in the course of suturing the anastomosis. If the lumen were free of viable cancer cells at the time the anastomosis was being constructed, they asserted, this complication could be eliminated. Cole et al. demon-

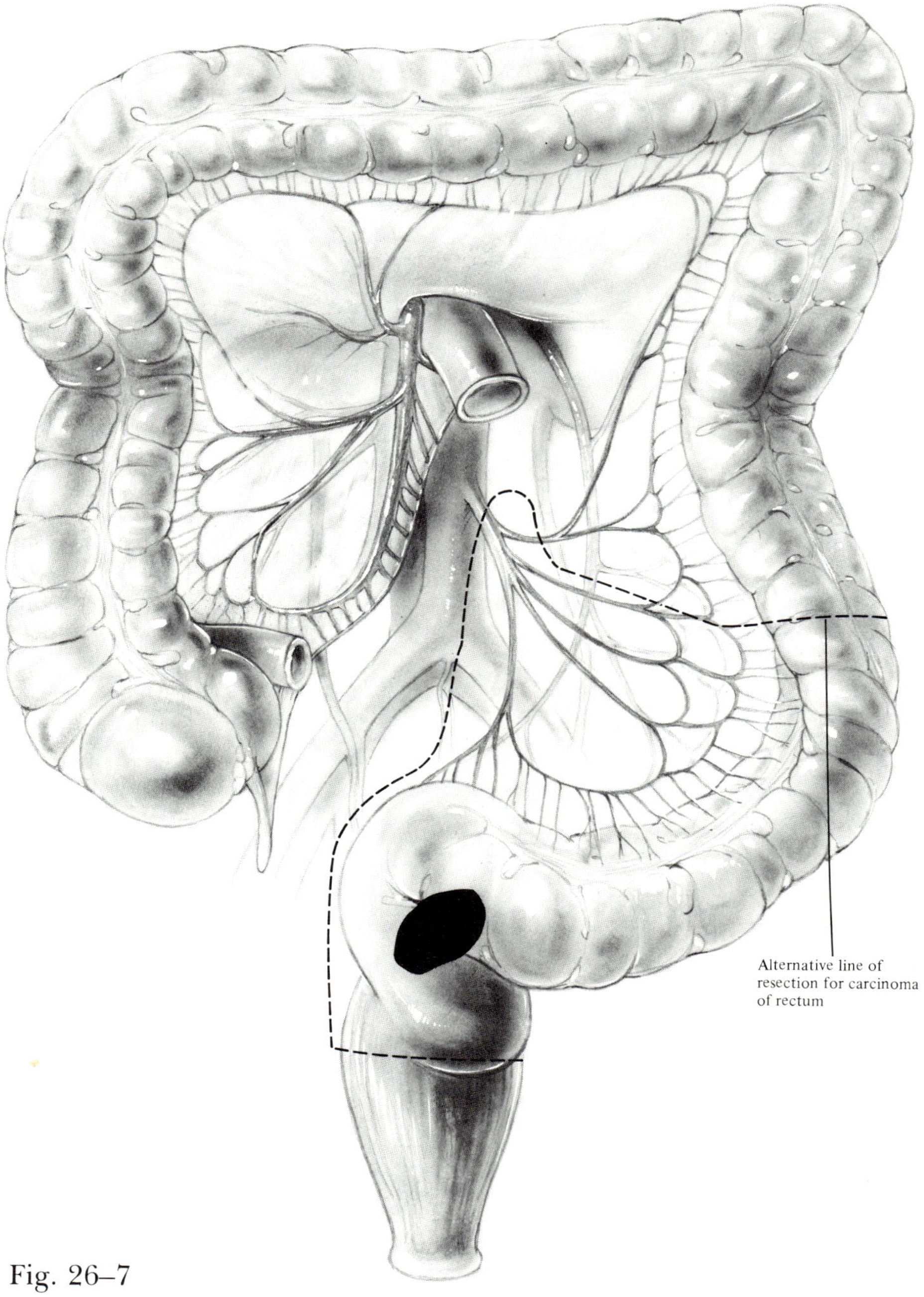

Fig. 26–7

strated that desquamated cancer cells did not survive in the intestinal lumen for more than 20 minutes. If the surgeon would occlude the lumen of the colon proximal and distal to the tumor by applying tight ligatures of 3 mm umbilical tape, they maintained, the lumen of the colon should be free of viable cancer cells 20 minutes later, when the anastomosis was being initiated. Since the application of umbilical tape ligatures requires only a few seconds, we use them in all cases of colon malignancy.

Other data suggest that the use of the closed type of anastomosis reduces the incidence of suture-line recurrence. Perhaps this is because the mucosal sutures are omitted. If the needle never passes into the lumen in the course of the anastomosis, it eliminates one method by which cells are implanted.

The use of iodized catgut for the mucosal layer caused a reduction in suture-line implantation of cancer in experimental animals, according to Cohn et al. Using iodized catgut instead of the chromic variety does not impose any additional burden on the surgeon or the patient. Consequently, for those patients in whom ligature of the lumen of the colon or rectum distal to the cancer can not be accomplished (e.g. in the lower rectum), the use of iodized catgut may be advisable.

In treating lesions of the lower rectum where the lumen can not be occluded 20 minutes before the anastomosis, it is advisable to apply an occluding clamp distal to the tumor after the dissection is complete. The rectal ampulla should then be irrigated through a previously placed Foley catheter. A 1:1000 solution of bichloride of mercury, 40% ethyl alcohol, sterile water, or other cytotoxic agent may be used. Finally, the rectum should be transected distal to the occluding clamp.

References

Barnes JP (1952) Physiological resection of the right colon. Surg Gynecol Obstet 94:723

Cohn I Jr et al. (1963) Control of tumor implantation during operations on the colon. Ann Surg 157:825

Cole WH et al. (1954) Carcinoma of the colon with special reference to prevention of recurrence. JAMA 155:1549

Goligher JC (1975) Surgery of the anus, rectum and colon, 3rd ed. Bailliere Tindall, London

Stearns MW, Schottenfeld D (1971) Techniques for the surgical management of colon cancer. Cancer 28:165

Turnbull RB Jr et al. (1967) Cancer of the colon: the influence of the no-touch isolation technique on survival rates. Ann Surg 166:420

27 Right Colectomy for Cancer

Indications

A right colectomy is indicated for malignancies of the ileocecal region, ascending colon, and transverse colon.

Preoperative Preparation

(See Chap. 25.)

Pitfalls and Danger Points

- Injury or inadvertent ligature of superior mesenteric vessels
- Laceration of retroperitoneal duodenum
- Trauma of right ureter
- Avulsion of branch between inferior pancreaticoduodenal and middle colic veins
- Failure of anastomosis

Operative Strategy

A dissection initiated at the origins of the middle colic and ileocolic vessels makes it possible to perform a more complete lymph node dissection in these two critical areas. In addition, by devoting full attention to the lymphovascular pedicles early in the operation, before the anatomy has been distorted by traction or bleeding, the surgeon will gain thorough knowledge of the anatomical variations that may occur in the vasculature of the colon. In addition, the surgeon will become adept at performing the most dangerous step of this procedure—high ligation of the ileocolic vessels—without traumatizing the superior mesenteric artery and vein.

In most cases, when the vascular pedicles are ligated close to their points of origin, it can be seen that the right colon is supplied by two vessels: the ileocolic trunk and the middle colic artery. The middle colic artery generally divides early in its course into a right and left branch. The left branch forms a well-developed marginal artery, which connects with the left colic artery at the splenic flexure. When the proximal half of the transverse colon is removed, the left colic connection of this marginal artery supplies the remaining transverse colon.

Very rarely a patient may not have good arterial flow from the divided marginal artery. In such a case the splenic flexure, and sometimes the descending and sigmoid colon, may have to be resected.

After the two major lymphovascular pedicles have been divided and ligated, the remainder of the mesentery to the right colon and the mesentery to the distal segment of the ileum should be divided.

At this time, if occluding clamps are applied to the anticipated points of transection of the transverse colon and of the ileum, the entire specimen can be seen to be isolated from any vascular connection with the patient. This is all done before there is any manipulation of the tumor—hence the "no-touch" technique. The specimen may now be removed by the traditional method of incising the peritoneum in the right paracolic gutter and elevating the right colon.

(See the discussion of operative strategy for the colon anastomosis in Chap. 25.)

Operative Technique of Right and Transverse Colectomy

Incision

Make a midline incision from the midepigastrium to a point about 8 cm below the umbilicus. Explore the abdomen for hepatic, pelvic, peritoneal, and nodal metastases. A solitary hepatic metastasis may well be resected at the same time the colectomy is performed. A moderate degree of hepatic metastasis is not a contraindication to the removal of a locally resectable colon carcinoma. The primary tumor should be inspected but manipulation of it should be avoided at this stage.

Ligature of Colon Proximal and Distal to Tumor

Insert a blunt Mixter right-angle clamp through an avascular portion of the mesentery close to the colon, distal to the tumor, and draw a 3 mm umbilical tape through this puncture in the mesentery. Tie the umbilical tape firmly, to completely occlude the lumen of the colon. Carry out an identical maneuver at a point on the terminal ileum, thus accomplishing complete occlusion of the lumen proximal and distal to the tumor.

Omental Dissection

For a carcinoma located in the hepatic flexure, divide the adjacent omentum between serially applied Kelly hemostats just distal to the gastroepiploic arcade of the stomach (**Fig. 27–1**). If the neoplasm is located in the area of the cecum, however, there does not appear to be any merit in resecting the omentum, except for the portion of the omentum that may be adherent to the actual tumor. Otherwise, when a tumor is located in the cecum, the omentum may be dissected—with scalpel and Metzenbaum scissors—off the right half of the transverse colon through the avascular plane. After this has been accomplished, with the transverse colon drawn in a caudal direction the middle colic vessels can be seen as they emerge from the lower border of the pancreas to cross over the retroperitoneal duodenum.

Division of Middle Colic Vessels

In operations for carcinoma of the cecum and the proximal 5–7 cm of ascending colon, it is not necessary to divide the middle colic vessels before they branch.

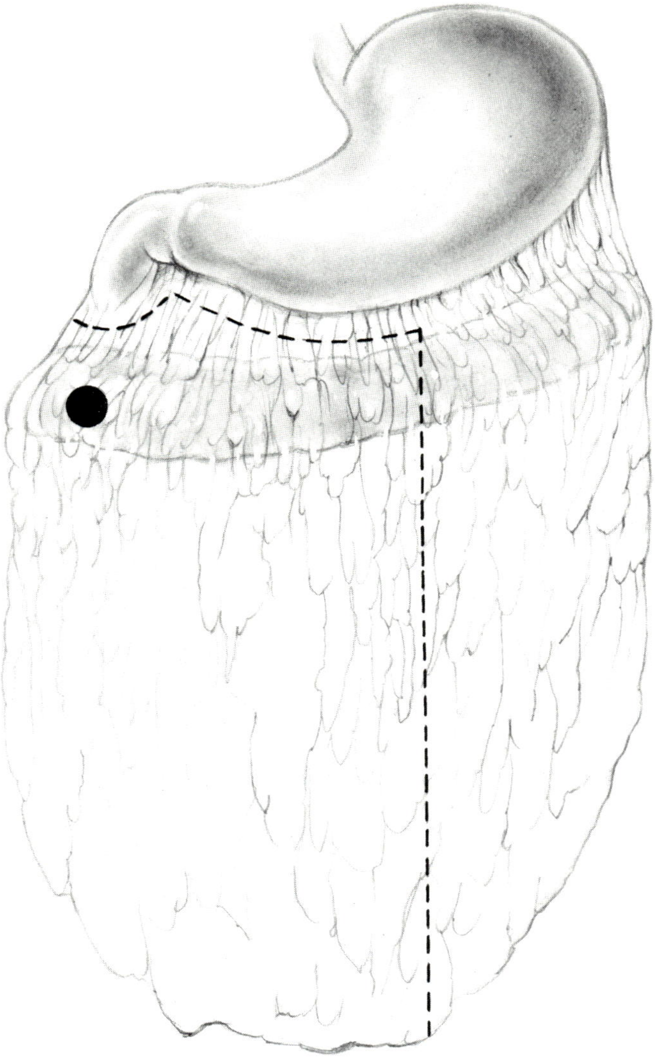

Fig. 27–1

The left branch of the middle colic may be preserved and the right branch divided and ligated just beyond the bifurcation (**Fig. 27–2**).

In operations for tumors near the hepatic flexure of transverse colon, dissect the middle colic vessels up to the lower

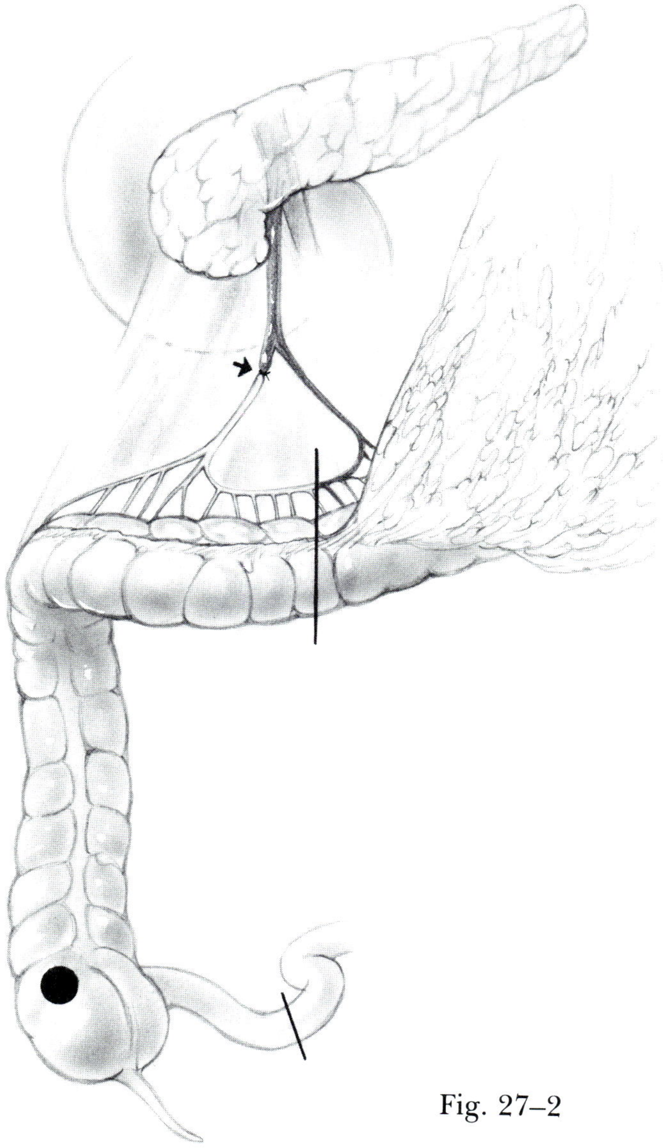

Fig. 27–2

border of the pancreas (**Fig. 27–3**). Be careful not to avulse a fairly large collateral branch that connects the inferior pancreaticoduodenal vein with the middle colic vein (**Fig. 27–4**). If this is torn considerable bleeding follows, for the proximal end of the pancreaticoduodenal vein retracts and is difficult to locate. As these structures are fragile, gentle dissection is necessary. Place a Mixter clamp deep to the middle colic vessels at the appropriate point, draw a 2–0 cotton ligature around the vessels, and ligate them. Sweep any surrounding lymph nodes down toward the specimen and place a second ligature 1.5 cm distal to the first. Divide the vessels 1 cm beyond the proximal ligature. Divide the mesocolon toward the point on the transverse colon already selected for division. Divide and ligate the marginal artery and clear the transverse colon of fat and areolar tissue in preparation for an anastomosis. Now apply an Allen clamp to the transverse colon, but to minimize bacterial contamination of the abdominal cavity do not transect the colon at this time.

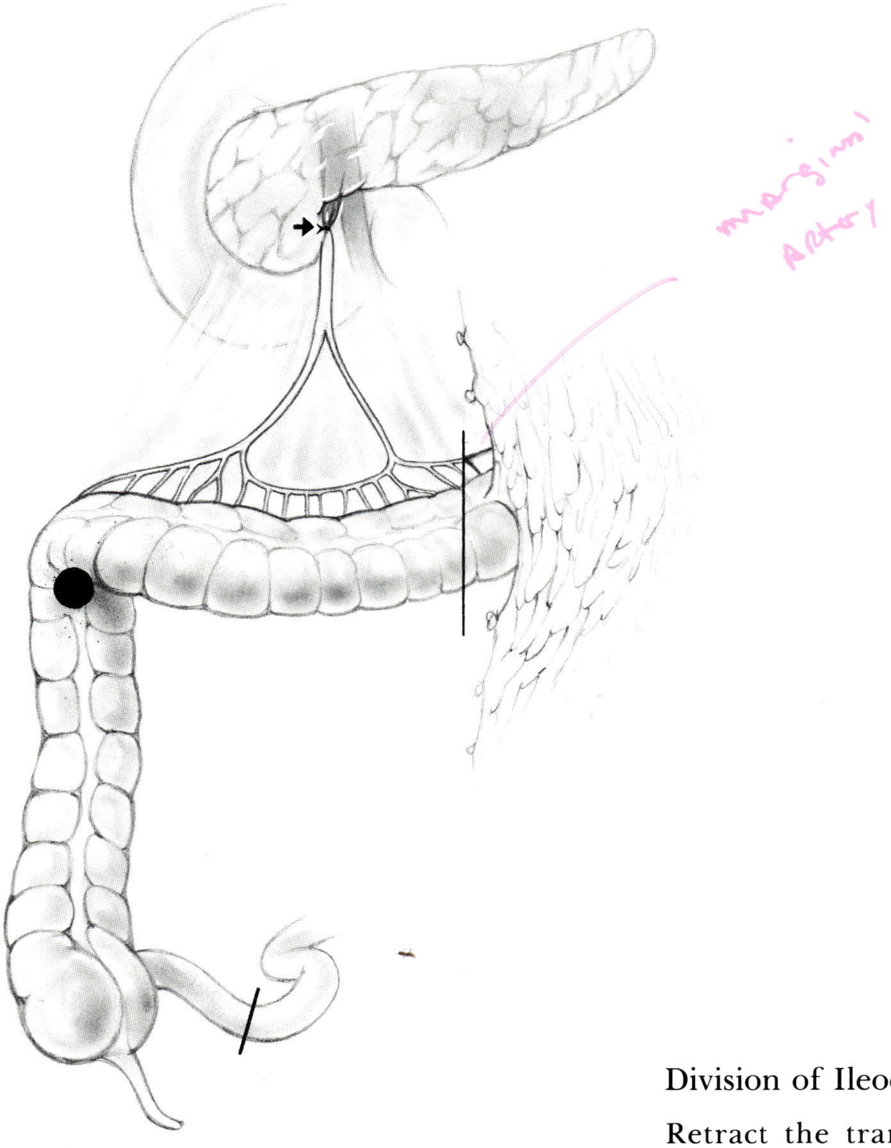

Fig. 27–3

Division of Ileocolic Vessels

Retract the transverse colon in a cephalad direction. Pass the left index finger deep to the right mesocolon (Fig. 27–5) by inserting the finger through the incision already made in the transverse mesocolon. Gentle finger dissection should disclose, in front of the fingertip, a fairly large artery with vigorous pulsation. This is the ileocolic arterial trunk (**Fig. 27–5**). If the surgeon's index finger is slid toward the patient's left, it will palpate the adjacent superior mesenteric artery. After identifying these two major vessels, it is a simple matter to incise the peritoneum overlying the ileocolic artery with a Metzenbaum scissors. By gentle dissection, remove areolar and lymphatic tissue from

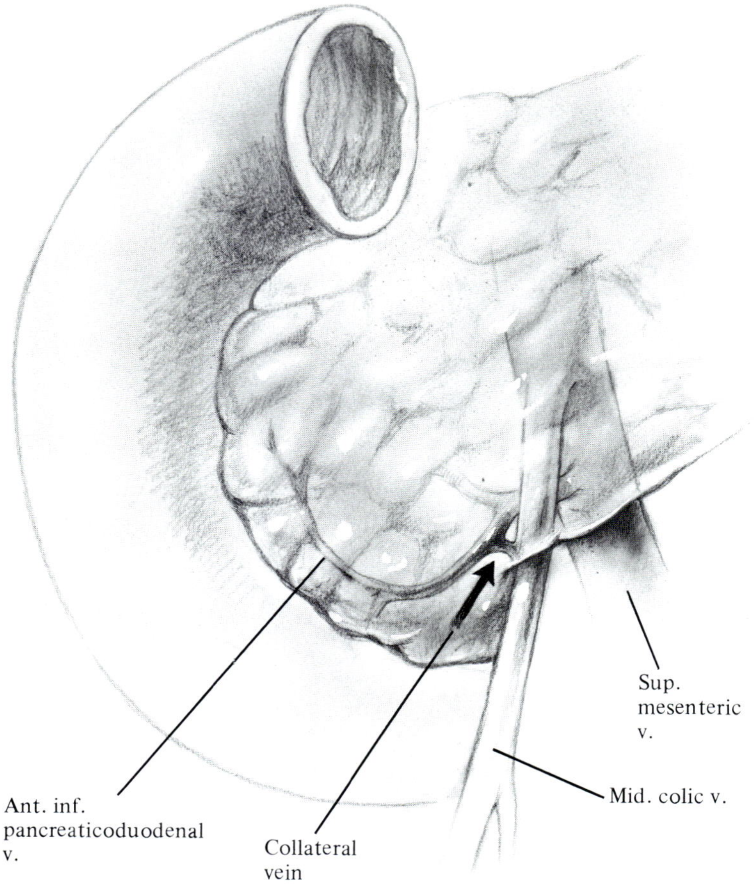

Fig. 27–4

the circumference of the ileocolic artery and vein. After rechecking the location of the superior mesenteric vessels, pass a blunt Mixter right-angle clamp beneath the ileocolic artery and vein. Ligate the vessels individually with 2–0 cotton ligatures and divide them at a point about 1.5 cm distal to their junctions with the superior mesenteric vessels.

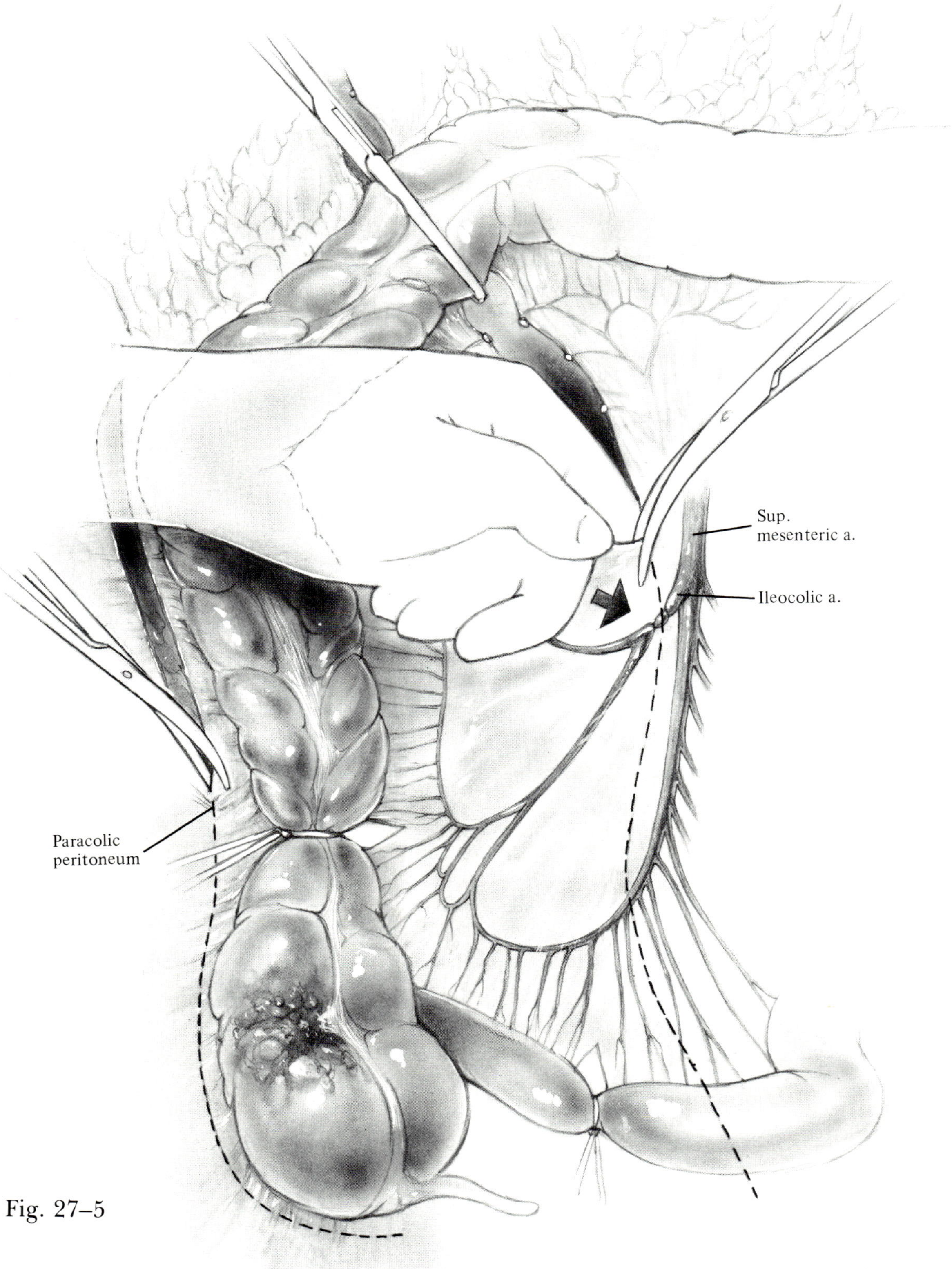

Fig. 27–5

Division of Ileal Mesentery

Pass the left index finger behind the remaining right mesocolon into an avascular area of 3–4 cm. This can be divided, and leads to the mesentery of the terminal ileum. For neoplasms close to the ileocecal junction, include 10–15 cm of ileum in the specimen. For tumors near the hepatic flexure, no more than 8–10 cm of ileum need be resected. In any case, divide the ileal mesentery between Crile hemostats, serially applied until the wall of the ileum has been encountered. After ligating each of the hemostats with 3–0 or 2–0 cotton, clear the areolar tissue from the circumference of the ileum in preparation for an anastomosis and apply an Allen clamp to this area. At this point the specimen has been isolated from any vascular connection with the host.

Division of Right Paracolic Peritoneum

Retract the right colon in a medial direction and make an incision in the peritoneum of the paracolic gutter (**Fig. 27–5**). The left index finger may be inserted deep to this layer of peritoneum, which should then be transected over the index finger, either with Metzenbaum scissors or with electrocautery. Continue this dissection until the hepatic flexure is free of lateral attachments. Rough dissection around the retroperitoneal duodenum may lacerate it inadvertently, so be aware of its location. Next, identify the right renocolic ligament and divide it by Metzenbaum dissection. When this is accomplished, the fascia of Gerota, with perirenal fat, may be gently swept from the posterior aspect of the right mesocolon. Continue this dissection caudally and the ureter and gonadal vessel will be unroofed.

Identification of Ureter

If the location of the ureter is not immediately evident, identify the right common iliac artery. The undisturbed ureter generally crosses the common iliac artery where it bifurcates into its internal and external branches. If the ureter is not in this location, the lateral leaflet of peritoneum should be elevated, as the ureter may be adhering to the undersurface of this peritoneal flap. The ureter is often displaced by the retraction of the peritoneal flap to which it adheres. If the ureter is not present on the lateral leaflet of peritoneum, a similar maneuver should be carried out, elevating the medial leaflet of peritoneum in the search for it. Typical ureteral peristalsis should occur when the ureter is compressed with forceps.

The right colon remains attached to the peritoneum now only at the inferior and medial aspects of the cecum and ileum. There should be no difficulty in dividing this.

Insertion of Wound Protector Drape

Now that the dissection is complete, with the exception of the division of the bowel, insert a plastic ring-drape into the abdominal incision to protect the incision and subcutaneous fat from contamination during construction of the anastomosis.

Division of Ileum and Colon

Protect the abdomen with large gauze pads and remove the specimen, together with the Allen clamps that already have

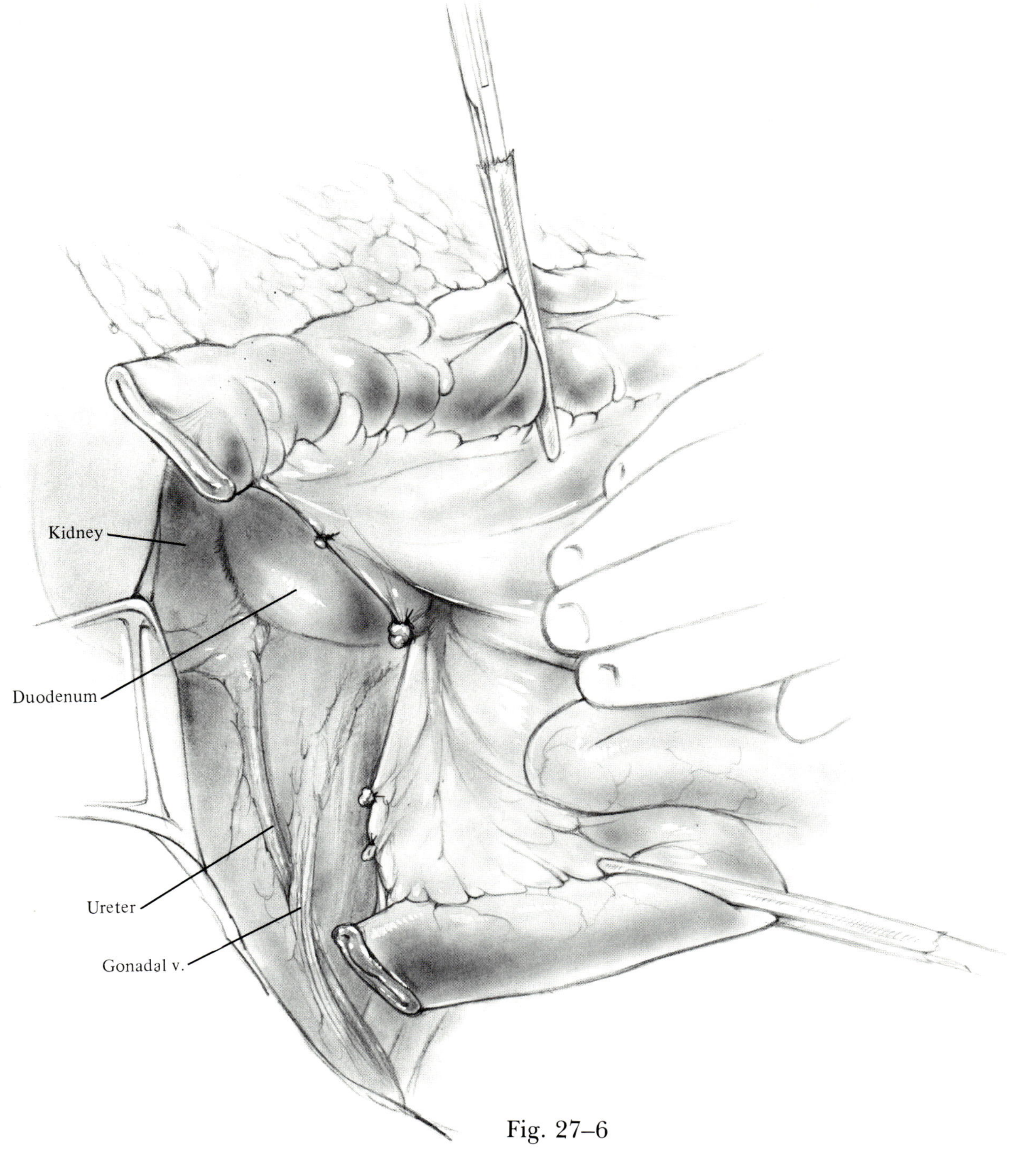

Fig. 27–6

been applied to the ileum and transverse colon. If necessary, linen-shod Doyen noncrushing intestinal clamps may be applied to occlude the ileum and transverse colon at a point at least 10 cm from their cut edges, in preparation for an open, two-layer end-to-end anastomosis (**Fig. 27–6**).

Before any anastomosis is begun, the blood supply should be carefully evaluated. Generally there will be no problem with the terminal ileum if no hematoma has been induced. Evaluate the adequacy of the blood supply to the cut end of the colon by palpating the pulse in the marginal artery. For additional data about the blood supply, divide a small arterial branch near the cut end of colon and observe the pulsatile arterial flow. If there is any question about the vigor of the blood supply, additional transverse colon must be resected.

Ileocolon Two-Layer End-to-End Anastomosis

Align the cut ends of the ileum and transverse colon facing each other so that their mesenteries are not twisted. Since the diameter of ileum will be narrower than that of colon, a Cheatle slit is made with a Metzenbaum scissors on the antimesenteric border of the ileum for a distance of 1–2 cm, to help equalize these two diameters (**Fig. 27–7**). The corners of the slit should not be rounded off.

Insert the first seromuscular layer of interrupted sutures, using 4–0 cotton on atraumatic or French needles. Initiate this layer by inserting the first Lembert suture at the antimesenteric border and the second at the mesenteric border to serve as guy sutures. Attach hemostats to each of these sutures. Drawing the two hemostats apart will make insertion of additional su-

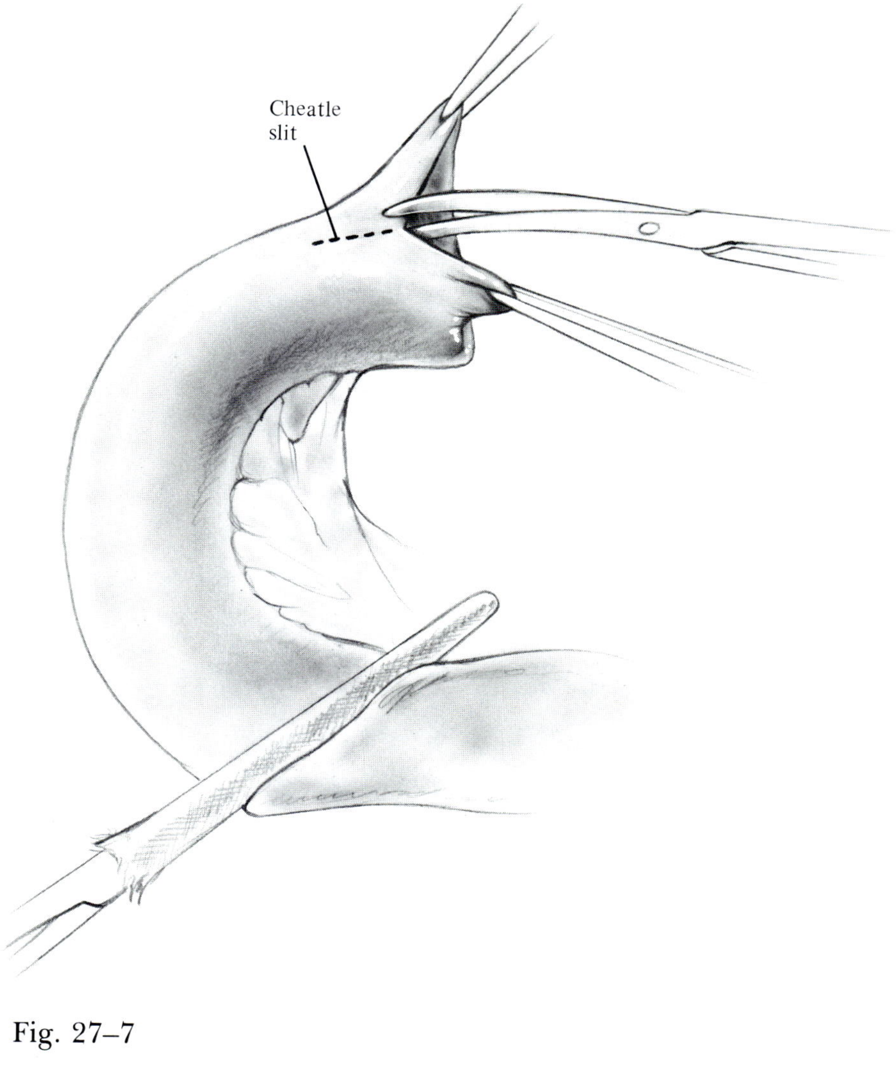

Fig. 27–7

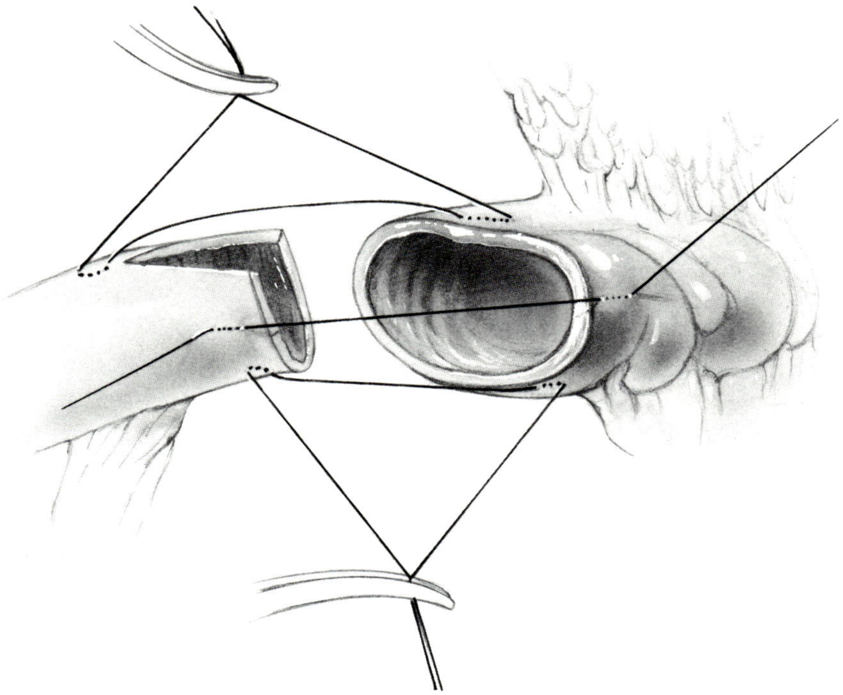

Fig. 27–8

tures by successive bisection more efficient (**Fig. 27–8**). Now complete the *anterior seromuscular layer* of the anastomosis by inserting interrupted Lembert seromuscular sutures (**Fig. 27–9**). After the entire anterior layer has been inserted and tied, cut the tails of all the sutures except for the two guy sutures.

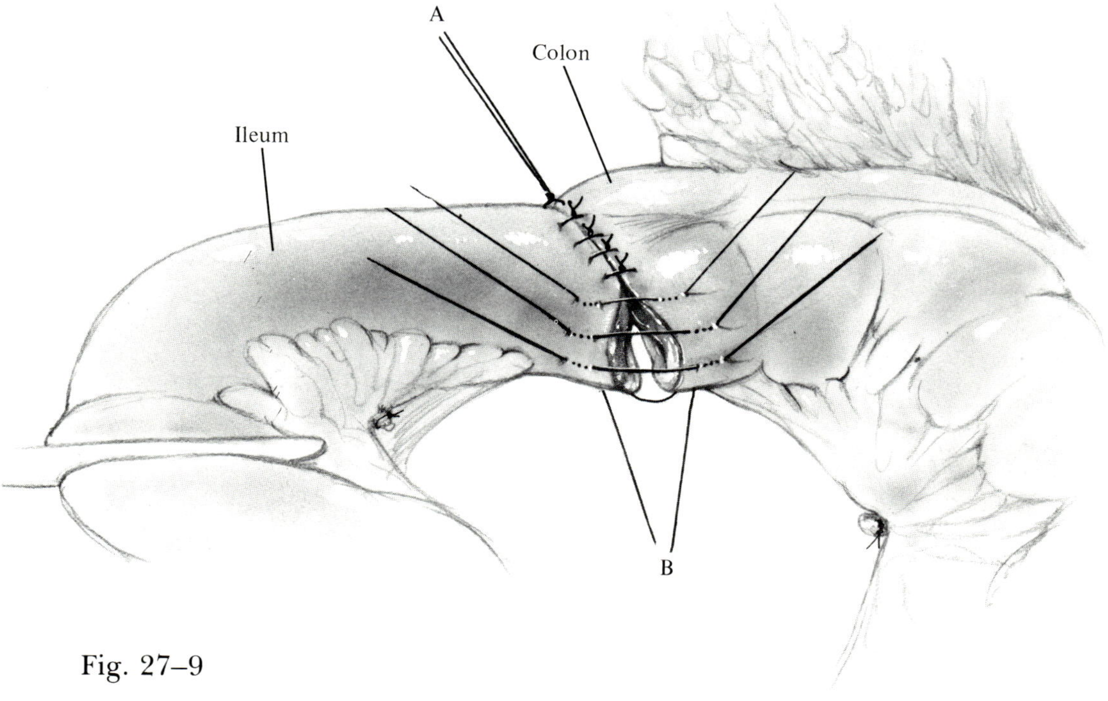

Fig. 27–9

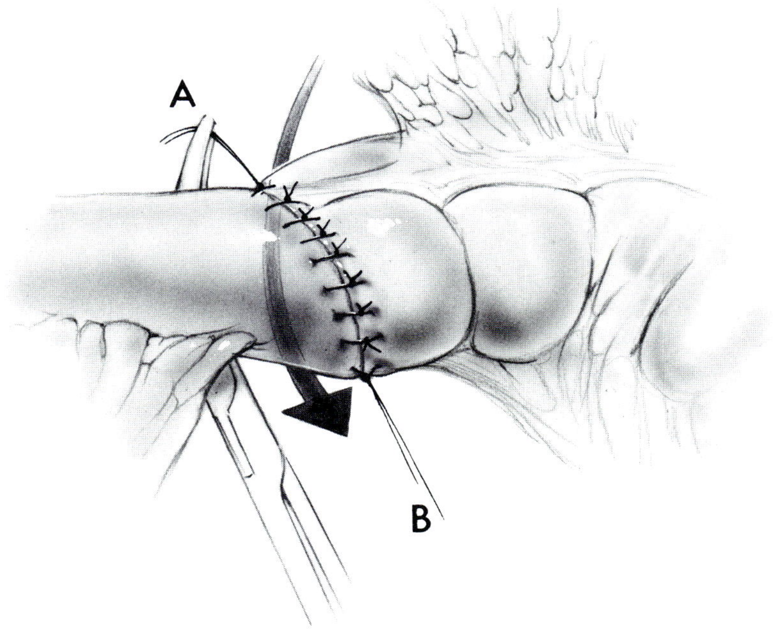

Fig. 27–10

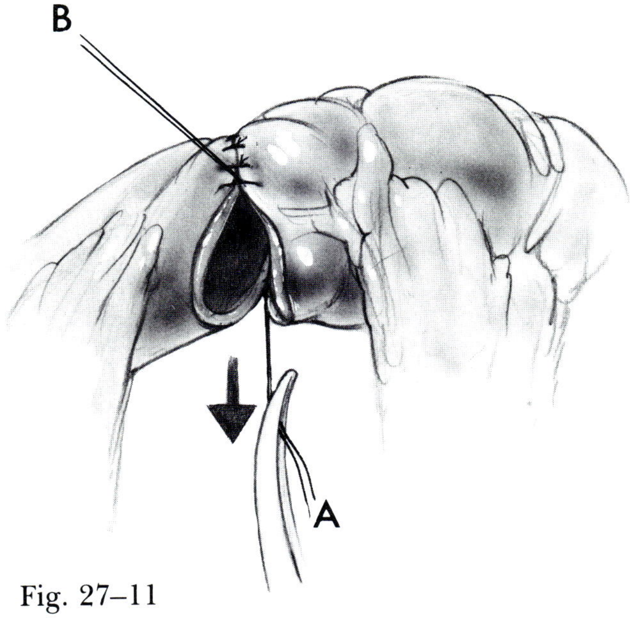

Fig. 27–11

To provide exposure for the mucosal layer, invert the anterior aspect of the anastomosis by passing the hemostat containing the antimesenteric guy suture (labeled *A* in **Fig. 27–10**) through the rent in the mesentery deep to the ileocolonic anastomosis. Then draw the mesenteric guy suture (labeled *B*) in the opposite direction and expose the mucosa for the application of the first layer of mucosal sutures (**Fig. 27–11**).

Use 4–0 chromic catgut, double armed with straight needles. Begin the first suture at the midpoint (**Fig. 27–12a**). Then pass the straight needle in a continuous fashion toward the patient's right so as to lock each suture. Take relatively small bites (4 mm). When the right margin of the suture line is reached, tag the needle with a hemostat, and with the second needle initiate the remainder of the mucosal approximation, going from the midpoint of the anastomosis toward the patient's left in a continuous locked fashion (**Fig. 27–12b**). When this layer has been completed (**Fig 27–12c**) close the superficial mucosal layer of the anastomosis with

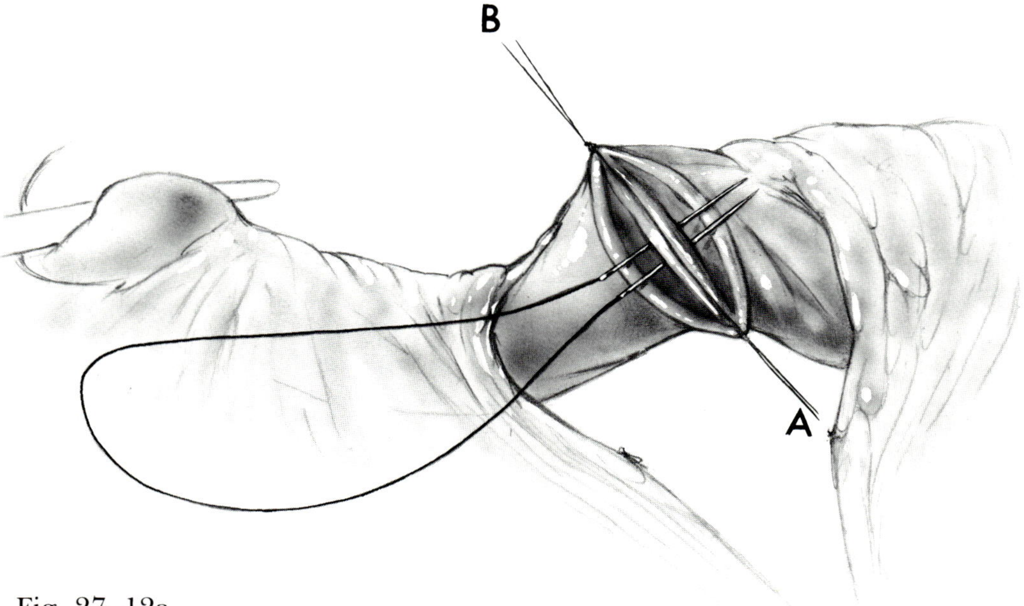

Fig. 27–12a

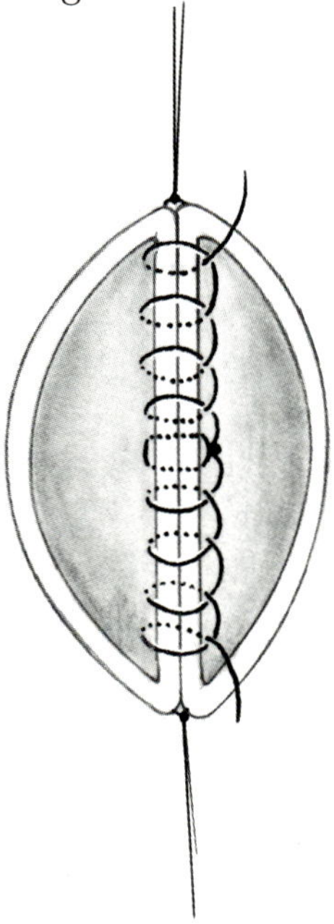

Fig. 27–12b

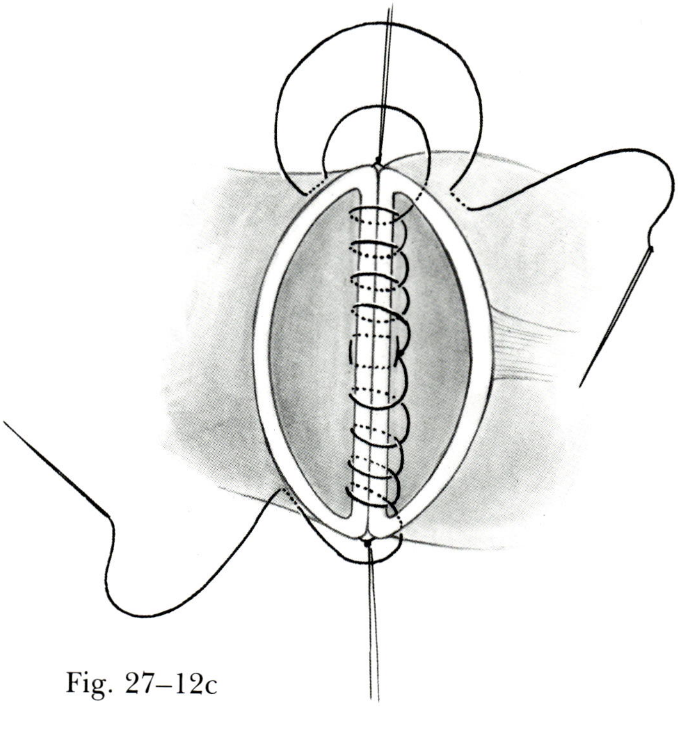

Fig. 27–12c

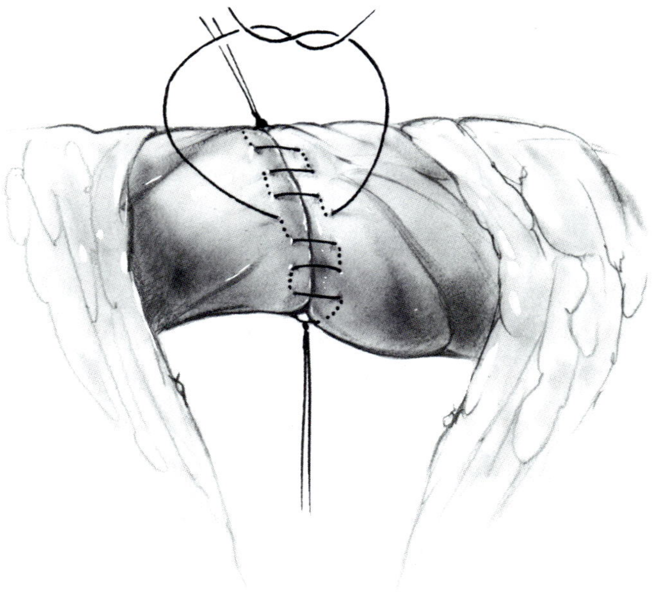

Fig. 27–13

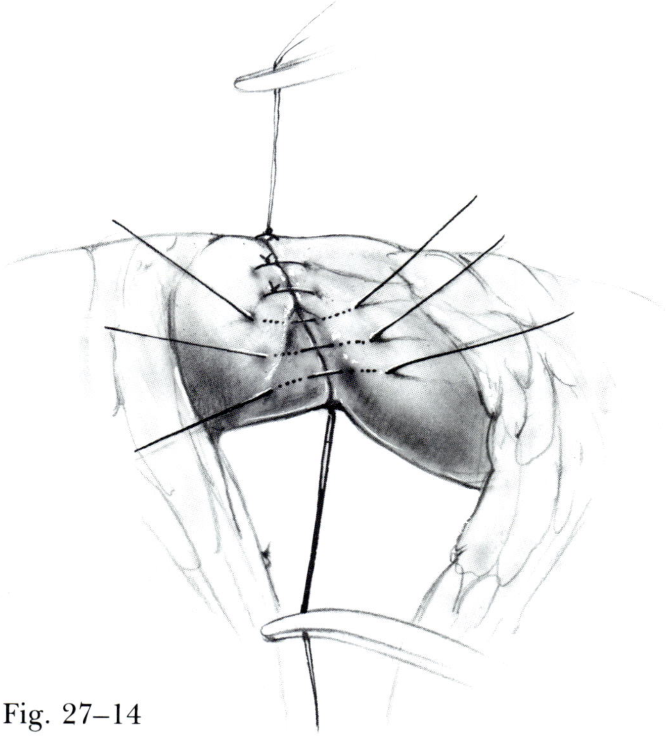

Fig. 27–14

continuous Connell or Cushing sutures beginning at each end of the anastomosis. Terminate the mucosal suture line in the midpoint of the superficial layer by tying the suture to its mate (**Fig. 27–13**).

Accomplish the final seromuscular layer by inserting interrupted 4–0 cotton Lembert sutures (**Fig. 27–14**). Devote special attention to ensuring a secure closure at the mesenteric border. Then cut all the cotton sutures and test the lumen with thumb and forefinger to gauge the width of the anastomotic stoma. It should easily admit the tip of the thumb.

Close the defect in the mesentery by continuous suture of 2–0 PG. Take care to avoid occluding important vessels running in the mesentery in the course of the continuous suture.

If desired, a one-layer anastomosis can be constructed by the technique described above, simply by omitting the mucosal suture. If it is accomplished without error, the result will be as successful as after the two-layer method.

Anastomosis by Stapling, Steichen Technique (Functional End-to-End)

To perform a stapled anastomosis, clear an area of mesentery and apply the TA–55 Auto Suture stapler transversely across the colon. Staples of 3.8 mm size are generally used. Transect the colon flush with the TA–55, using a scalpel. Carry out the identical procedure at the selected site on the ileum. Some oozing of blood should be evident despite the double row of staples. Control excessive bleeding by carefully applying electrocoagulation or by using chromic sutures. Then align the ileum and colon side-by-side and, with a heavy scissors, excise a triangular 8 mm wedge from the antimesenteric margins of both the ileum and colon (**Fig. 27–15**).

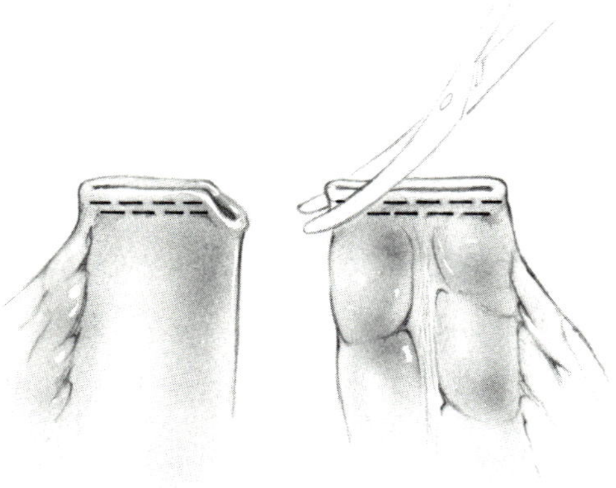

Fig. 27–15

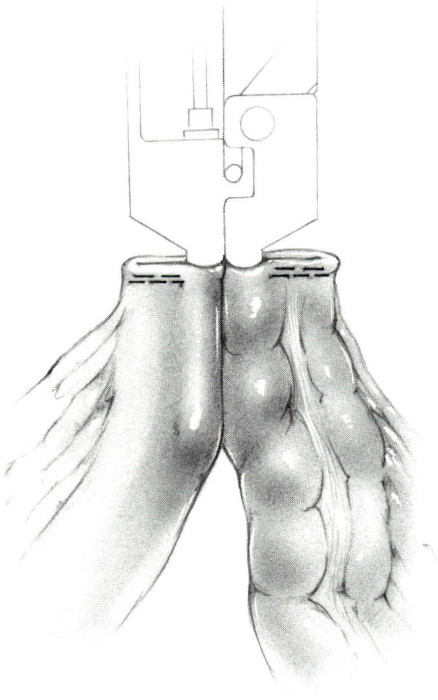

Fig. 27–16

Insert one of the two forks of the GIA anastomosing instrument into the lumen of the ileum and the other into the colon, *hugging the antimesenteric border* of each (**Fig. 27–16**). Neither segment of intestine should be stretched, as this may result in excessive thinning of the bowel, leaving inadequate substance for the staples to grasp. After ascertaining that both segments of the bowel are near the hub of the GIA instrument, fire the device; this should result in a side-to-side anastomosis 4–5 cm long. Unlock and remove the device and inspect the staple line for bleeding as well as for possible technical failure in the closing of the staples.

Now apply Allis clamps to the remaining defect in the anastomosis and close it by a final application of the TA–55

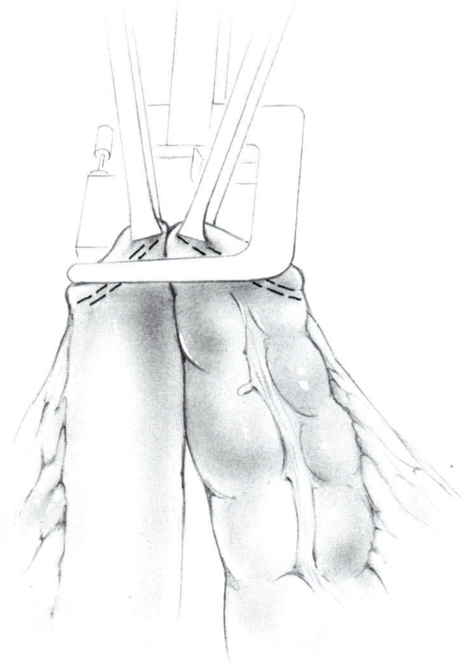

Fig. 27–17

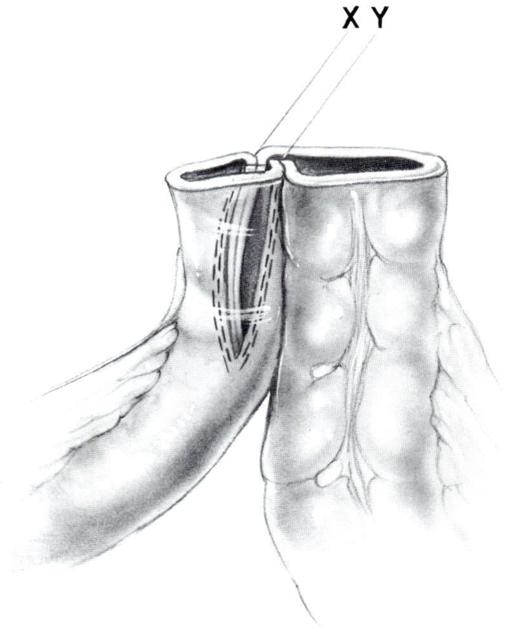

Fig. 27–18

instrument (**Fig. 27–17**). Take care to include a portion of *each of the previously applied staples lines* in the final application of the stapler. However, in applying the Allis clamps, do not align points *X* and *Y* (**Fig. 27–18**) exactly opposite each other, as this will result in six staple lines meeting at one point. The alignment of these two points, as shown in **Fig. 27–19**, produces the best results. Check the patency of the anastomosis by invaginating the colon through the anastomosis, which should admit the tips of two fingers. Then lightly touch the everted mucosa with the electrocoagulator. During closure of the mesentery, cover the everted staple lines with adjoining mesentery or omentum if convenient.

We have modified Steichen's method of anastomosing ileum to colon, making it simpler by eliminating two applications of the stapler. In our technique the first step is to insert the GIA device, one fork into the open end of ileum and the other fork into the open colon. Fire the GIA, establishing a partial anastomosis between the antimesenteric borders of ileum and colon as seen in Fig. 27–18.

Apply four or five Allis clamps to approximate the lips of the ileum and colon

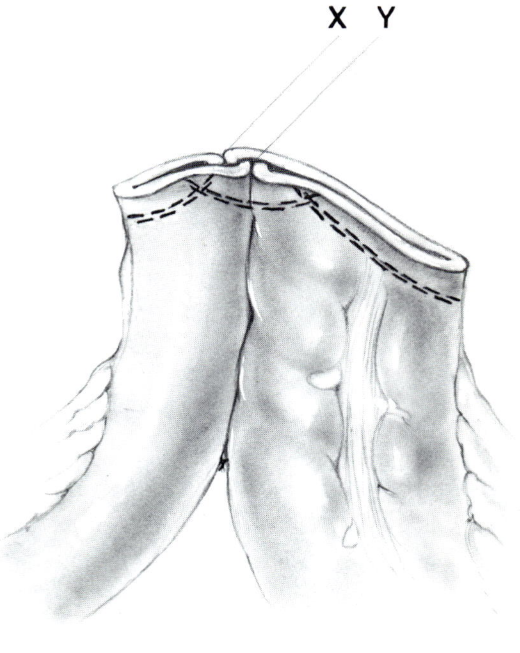

Fig. 27–19

(in eversion) taking care that points X and Y are not in apposition. Then apply a TA–90 stapler beneath the Allis clamps, tighten the alignment pin, and fire the staples. The end result is illustrated in **Fig. 27–20**. In our experience this is the most efficient and reliable method of constructing an ileocolonic anastomosis.

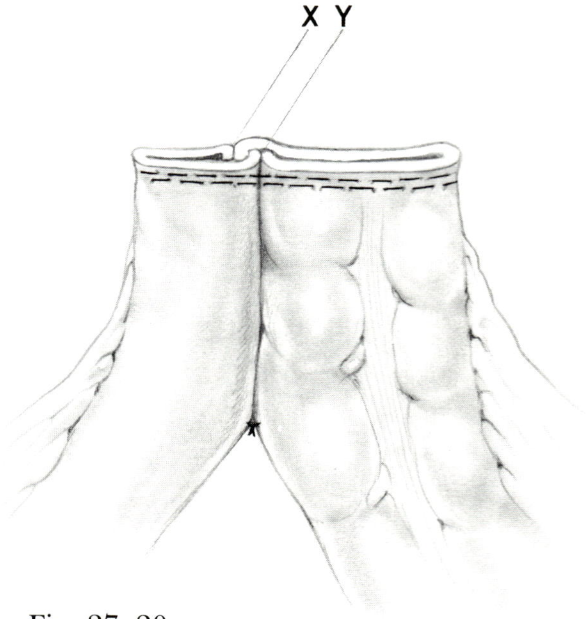

Fig. 27–20

Another stapling technique for the ileocolonic anastomosis is Weakley's side-to-side technique (see Figs. 28–30 through 28–32). Take special care so that the "blind" end of the ileum extends no more than 1 cm beyond the anastomosis.

Wound Closure

Remove the Wound Protector drape. The surgical team should now change gloves and discard all instruments used up to this point. Irrigate the operative field with saline and then with a dilute antibiotic solution. Cover the anastomosis with omentum if possible. Carry out closure of the wound in routine fashion. Finally, close the skin over a subcutaneous closed-suction catheter (see Chap. 2).

Postoperative Care

Continue nasogastric suction until the patient is passing flatus freely per rectum and until there is no abdominal distention.

Delay oral intake of liquid and food until the seventh postoperative day. If the patient is suffering from paralytic ileus, delay oral intake further, and take steps, such as diagnostic X rays, to rule out mechanical obstruction of the small bowel.

In the absence of preoperative intra-abdominal sepsis, discontinue antibiotics the day after the operation.

Complications

Leakage from an ileocolonic or colocolonic anastomosis may be manifested by peritonitis, colocutaneous fistula, or localized intraperitoneal abscess. The surgical team must keep alert at all times for any sign of localized or spreading peritonitis, as this complication should be managed by prompt relaparotomy and exteriorization of both ends of the anastomosis.

Sepsis in the subhepatic, subphrenic, or pelvic areas are occasional complications of anastomoses of the colon, even in the absence of leakage. Each of these requires local drainage.

Wound infection generally requires prompt removal of all overlying skin sutures to permit wide drainage of the entire infected area.

28 Left Colectomy for Cancer

Indications

Whereas malignancies of the proximal three-quarters of the transverse colon require the excision of the right and transverse colon, cancers of the distal transverse colon, splenic flexure, descending colon, and sigmoid are treated by left hemicolectomy (see Chap. 26).

Preoperative Preparation

(See Chap. 25.)

Pitfalls and Danger Points

- Injury to spleen
- Failure of anastomosis
- Injury to ureter

Operative Strategy

Extent of Dissection

Lymph draining from malignancies of the left colon flows along the left colic or sigmoidal veins to the inferior mesenteric vessels. In the usual case, the inferior mesenteric artery should be divided at the aorta and the inferior mesenteric vein at the lower border of the pancreas.

Except for the treatment of lesions situated in the distal sigmoid, the lower point of division of the colon is through the upper rectum, 2–3 cm above the promontory of the sacrum (see Fig. 26–5). No presacral elevation of the rectal stump need be carried out, and the anastomosis should be intraperitoneal. The blood supply of a rectal stump of this length, arising from the inferior and middle hemorrhoidal arteries, is almost invariably of excellent quality. The blood supply of the proximal colonic segment, arising from the middle colic artery, generally is also excellent, providing that care is exercised not to damage the marginal vessel at any point in its course.

Liberation of Splenic Flexure

The splenic flexure of the colon may be completely liberated without dividing a single blood vessel if the surgeon can recognize anatomical planes accurately. The only blood vessels going to the colon are those arising from its mesentery. Bleeding during the course of this dissection arises from three sources:

1) Frequently, *downward traction on the colon and its attached omentum* avulses a patch of splenic capsule to which the omentum adheres. It is worthwhile to inspect the lower pole of the spleen at the *onset* of this dissection and to divide such areas of adhesion with a Metzenbaum scissors under direct vision before applying traction.

2) Bleeding arises when the *surgeon does not recognize the plane* between the omentum and appendices epiploica attached to the distal transverse colon. The appendices may extend 1–3 cm cephalad to the transverse colon. When they are divided inadvertently, bleeding follows. Note that the character of the fat in the omentum is considerably different from that of the appendices. The former has the appearance of multiple small lobulations, each 4–6 mm in diameter, while the appendices epiploica contain fat that appears to have a completely smooth surface. If the proper plane between the omentum and appendices can be identified, the dissection will be bloodless.

3) Bleeding can arise from the *use of blunt dissection* to divide the renocolic ligament. This ruptures a number of veins along the surface of Gerota's capsule, which overlies the kidney. Bleeding can be prevented by accurately identifying the renocolic ligament, delineating it carefully, and then dividing it with a Metzenbaum scissors along the medial margin of the renal capsule. Although the classical anatomy books do not generally describe a "renocolic ligament," this can regularly be identified as a thin structure (see Figs. 28–2 and 28–3) extending from the anterior surface of the renal capsule to the posterior surface of the mesocolon.

There are three essential steps in the safe liberation of the splenic flexure. First, the obvious one, incise the parietal peritoneum in the left paracolic gutter going cephalad to the splenic flexure. Second, dissect the left margin of the omentum from the distal transverse colon as well as from the left parietal peritoneum near the lower pole of the spleen (in those patients who have this attachment). Third, the least well understood step, identify and divide the renocolic ligament between the renal capsule and the posterior mesocolon. Then pass the index finger deep to this ligament in the region of the splenic flexure (see Fig. 28–3); this plane leads to the lienocolic ligament, which is also avascular and may be divided by a Metzenbaum scissors, provided that this ligament is separated from underlying fatty tissue by finger dissection. The fatty tissue may contain an epiploic appendix with a blood vessel. After the lienocolic ligament has been divided, the index finger should lead to the next avascular "ligament," which extends from the pancreas to the transverse colon. This pancreaticocolic "ligament" comprises the upper portion of transverse mesocolon. Dividing this frees the distal transverse colon and splenic flexure, except for the mesentery. For all practical purposes the renocolic, lienocolic, and pancreaticocolic "ligaments" are one continuous avascular membrane with multiple areas of attachment.

No-Touch Technique

Turnbull's no-touch technique is more difficult to apply to lesions of the left colon than to those on the right. However, in many cases it can be accomplished by liberating the sigmoid colon early in the procedure, identifying and ligating the inferior mesenteric vessels, dividing the mesocolon, all before manipulating the tumor. In some cases the tumor's location or obesity of the mesocolon make this approach more cumbersome for the surgeon, unlike the situation on the right side where the anatomy lends itself to the adoption of the no-touch method as a routine procedure. Most surgeons content themselves with minimal manipulation of the tumor while they use the operative sequence of first liberating the left colon and then ligating the lymphovascular attachments.

Technique of Anastomosis

Because the anastomosis is generally intraperitoneal and because the rectal stump is largely covered by peritoneum, there should be a leakage rate in elective cases of less than 2%. Anastomosis may be done by the end-to-end technique or by the Baker side-to-end method, at the option of the surgeon.

If a stapling technique is desired, we prefer the functional end-to-end anastomosis (Figs. 28–33 through 28–36). An EEA end-to-end stapling device (Figs. 30–23 through 30–29) may also be used, although the internal diameter of the anastomosis (2.1 cm) resulting from this technique may be slightly narrow. On several occasions we have observed that a stapled anastomosis did not dilate with the passage of time, as is usually the case when sutures are used. Consequently, stapled anastomoses of the colon should probably be made larger in diameter than they would if sutures were used.

Operative Technique

Incision and Exposure

Make a midline incision from a point about 4 cm below the xiphoid to the pubis (**Fig. 28–1a**) and open and explore the abdomen. Insert a "chain" retractor to elevate the left costal margin. This improves the exposure for the splenic flexure dissection. Exteriorize the small intestine into a sterile plastic intestinal bag and retract it to the patient's right. Apply umbilical tape ligatures to occlude the lumen proximal and distal to the tumor.

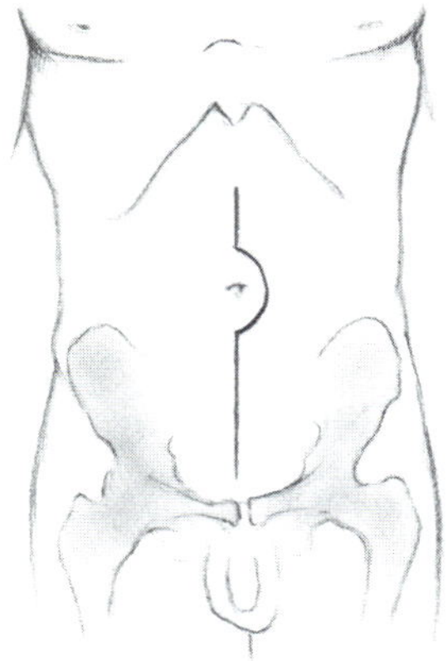

Fig. 28–1a

Liberation of Descending Colon and Sigmoid

Standing at the patient's left, make a long incision in the peritoneum of the left paracolic gutter between the descending colon and the white line of Toldt (**Fig. 28–1b**). Use the left index finger to elevate this peritoneal layer and continue the incision upward with a Metzenbaum scissors until the right-angle curve of the splenic flexure is reached. At this point, the peritoneal incision must be moved close to the colon; otherwise, the incision in the parietal peritoneum will tend to continue upward and lateral toward the spleen.

Similarly, with the index finger leading the way, use the Metzenbaum scissors to complete the incision in a caudal direction, liberating the sigmoid colon from its lateral attachments down to the rectosigmoid region.

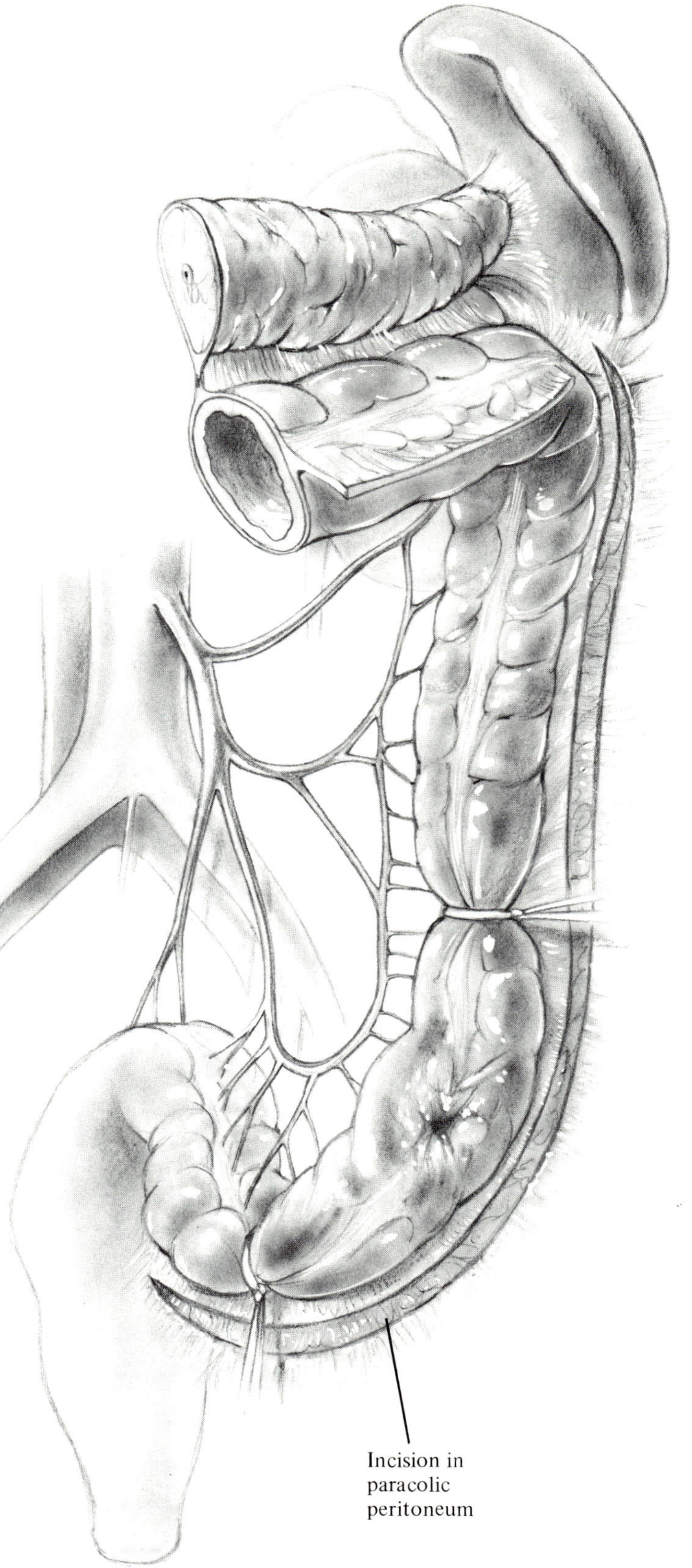

Fig. 28–1b

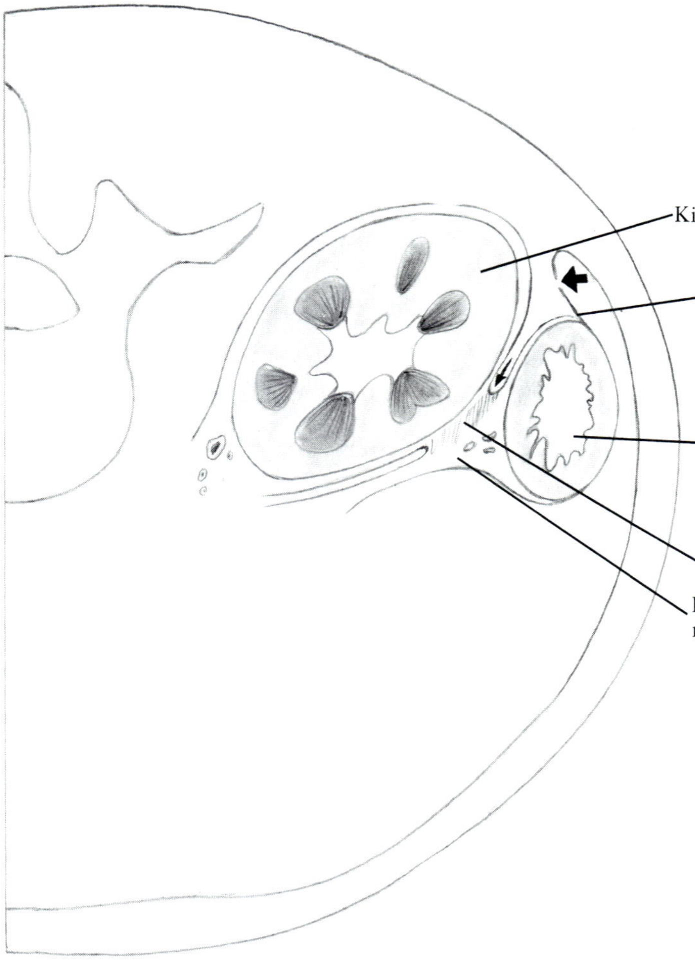

Fig. 28–2

Division of Renocolic Ligament

With the descending colon retracted toward the patient's right, a filmy attachment can be visualized covering the renal capsule and extending medially to attach to the posterior surface of the mesocolon (**Fig. 28–2**). Most surgeons bluntly disrupt this renocolic attachment, which resembles a ligament, by using a gauze pad in a sponge holder, but this maneuver often tears small veins on the surface of the renal capsule and causes unnecessary bleeding. Instead, the structure should be divided with a Metzenbaum scissors near the junction of the medial margin of the renal capsule and the adjacent mesocolon. Once the incision is initiated, the structure is best delineated by elevation over the index finger (**Fig. 28–3**). After the renocolic ligament has been divided, the upper ureter lies exposed, as does the gonadal vein. Trace the ureter down to its entrance into the pelvis and encircle it with a Vesseloop tag for future identification.

Splenic Flexure Dissection

The lower pole of the spleen can now be seen. If there are any adhesions between the omentum and the capsule of the spleen, divide them by sharp dissection in order to avoid the inadvertent avulsion of the splenic capsule that traction on the omentum can produce. If bleeding occurs because the splenic capsule has been torn, it can usually be controlled by applying a hemostatic patch of Surgicel or Avitene. Occasionally, sutures on a fine atraumatic needle are helpful.

At this stage identify and divide the attachments between the omentum and the lateral aspect of the transverse colon.

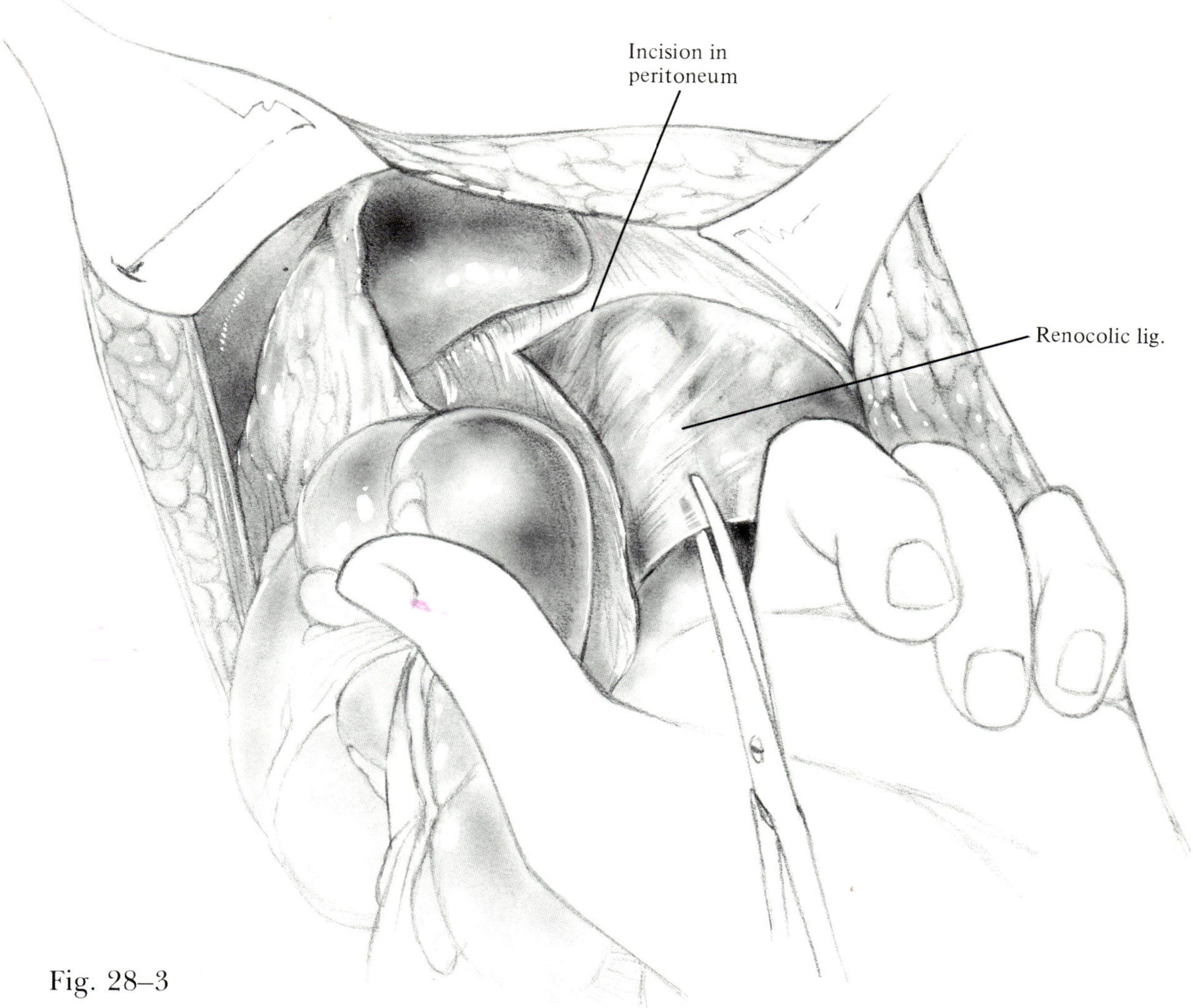

Fig. 28–3

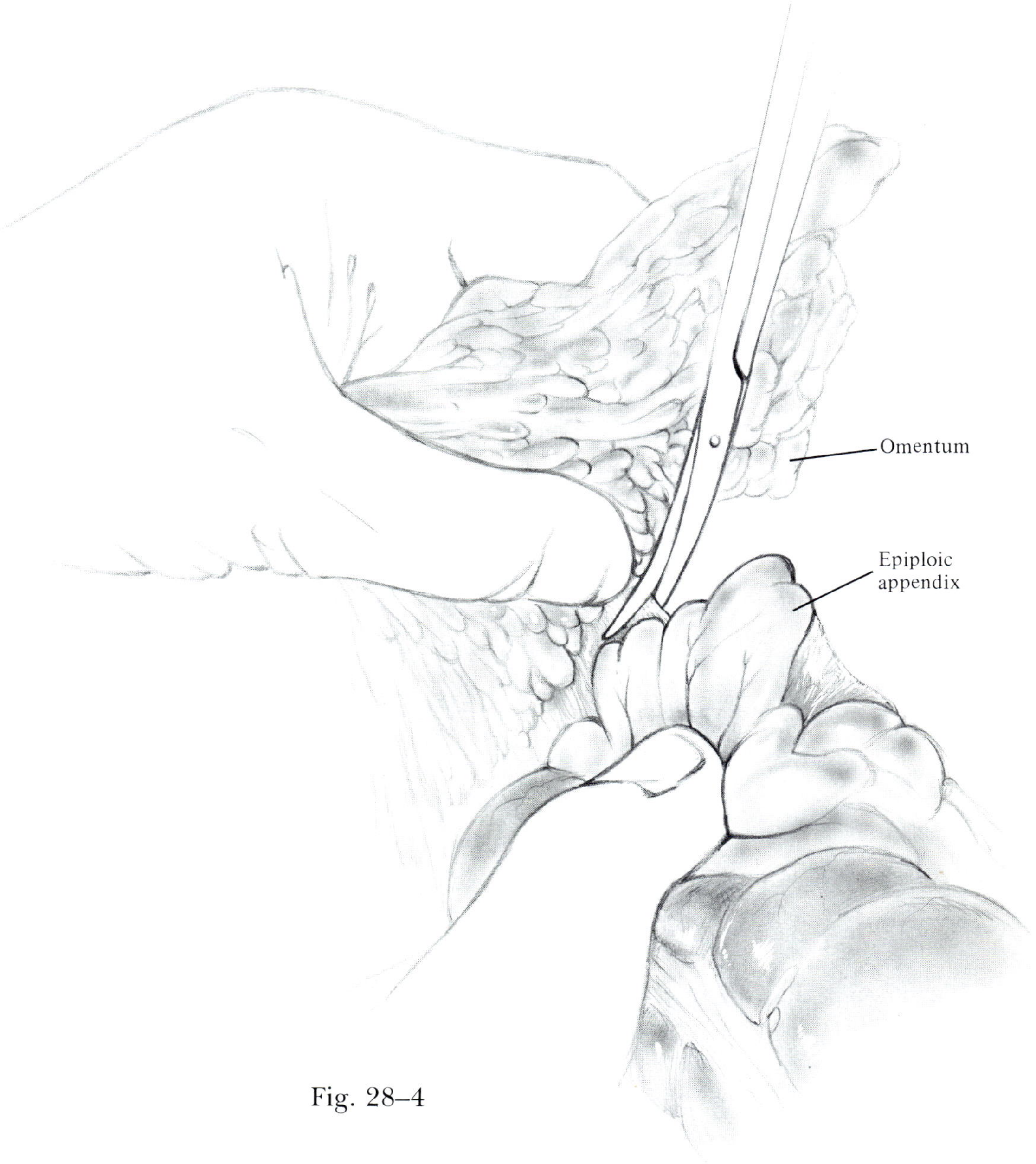

Fig. 28–4

Remember to differentiate carefully between the fat of the appendices epiploica and the more lobulated fat of the omentum (see "Operative Strategy," this chapter). Free the omentum from the distal 10–12 cm of transverse colon (**Fig. 28–4**). If the tumor is located in the distal transverse colon, leave the omentum attached to the tumor and divide the omentum just outside the gastroepiploic arcade.

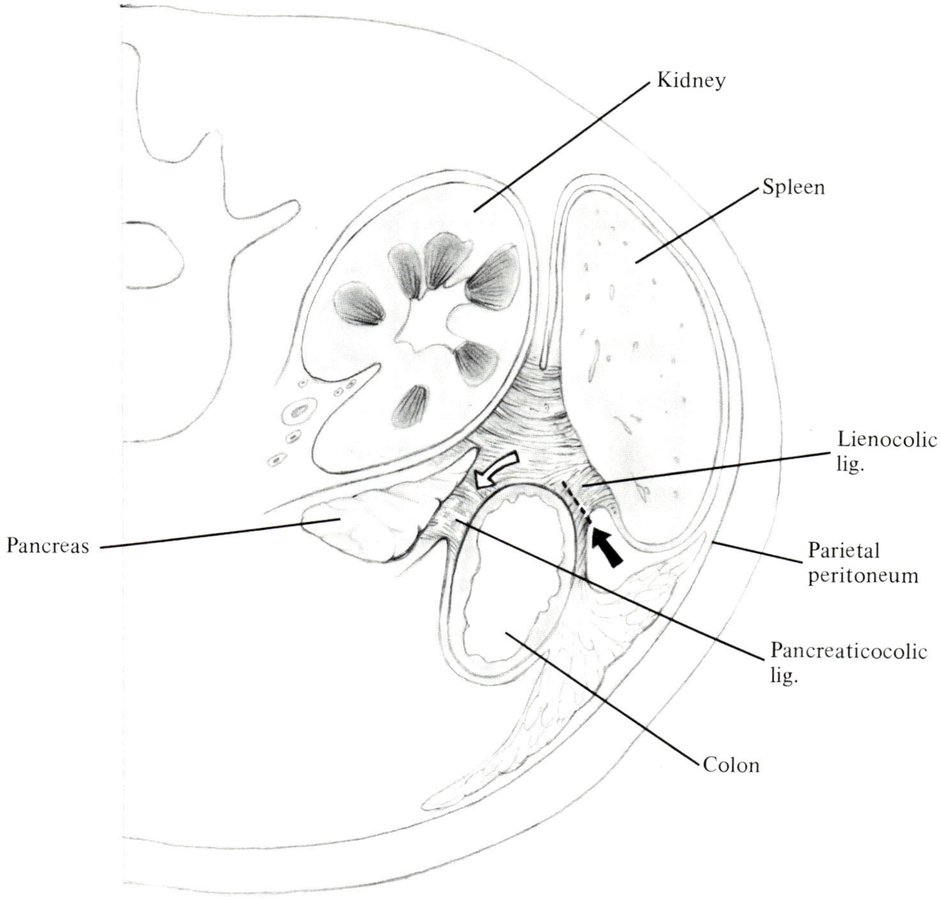

Fig. 28–5

Return now to the upper portion of the divided renocolic ligament. Insert the *right* index finger underneath the upper portion of this ligament and pinch it between the index finger and thumb; this localizes the lienocolic ligament (**Fig. 28–5**). This ligament should be divided by the first assistant, guided by the surgeon's right index finger. By inserting the index finger 5–6 cm farther medially, an avascular pancreaticocolic "ligament" (**Figs. 28–5 and 28–6**) can be identified. This is an upper extension of the transverse mesocolon. After this structure has been divided, the distal transverse colon and splenic flexure become free of all posterior attachments. If there is any bleeding in the area, correct it by using ligatures and electrocoagulation.

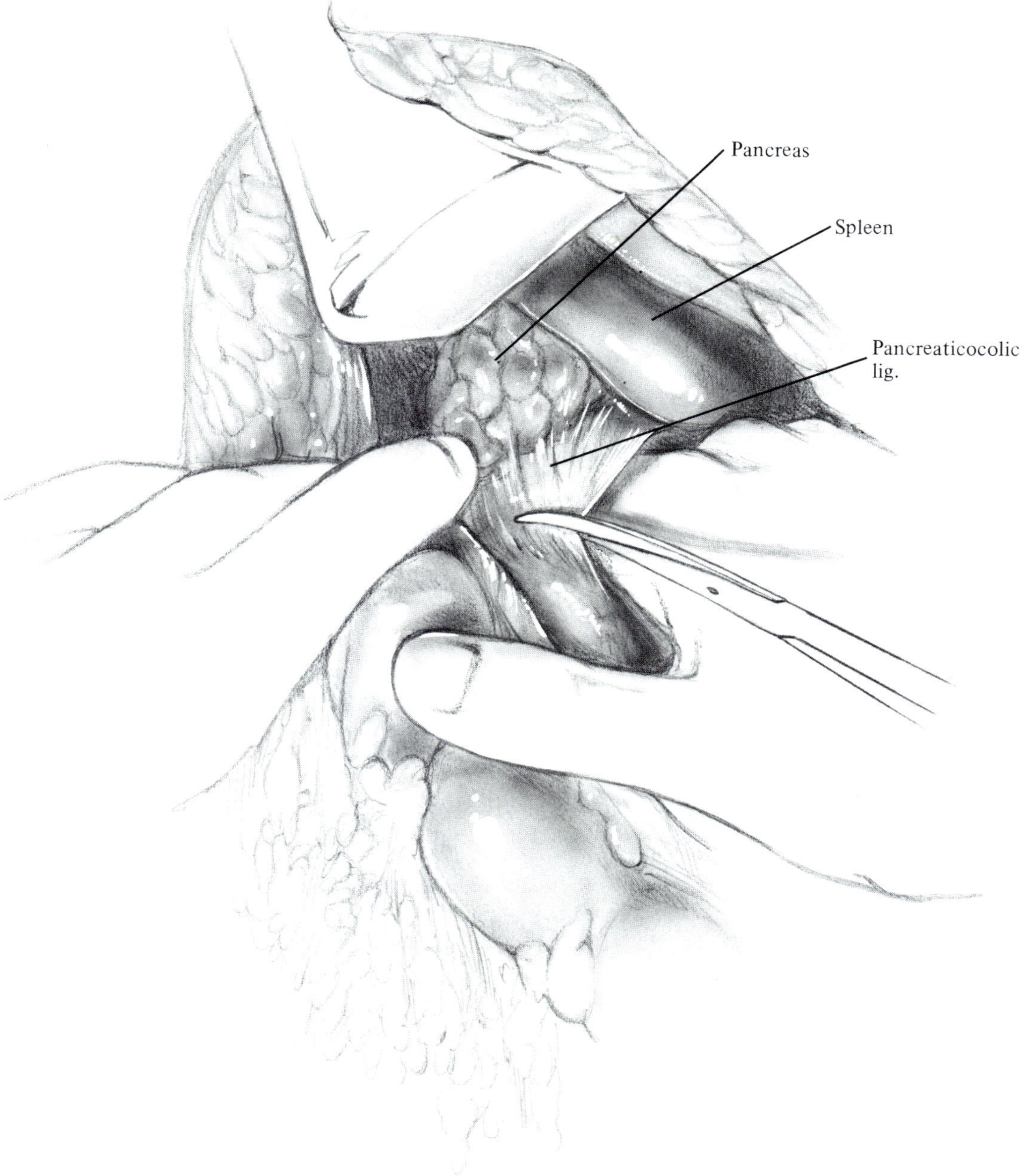

Fig. 28–6

Ligation and Division of Inferior Mesenteric Artery

Make an incision on the medial aspect of the mesocolon from the level of the duodenum down to the promontory of the sacrum. The inferior mesenteric artery is easily identified by palpation at its origin from the aorta. Sweep the lymphatic tissue in this vicinity downward,

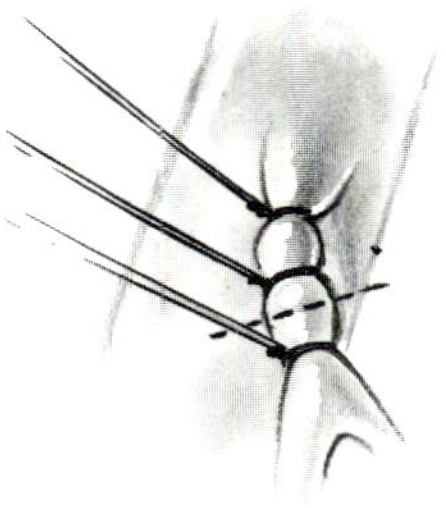

Fig. 28–7

skeletonizing the artery, which should be doubly ligated with 2–0 cotton at a point about 1.5 cm from the aorta (**Fig. 28–7**) and then divided. Sweep the preaortic areolar tissue and lymph nodes toward the specimen. It is not necessary to skeletonize the anterior wall of the aorta, as this could divide the preaortic sympathetic nerves, which would result in sexual dysfunction in the male. If the preaortic dissection is carried out by gently sweeping the glands laterally, the nerves will not be divided inadvertently. Now divide the inferior mesenteric vein as it passes behind the duodenojejunal junction and pancreas.

Division of Mesocolon

Depending on the location of the tumor, divide the mesocolon between clamps up to and including the marginal artery (**Fig. 28–8**).

Ligation and Division of Mesorectum

Separate the distal ligated pedicle of the inferior mesenteric artery and the divided mesocolon from the aorta and iliac vessels down to the promontory of the sacrum. Divide the vascular tissue around the rectum between pairs of hemostats sequentially until the wall of the upper rectum is visible. Then free the rectal stump of surrounding fat and areolar tissue at the point selected for the anastomosis. This point should be 2–3 cm above the promontory of the sacrum, where three-quarters of the rectum is covered anteriorly and laterally by peritoneum.

Insertion of Wound Protector

Insert a Wound Protector ring drape into the abdominal cavity to protect the subcutaneous panniculus from contamination when the colon is opened.

Division of Colon and Rectum

Expose the point on the proximal colon selected for division. Apply an Allen clamp to the specimen side. Divide the colon after applying a Doyen or other type of nontraumatic clamp to avoid contamination. To prepare for the anastomosis, completely clear the areolar tissue and fat from the distal centimeter of the proximal colon so that the serosa is exposed throughout its circumference. Handle the distal end of the specimen in the same manner by applying an Allen clamp to the specimen side. Now divide the upper rectum and remove the specimen. Suction the rectum free of any contents. Apply no clamp. Fine catgut ligatures may have to be used to control bleeding from the rectal wall. Completely clear surrounding fat and areolar tissue from a cuff of rectum 1 cm in width so that seromuscular sutures may be inserted accurately.

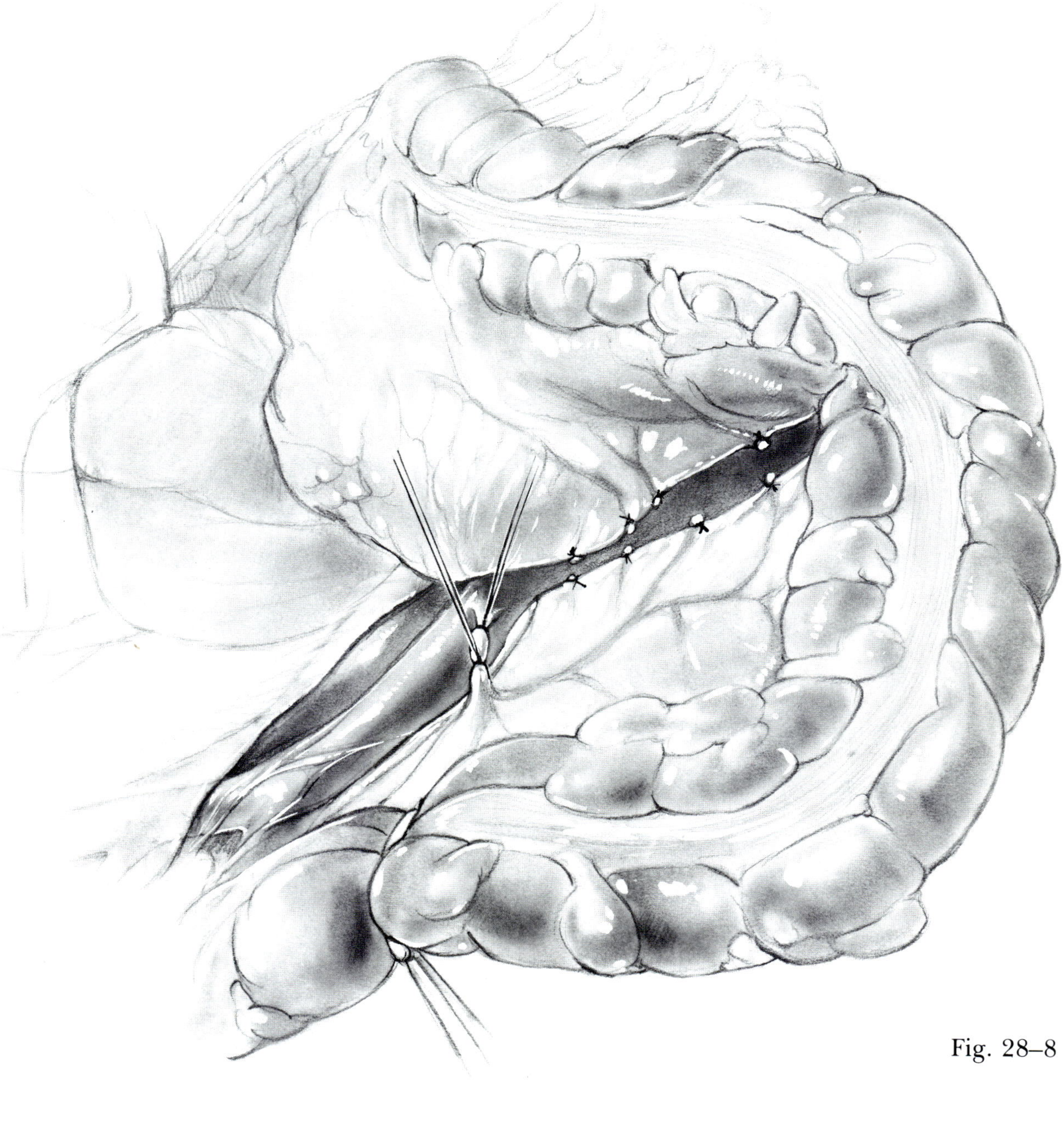

Fig. 28–8

End-to-End Two-Layer Anastomosis, Rotation Method

There are eight steps to the end-to-end two-layer anastomosis, rotation method:

1) Check the *adequacy of the blood supply* of both ends of the bowel.

2) Check whether a *cuff of at least 1 cm of serosa* has been cleared of areolar tissue and blood vessels at both ends of the bowel.

3) *Rotate the proximal colonic segment* so that the mesentery enters from the right lateral margin of the anastomosis. Leave the rectal segment undisturbed (**Fig. 28–9**).

4) If the diameter of the lumen of one of the segments of bowel is significantly narrower than the other, *make a Cheatle slit,* 1–2 cm long, on the antimesenteric border of the narrower segment of bowel (see Figs. 27–7 and 27–8).

5) *Insert the first layer of seromuscular sutures.* If the rectal stump is not bound down to the sacrum and if it can be rotated easily for 180°, it is more efficient to insert the anterior seromuscular layer as the first step in the anastomosis. Insert interrupted 4–0 cotton atraumatic Lembert seromuscular guy sutures, first to the lateral border of the anastomosis and then to the medial border. By the technique of successive bisection, place the third Lembert suture on the anterior wall halfway between the first two (Fig. 28–9). Each stitch takes about 5 mm of tissue, including the submucosa, of the rectum and then of the descending colon.

6) After all the anterior sutures have been inserted, *tie them and cut all the suture tails* except for those of the two end guy sutures, which should be grasped in hemostats (**Fig. 28–10**). Pass a hemostat beneath the suture line, grasp the right lateral stitch (labeled *A* in **Fig. 28–11**), and rotate the anastomosis 180° (**Fig. 28–12**).

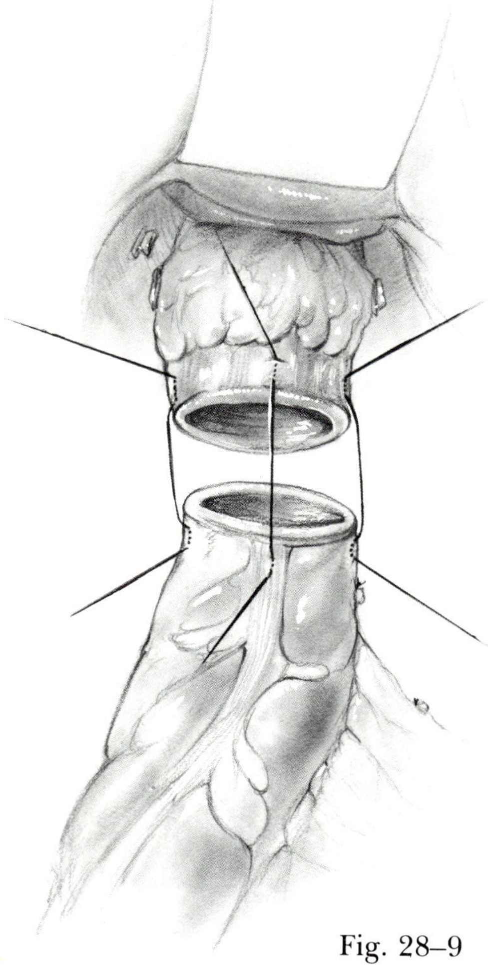

Fig. 28–9

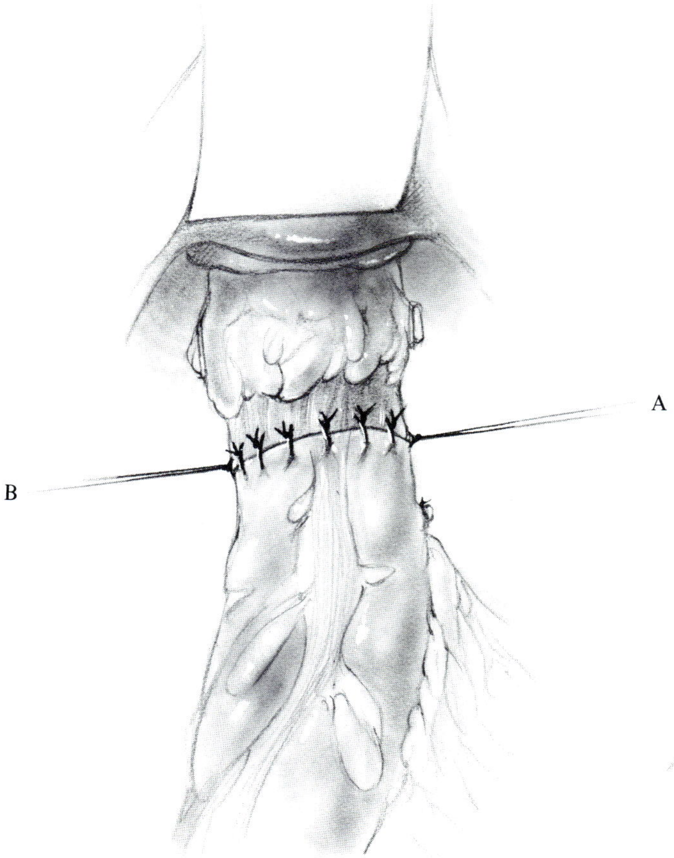

Fig. 28–10

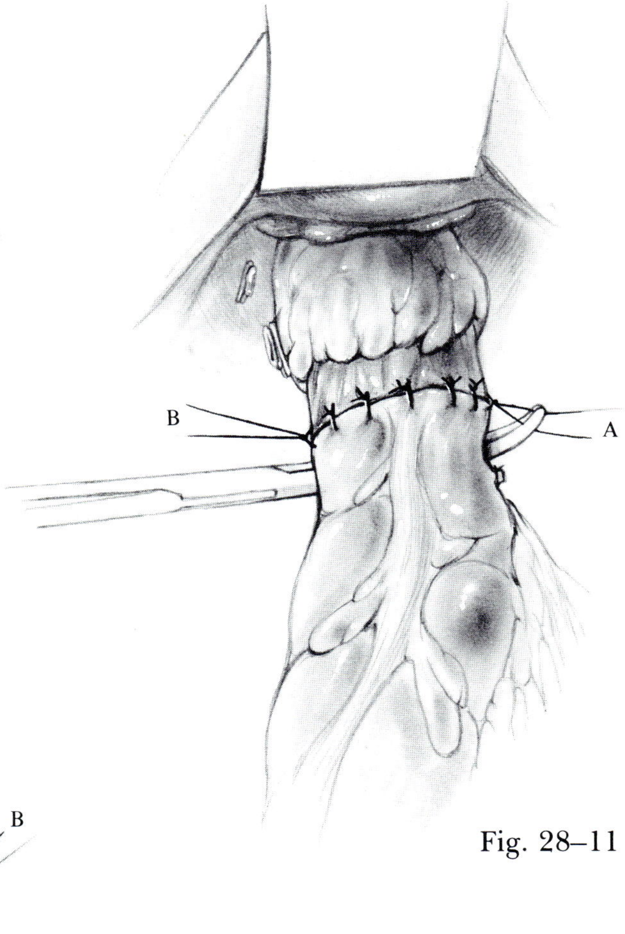

Fig. 28–11

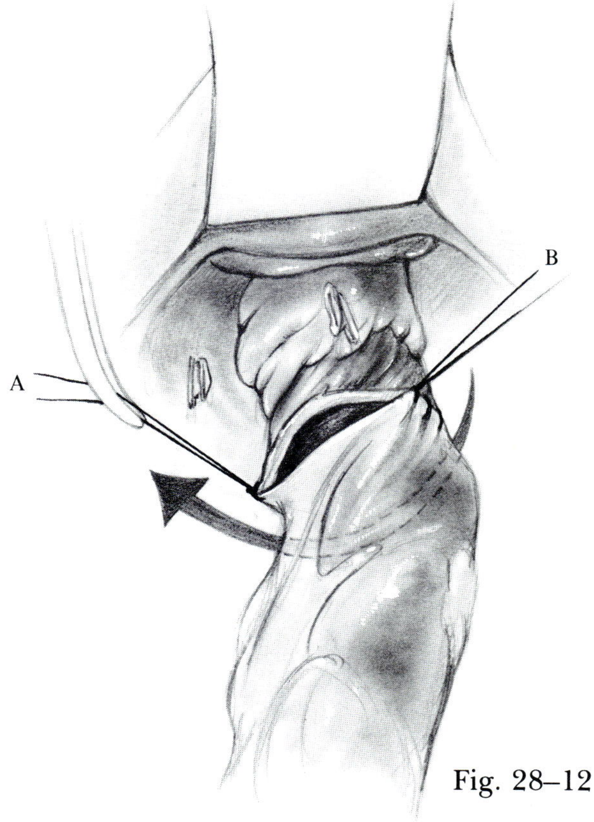

Fig. 28–12

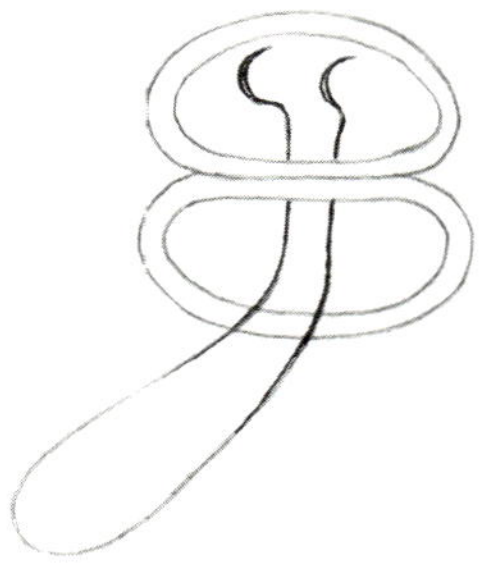

Fig. 28–13a

7) Place a double-armed 4–0 chromic catgut *suture in the middle of the deep mucosal layer* (**Fig. 28–13a**). Complete this layer with a continuous locked suture through the full thickness of the bowel (**Fig. 28–13b**). Then, with the same two needles, using a continuous Connell or Cushing suture complete the remainder of the mucosal approximation (**Fig. 28–14**).

8) Approximate the *final seromuscular layer* with interrupted 4–0 atraumatic Lembert cotton sutures (**Fig. 28–15**). After all the suture tails are cut, permit the anastomosis to rotate back 180° to its normal position.

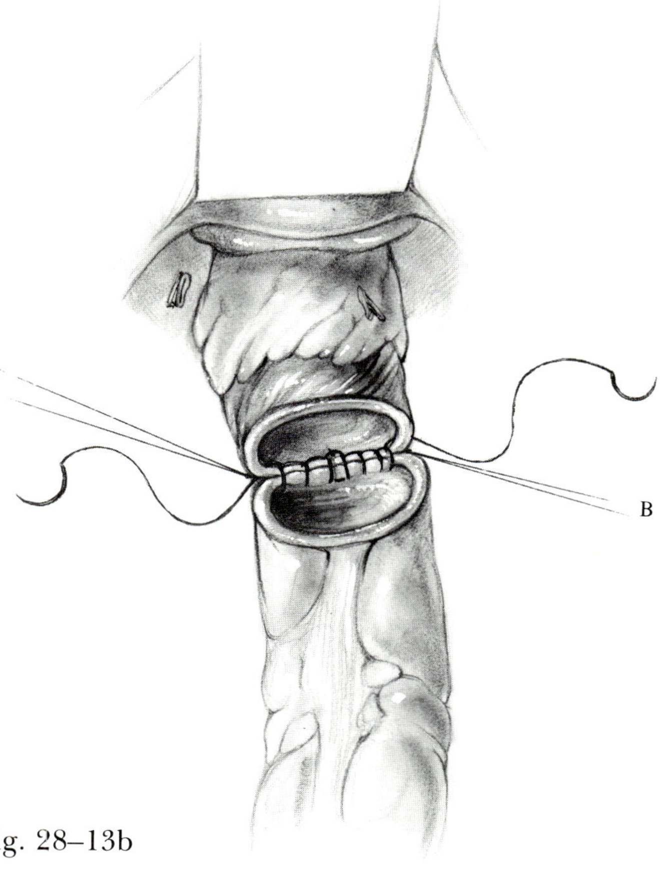

Fig. 28–13b

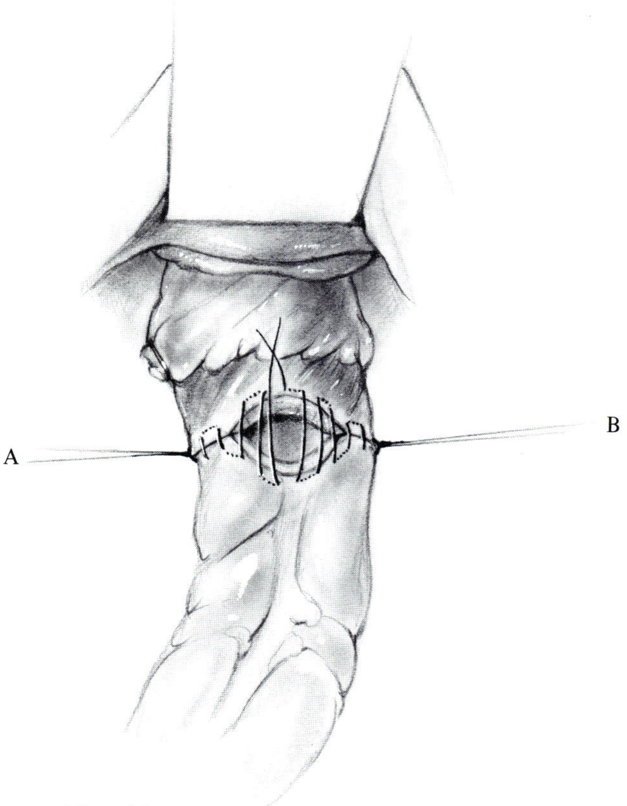

Fig. 28–14

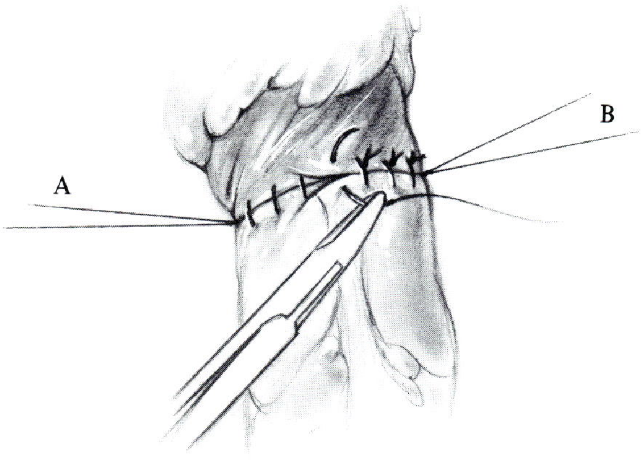

Fig. 28–15

End-to-End Anastomosis, Alternative Technique

When the rectum and colon cannot be rotated 180°, as required for the method described above, an alternative technique must be used, in which the posterior seromuscular layer is inserted first. To do this, insert a seromuscular suture of 4–0 cotton into the left side of the rectum and of the proximal colon. Do not tie this suture; grasp it in a hemostat; use it as the left guy suture. Place a second suture of the identical type on the right lateral aspects of the rectum and proximal colon and similarly hold it in a hemostat (**Fig. 28–16**).

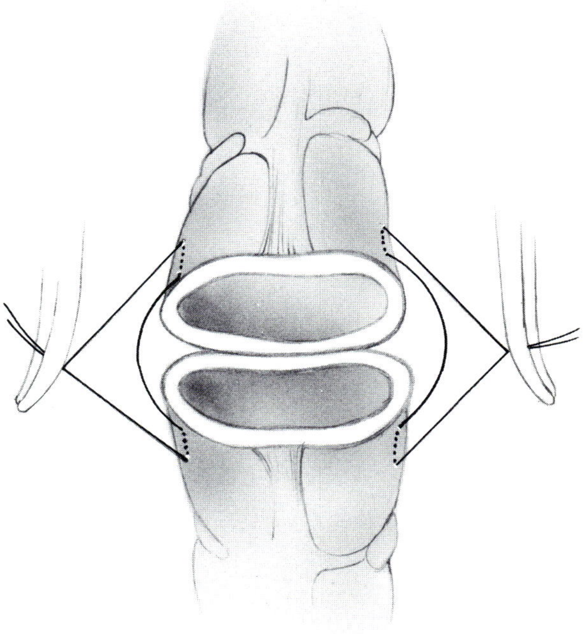

Fig. 28–16

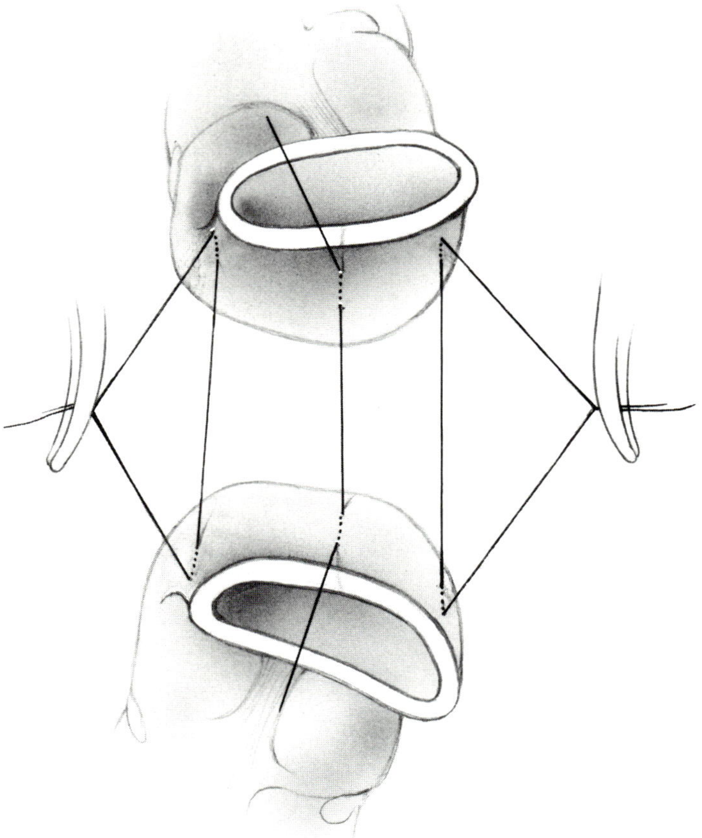

Fig. 28–17

Insert interrupted 4–0 cotton seromuscular Lembert sutures (**Fig. 28–17**) to complete the posterior layer. This is done preferably by the successive bisection technique. As each suture is inserted, attach it to a hemostat until the layer is completed. At the conclusion of the layer tie all the sutures and cut all the tails except for those of the two lateral guy sutures.

Initiate the posterior mucosal layer with a double-armed atraumatic suture of 4–0 chromic catgut. Insert the suture in mattress fashion in the midpoint of the posterior layer of mucosa and tie it (**Fig. 28–18**). If the exposure is good, straight

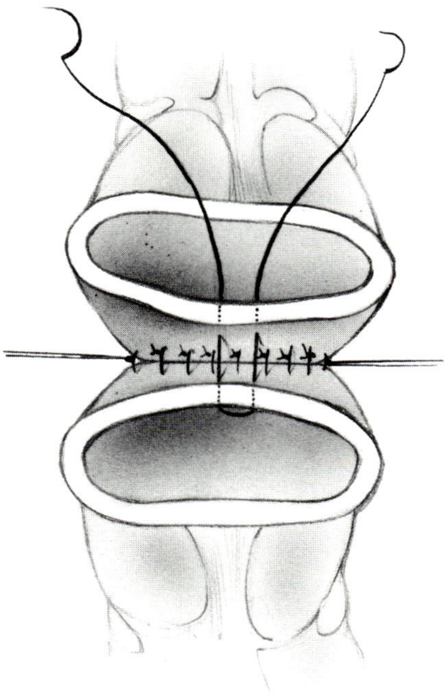

Fig. 28–18

needles may be used. In patients who have a deep pelvis, curved needles are preferable. In either case, use one needle to initiate a continuous locked suture, taking bites averaging 5 mm in diameter and going through all the coats of bowel (**Fig. 28–19**). Continue this in a locked fashion until the left lateral margin of the anastomosis is reached (**Fig. 28–20**). At this point pass the needle from inside to the outside of the rectum and hold it temporarily in a hemostat.

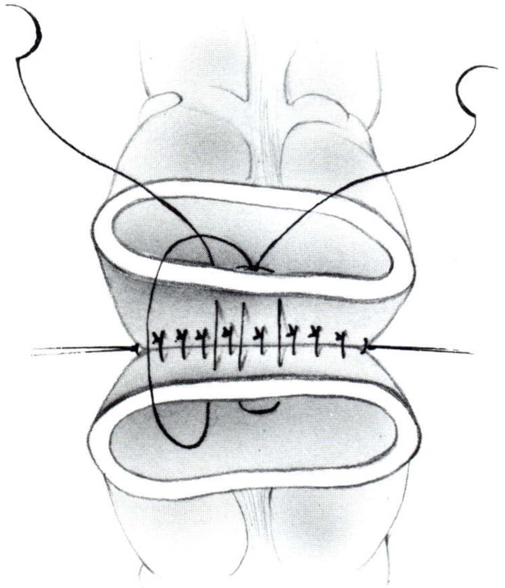

Fig. 28–19

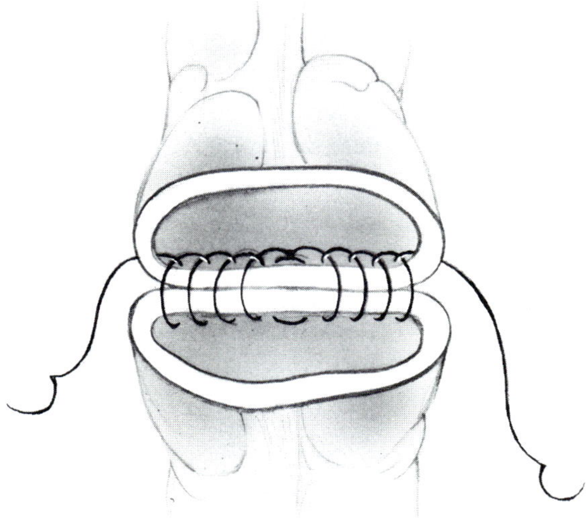

Fig. 28–21

Grasp the remaining needle and insert a continuous locked suture of the same type, beginning at the midpoint and continuing to the right lateral margin of the bowel. Here, pass the needle through the rectum from inside out (**Fig. 28–21**).

Standing on the left side of the patient, use the needle on the right lateral aspect of the anastomosis to initiate the anterior mucosal layer. Insert continuous sutures of either the Cushing or Connell type to a point just beyond the middle of the anterior layer. Then grasp the needle emerging from the left lateral margin of the incision and insert a similar continu-

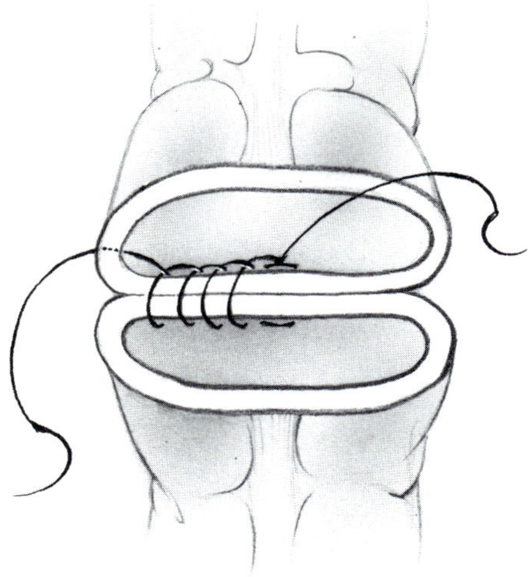

Fig. 28–20

ous Connell or Cushing stitch. Complete the anterior mucosal layer by tying the suture to its mate and cutting the tails of these sutures (**Figs. 28–22 and 28–23**).

Complete the anterior seromuscular layer by inserting interrupted 4–0 cotton atraumatic Lembert sutures (**Fig. 28–24**).

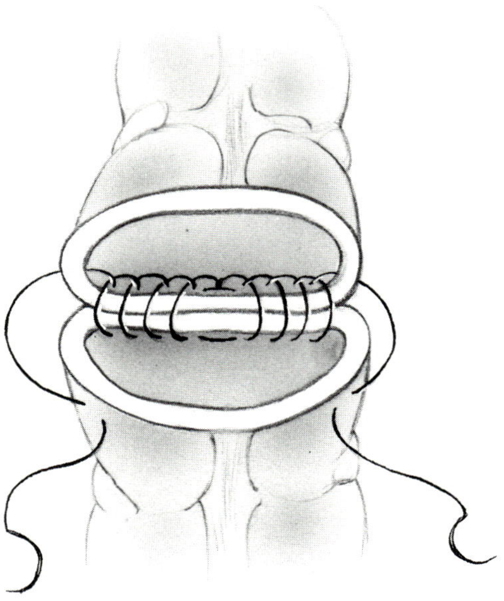

Fig. 28–22

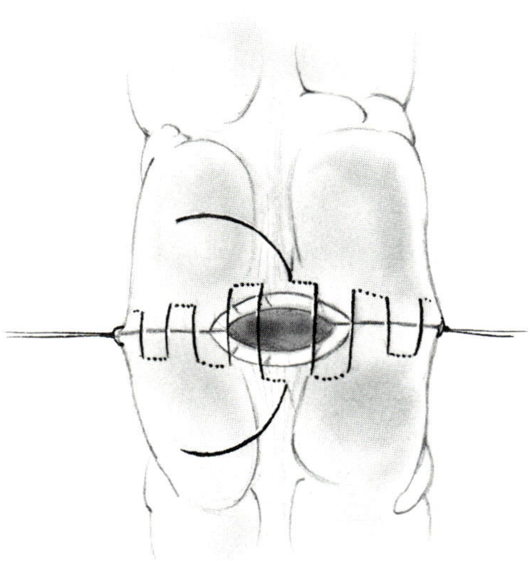

Fig. 28–23

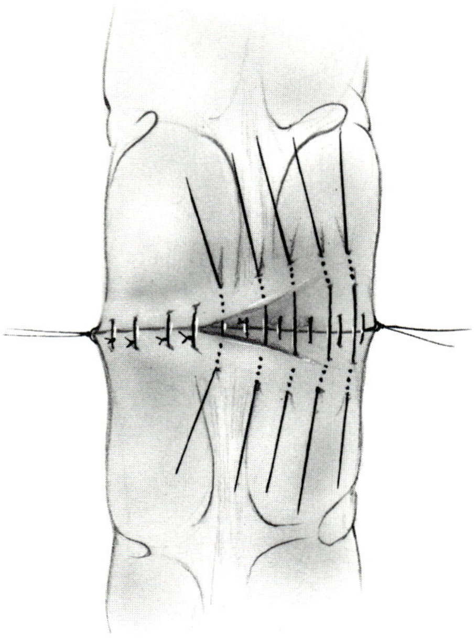

Fig. 28–24

Now carefully rotate the anastomosis to inspect the integrity of the posterior layer. Test the diameter of the lumen before closing the mesentery by invaginating the colon through the lumen gently with the thumb and forefinger. Then close the mesentery with a continuous 2–0 PG suture (**Fig. 28–25**). Leave the peritoneal defect in the left paracolic gutter unsutured.

Stapled Colorectal Anastomosis, Technique of Weakley

In the Weakley technique of stapled colorectal anastomosis, step 1 of the rotation method is modified in that the proximal descending colon is stapled closed by the TA–55 stapling device (**Fig. 28–26**). To carry out this procedure, apply an Allen clamp to the specimen side and divide the colon flush with the stapler. Remove the stapler (**Fig. 28–27**). Replace the Allen

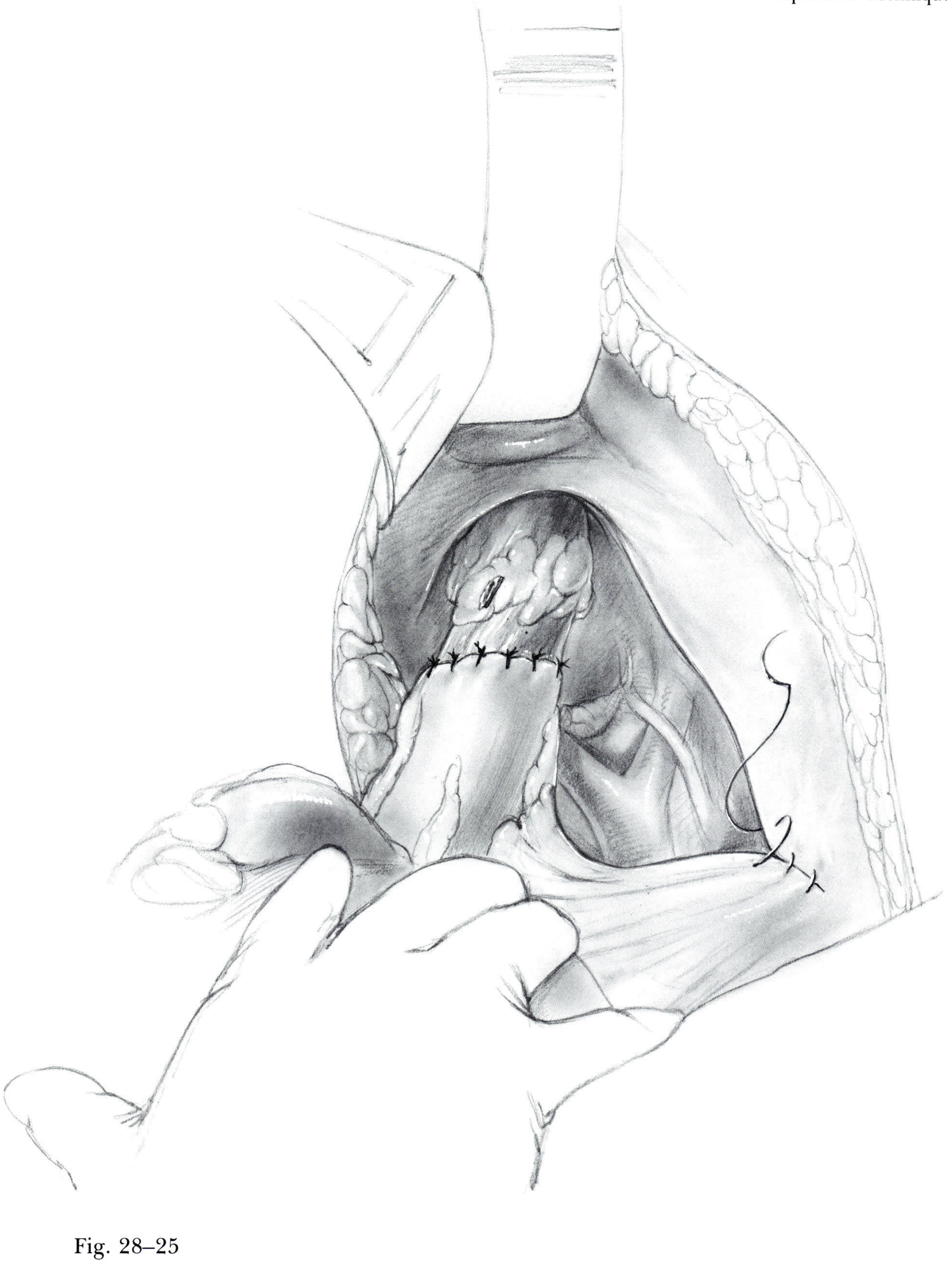

Fig. 28–25

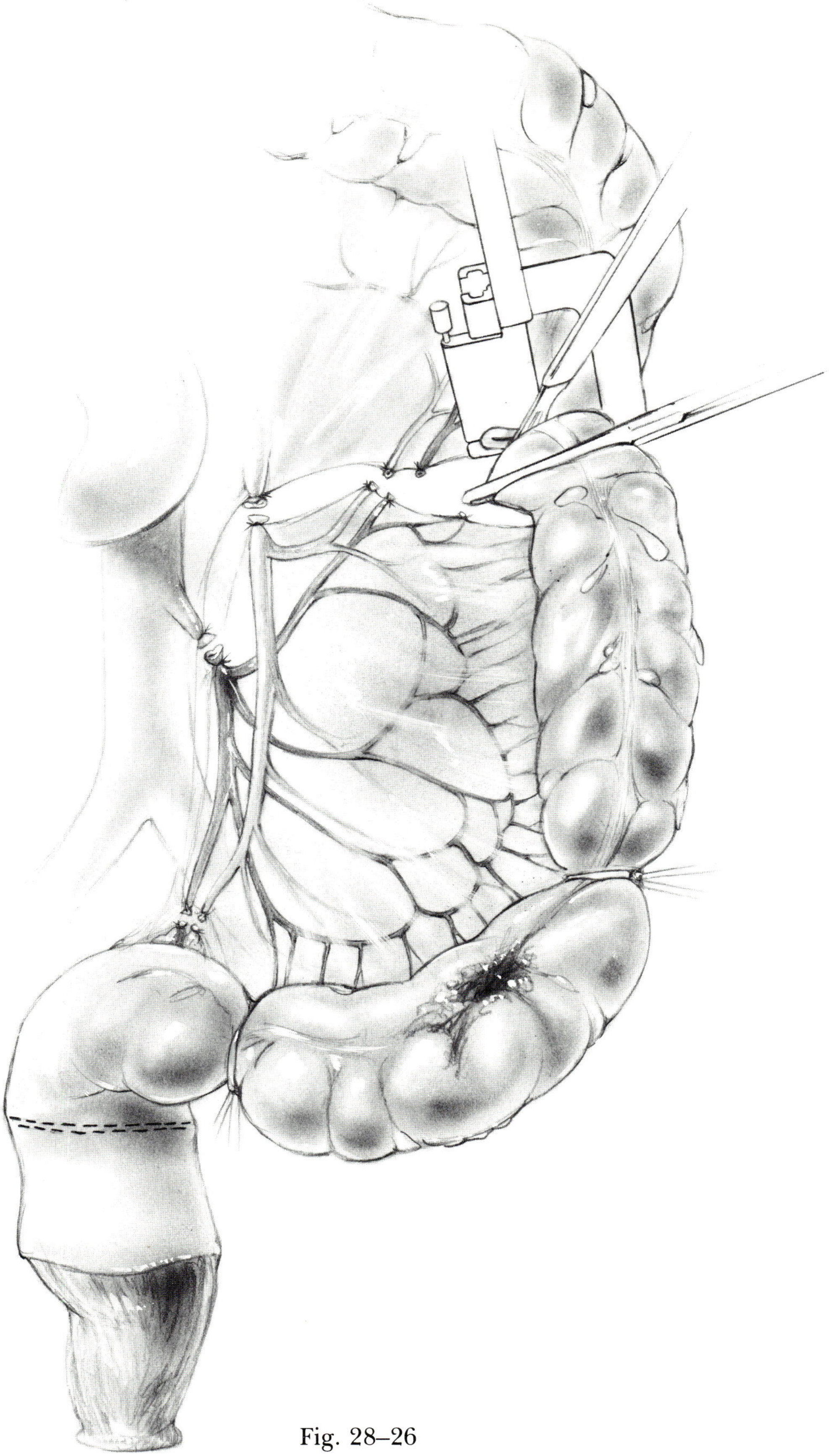

Fig. 28–26

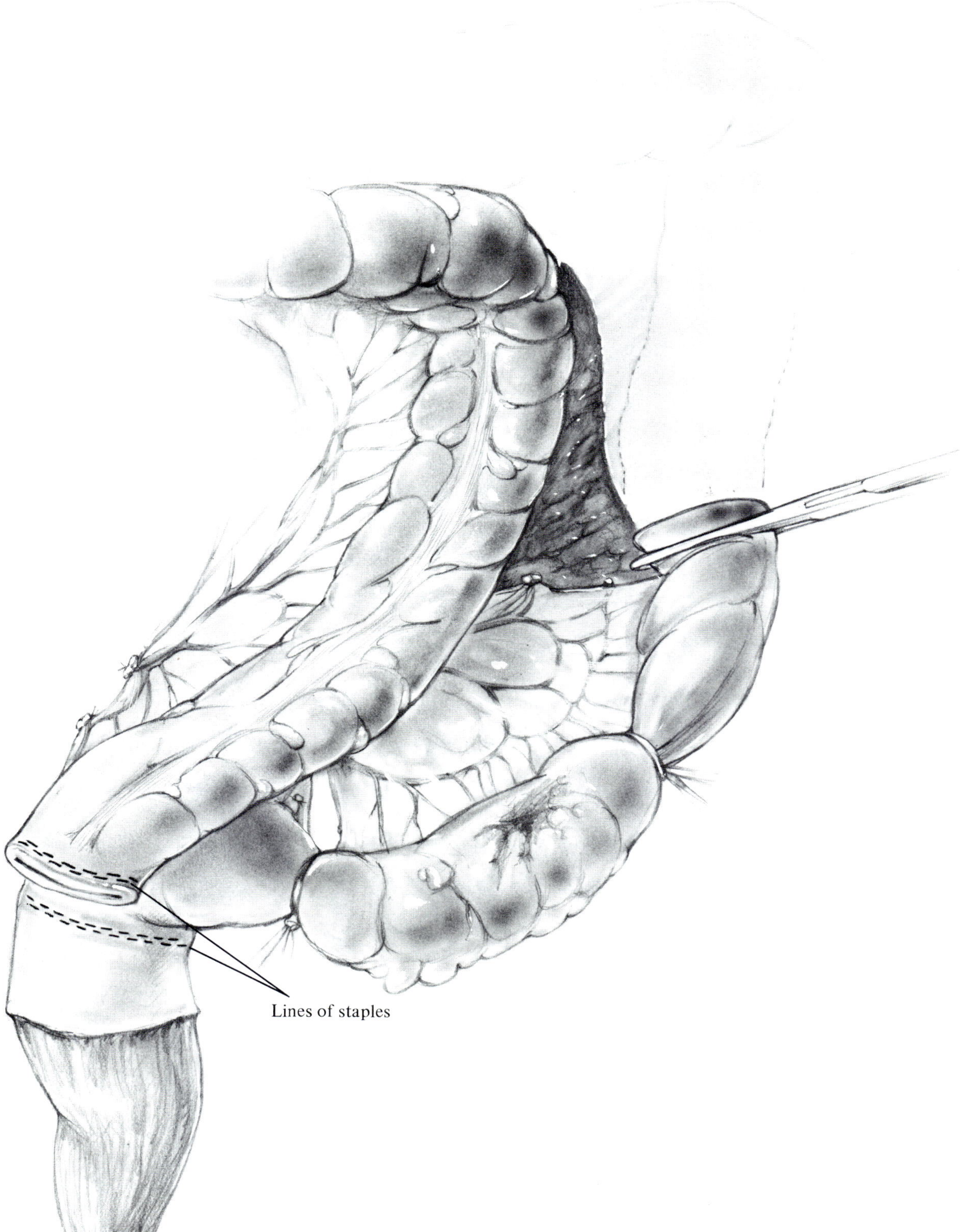

Fig. 28–27

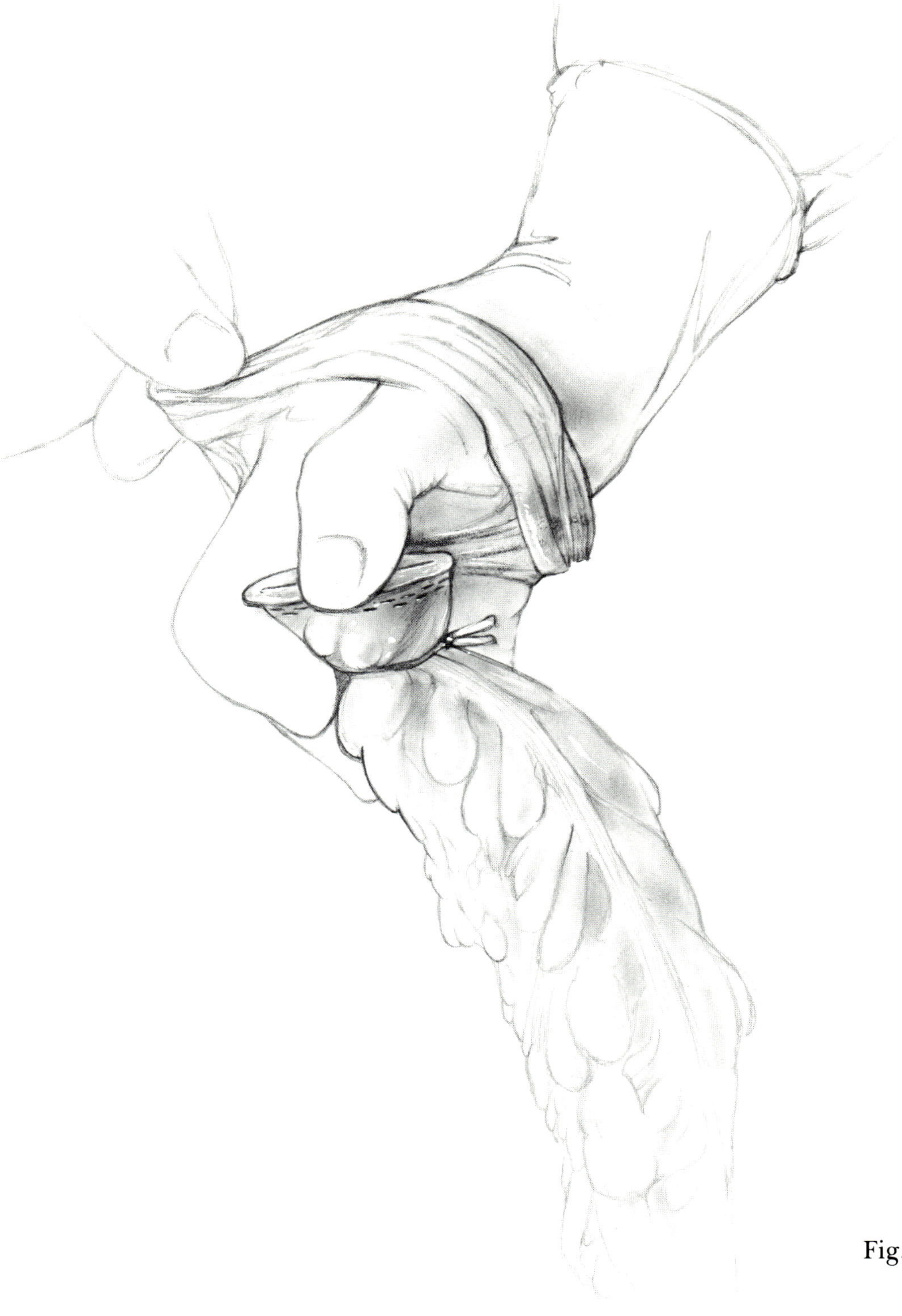

Fig. 28–28

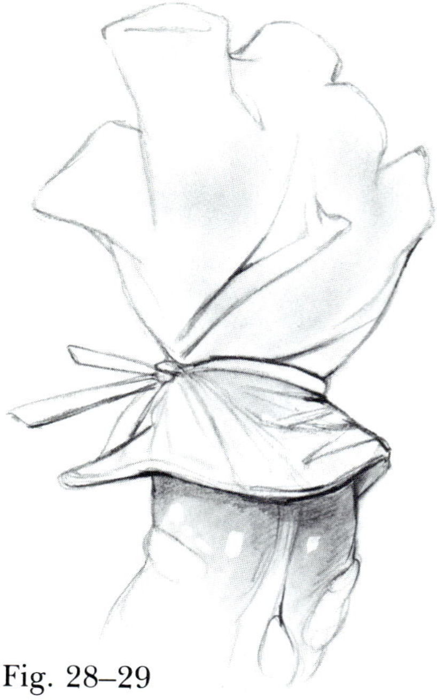

Fig. 28–29

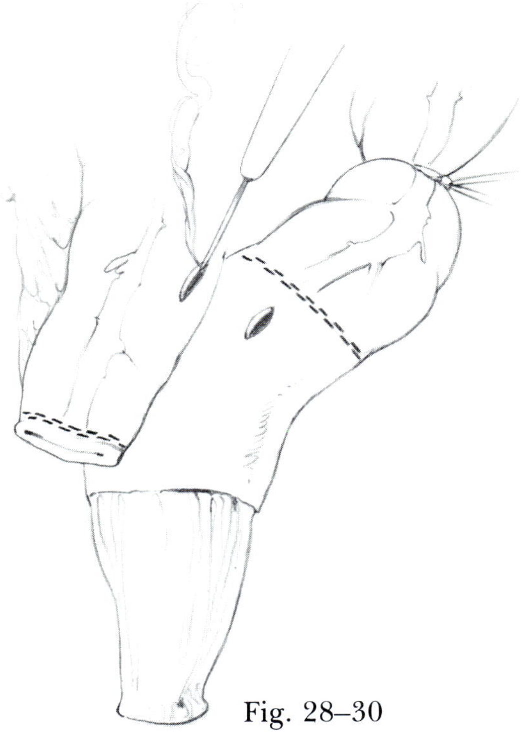

Fig. 28–30

clamp with an umbilical tape ligature covered with a sterile rubber glove (**Figs. 28–28 and 28–29**). Then direct attention to the rectum, a segment of which previously has been cleared of surrounding fat and vascular tissue. Use the TA–55 device, generally with 3.5 mm staples (Fig. 28–26), to apply a layer of staples to this segment of rectum. Do not remove the specimen; retain it so that mild upward traction on it can stabilize the rectum during the application of the stapling device (Fig. 28–27).

Make a stab wound on the antimesenteric border of the proximal colon at a point 5–6 cm proximal to the staple line. Either a scalpel blade or electrocautery may be used to make this incision. Make a second stab wound in the anterior wall of the rectal stump at a point 1 cm distal to the staple line already in place (**Fig. 28–30**). Approximate the two stab wounds opposite each other, placing the proximal colonic segment anterior to the rectal stump. Insert the GIA device, one fork

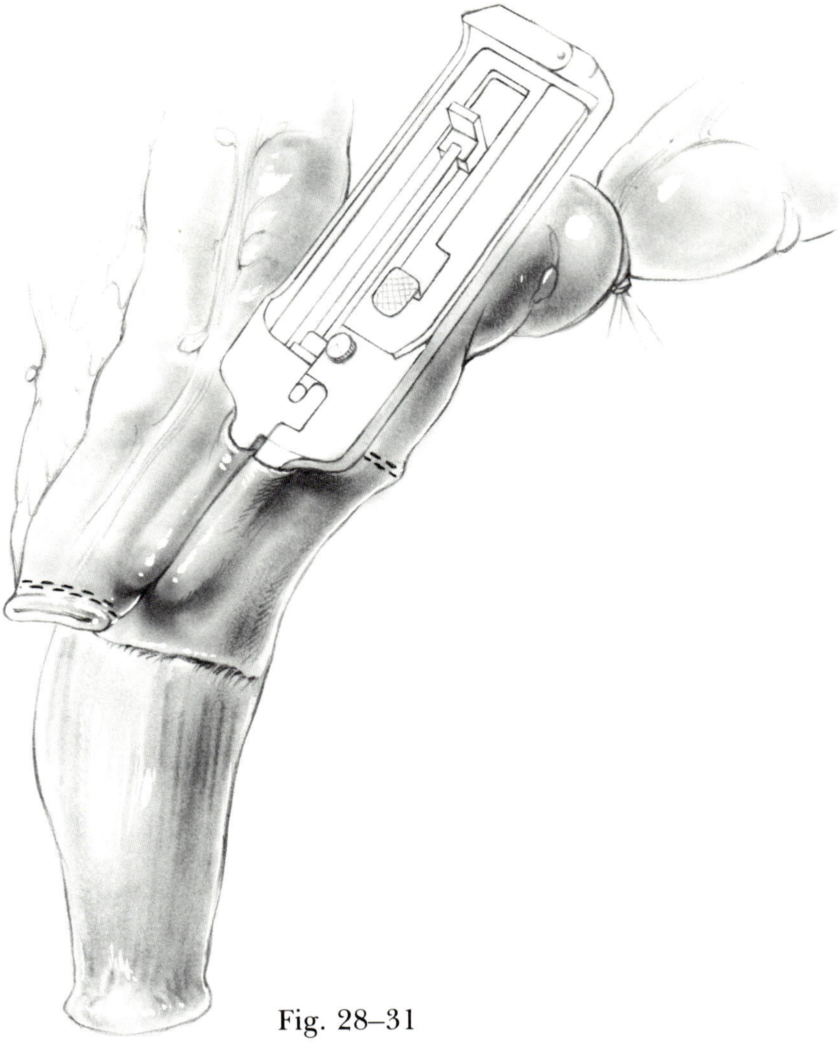

Fig. 28–31

into the rectal stump and the other into the proximal colonic segment (**Fig. 28–31**). Allis clamps or guy sutures may be used to approximate the rectum and colon in the crotch of the GIA device. Fire and remove the GIA stapler; then carefully inspect the staple line for any defects or bleeding. Close the remaining defect with a continuous inverting 4–0 PG atraumatic suture to the mucosa. Reinforce this closure with a layer of interrupted 4–0 cotton atraumatic seromuscular Lembert sutures (**Fig. 28–32**). Carefully inspect all the staple lines to ascertain that the staples have closed properly into the shape of a B. Bleeding points may require careful electrocoagulation or fine suture-ligatures. The rectosigmoid is transected just above the rectal staple line (Fig. 28–32) with the removal of the specimen.

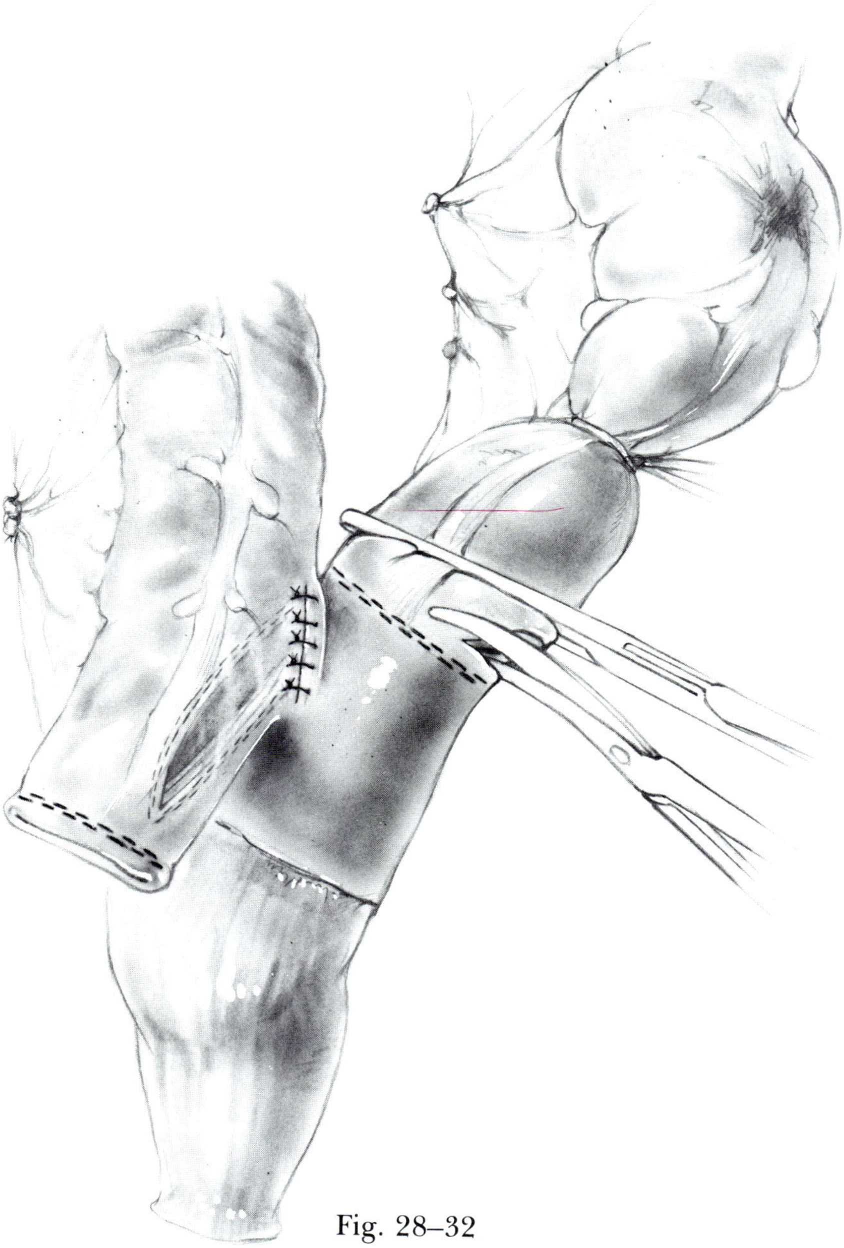

Fig. 28–32

Stapled Colocolonic Functional End-to-End Anastomosis, Chassin's Method

When the lumen of one segment of bowel to be anastomosed is *much* smaller than the other, as in many ileocolonic anasatomoses, the stapling technique illustrated in Figs. 27–18 and 27–20 is the simplest method, although the technique of Weakley is also suitable. When a stapled anastomosis is constructed distal to the sacral promontory, the EEA technique (see Chap. 30) is much preferred. However, for all other intraperitoneal anastomoses of small and large bowel, we have developed a modification of the end-to-

Antimesenteric side not on tenia

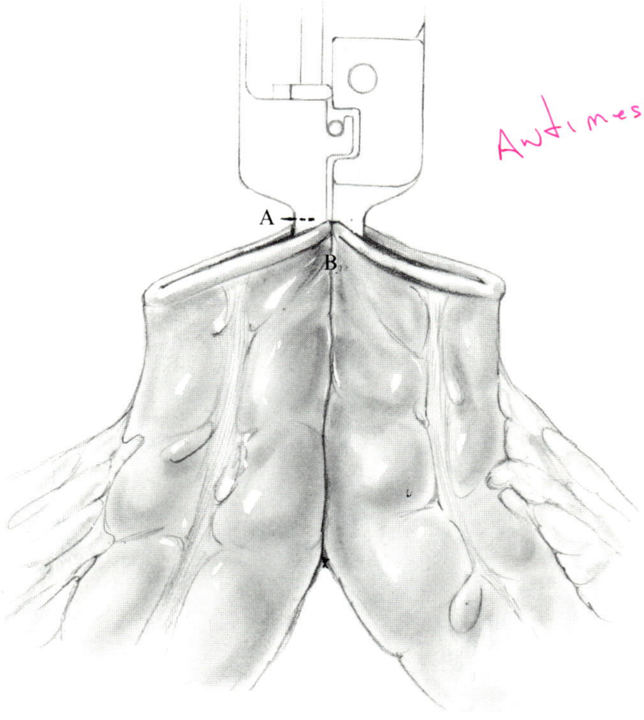

Fig. 28–33

end anastomosis. This modification, described in the following steps, avoids the possibility that six rows of staples may be superimposed, one upon the other, as may happen in the Steichen method:

1) Align the two open ends of bowel to be anastomosed side by side, with the antimesenteric borders of each in contact.

2) Insert the GIA instrument, placing one fork in each lumen (**Fig. 28–33**). Draw the mesenteric borders of the bowel in the direction opposite to the location of the GIA device. Avoid bunching too much tissue in the crotch of the GIA. Lock and fire the instrument.

3) After unlocking the GIA instrument and removing the knife assembly, withdraw the GIA from the bowel. Apply an Allis clamp to one extremity of the GIA staple line (point *A* in Fig. 28–33). Apply a second Allis clamp to the opposite end of the GIA staple line (point *B* in Fig. 28–33). These two Allis clamps should then be drawn apart as shown in **Fig. 28–34**.

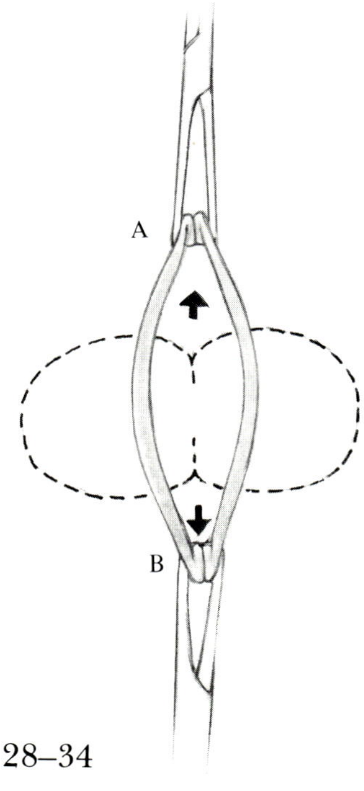

Fig. 28–34

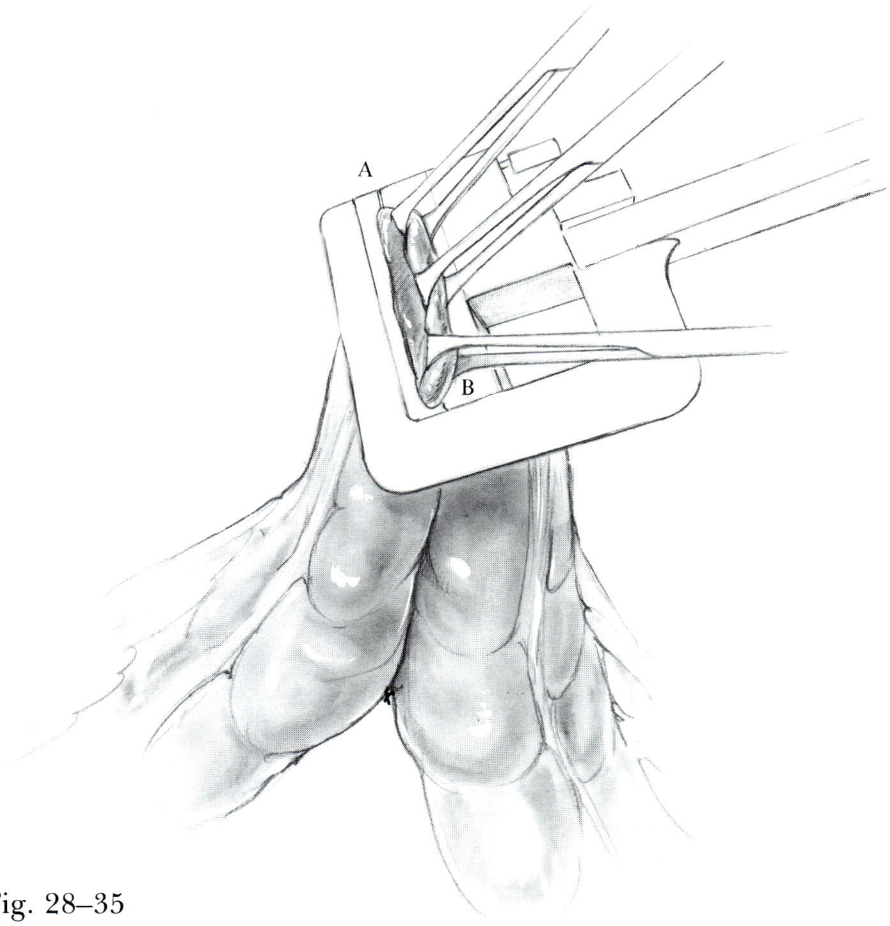

Fig. 28–35

4) Apply additional Allis clamps to close the remaining defect in the anastomosis by approximating mucosa to mucosa, as in **Fig. 28–35**.

5) Close the remaining defect in an everting fashion by either a single application of the TA–90 device or by two applications of the TA–55. Fig. 28–35 illustrates the complete closure of the defect with one application of the TA–90 just deep to the Allis clamps. Be sure that the TA–90 staple line includes both point *A* and point *B*, which mark respectively the near and far terminations of the GIA staple line. Unless the GIA and the TA–90 staple lines overlap, there exists the possibility of a gap in the stapled closure.

6) After the TA–90 device has been placed in the proper position, drive home and tighten the alignment pin. Then rotate the wing nut of the TA–90 until the narrow black band falls within the confines of the wide black band on the handle. When it does, fire the device. Excise the redundant bowel with a Mayo scissors and

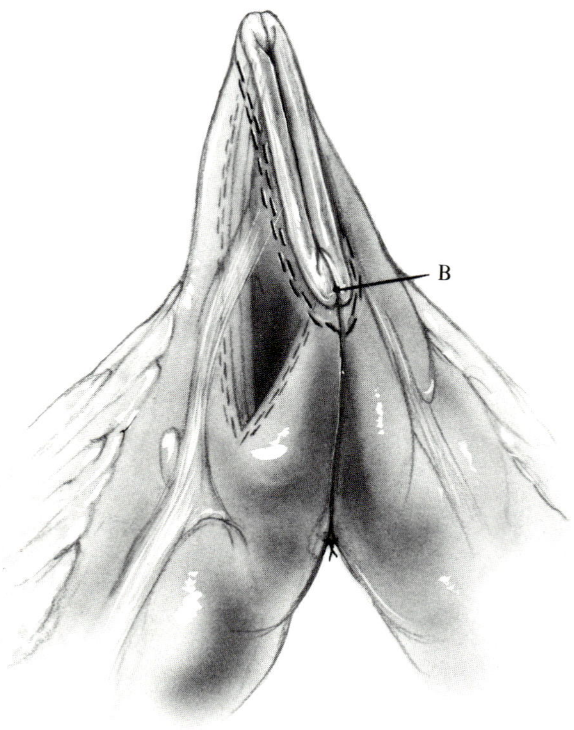

Fig. 28–36

lightly electrocoagulate the everted mucosa. Remove the TA–90 (**Fig. 28–36**) and carefully inspect the entire anastomosis for the proper B formation of staples.

Finally, insert a single 4–0 atraumatic cotton seromuscular Lembert suture at the base of the GIA staple line (Fig. 28–36). This prevents any undue distracting force from being exerted on the stapled anastomosis.

Antibiotic Irrigation

After the surgical team removes the Wound Protector drape and discards all surgical gloves and instruments, the abdominal cavity and the subcutaneous panniculus should be irrigated with an antibiotic solution.

Wound Closure

Most surgeons prefer to close the defect in the mesocolon (Fig. 28–25). A continuous suture of 2–0 PG is suitable for this purpose. However, the defect is usually so large that omitting this step does not seem to lead to internal bowel herniation. Close the abdominal incision in routine fashion without placing any drains into the peritoneal cavity; subcutaneous closed-suction catheters, however, are generally used (see Chap. 2).

Postoperative Care

(See Chap. 27.)

Complications

(See Chap. 27.)

29 Operations for Rectal Cancer

Concept: Selection of Operation for Cancer 0–6 cm from Anal Verge

Method of Measuring Length from Anal Verge

Measurements of the location of malignancies in the rectum are generally made by placing the patient in the knee-chest position, inserting a proctosigmoidoscope, and reading off the number of centimeters indicated by the markers on the outside of the scope at the point where the perianal skin meets the scope. This measures the distance between the anal verge and the lower border of the tumor where the tip of the proctoscope has been inserted. Remember that when a measurement is cited taking the anal verge as the point of reference, it does not refer to the rectum alone but includes the length of the anal canal in the calculation. The rectal mucosa meet the squamous epithelium of the anal skin at the "dentate line." This line is 2–3 cm above the anal verge and about 1 cm below the upper border of the sphincter muscles of the anal canal. The length of the anal canal is about 4 cm. All the measurements cited below are made from the reference point of the anal verge.

Electrocoagulation

To treat a malignancy in the distal rectum (0–6 cm), the surgeon's choice lies between performing an abdominoperineal proctectomy and some local procedure such as electrocoagulation or excision. Coagulation is effective and has been followed by minimal mortality when applied to lesions that are anatomically suited to this technique. Unfortunately, even in cases when fulguration may eliminate the primary carcinoma, there is no way of ascertaining that the lymph nodes are free of metastases. For this reason, a large body of follow-up data will have to be accumulated before fulguration can be recommended as the treatment of choice for patients in whom abdominal surgery is not contraindicated by severe systemic illness. If on digital rectal examination, metastatic lymph nodes can be palpated in the presacral space, fulguration for cure is contraindicated. When one excludes operations for palliation, abdominoperineal proctectomy is the operation of choice for tumors at the 0–6 cm level.

If electrocoagulation is to be used to manage rectal cancer, the ideal lesion for treatment would be a non-fixed tumor of small size (3–5 cm diameter) with a well-differentiated cell type, located preferably on the posterior wall of the lower rectum. For the rare patient whose medical condition really contraindicates major surgery, and for those who already have an identifiable distant metastasis, electrocoagulation may be used to treat tumors that are less than ideal in size and location.

This modality should never be applied to malignancies that are circumferential in location, as this will result in complete stenosis during the healing process. Nor should it be used in tumors above the 9–10 cm level especially on the anterior aspect of the rectum.

Local Excision

By intussuscepting a small tumor or villous adenoma through the anus, local excision with suture of the defect is sometimes feasible. Parks and Thompson recommend dissection through the intersphincteric plane for small lesions of this type, using the Parks self-retaining anal retractor. This method gives the pathologist a specimen suitable for thorough analysis by serial microscopic sections, which is important when there is doubt about the presence of invasive cancer—as, for example, in some villous adenomas.

Radiotherapy for Cure

Another promising modality for managing rectal lesions no larger than 3 cm wide is Papillon's technique of intensive intralumenal irradiation of non-fixed, well-differentiated adenocarcinomas of the rectum. This therapy is administered through a proctoscope. Preliminary studies show good results in selected cases. Papillon's findings are being tested in this country by Sischy.

Preoperative Adjuvant Radiotherapy

Although considerable data have been accumulated, it is not yet clear whether preoperative radiation therapy improves the prognosis of patients suffering from rectal cancer. Dosages of 2000–5000 rads have been given before surgery is undertaken, and some tumors do shrink following therapy. For lesions that on preoperative physical examination appear to be fixed to the presacral space posteriorly or to the prostate anteriorly, preoperative radiation may occasionally result in sufficient shrinkage to convert what would be an inoperable lesion into a resectable one. This course should be followed for patients who have such lesions. Even though the supporting evidence is not conclusive, it is our policy to recommend preoperative radiation for patients who have large or fixed lesions. For patients with Duke's C lesions we believe that postoperative radiotherapy may reduce the incidence of local recurrence.

Abdominoperineal Proctectomy

With rare exceptions, abdominoperineal proctectomy is the operation of choice for cancer of the lower third of the rectum, 0–6 cm above the anal verge. Using proper technique the mortality rate should be no more than 1%–2% following operations done for cure.

Concept: Selection of Operation for Carcinoma 6–11 cm from Anal Verge

Requirements for Maintaining Normal Fecal Continence

Using the abdominosacral or the EEA stapler operation, it is often technically possible to resect lesions of the lowermost rectum and to perform an anastomosis at the mucocutaneous junction of the anus. However, normal fecal continence seems to require 1–2 cm of residual rectal wall above the dentate line, as well as normally functioning internal sphincter and puborectalis muscles. Following "pull-through" operations of the Bacon or Cutait-Turnbull type, the patient may lose the proprioceptive sensation that warns of an impending movement of stool or flatus. A normal individual, if a toilet is not immediately at hand, can occlude the anus by tensing the voluntary external sphincter muscle. This voluntary constriction can last for 40 to 60 seconds, until fatigue sets in. But usually, before that time elapses, the crest of the peristaltic wave ebbs and the rectum undergoes a period of relaxation before the next peristaltic contraction. True fecal continence thus requires the presence of a sense of proprioception as well as the ability to contract the external sphincter. After a pull-through operation, however, sometimes the patient's first hint that the colon is about to evacuate stool comes when liquid stool or flatus touches the perianal skin. It is only at this point that the patient is aware of the need to constrict the voluntary sphincter. As a consequence, control of liquid stool or flatus is often defective. Defective control will also follow complete excision of the internal sphincter, which has the function of keeping the rectum closed except when peristalsis propels a bolus of stool.

Carcinomas above the 6 cm level are often amenable to low anterior resection or abdominosacral resection, which are accompanied by satisfactory fecal continence. But it should be noted that for many months following resection, patients who undergo this procedure do not possess a real rectal reservoir function. In the normal rectum, peristaltic contraction in the process of evacuation is accompanied by a *reflex relaxation in the tone of the internal sphincter* and puborectalis muscles. Following resection of the rectal wall in the region 3–6 cm above the anal verge, this reflex relaxation fails, according to Bennett et al. After the operation, patients complain of incomplete evacuation and of having many small formed stools during the course of the day. In some cases severe constipation ensues. However, within 6 months to a year following surgery almost all these patients develop quite satisfactory function in evacuating the rectum and in control of flatus or liquid stool. Since postoperative survival following resection of a carcinoma of the midrectum is no worse than that following total proctectomy, resection and anastomosis is the preferable alternative if these are feasible technically. A margin is needed of 4 cm of rectum distal to the tumor and an additional 1–2 cm of residual rectal wall above the dentate line to assure proprioception and fecal continence.

Anterior Resection

Skilled and experienced surgeons can accomplish anterior resection with anastomosis for cancer as low as 6 cm from the anal verge in women and 8 cm in some men. This technique requires complete dissection of the rectum down to the levator diaphragm and to the distal margin of the prostate anteriorly in males. Anastomosis is contraindicated for patients who have a narrow pelvis or are obese. It is also contraindicated in any case in which the exposure is inadequate to insert sutures with accuracy. Under these conditions, the surgeon must turn to an alternative method. A stapled anastomosis using the EEA device can often be accomplished at a level 2–3 cm lower than can be achieved by suturing from the anterior approach. If this alternative is not suitable, abdominoperineal proctectomy may be performed.

It should be recognized that the postoperative five-year survival of patients who are operated on for lesions above the 6 cm level appears to be the same whether abdominoperineal proctectomy is performed or resection and anastomosis is accomplished. Malignancies located 0–6 cm from the anus may have lymphatic extension in both cephalad and caudal directions. Above the 6 cm level, extension is exclusively cephalad unless the proximal lymph channels are already blocked with cancer.

Akwari and Kelly found that, 2 years after the resection and anastomosis of tumors at the 6–10 cm level, the results were just as good as those following the same operation for cancers at the 10–20 cm and over 20 cm levels.

Low Colorectal Anastomosis Using EEA Stapling Technique

The recently introduced Auto Suture EEA stapling apparatus enables the surgeon to construct an end-to-end anastomosis at a level much lower than is practicable by hand suturing. Results with this technique have been highly promising. This device permits a safe anastomosis after resection of tumors situated as low as 6 cm from the anal verge. However, there are many pitfalls of a technical nature in the EEA method, and the technique must be mastered before consistent success can be achieved.

The EEA technique is admirably suited to low colorectal anastomosis—those at or below the peritoneal reflection, where suturing may be difficult. For higher colon anastomoses, other stapling or suture techniques provide an anastomotic stoma larger in diameter than the 2.2 cm that follows the use of the EEA stapler. Also, it has not yet been demonstrated that the stoma made with two layers of staggered staples will dilate with the passage of stool, as does the usual anastomosis made with interrupted nonabsorbable and continuous catgut sutures.

Low Colorectal Anatomosis Using Combined Abdominal and Sacral Approaches

Localio et al. have reported excellent results after resecting lesions in the 6–11 cm range by mobilizing the rectum through the abdominal approach and then performing the colorectal anastomosis through a posterior incision with coccygectomy. However, this is a complex operation, not suitable for the occasional operator. The same low resection and anastomosis can be accomplished with greater efficiency by proper use of the EEA stapling technique.

References

Akwari OE, Kelly K (1980) Anterior resection for adenocarcinoma of the distal large bowel. Am J Surg 139:88

Bennett RC et al. (1973) The physiologic status of the anorectum after pull-through operations. Surg Gynecol Obstet 136:907

Localio SA et al. (1978) Abdominosacral resection for carcinoma of the midrectum: ten years' experience. Ann Surg 188:475

Parks AG, Thomson JPS (1977) Per-anal endorectal operative techniques. In: Rob C, Smith R (eds) Operative surgery, colon, rectum and anus, 3rd edn. Butterworth, London, p. 157

30 Low Anterior Resection for Rectal Cancer

Indications

Low anterior resections are performed to treat malignant tumors of the middle and upper thirds of the rectum, 6–14 cm from the anal verge.

Preoperative Preparation

(See Chap. 25.)

Pitfalls and Danger Points

- Anastomotic failure
- Presacral hemorrhage
- Trauma to rectal stump during presacral dissection
- Ureteral damage

Operative Strategy

Prevention of Anastomotic Complications

When a high anterior resection is performed in conjunction with an intraperitoneal colorectal anastomosis, the incidence of postoperative complications of the anastomosis is minimal. On the other hand, a low anterior resection with a colorectal anastomosis below the peritoneal reflection reportedly is followed by *clinical* leakage rates of 10.4% (Schrock et al.) and 27% (Goligher et al.). When Goligher et al. tested the low anastomosis radiographically by performing a Hypaque enema on the 14th postoperative day, they found a leakage rate of 69%.

The numerous factors that contribute to anastomotic failure are discussed in Chap. 25. For several reasons, the low colorectal anastomosis offers additional difficulty.

1) *Anatomical exposure is often difficult.* This is especially true of males whose pelvis is narrow and of obese patients. Consequently, it is easy to make small tears in the rectum when inserting sutures, especially as the difficulty in exposure often requires the surgeon's hand to be held at an awkward angle.

2) Due to the lack of serosal cover over the retroperitoneal rectum, *it is very easy to mistake mucosa for the muscular layer.* If sutures are erroneously inserted into the mucosal instead of the submucosal-muscular layers, the anastomosis will leak because the mucosa itself possesses little tensile strength. Identify the longitudinal muscle covering the rectum and be sure to incorporate this layer in the suture line!

3) The *diameter of the rectal ampulla frequently measures in excess of 5–6 cm,* while the lumen of the proximal colon, after proper bowel preparation, is often half this size. The anastomotic technique used must be capable of correcting this disparity.

4) When the surgeon has not achieved perfect hemostasis in the pelvis, the *presacral space frequently becomes the site of a postoperative hematoma* that becomes infected and develops into an abscess. This abscess may erode through the colorectal suture line.

5) If the pelvic peritoneal floor is closed above the colorectal anastomosis, dead space may surround the anastomosis. This is especially conducive to leakage in the anastomosis.

We have virtually eliminated leakage by adopting the side-to-end colorectal technique of anastomosis advocated by Baker, and by Zollinger and Sheppard. This permits the anastomosis to be exactly equal in diameter to the lumen of the commodious rectal ampulla. Healthy-sized bites of tissue may be enclosed in the sutures without any danger that postoperative stenosis will result. In effect, at the conclusion of the anastomosis, *the rectal ampulla has been invaginated into the side of the proximal colon* (see Fig. 30–21). Placing the anastomosis within 1 cm of the closed end of proximal colon, eliminates the danger the patient will develop a blind-loop syndrome.

Following a low anastomosis we routinely insert one or two multiperforated plastic tubes for closed-suction drainage into the presacral space. Six millimeter diameter Jackson-Pratt Silastic tubes are brought out retroperitoneally through puncture wounds in the left lower quadrant or the perineum and are attached to a sterile, closed plastic container for continuous suction. To help prevent an infected hematoma from developing in the pelvis, 50 mg of kanamycin in 50 ml of sterile saline is injected through the suction catheters every 6 hours for 5 days.

The peritoneal pelvic floor is not resutured after the colorectal anastomosis is completed.

Some authorities believe that wrapping an anastomosis with omentum is important to prevent leakage. While we use this technique when the omentum is easily available, we do not perform complex omental-lengthening maneuvers to accomplish an omental wrap. A properly constructed anastomosis does not require the contiguity of the omentum to heal without leaking.

The data are still insufficient to determine the complication rate following performance of an EEA stapled colorectal anastomosis. However, our preliminary results appear to be *highly promising.* We have used this technique successfully to resect malignant tumors including a 4 cm distal margin and located as low as 6 cm from the anal verge. Because the EEA technique simplifies and accelerates an otherwise difficult anastomosis, it is particularly suitable for the aged patient suffering from a serious systemic disease, but it has many technical pitfalls that must be avoided.

Extent of Lymphovascular Dissection

Goligher (1975) advocated the routine ligation of the inferior mesentery artery at the aorta not only for lesions of the descending colon but for rectal cancer also. When this is done, the entire blood supply of the proximal colon must come through the marginal artery all the way from the middle colic artery. Although this proves adequate in the majority of patients, there is a danger that the surgeon may not recognize those patients whose blood supply is not quite sufficient.

We believe the risk of this occurring is greater than the benefits that may accrue to the patient by routinely amputating the extra 3 cm of inferior mesenteric artery. It is important that the blood supply to the proximal colon undergoing anastomosis not only be adequate but be optimal before this segment is used in a low colorectal anastomosis. Consequently, in the usual case of rectal cancer we transect the inferior mesenteric artery just distal to the origin of the left colic vessel (see Fig. 26–6). Even if only the ascending branch of the left colic is preserved, there usually is vigorous arterial pulsation in the mesentery of the descending colon. For obese patients, transillumination of the mesentery is helpful in identifying the junction between the inferior mesenteric and left colic arteries.

If the inferior mesenteric artery is ligated proximal to the take-off of the left colic artery, be sure always to liberate the splenic flexure and resect the majority of the descending colon unless it can be proven that the circulation through the marginal artery at a lower level is vigorous. This can be accomplished only by demonstrating pulsatile flow from a cut arterial branch at the proposed site of the transection of the colon. *Poor blood flow leads to poor healing.*

In the usual rectal cancer case the sigmoid colon is removed and the descending colon is used for anastomosis. This generally requires the liberation of the splenic flexure, which can be accomplished in a few minutes once the surgeon has mastered the technique.

Goligher et al. (1970) found that 51% of the patients in their series of 73 anterior resections (both high and low) experienced postoperative leakage, as determined by radiological examination. In 62 consecutive colorectal anastomoses following anterior resection done under our supervision at Booth Memorial Hospital in accordance with the principles outlined in this chapter, only two leaks were detected radiographically when routine Hypaque enema X rays were done in each case on the tenth postoperative day.

Indications for Complementary Colostomy

When there is difficulty in constructing a low colorectal anastomosis and it is likely the surgeon has created a less-than-perfect anastomosis, a complementary right transverse colostomy should be constructed. If this is immediately matured by suturing the mucosa to the subcuticular layer of the skin, it is possible to close the colostomy about 2 weeks after the tumor has been resected if a barium colon enema shows a normal anastomosis. Thus, closure of the colostomy can be accomplished during the same hospital admission as the anterior resection.

Presacral Dissection: Prevention of Hemorrhage

Contrary to what apparently is a widely held perception, radical cancer surgery does *not* require stripping the tissues off the sacrum down to the periosteum. The dissection of the perirectal tissues proximal to the carcinoma is necessary for the removal of *tumor emboli* within the lymph nodes and lympathic channels. If tumor has invaded widely into the mesorectum and presacral tissues, the lesion is generally beyond cure by radical surgery.

There is a network of veins lying on the presacral periosteum that drain into the sacral foramina (see Fig. 30–6b). When these are torn by blunt dissection, clamping or ligation, to control the hemorrhage that results, often is impossible, since the torn vessel retracts into the foramen. The massive venous hemorrhage that can follow may not be stemmed even by ligating the hypogastric arteries. Most intraoperative fatalities during total proctectomy are caused by this type of presacral venous hemorrhage.

If the surgeon cannot very quickly control lacerated presacral veins with a hemostat or bone wax, the bleeding area should be covered with a sheet of Surgicel over which a large gauze pack should be placed, filling the sacral hollow. This almost always controls the hemorrhage.

Unless the presacral vessels are directly invaded by a bulky tumor of the midrectum, massive presacral venous hemorrhage is entirely preventable. Blunt hand dissection of the presacral space is not a desirable technique. The surgeon's hand does not belong in this area until scissors dissection under direct vision has freed all the perirectal tissues from any posterior attachments to the sacrum. This should be done with a long Metzenbaum scissors, combined with gentle upward traction on the rectum. As the scissors are inserted on each side of the midline, the perirectal tissues can easily be lifted in an anterior direction *without removing the thin layer of endopelvic fascia that covers the presacral veins.* When the presacral dissection stays in the proper plane, the presacral veins are hidden from view by this layer of fascia, as Fig. 30–6a shows. Occasionally, branches of the middle sacral vessels enter the perirectal tissues from behind. These may be divided between Hemoclips.

This dissection is easily continued down to the area of the coccyx, where the fascia of Waldeyer becomes somewhat dense as it goes from the anterior surfaces of the coccyx and sacrum to attach to the lower rectum (see Fig. 30–8). Attempts to penetrate this fascia by blunt finger dissection may rupture the rectum rather than the fascia, which is strong. This layer must be incised sharply with a scissors or scalpel, after which one can see the levator diaphragm. When the posterior dissection has for the most part been completed, only *then* should the surgeon's hand enter the presacral space to sweep the dissection toward the lateral pelvic walls. This maneuver helps define the lateral ligaments. The dissection should be bloodless.

Other points of hemorrhage in the pelvic dissection may occur on the lateral walls. These can usually be readily identified and occluded by ligature or Hemoclips. Close attention should also be paid to the left iliac vein, which may be injured in the course of the dissection. As most serious bleeding in pelvic dissections is of venous origin, ligation of the hypogastric arteries is rarely indicated.

Presacral Dissection: Preservation of Hypogastric Nerves

As the rectum is elevated from the presacral space and the anterior surface of the aorta cleared of areolar and lymphovascular tissue, a varying number of preaortic sympathetic nerves of the superior hypogastric plexus can be identified. These are the contribution of the sympathetic nervous system to the bilateral inferior hypogastric (pelvic) plexuses. In males their preservation is necessary for normal ejaculation. After they cross the region of the aortic bifurcation and sacral promontory, they coalesce into two major nerve bundles, called the hypogastric nerves. Each nerve, which may have 1–3 strands, runs toward the posterolateral wall of the pelvis in the vicinity of the hypogastric artery (see Figs. 30–2c and 30–4). We agree with Goligher (1975) that in most malignancies of the distal rectum, these nerves can be preserved without compromising the patient's chances of cure.

After the inferior mesenteric artery and vein are divided and the lymphovascular tissues elevated from the bifurcation of the aorta by blunt dissection, the sympathetic nerves remain closely attached to the aorta and need not be damaged if the dissection is gently performed. At the promontory of the sacrum, if the rectum is dissected as described above, the right and left hypogastric nerves can be seen posterior to the plane of dissection and can be preserved—provided there is a sufficient distance separating them from the tumor. There also seems to be a diminution in the incidence of bladder dysfunction after nerve preservation.

Ureteral Dissection

To prevent damage to the ureters, these delicate structures must be identified and traced well down into the pelvis. The normal ureter crosses the common iliac artery at the point this structure bifurcates into its external and internal branches. Because the ureter and a leaf of incised peritoneum are often displaced during the course of dissection, if the ureter is not located in its usual position the undersurfaces of both the lateral and medial leaves of peritoneum should be inspected. The identity of the ureter can be confirmed if pinching or touching the structure with a forceps results in typical peristaltic waves. If doubt exists, the anesthesiologist may be instructed to inject indigo carmine dye intravenously; this stains the ureter blue, unless the patient is oliguric at the time of injection. The ureter should be traced into the pelvis beyond the point at which the lateral ligaments of the rectum are divided.

Operative Technique

Incision and Position

Patients who have lesions within 14 cm of the anal verge should be placed in the same modified lithotomy position, utilizing Lloyd-Davies leg rests, as is described in Chap. 31 for the abdominal-perineal proctectomy (**Figs. 30–1a and 30–1b**). The second assistant should stand between the patient's abducted thighs for the pelvic portion of the operation while the surgeon works from the patient's left. Using this position, the surgeon may judge, after the tumor is mobilized, whether the patient is suitable for an anterior anastomosis, abdominal-perineal proctectomy, or end-to-end anastomosis with the EEA stapling device. All these techniques are best done with the patient in this position. The only operation that cannot be done in this position is the abdominosacral resection and anastomosis. If the surgeon elects to perform the latter procedure, the abdominal part of the operation should be completed first, the abdominal incision closed, and the patient turned to the prone position for the posterior Kraske incision and anastomosis.

For the anterior resection, a midline incision is preferable, extending from a point about 6 cm below the xiphoid process down to the pubis.

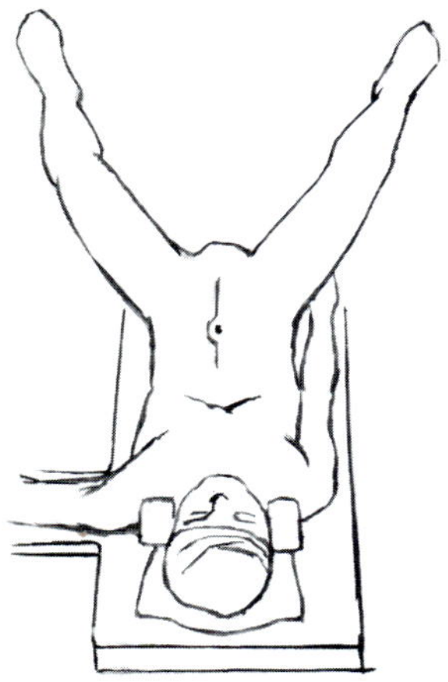

Fig. 30–1a

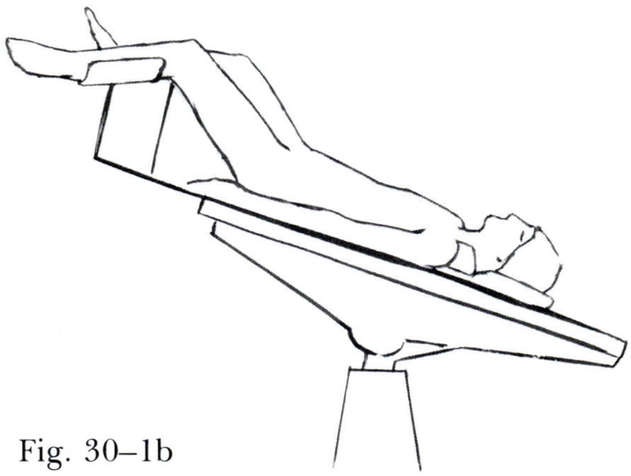

Fig. 30–1b

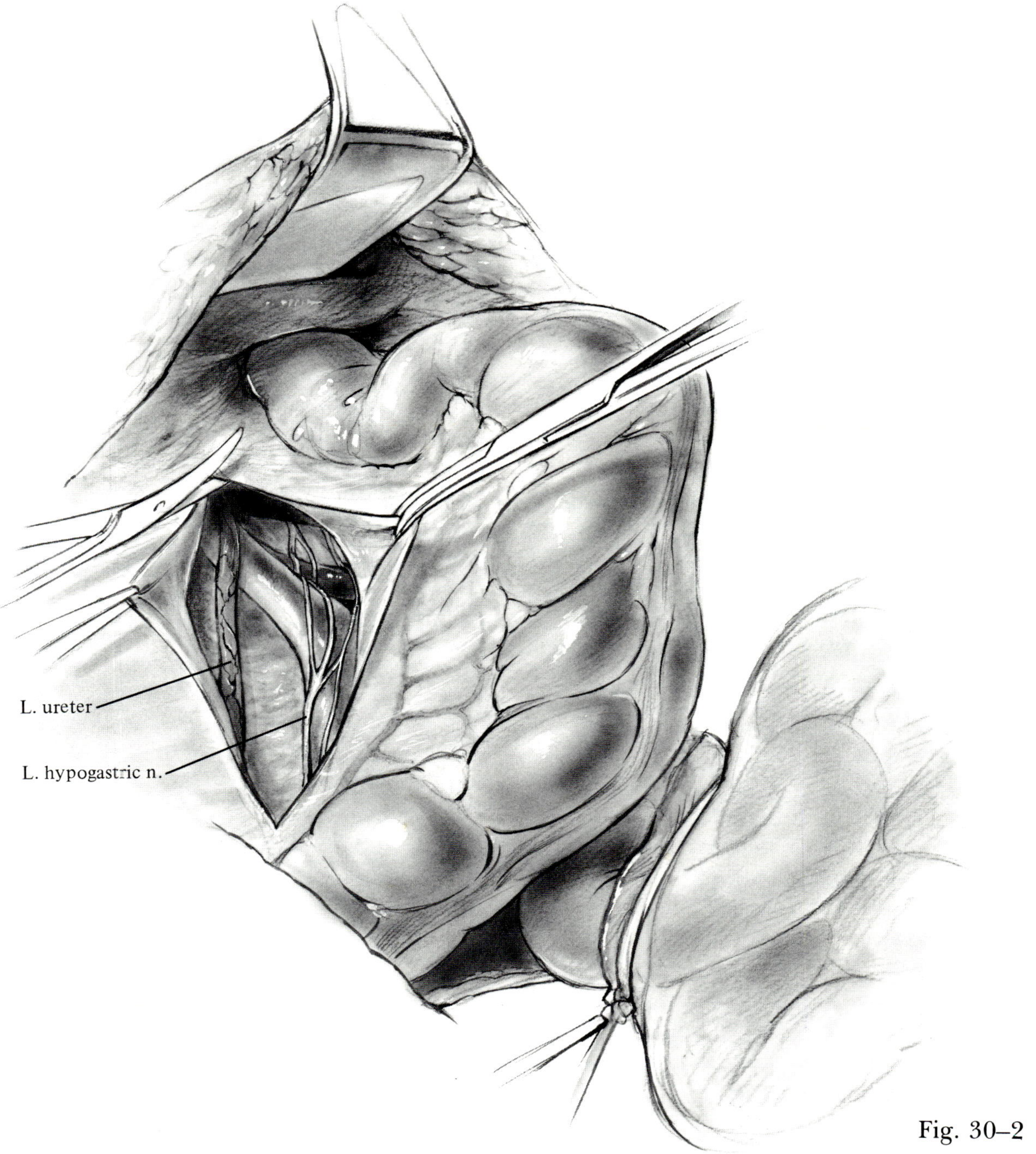

Fig. 30–2

Exploration and Evisceration of Small Bowel

Palpate and inspect the liver. A moderate amount of metastasis is not a contraindication to a conservative version of the anterior resection. Explore the remainder of the abdomen and then eviscerate the small bowel into a Vi-Drape plastic intestinal bag.

Mobilization of Sigmoid

Expose the left lateral peritoneal gutter. Occlude the lumen of the colon by ligating the distal sigmoid with umbilical tape. By drawing the sigmoid colon medially, several congenital attachments between the mesocolon and the posterolateral parietal peritoneum can be divided with a scissors (**Fig. 30–2**). Extend the incision in the peritoneum cephalad as far as the splenic flexure.

Identify the left ureter and tag it with a Vesseloop for later identification.

Use a scissors to continue the peritoneal incision along the left side of the rectum down to the rectovesical pouch. Identify the course of the ureter well down into the pelvis. Now retract the sigmoid to the patient's left and make an incision on the right side of the sigmoid mesocolon. The incision should begin at a point overlying the bifurcation of the aorta and should continue in a caudal direction along the line where the mesosigmoid meets the right lateral leaf of peritoneum in the presacral space. After the right ureter has been identified, carry the incision down toward the rectovesical pouch (**Figs. 30–3 and 30–4**).

If exposure is convenient, incise the peritoneum of the rectovesical pouch, or rectouterine pouch in the female (Fig. 30–3). If exposure is not convenient, this step should be delayed until the presacral dissection has elevated the rectum sufficiently to bring the rectovesical pouch easily to the field of vision.

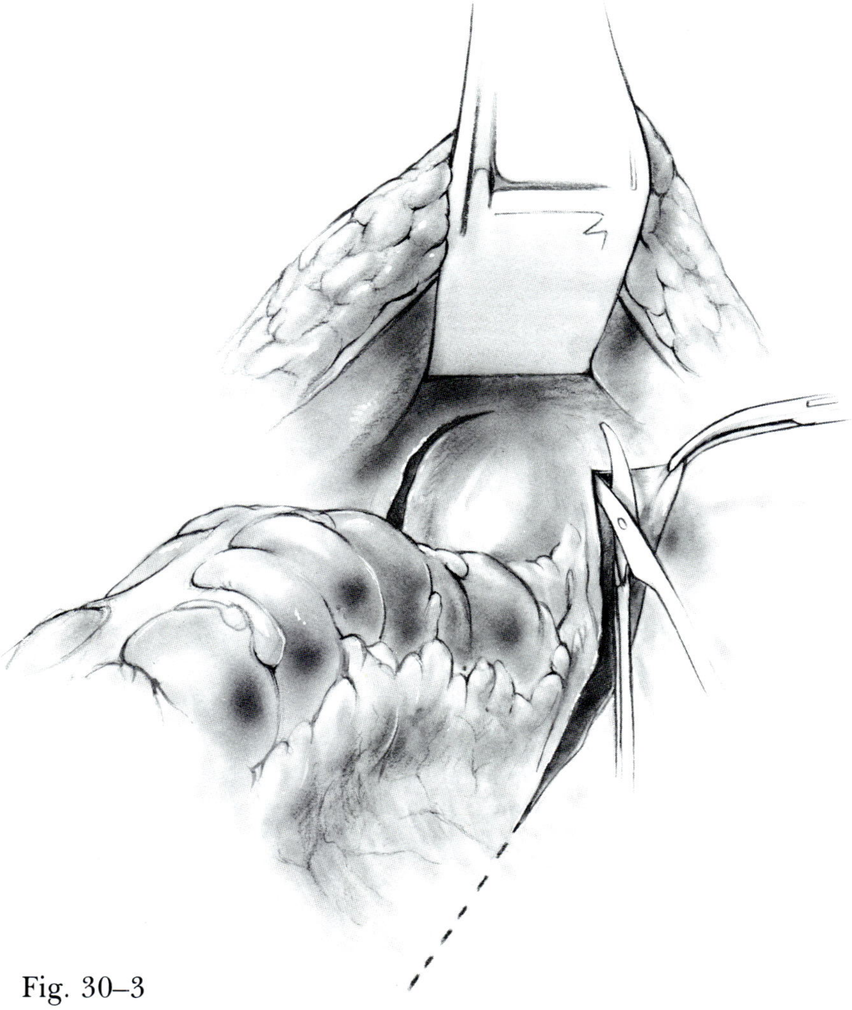

Fig. 30–3

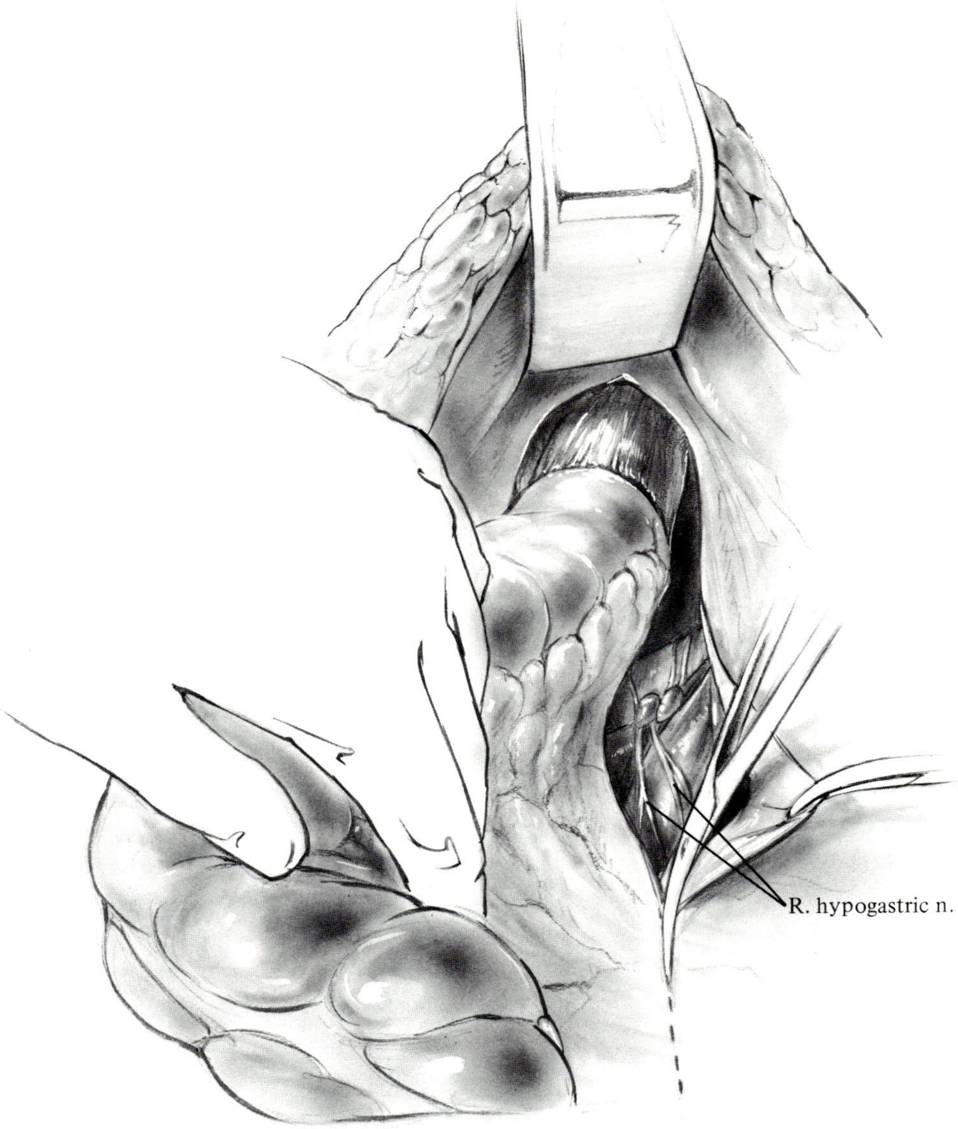

Fig. 30–4

Lymphovascular Dissection

Apply skyward traction to the colon, gently separate the gonadal vein from the lateral leaf of the mesocolon, and allow it to fall to the posterior. Insert an index finger between the deep margin of the mesosigmoid and the bifurcation of the aorta to feel the pulsation of the inferior mesenteric artery lying superficial to the finger. In patients who are markedly obese, this vessel may be divided and ligated at the level of the aortic bifurcation without further dissection. In most patients, however, it is quite simple to incise the peritoneum overlying the origin of the inferior mesenteric artery, and to sweep the areolar and lymphatic tissue downward until one sees the point at which the inferior mesenteric artery gives off the left colic branch (Fig. 30–5).

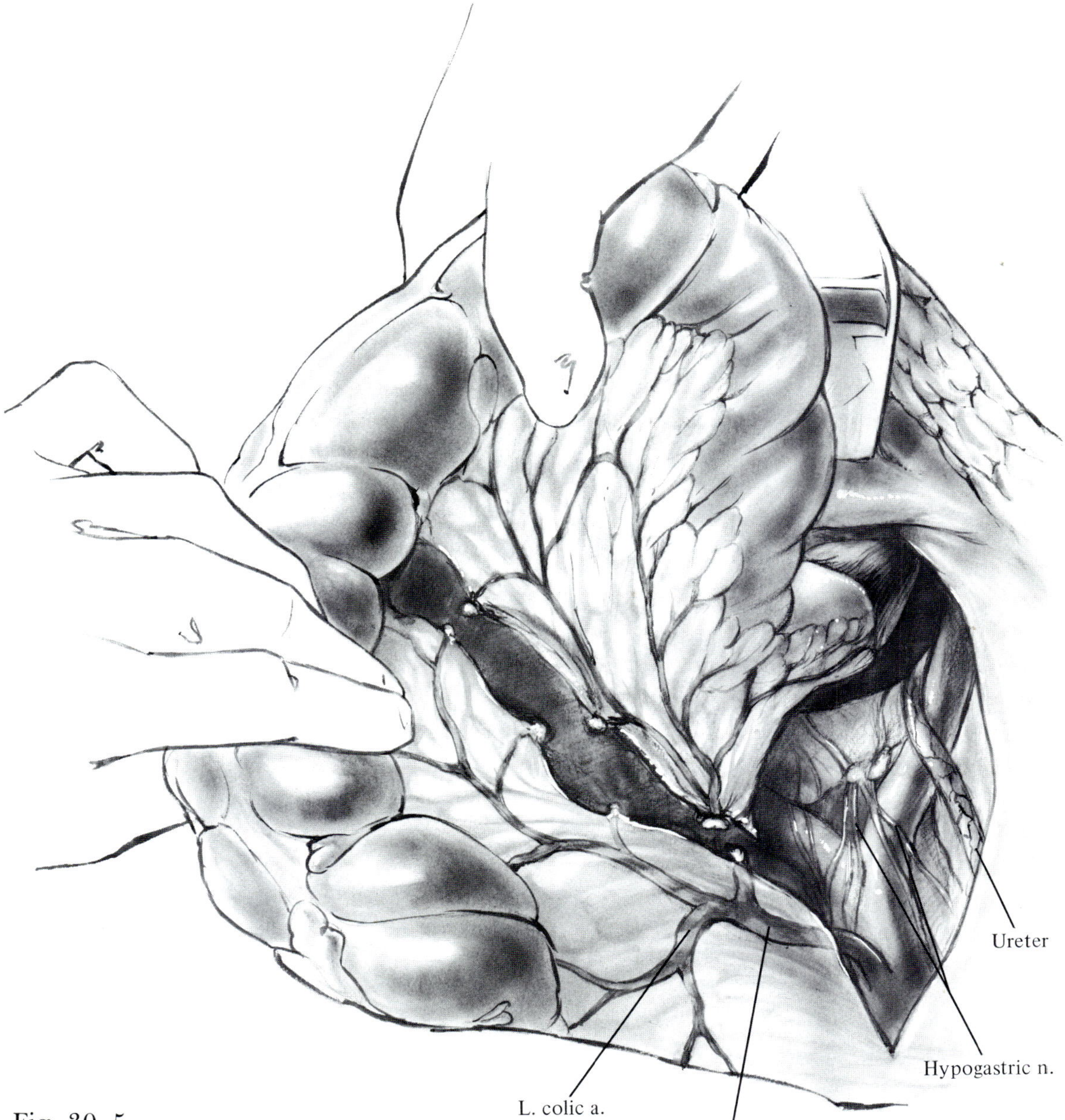

Fig. 30–5

In routine cases divide the inferior mesenteric vessels between 2–0 ligatures just distal to this junction. Then make a superficial scalpel incision along the surface of the mesocolon: begin at the point where the inferior mesenteric vessels were divided and continue to the descending colon or upper sigmoid. Complete the division of the mesentery along this line by dividing it between serially applied Kelly hemostats and then ligating with 2–0 cotton or PG (**Fig. 30–5**). In nonobese patients it is feasible to incise the peritoneum up to the point where a vessel is visualized and then to apply hemostats directly to each vessel as it is encountered. With this technique, the surgeon will encounter only one or two vessels on the way to the marginal artery of the colon.

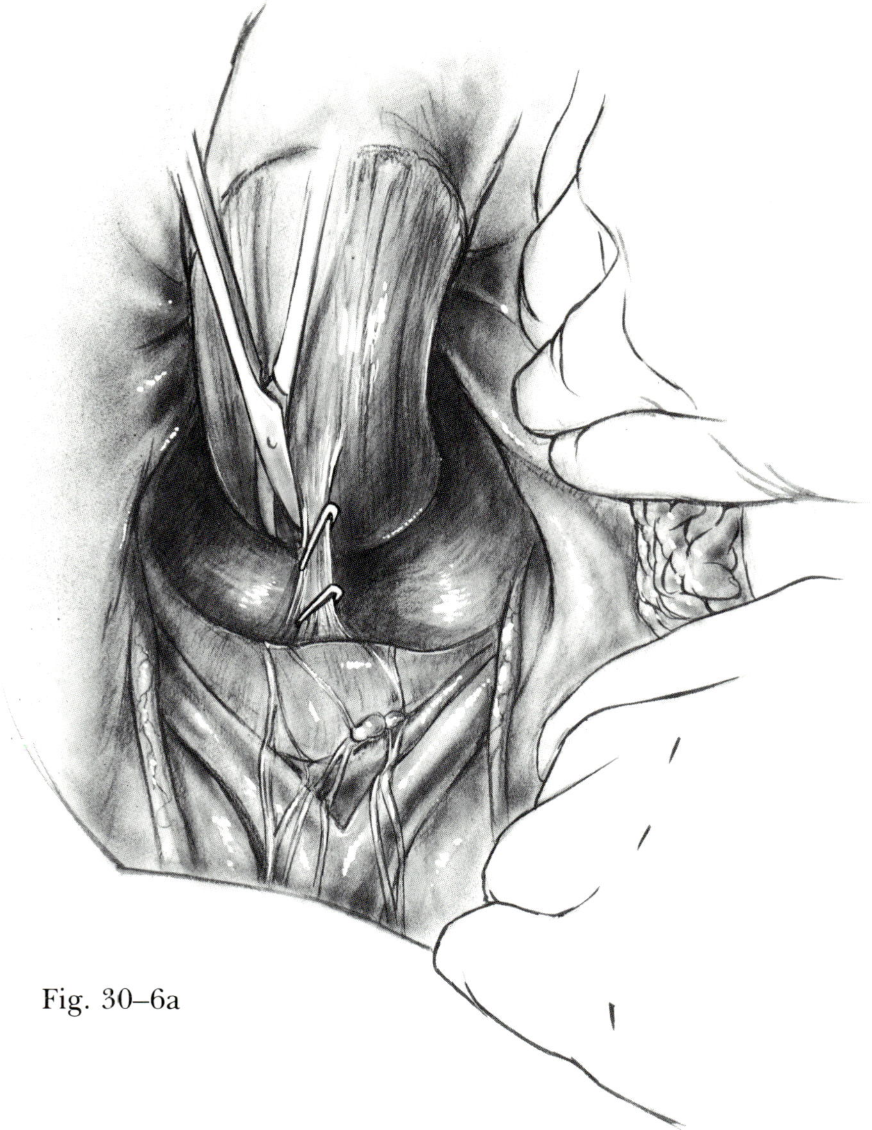

Fig. 30–6a

Sweep the mesosigmoid and the lymphovascular bundle distal to the ligated inferior mesenteric vessels off the anterior surfaces of the aorta and common iliac vessels by blunt dissection. Leave the preaortic sympathetic nerves intact. To minimize the time during which the patient's abdomen is exposed to possible fecal contamination, do not divide the descending colon at this stage.

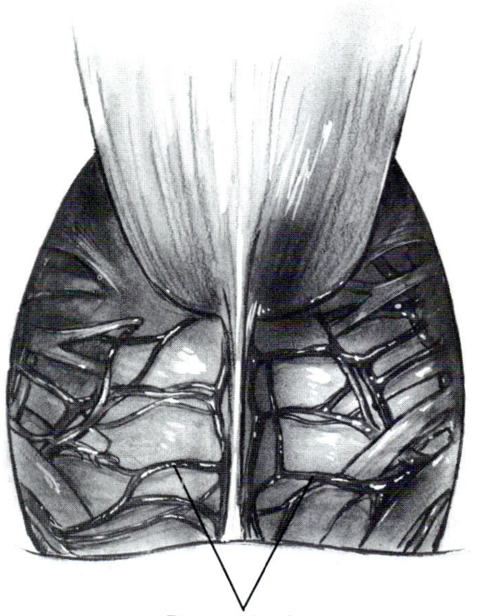

Fig. 30–6b

Presacral Dissection

With the lower sigmoid on steady upward retraction, it becomes evident that there is a band of tissue extending from the midsacral region to the posterior rectum and mesorectum. On either side of this dense band there is only areolar tissue. Any tendency on the part of the surgeon to insert a hand into the presacral space should be stoutly resisted. Instead, a long, closed Metzenbaum scissors should be used as a blunt dissector (Fig. 30–6a). Insert it first to the right of the midline behind the rectum, and by gently elevating the mesorectum the proper presacral plane will be entered. Repeat this maneuver identically on the left side of the midsacral line. Then direct attention to the remaining band of tissue, which contains branches of the middle sacral artery, and divide it with scissors after applying large Hemoclips (**Fig. 30–6a**).

At this time the surgeon will see a thin layer of fibroareolar tissue covering the sacrum. If a shiny layer of sacral periosteum, ligaments, or the naked presacral veins can be seen (**Fig. 30–6b**), the plane of dissection is *too deep*, presenting the danger of major venous hemorrhage.

Elevate the *distal* rectum from the lower sacrum with gauze in a sponge holder. If the dissection has been completed properly, as described, note that the preaortic sympathetic nerves divide into two major trunks in the upper sacral area and then continue laterally to the right and left walls of the pelvis (see Figs. 30–2 and 30–4). Gently dissect these nerves off the posterior wall of the specimen, unless the nerves have been invaded by tumor.

Now the surgeon may insert a hand into the presacral space, with the objective not of penetrating more deeply toward the coccyx, but rather of extending the presacral dissection laterally to the right and to the left, so that the posterior aspect of the specimen is elevated from the sacrum as far as the lateral ligaments on each side. Place the lateral ligament on the left side on stretch by applying traction to the rectum toward the right. Apply large Hemoclips and divide the ligament between them (**Fig. 30–7**). In some cases the ligament may be 2 cm or more in width, so that additional pairs of Hemoclips may be needed.

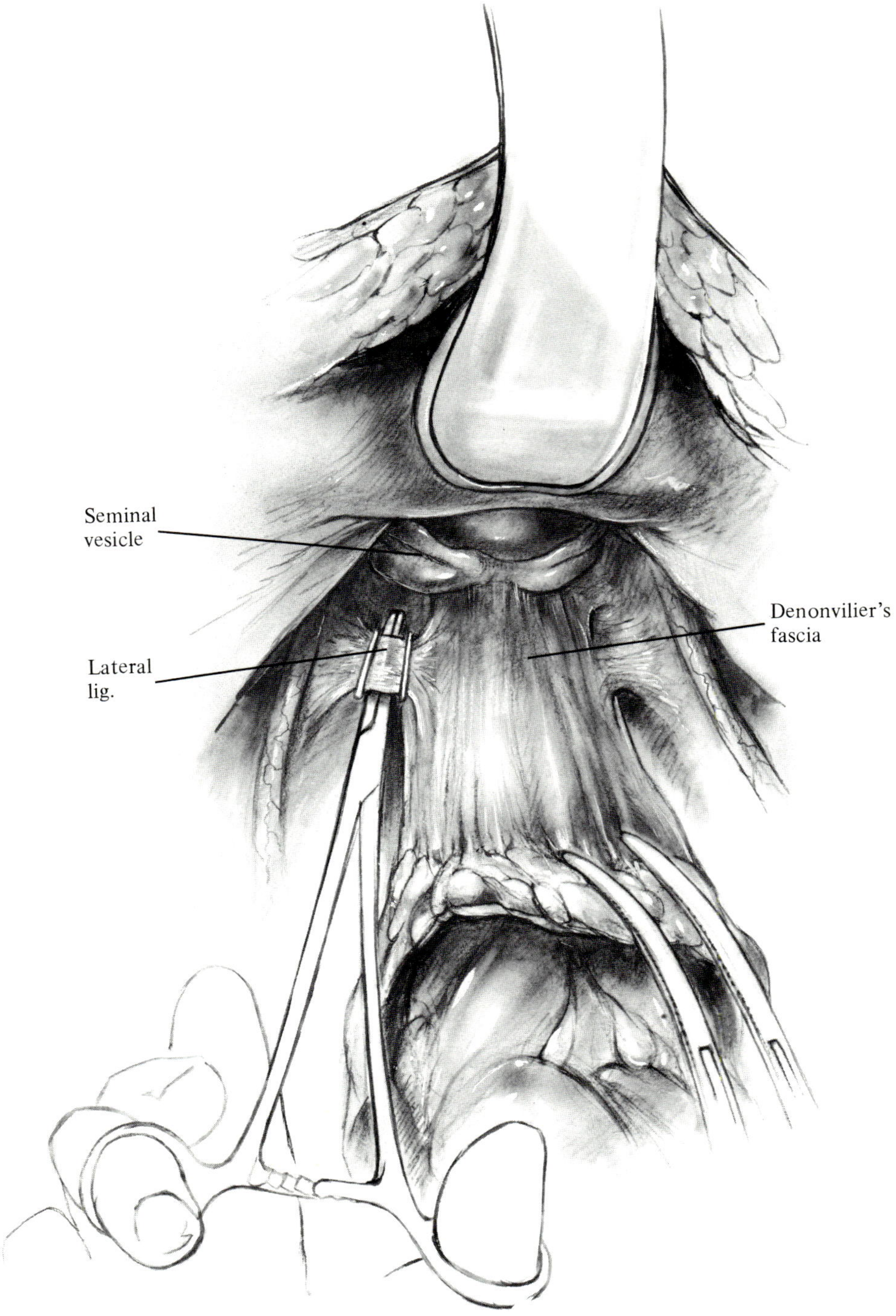

Fig. 30–7

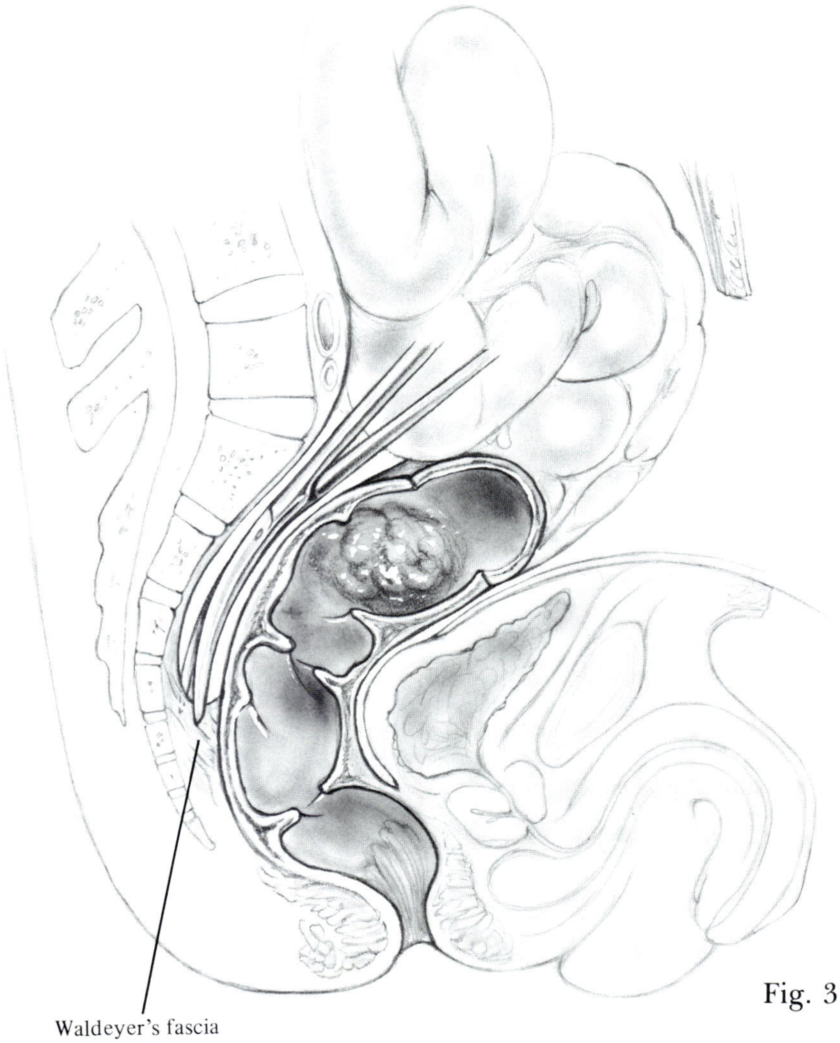

Fig. 30–8

Carry out a similar maneuver to divide the right lateral ligament. Before dividing each lateral ligament, recheck the position of the respective ureter and hypogastric nerve to be certain they lie lateral to the point of division. Then divide the fascia of Waldeyer, which extends from the coccyx to the posterior rectal wall (**Fig. 30–8**).

Now direct attention to the anterior dissection. Use a Lloyd-Davies bladder retractor to pull the bladder (in women, the uterus) in an anterior and caudal direction. If the peritoneum of the rectovesical pouch has not already been incised, per-

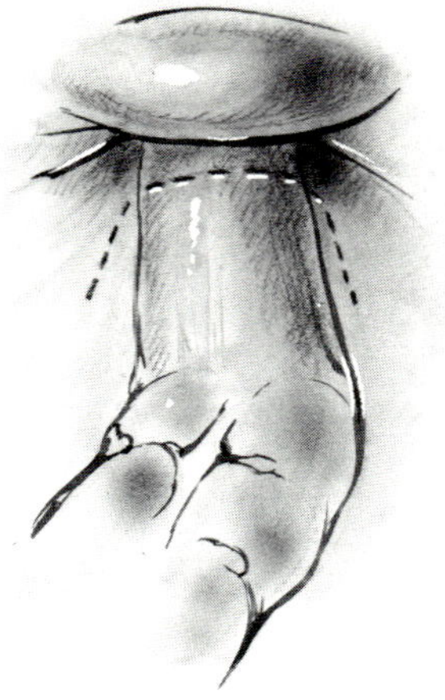

Fig. 30–9a

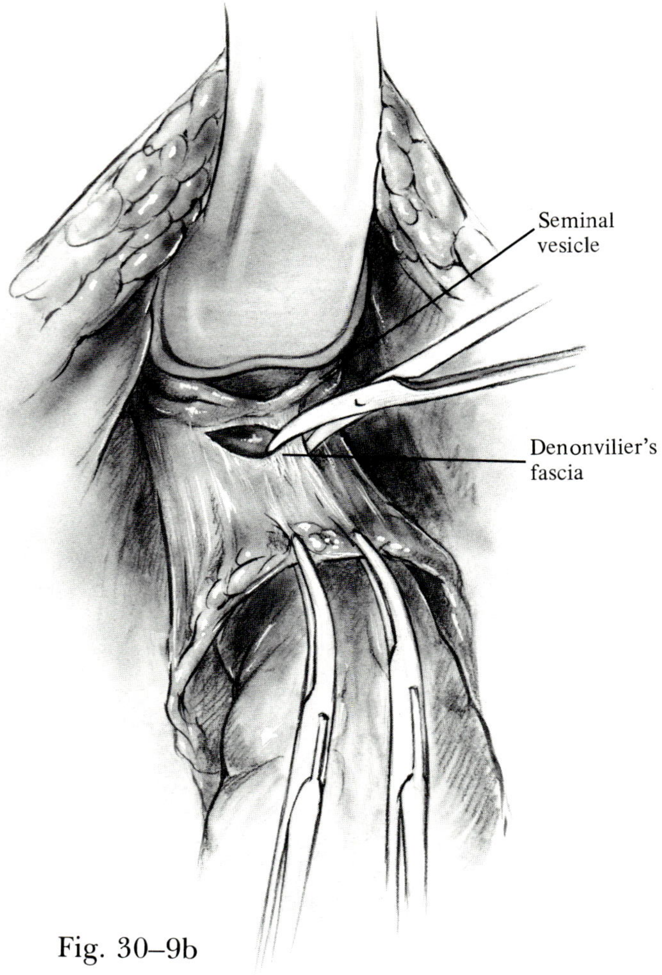

Fig. 30–9b

form this maneuver now, thereby connecting the incisions in the pelvic peritoneum previously made on the right and left sides of the rectum (**Fig. 30–9a**). Apply one or more long hemostats or forceps to the posterior lip of the incised peritoneum of the rectovesical pouch. Place traction on these hemostats to draw the peritoneum and Denonvillier's fascia in a cephalad and posterior direction, and use Metzenbaum scissors dissection to separate the rectum from the seminal vesicles and prostate (**Fig. 30–9b**). Use blunt finger dissection to further separate the rectum from the posterior wall of the prostate. Finally, secure hemostasis in this region by electrocoagulating multiple bleeding points.

In female patients the anterior dissection is somewhat simpler. With a Harrington retractor elevating the uterus, use scalpel dissection to initiate the plane of dissection separating the peritoneum and fascia of Denonvillier from the posterior lip of the cervix until the proximal vagina has been exposed. Some surgeons routinely perform bilateral salpingo-oophorectomy in women who have rectal and sigmoid cancer, because the ovaries are sometimes a site of metastatic deposit. Whether this step is of value has not been ascertained. We do not perform this maneuver in the absence of visible metastasis to the ovaries.

Pelvic Hemostasis

The entire pelvic dissection, if properly performed, should entail minimal blood loss. While Hemoclips may control clearly identified vessels along the lateral wall of the pelvis, they are rarely useful in the presacral area. Here the vessels consist of thin-walled veins, which are easily torn by metallic clips either at the time of application or during the act of sponging the area later.

Except in the case of a small, clearly defined bleeding point that can be held in a forceps, electrocoagulation may also be hazardous, as the coagulating tip may act as a scalpel and convert the bleeding point into a major venous laceration. Here a ball-tipped electrode is safer than those with sharp tips.

Almost invariably, presacral bleeding results from a tear in one of the veins that drain into a sacral foramen. When hemorrhage occurs, the area of bleeding should be covered by a sheet of oxidized cellulose (Surgicel) over which pressure is applied with a large gauze pack. Place omentum between the pack and the anastomosis. If the area of bleeding is only 1–2 cm in diameter, at a later stage in the operation an attempt may be made to remove the gauze pack, leaving the small patch of Surgicel. Alternatively, microfibrillar collagen (Avitene) may be used in this situation. Unless the Surgicel or Avitene produces complete hemostasis, replace the gauze pack in the presacral space and leave it there for 24–48 hours. Then remove it by relaparotomy under general anesthesia. If the pack is not removed within 24–48 hours, the risk of pelvic sepsis increases, and complementary colostomy should be performed.

Mobilization of Proximal Colon

If the previously selected point on the descending colon does not easily reach down into the pelvis, mobilize the remainder of the descending colon by incising first the peritoneum in the paracolic gutter and then the "renocolic" ligament. Liberate the entire splenic flexure according to the steps described in Chap. 28. By dividing the transverse branch of the left colic artery (see Fig. 30–1) and retaining the cephalad branch, considerable additional length may be obtained. Completely clear the fat and mesentery from a 1 cm width of serosa at the point selected for division of the descending colon.

Insertion of Wound Protector Drape

At this point insert the plastic ring drape into the abdominal incision to protect the subcutaneous panniculus from contamination.

Preparation of Rectal Stump

When the rectum is divided at a low level, the mesorectum is no longer a single pedicle traveling along the posterior surface of the rectum. Rather, it fans out into multiple branches. Select a point 4–5 cm distal to the lower border of the tumor and seek the plane between the muscularis of the rectum and the surrounding blood vessels. This plane can sometimes be palpated with the finger; at other times a large blunt-nosed hemostat can be insinuated into it.

Grasp the fat and vascular tissues in a series of hemostats. After dividing the tissue between hemostats, ligate each of them with 2–0 PG. Well-delineated longitudinal muscle fibers should now be visible all around the lower rectum at the site selected for the anastomosis. At this time place a large right-angle clamp across the entire lumen of the rectum below the tumor.

Irrigation of Rectal Stump

Insert a Foley catheter with a 5 ml bag into the rectum. Attach the catheter to plastic tubing so as to permit the intermittent inflow and drainage of 500 ml of sterile water. Other tumoricidal solutions such as 1:1,000 mercuric bichloride or 40% alcohol may be used at the surgeon's option. After the irrigation is completed and the rectum emptied, remove the catheter.

Selection of Technique for Anastomosis

The side-to-end suture technique should be elected if a low colorectal anastomosis is attempted where the suture line is below the peritoneal reflection. Alternatively, an EEA stapling device may be used. At higher levels, the techniques described in Chap. 28 are also suitable.

Side-to-End Low Colorectal Anastomosis (Baker)

Turn to the previously cleared area on the descending colon that will be used for the anastomosis. Apply a TA–55 stapler across this cleared area and fire the

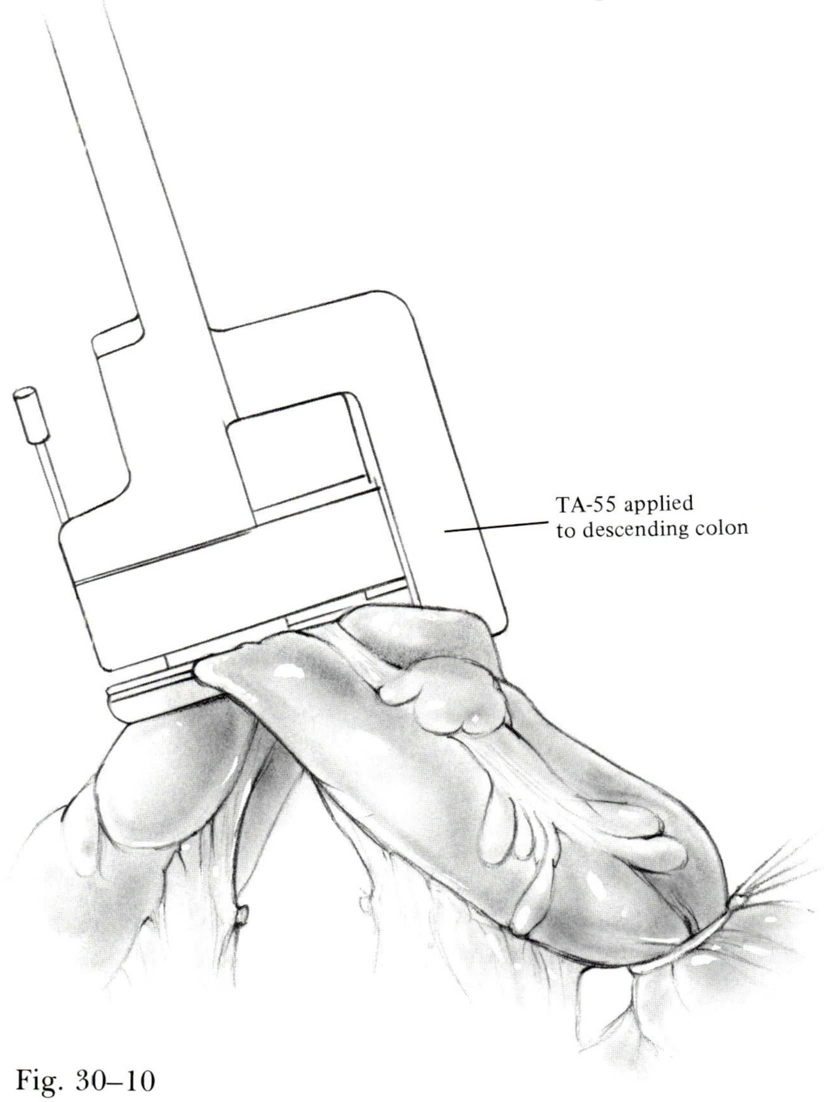

Fig. 30–10

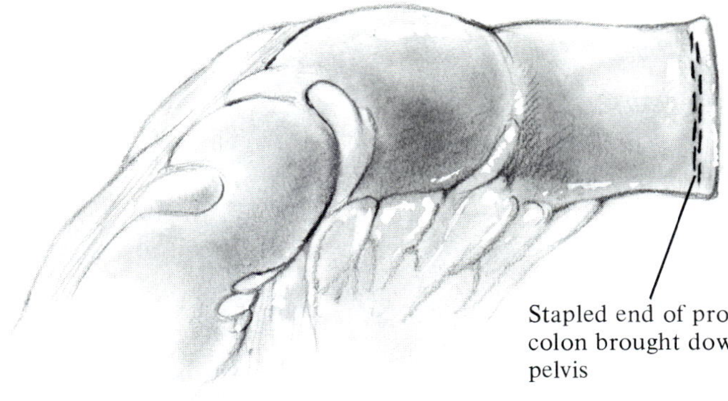

Fig. 30–11

staples (**Fig. 30–10**). Place an Allen clamp 1 cm distal to the TA–55 to occlude the specimen side. Divide the colon flush with the stapling device, using a scalpel, and lightly electrocoagulate the everted mucosa (**Fig. 30–11**). Ligate the specimen side with umbilical tape. After the Allen clamp is removed, apply a sterile rubber glove over the ligated end and tie the rubber glove in place with another umbilical tape ligature (**Figs. 30–12a and 30–12b**). Retain this segment of colon, containing the specimen, temporarily to provide traction on the rectal stump.

Bring the stapled end of the proximal colon down into the pelvis and line it up tentatively with the rectal stump 4–5 cm beyond the tumor. Place a scratch mark along the antimesenteric border of the descending colon beginning at a point 1 cm proximal to the stapled end and continuing cephalad for a distance equal to the diameter of the rectal stump.

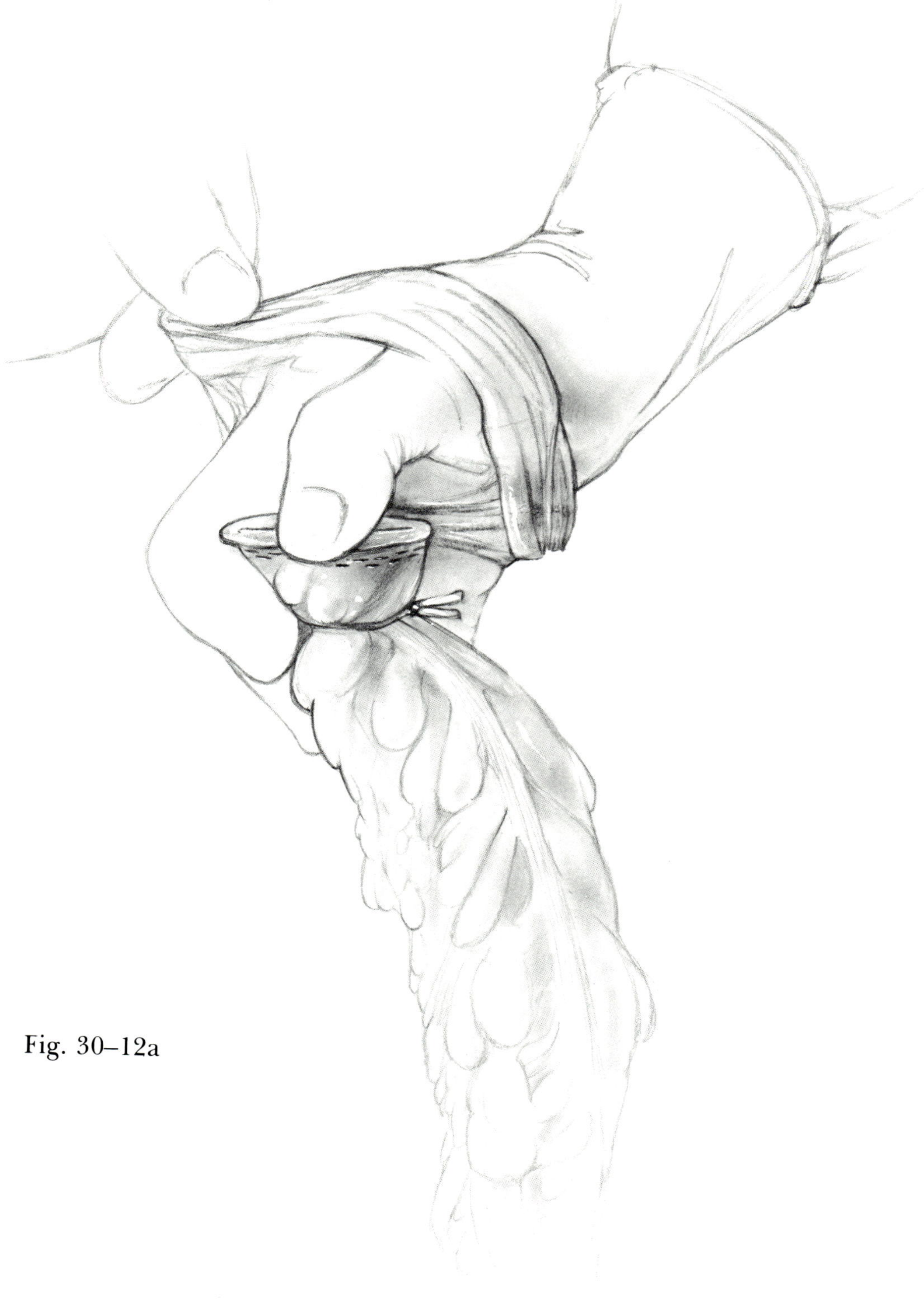

Fig. 30–12a

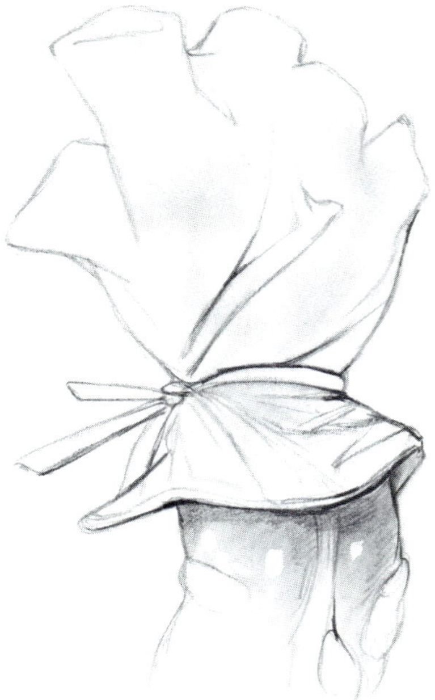

Fig. 30–12b

Now insert a lateral guy suture into the left lateral margin of the rectal stump and the proximal colon and hold this suture in a hemostat. Place a second guy suture in a similar fashion between the right lateral margin of the rectum and the colon and hold it in a hemostat too (**Fig. 30–13**).

Approximate the posterior muscular layer with interrupted 4–0 cotton Cushing sutures, taking bites, 5 mm wide, of colon and of rectum. Use a Stratte or a Finochietto angled needle-holder (see Glossary) when sewing deep in the pelvis—this will enhance the smooth insertion of the curved needle. Insert these sutures 6–7 mm behind the anticipated lines of tran-

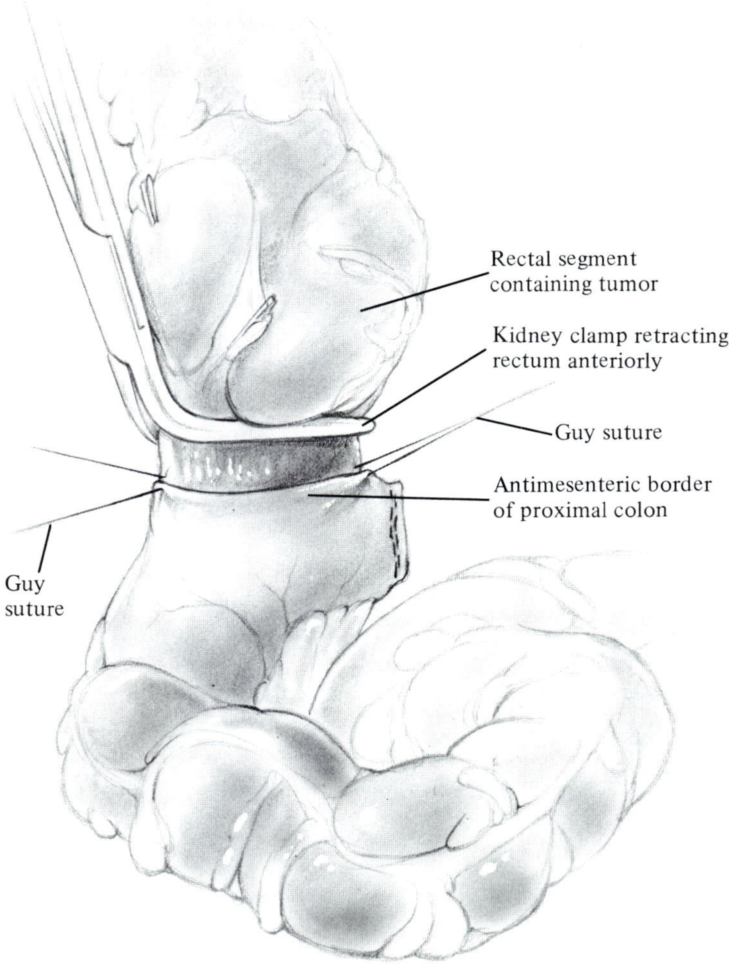

Fig. 30–13

section of the colon and rectum. The preferred technique is the one of successive bisection (**Figs. 30–14 and 30–15**). Tie none of these sutures until all have been placed. When the anastomosis is at a very low level, it is convenient to keep the proximal colonic segment well above the promontory of the sacrum until all the posterior seromuscular sutures have been inserted. Be sure that these stitches catch the longitudinal muscle of the rectum. If only mucosa is used for the anastomosis, failure is likely.

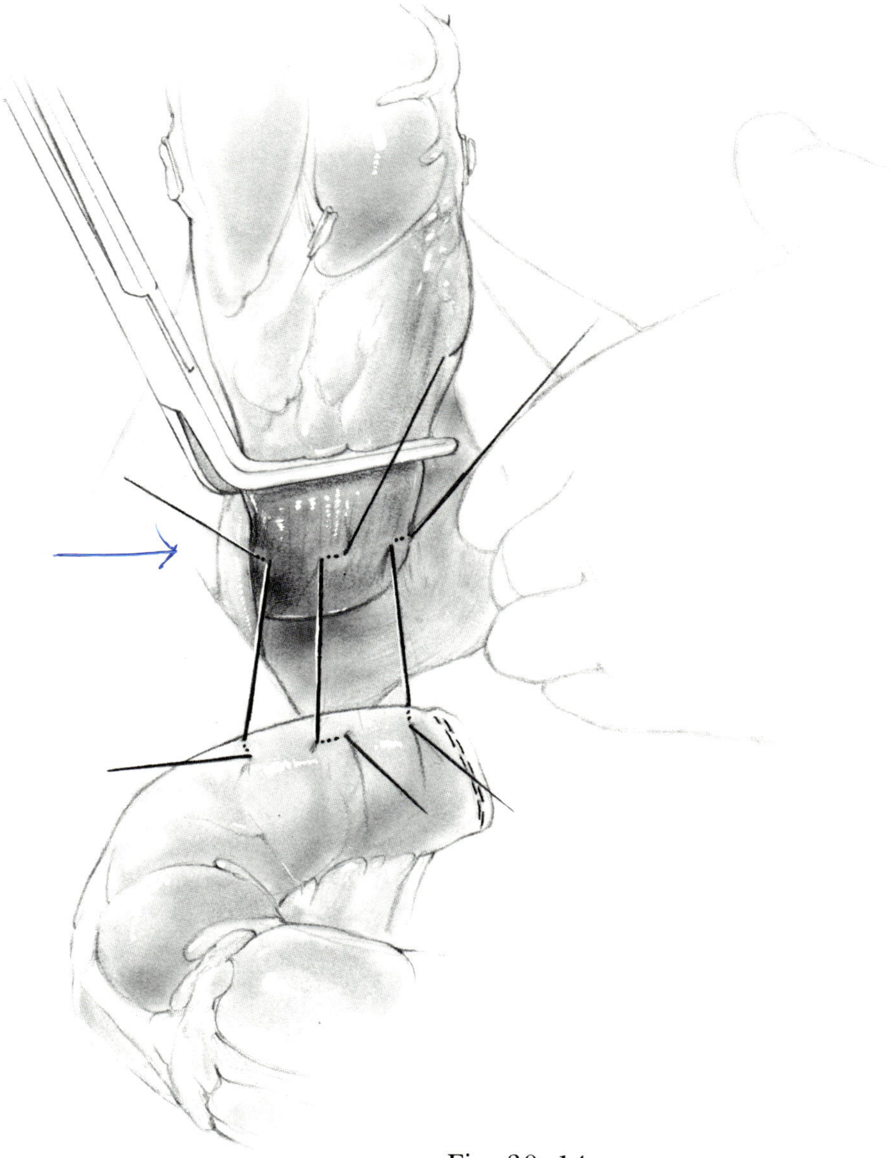

Fig. 30–14

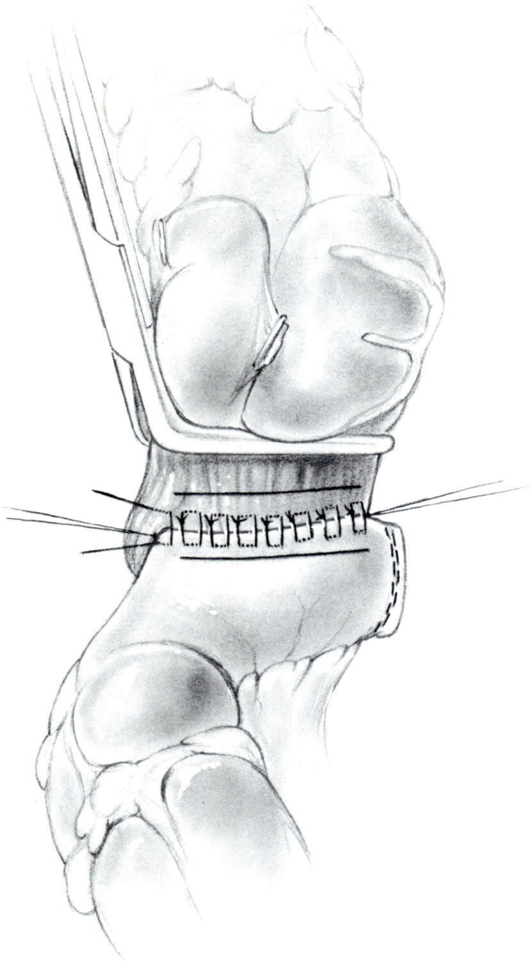

Fig. 30–15

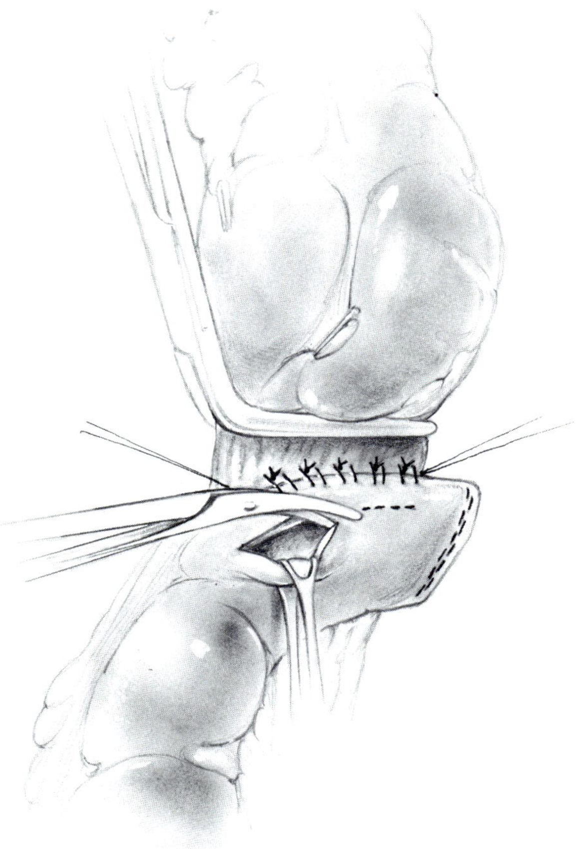

Fig. 30–16

Incise the previous scratch mark in the proximal colonic segment with a scalpel and a Metzenbaum scissors (**Fig. 30–16**). Make a similar incision along a line 6–7 mm proximal to the sutures already placed in the rectum.

If exposure is difficult, it is sometimes helpful to maintain gentle traction on the tails of the Cushing sutures to improve exposure while suturing the mucosa. Then cut the tails of the Cushing sutures successively as the mucosal sutures are inserted. Otherwise, cut all the Cushing sutures at one time, except for the two lateral guy sutures, which should be retained for the moment.

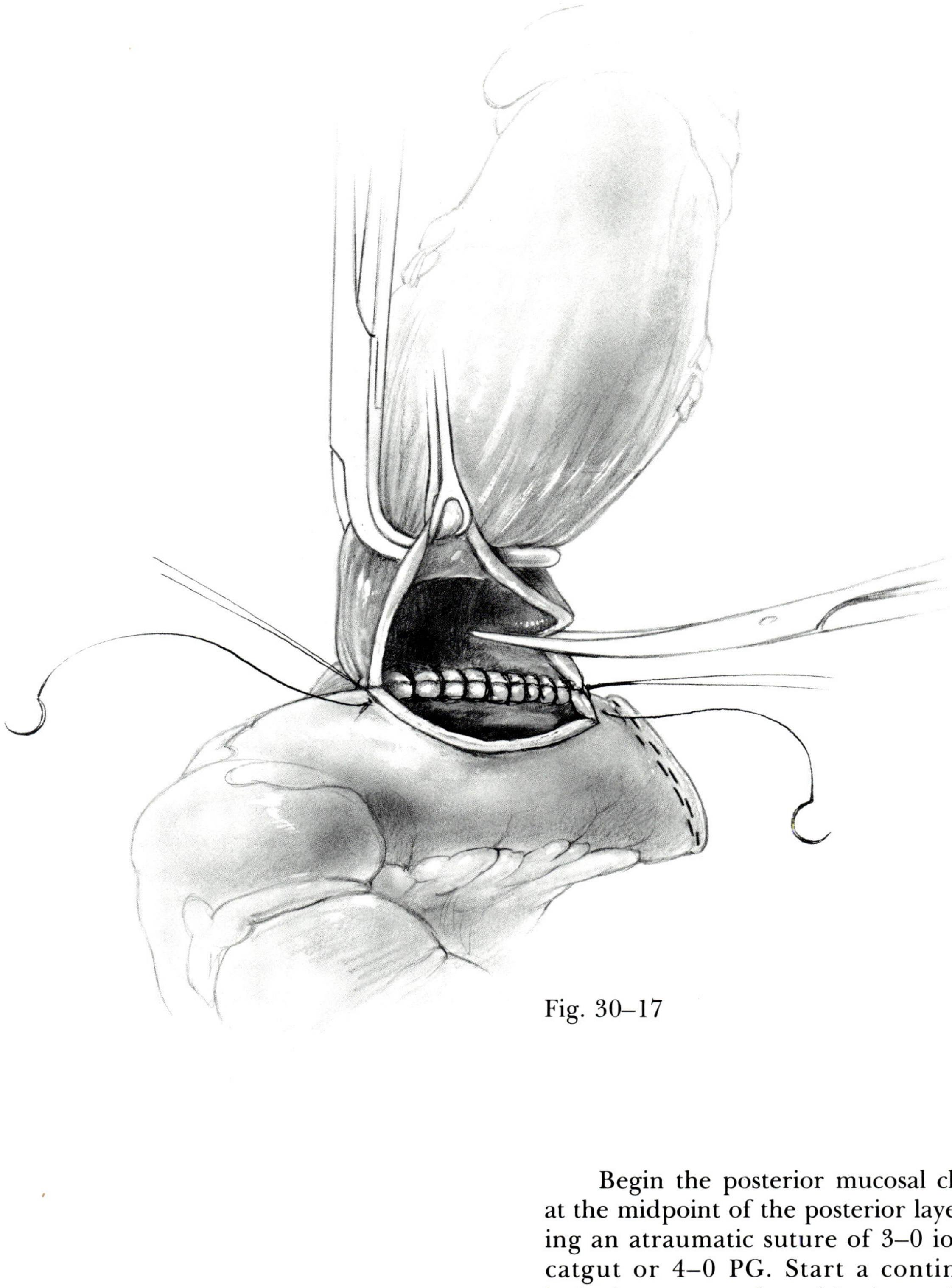

Fig. 30–17

Begin the posterior mucosal closure at the midpoint of the posterior layer, using an atraumatic suture of 3–0 iodized catgut or 4–0 PG. Start a continuous locked suture at the midpoint and continue it to the right lateral margin. The second suture of the same material should progress from the midpoint toward the left lateral margin of the suture line (**Fig. 30–17**).

Divide the anterior wall of the rectum just below the large right-angle clamp and remove the specimen. Request an immediate frozen-section histological examination of the distal margin of the specimen to rule out the presence of cancer. If tumor cells are found at the margin, resection of additional rectum is indicated.

Now approximate the anterior mucosal layer by a continuous suture of the Connell or Cushing type (**Fig. 30–18**). Accomplish this by grasping the needle, which has completed the posterior mucosal layer and is now in the lumen at the right margin of the anastomosis, and passing it from inside out through the rectum. The suture line should progress from the right lateral margin toward the midpoint of the anterior layer. When this has been reached, grasp the second needle, located at the left lateral margin of the posterior mucosal layer. Use this needle to complete the anterior mucosal layer from the left lateral margin to the midpoint where the anterior mucosal layer is terminated with the mucosa completely inverted (Fig. 30–18).

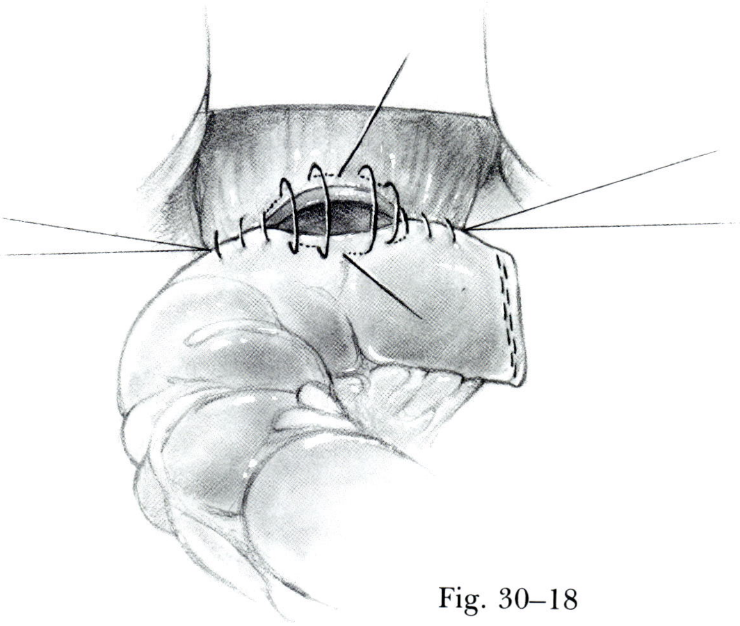

Fig. 30–18

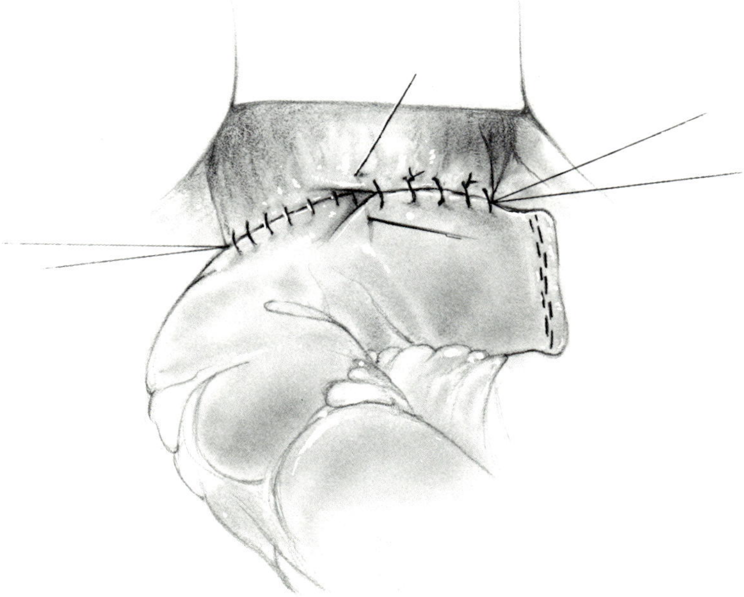

Fig. 30–19

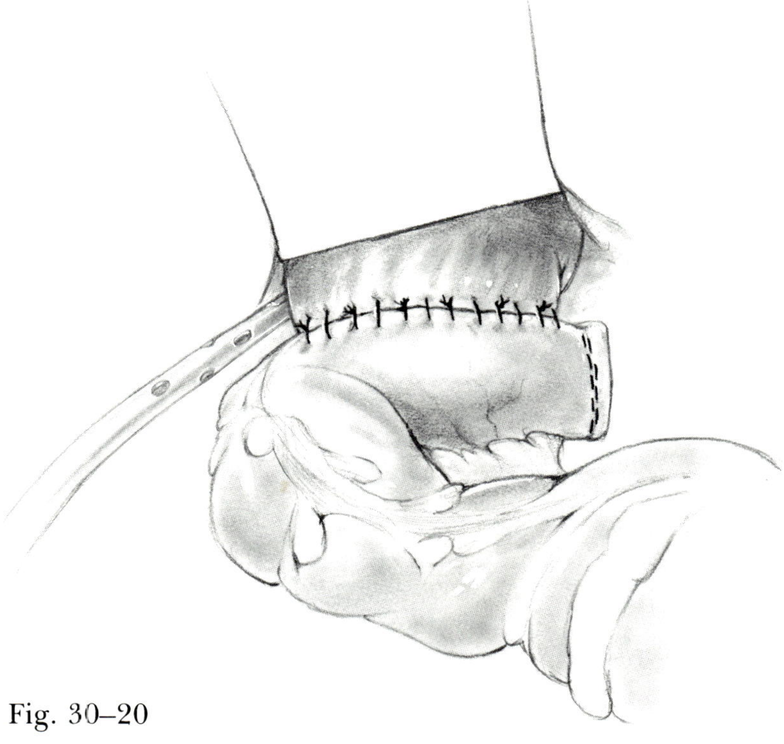

Fig. 30–20

Close the anterior muscular layer with interrupted 4–0 atraumatic cotton Lembert or Cushing sutures (**Figs. 30–19 and 30–20**). Insert this row of sutures about 6 mm away from the mucosal suture line to accomplish a certain amount of invagination of the rectum into the colon. Because the side-to-end lumen is large in dimension, narrowing will not result. A sagittal section of the anastomosis in **Fig. 30–21** illustrates this point. After the anastomosis is completed, carefully inspect the posterior suture line for possible defects, which can be corrected by additional sutures.

Fig. 30–21

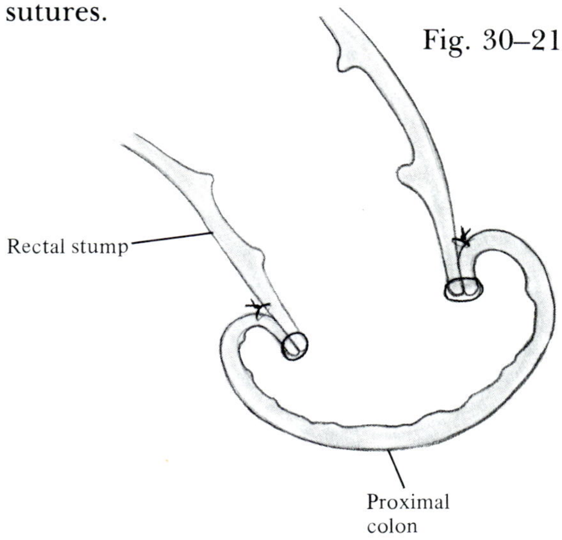

At this point cut the sutures and thoroughly irrigate the pelvis with a dilute solution of antibiotics.

The large defect in the preaortic peritoneum, which constitutes the medial aspect of the mesocolon, may be closed by a continuous suture of 2–0 PG on a fine curved needle. Carry this continuous suture down along the right side of the pelvis. Do not close the peritoneum anterior and to the left of the colorectal anastomosis. On many occasions, closure of the defect in the mesentery has been omitted. This omission has brought no noticeable ill effect, probably because the defect is so large as not to permanently entrap any small intestine. The lateral paracolic peritoneal defect should never be resutured.

Make a final check to ensure there is no tension on the colorectal suture line. If there is, additional proximal colon must be liberated. There must be sufficient slack so that the colon *fills up the hollow of the sacrum* on its way to the anastomosis, thus eliminating any dead space.

Alternative Method of Colorectal Side-to-End Anastomosis

When the surgeon does not find it practicable to leave the specimen attached to the rectal stump for purposes of traction, the preferred technique that is described above, then an alternative method may be used for the anastomosis.

After the first step in the Baker method (see Fig. 30–10) has been completed, remove the specimen by a scalpel incision across the rectum distal to the right-angle clamp. This leaves the rectal stump wide open. To prevent the short rectal stump from retracting beyond the prostate, apply long (30 cm) Allis clamps to the right and left corners of the rectal stump. Insert a Lloyd-Davies bladder retractor deep to the prostate for purposes of exposure.

Bring the previously prepared segment of descending colon down to the sacral promontory. The end of this segment of colon should have already been occluded by an application of the TA–55 stapling device. Make an incision on the antimesenteric border of the colon beginning 1 cm from the stapled end and continuing proximally for 4–5 cm, which is the approximate diameter of the rectal ampulla.

Insert a guy suture of atraumatic 4–0 cotton from the left lateral wall of the rectal stump to the termination of the incision in the colon. Grasp this suture in a hemostat without tying it. Place a similar suture in the right lateral walls of the rectal stump and colon.

Close the remainder of the posterior wall with interrupted horizontal mattress sutures of atraumatic 4–0 cotton. Place the first suture at the midpoint of the posterior layer. Using a curved needle, begin the stitch on the mucosal side of the proximal colon and go from inside out through all the layers of colon. Then pass the needle from outside in into the rectal stump. It is vitally important that the muscularis of the rectum be included in this bite. Often the muscularis retracts 1 cm or more beyond the protruding rectal mucosa.

Bring the same needle back from inside out on the rectal stump and then from outside in on the proximal colon. Leave this suture untied but grasp it in a hemostat. When it is tied at a later stage in the procedure, the knot will lie on the mucosa of the colon.

Place the second horizontal mattress suture halfway between the first suture and the *left* lateral guy suture by the same technique. Place the third suture so that it bisects the distance between the midpoint of the posterior layer and the *right* lateral guy suture. Place the remaining stitches by the technique of successive bisection until this layer is complete (**Fig. 30–22**).

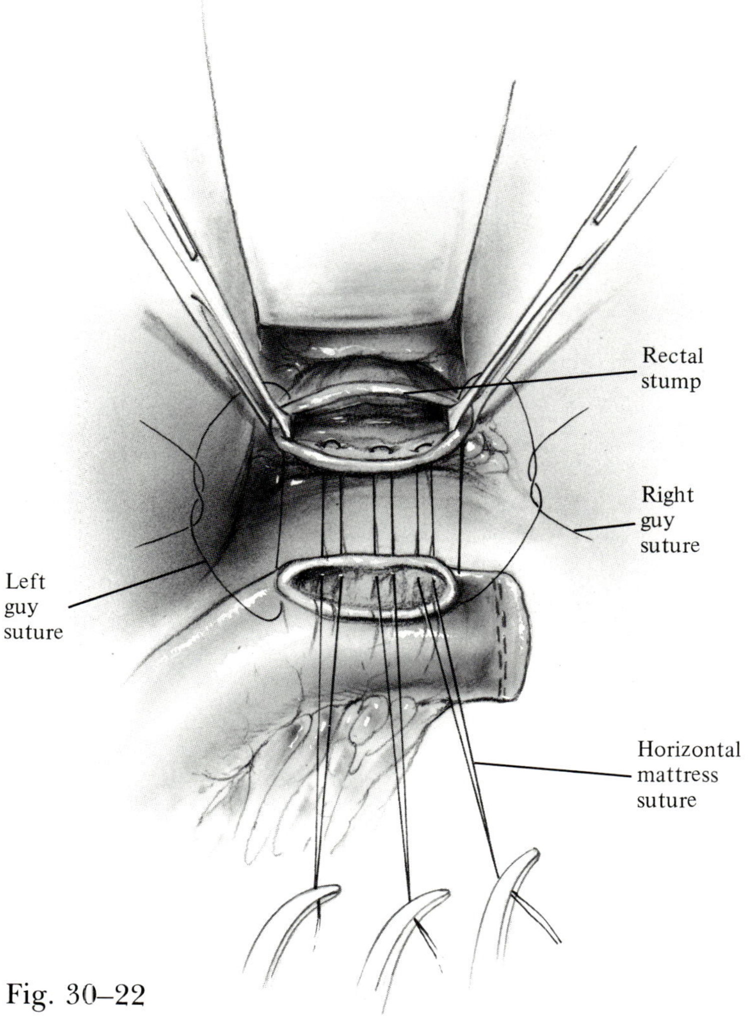

Fig. 30–22

The colon should slide down against the rectal stump while the assistant holds the ends of all the sutures taut. Tie the sutures and leave the tails long, grasping each again in a hemostat. Retaining the long tails of these stitches and applying mild upward traction improves the exposure for insertion of the mucosal sutures.

The remainder of the anastomosis is similar to that described above in the Baker technique.

EEA Stapled Low Colorectal Anastomosis

In the EEA stapling technique for low colorectal anastomosis, place the patient in the Lloyd-Davies position, with thighs abducted, anus exposed, and sacrum elevated on a small sandbag.

For tumors situated 6–9 cm above the anal verge, it will be necessary to dissect the rectum down to the levator diaphragm. This requires complete division of Waldeyer's fascia posteriorly, dissection of the anterior rectum away from the prostate to the level of the urethra, and division of the lateral ligaments down to the levators.

Unless the patient has a narrow pelvis the entire levator diaphragm comes into view (**Fig. 30–23**). All of the perirectal lymphatics will readily peel off from the levator musculature. Then, follow the posterior wall of the rectum down to puborectalis muscle, which marks the cephalad

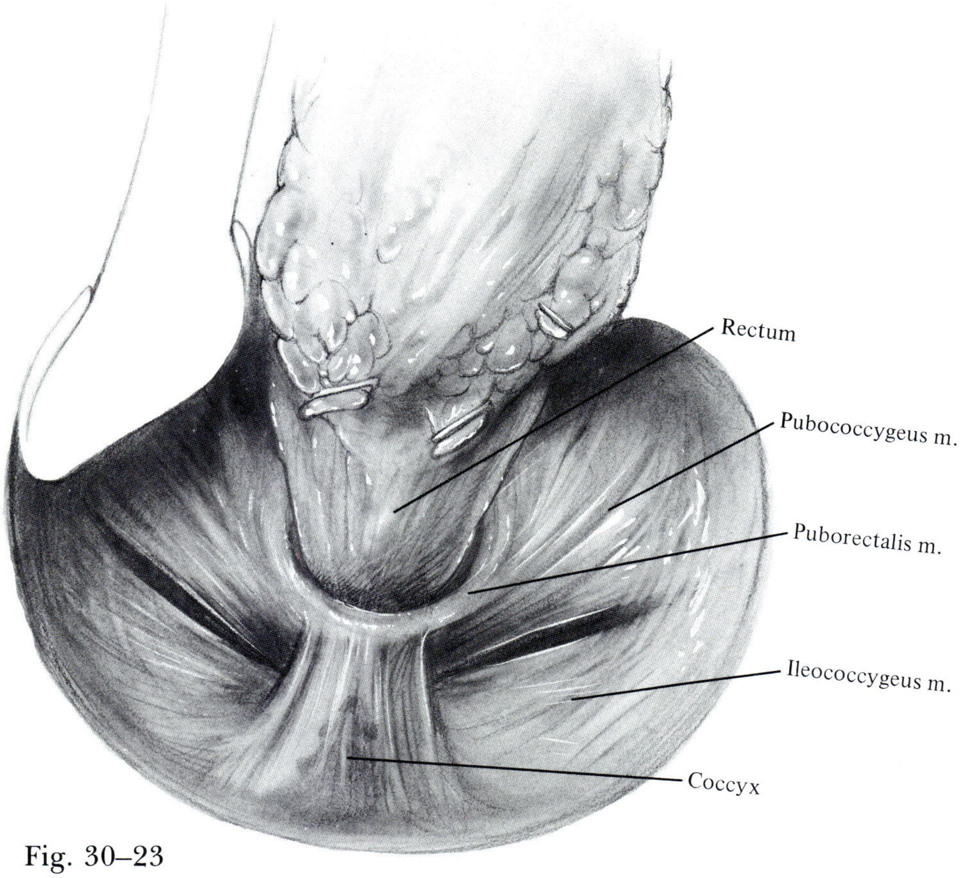

Fig. 30–23

margin of the anal canal. Take care not to continue dissecting beyond the puborectalis as it is easy to enter the intersphincteric plane and to liberate the rectum down to the anal verge. An anastomosis to the skin of the anal canal is technically feasible but would result in excision of the internal sphincter together with the specimen, because the intersphincteric space is the natural plane of dissection which one enters from above.

Place a large right-angle renal pedicle clamp across the rectum about 1 cm beyond the lower edge of the tumor.

Then divide the upper colon between Allen clamps at the site previously selected for this purpose. Ligate the cut distal end of the descending colon with umbilical tape and cover it with a sterile rubber glove (see Fig. 30–12a and b).

Bring the proximal colon down into the pelvis. There should be sufficient slack in the colon to fill the hollow of the sacrum on its way to the site of the anastomosis. If there is not, then liberate the transverse colon to achieve sufficient slack.

Next, remove the Allen clamp and gently dilate the colon to 3.2 cm, which is the outer diameter of the EEA cartridge. This may be accomplished by digital dilatation or by gentle stretching with a rectal speculum, a Foley catheter, or the "sizing" device offered by the manufacturer. Sometimes, dilating the colon may prove the most frustrating step in the entire operation. Be careful *not to produce any serosal tears* by this maneuver. If dilatation to a 3.2 cm diameter cannot be achieved, abandon the stapling technique and construct a suture-anastomosis. Use of EEA cartridges of sizes smaller than 3.2 cm may not be advisable because the diameter of the anastomotic lumen (1.8 cm) produced by the next smaller cartridge may be too small for optimal function of the rectum.

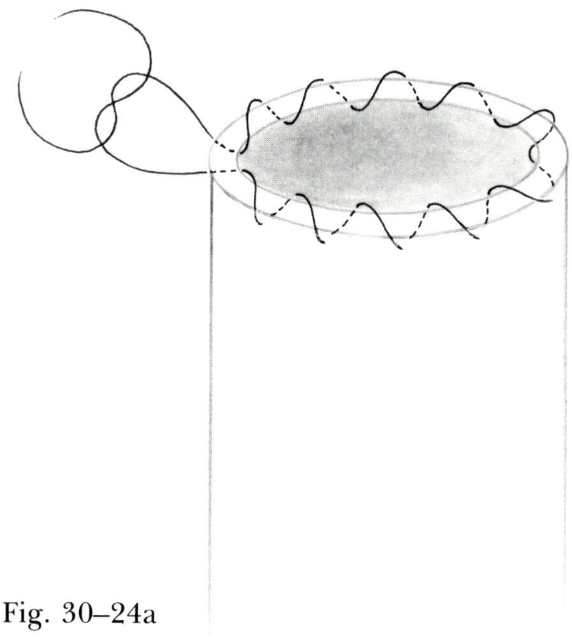

Fig. 30–24a

Then insert a 2–0 Prolene continuous over-and-over whip-stitch starting at the left margin of the proximal cut end of the colon (**Fig. 30–24a**). Ascertain that all fat and mesentery have been dissected off the distal 1.5–2.0 cm of colon so that there will be no fat or blood vessels interposed between the layers of bowel that will be included in the staple line. If blood vessels are trapped in the staple line, firing the EEA may produce significant bleeding in the rectal lumen. This will be difficult to control. Alternatively, the Auto Suture purse-string intrument (see Fig. D–33) may be used instead of a whip-stitch.

Insert a sterile short proctoscope into the anal canal and aspirate the rectum of its contents. Thoroughly irrigate the rectum with sterile water to wash out any desquamated tumor cells, and remove the proctoscope.

Next, insert an over-and-over whip-stitch into the rectal stump. To accomplish this, make an incision through the full thickness of the rectal wall on its left anterolateral aspect, leaving a margin of 4 cm beyond the tumor. Place traction on the right-angle clamp to maintain exposure of the lower rectum. Initiate a 2–0 atraumatic Prolene over-and-over whip-stitch at the left lateral corner of the rectal stump (**Fig. 30–24b**). As this stitch progresses along the anterior wall of the rectum toward the patient's right, divide more and more rectal wall (**Fig. 30–24c**). Continue the same suture circumferentially along the posterior wall of the rectum until the point of origin at the left lateral wall is reached and the specimen is completely detached (**Figs. 30–24d and 30–24e**). Do not attempt to insert the whip-stitch *after* the specimen has been detached because the rectal stump will retract beyond the prostate and suturing from above will be impossible in the case of tumors of the mid-rectum (6–10 cm above the anal verge). Each bite should contain 4 mm of full thickness of rectal wall, and the stitches should be no more than 6 mm apart to prevent gaps when the suture is tied. A 1.5–2.0 cm width of muscular wall of rectum behind the whip-stitch should be cleared of fat, blood vessels, and areolar tissue. When the staples

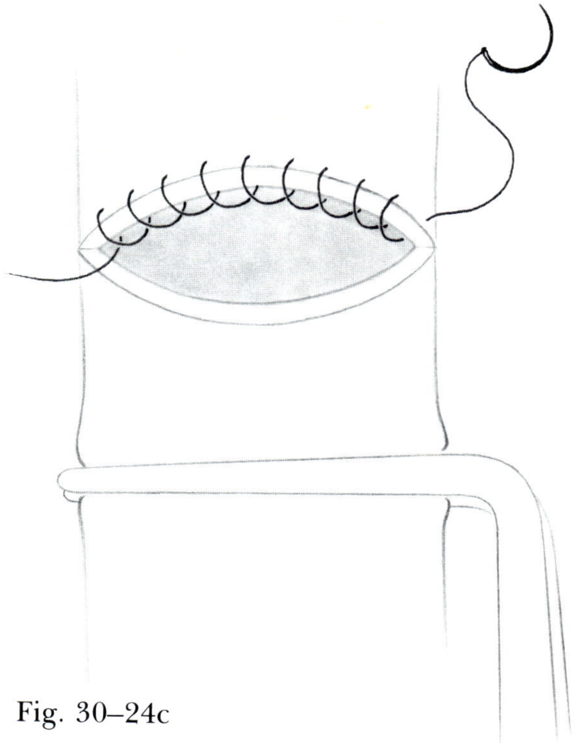

Fig. 30–24c

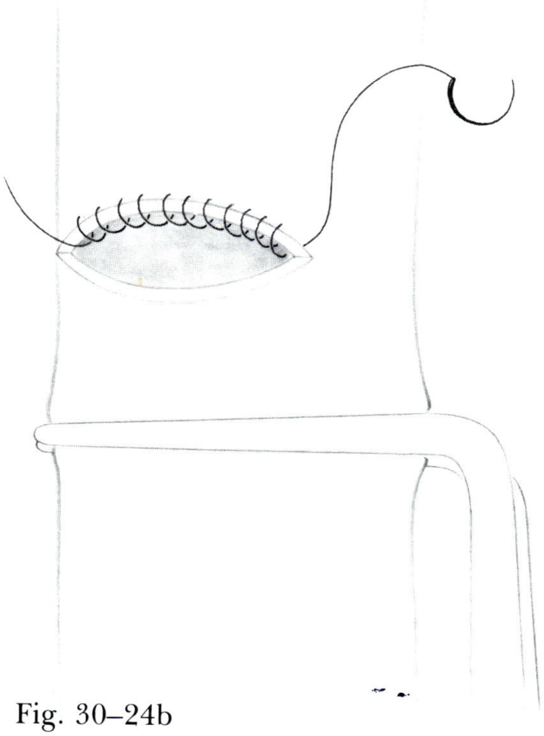

Fig. 30–24b

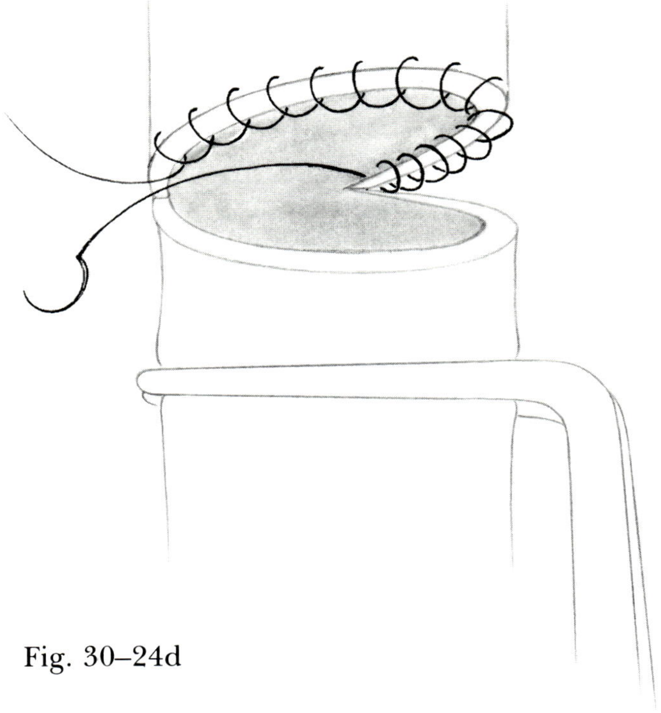

Fig. 30–24d

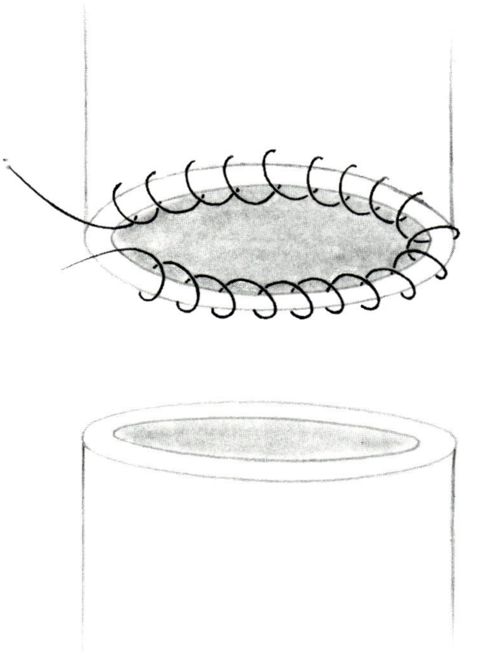

Fig. 30–24e

are fired, there should be no fat or mesentery between the muscular wall of the rectum and seromuscular wall of proximal colon. Grasp both ends of the Prolene purse-string suture in a hemostat. Irrigate the pelvis with a dilute antibiotic solution.

Now move to the perineal portion of the operative field. Check to be sure the screw that caps the anvil is on tightly. If it is not, there will be too much space between the anvil and the staples. This will prevent the staples from closing properly. Lubricate the tip of the EEA device with sterile surgical jelly. Insert the device into the anal canal and into the rectum with the trigger handles pointing anteriorly (**Fig. 30–25**). Slowly push the anvil of the EEA device through the lower rectal purse-string, then rotate the wing nut at the end of the EEA counterclockwise until the device is wide open. Tie the rectal purse-string firmly around the shaft of the EEA (**Fig. 30–26**) and cut the tails 5 mm from the knot.

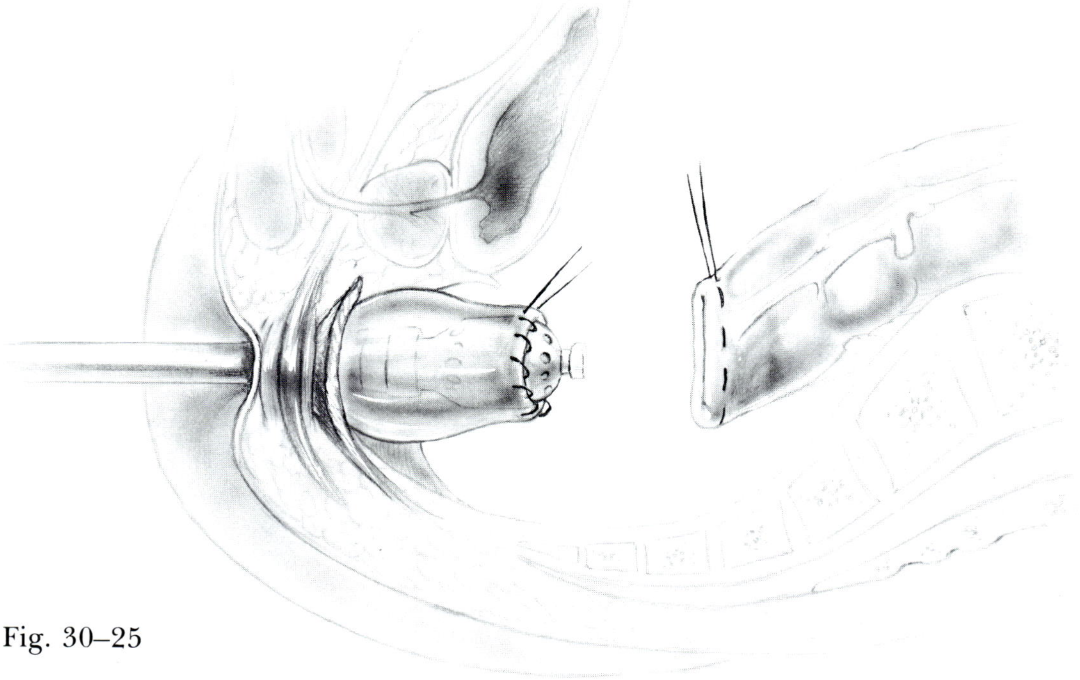

Fig. 30–25

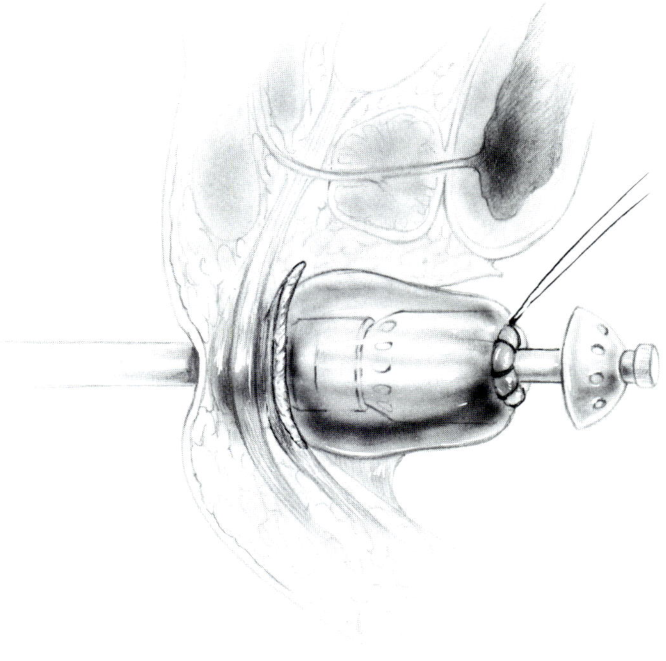

Fig. 30–26

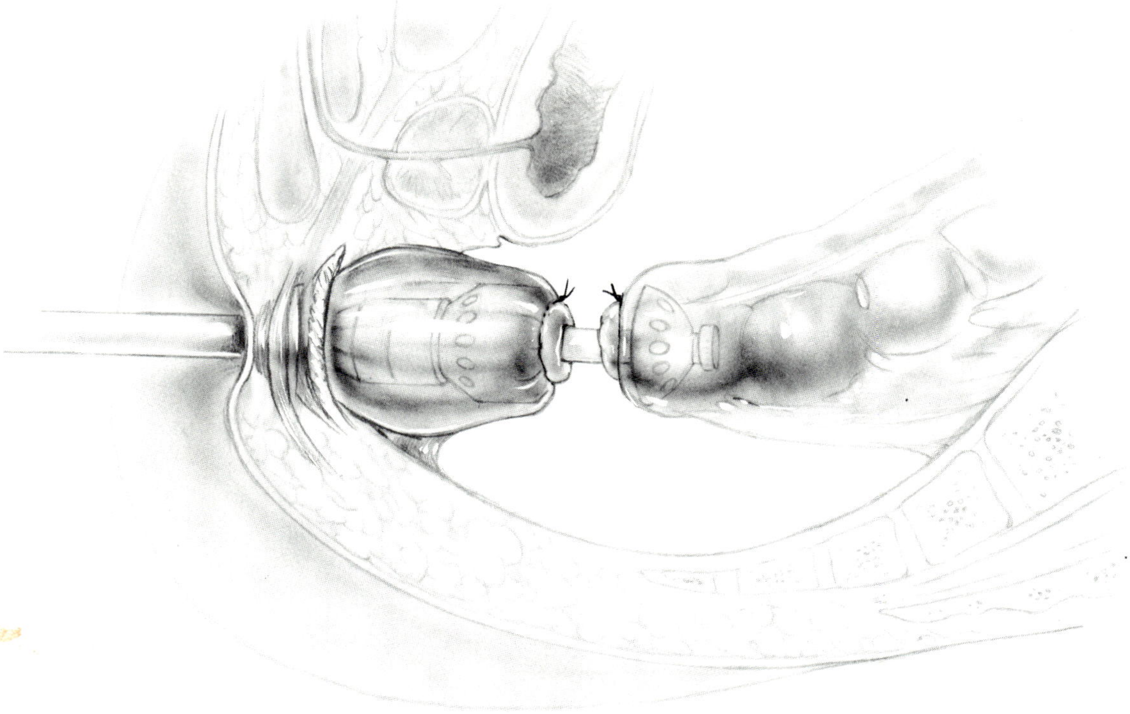

Fig. 30–27

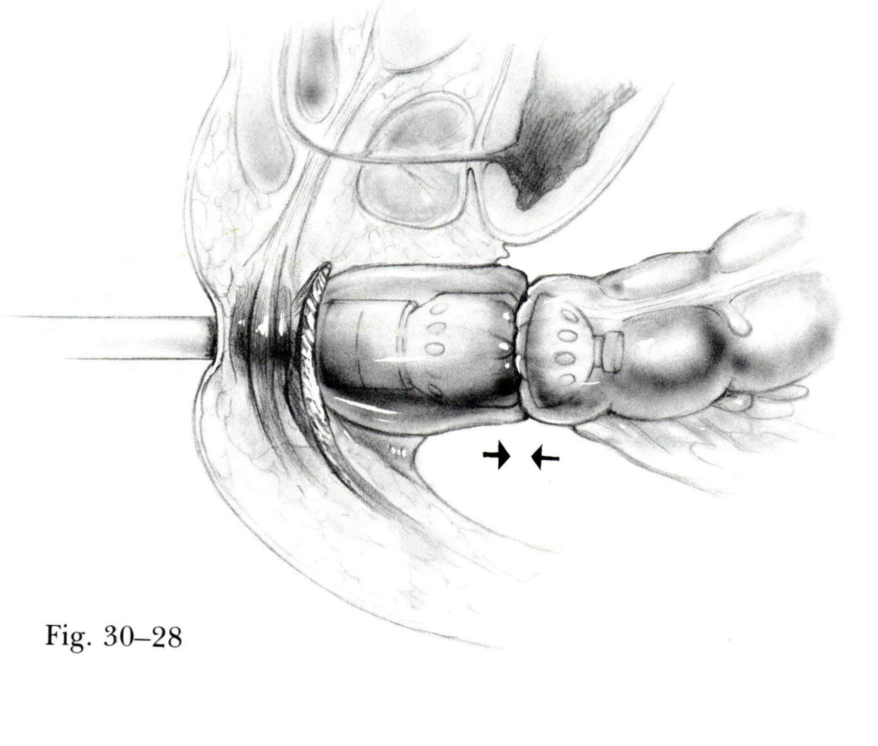

Fig. 30–28

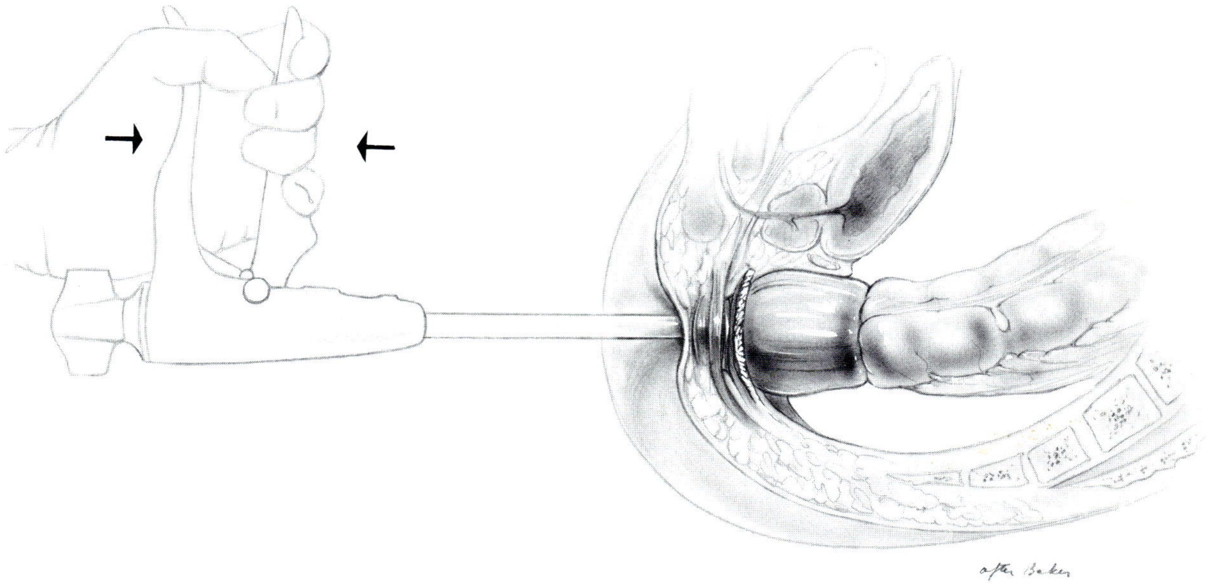

Fig. 30–29

Apply three Allis clamps in triangular fashion to the cut end of the proximal colon, the lumen of which has been dilated so that the colon may be brought over the cap of the EEA. When this has been accomplished, tie the colonic purse-string suture and cut its tails 5 mm from the knot (**Fig. 30–27**).

It is vital to observe the integrity of the two purse-string sutures, as any gap in the purse-string closures will cause a defect in the anastomosis.

Now *completely* close the EEA by rotating the wing nut in a clockwise fashion (**Fig. 30–28**). Check the vernier marks to confirm complete closure. This approximates the anvil to the staple cartridge. If closure is not complete, the staples will be too far from the anvil and will not close to form the B shape. Be sure that the vagina, the bladder, and the ureters are not grasped between the anvil and the cartridge during this step.

Unlock the trigger handles, then strongly compress them by applying a very firm grip (**Fig. 30–29**). Check the strength of the compression by observing if the black mark on the shaft of the instrument is in the proper location. If this step is done properly, two circular concentric rows of staples are fired against an anvil while a circular scalpel blade excises the tissues compressed by the two purse-string sutures in the rectum and colon. This results in a circular anastomosis with an internal diameter of 2.1 cm.

Now rotate the wing nut counterclockwise for seven half turns to separate the anvil from the cartridge. Rotate the EEA at least 180° to the right and then to the left. Remember that the anvil-cap measures 3.2 cm in diameter and that it must be extracted through a stapled anastomosis that has a diameter of only 2.1 cm. Accomplish this by depressing the EEA handle toward the floor, which will elevate the anterior lip of the anvil. This lip should be extracted first. Then the posterior lip can be delivered by elevating the EEA handle. It is sometimes helpful if the assistant grasps the anterior rectal stump with a gauze pad or inserts a Lembert suture to stabilize the staple line while the anvil is being extracted (**Figs. 30–30 and 30–31**).

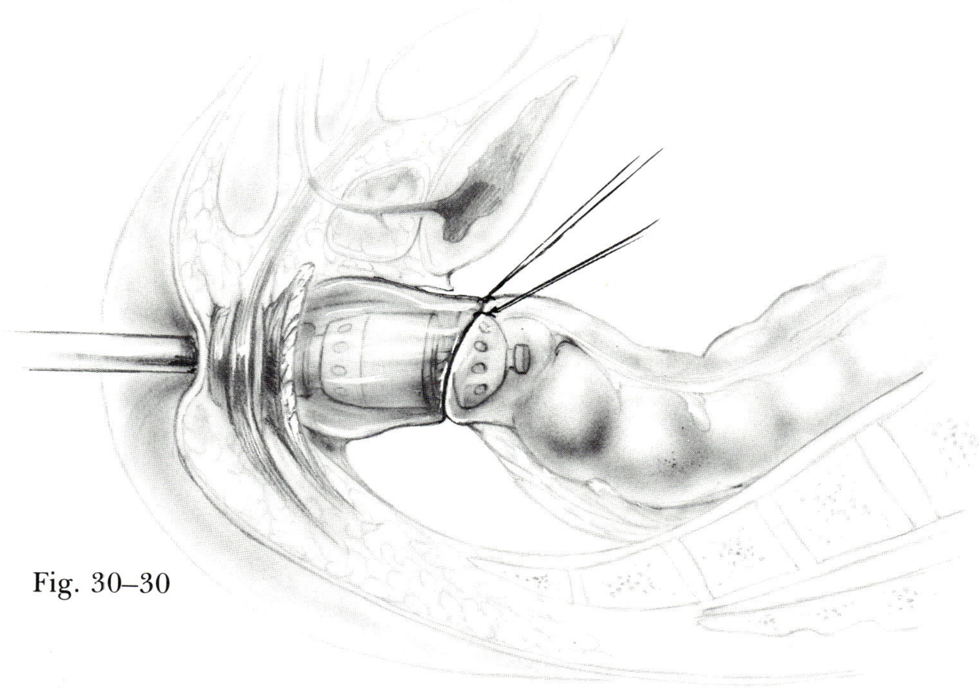

Fig. 30–30

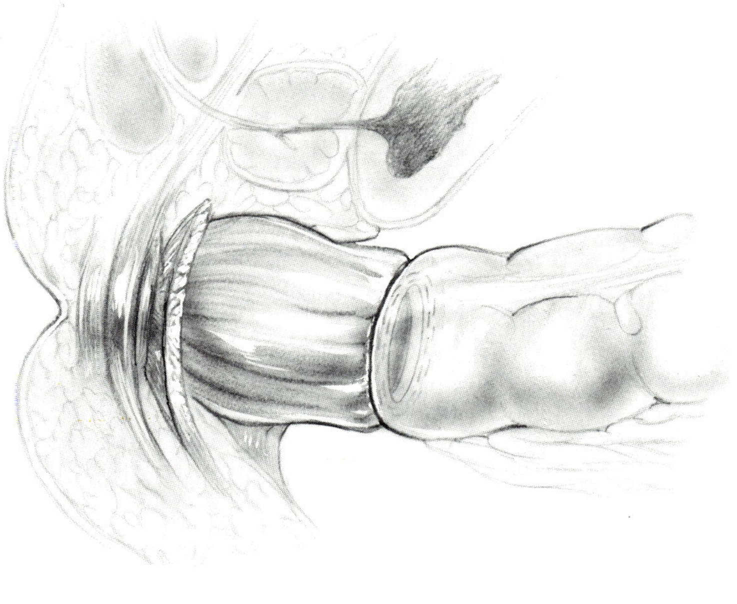

Fig. 30–31

After the instrument has been removed, turn the thumb screw on the cap of the staple cartridge counterclockwise, and remove the cap containing the anvil to reveal the segments of rectum and colon that have been amputated. The cartridge should contain two complete circles, each resembling a small doughnut. One represents the proximal margin of the rectum, and the other represents the distal margin of the proximal colon. Any gap in either of the two circles of bowel indicates a defect in the stapled anastomosis, caused by the bowel pulling out of the purse-string before being stapled. The surgeon should seek to locate and repair such defects. A complementary colostomy should also be considered.

The integrity of the stapled anastomosis should now be checked by digital examination and by proctoscopy. Occasionally, a bleeding point may require cautious electrocoagulation. Finally, insert a Foley catheter into the rectum and, through it, instill a sterile solution of methylene blue dye. Inspect the anastomosis for leakage of the dye. Use a sterile angled dentist's mirror to help observe the posterior aspect of the anastomosis. If a defect is detected, repair it with inverting sutures. Make a transverse colostomy (see Chap. 39) if there is any doubt about the security of the repair.

Pitfalls and Danger Points of EEA Colorectal Anastomosis

Most defects in the staple line are the result of an imperfect purse-string suture. If the purse-string does not hold the entire cut end of the bowel close to the shaft of the EEA instrument, then the staples cannot catch the complete circumference of the colon or rectum. This results in a defect and postoperative leakage. We prefer a whip-stitch to the purse-string to avoid this complication. If complete doughnut-like circles of full thickness of rectum as well as of colon can be identified after the device has been fired, this indicates that the staples have passed through complete circles of bowel and that there should be no defect.

Low colorectal EEA anastomoses fail also when too much bowel is left beyond the purse-string sutures. When an excessive volume of tissue is admitted into the cartridge, the capacity of the cartridge is exceeded. This results in extrusion of tissue when the cartridge is compressed against the anvil. The devitalized extruded tissue may emerge between the two walls of stapled bowel and interfere with healing. If instead of the usual purse-string, a whip-stitch (see Fig. 20–23) is used on the rectal and colonic segments, the possibility of this complication will be diminished. It is also essential to remove fat from the two bowel walls in the area where the staples are to be inserted.

One important exception to the use of the whip-stitch is in the case of a colorectal anastomosis high in the rectum where the rectal diameter is quite large. When a whip-stitch is used to compress a large rectum, it is sometimes impossible to snug the entire diameter up close to the shaft of the EEA. In this case a true purse-string suture works better than the whip-stitch (**Fig. 30–32**).

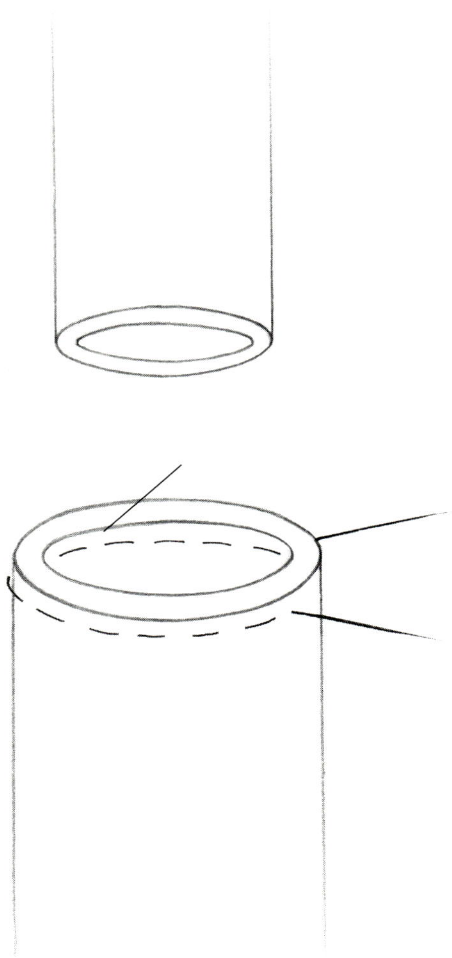

Fig. 30–32

An additional pitfall should be noted. If the trigger handles of the instrument are not compressed fully, the circular scalpel blade fires incompletely. The staples may be driven home, but the redundant colon and rectum within the anvil *do not get cut.* Forceful removal of the EEA device under these conditions will disrupt the entire anastomosis.

Incomplete firing of the circular blade occurs also when the tails of the Prolene purse-string or whip sutures have not been cut short. This happens because the circular blade is not powerful enough to transect the 2–0 Prolene suture tails. When the anvil cannot be disengaged easily, do not use force as this will disrupt the entire anastomosis. Rather, make a colotomy incision on the antimesenteric border of the upper colon 3–4 cm above the staple line. Then, unscrew and remove the anvil through the colotomy. Extracting the EEA device from the anus will now be a simple matter. Inspect the interior of the anastomosis through the colotomy opening. If a septum of inverted bowel remains in the lumen inside the circle of staples, excise the septum using a Potts angled scissors. Close the colotomy with the TA–55 stapler.

An obvious cause of EEA failure is the erroneous use of a cartridge that has been fired already. In this case the circular blade may function, but there are no staples; the surgeon is left with two cut ends of bowel, but no anastomosis. To avoid this error, before attaching the anvil look closely into the cartridge to be certain that it is properly loaded with staples and a circular blade. Unless the wing nut is loosened by seven counterclockwise half turns, the EEA cannot be removed from the rectum after firing the staples. This mishap occurs because the anastomosed bowel is still being grasped between the staple cartridge and the anvil, and forceful attempts to dislodge the EEA will disrupt the anastomosis.

As mentioned above, if the screw that caps the anvil is not screwed on tightly, or if the wing nut near the handle is not completely closed before the staples are fired, then the space between the staple cartridge and the anvil will be excessive. This will prevent proper closure of the legs of the staples, in which case the anastomosis may pull apart at the slightest stress.

Never use Hemoclips on any part of the colon or rectum that may possibly be included in the stapled anastomosis because these metal clips will prevent proper function of the staples and the EEA blade.

Intralumenal hemorrhage following an EEA anastomosis occurs if mesenteric blood vessels have been trapped in the staple line and are transected by the blade. Control of bleeding may be achieved by cautious electrocoagulation through a proctoscope or by inserting sutures through a proximal colotomy.

When the stapled anastomosis is situated at or above the cephalad margin of the anal sphincter muscles, i.e., at or above the puborectalis component of the levator muscle, fecal continence will not be lost. However, because the proximal colon segment does not function as a reservoir, the patient will defecate frequently during the first few months. Each peristaltic contraction results in the evacuation of a small, formed stool, but there is no inadvertent loss of stool or liquid.

On the other hand, if the anastomosis is at or below the dentate line, the loss of the internal sphincter results in fecal incontinence for 3–6 months and *sometimes permanently.*

Goligher (1979) described the insertion of the purse-string suture into the rectal stump by a transanal approach after dilating the anus and inserting a self-retaining bivalve Parks rectal retractor. Goligher recommends this maneuver in cases where the purse-string suture cannot be inserted from the abdominal approach. If the specimen is *not* detached until after the rectal purse-string suture is inserted, we have been able to resect tumors situated as low as 6 cm from the anal verge by the technique described in this chapter. If the specimen has been removed, then in men with tumors at 6–9 cm it will often not be possible to place the rectal purse-string stitch from above. Unfortunately, the technique of Goligher (1979) results in the excision of the internal sphincter muscle and produces some degree of fecal incontinence if the stapled anastomosis is placed at or below the dentate line. If the transanal approach is used, make every effort to insert the purse-string or whip-stitch into the rectal stump at least 1 cm above the anal canal so as to insure retention of the internal sphincter muscle. If proper application of the rectal stitch cannot be achieved, then one can perform a transanal end-to-end sutured anastomosis by the method of Parks, which makes a point of preserving the internal sphincter muscle. Otherwise either a pull-through operation or a permanent colostomy will be necessary.

A late complication that may take place is recurrent fecal impaction. This happens because the internal diameter of the stoma after an EEA stapled anastomosis is accurately fixed at 2.1 cm. The two staggered rows of staples are inert, however, and remain in place for an undetermined length of time following the operation, so the size of the stoma cannot readily be enlarged by bouginage. Unless they suffer from severe chronic constipation, most patients tolerate this size stoma without symptoms. However, the relatively small stoma does constitute one minor drawback to the use of the EEA. At this time we are quite enthusiastic about the EEA device for colorectal anastomoses that are so low that it would be difficult to use sutures without a posterior transsacral exposure. We have resected tumors 6 cm from the anal verge, using the EEA with a 4 cm margin of normal tissue, doing a successful stapled anastomosis flush with the upper margin of the anal canal.

Complementary colostomy and presacral drainage should be used following an EEA stapled anastomosis under the same conditions that would lead the surgeon to use these modalities following a sutured colorectal anastomosis. In general, we have not performed complementary colostomy, but routinely employ closed-suction presacral drainage for low extraperitoneal anastomoses.

For stapled intraperitoneal anastomoses at or above the sacral promontory, we prefer a functional end-to-end (see Figs. 28–33 through 28–36) or a Weakley (see Figs. 28–26 through 28–32) anastomosis rather than the EEA procedure. The latter often takes more time and is prone to more technical complications than the functional end-to-end or the Weakley method.

Wound Closure and Drainage

Remove the Wound Protector drape. The surgical team should change its gloves and discard all contaminated instruments. Thoroughly irrigate the abdominal cavity and wound with an antibiotic solution.

Close the incision in the usual fashion. Manage the subcutaneous layer and skin with a closed-suction catheter.

Postoperative Care

Nasogastric suction until bowel activity returns

No oral intake for the first 7 days

Continuation of perioperative antibiotics for 24 hours

Constant bladder drainage via Foley catheter for 6–7 days

Presacral suction catheters attached to closed suction drainage

Injection into catheters of 50 ml sterile saline solution containing 50 mg kanamycin every 6 hours

Drainage catheters removed after 5 days unless there is significant volume of drainage

Radiation therapy for Duke's B and C cases

Complications

1) *Bladder dysfunction* following low anterior resection may take place, especially in males with prostatism, but it is much less common than after abdominoperineal proctectomy. Generally, after 6–7 days of bladder drainage, function will resume.

2) *Pelvic sepsis* secondary to anastomotic leakage is the most common serious complication following low colorectal anastomosis. Any patient who has fever, leukocytosis, and ileus following low anterior resection should be assumed to have a leaking anastomosis and a pelvic abscess. Clinical manifestations of this complication commonly occur between the sixth and ninth postoperative days. Cautious digital examination of the rectum by the surgeon may prove to be diagnostic if the finger discloses a defect in the suture line, generally on its posterior aspect. Careful proctoscopic examination may disclose evidence of a defect in the suture line.

A patient may have sustained a pelvic abscess even in the absence of a definite defect in the suture line. Consequently, a patient who is febrile and toxic should undergo exploratory laparotomy and drainage of any septic process. In most cases the patient will also require a transverse colostomy.

Patients who have mild systemic symptoms and who are suspected of having pelvic infection may be treated by withdrawing food, administering intravenous antibiotics, and hyperalimentation. Occasionally, a presacral abscess drains into the rectum through the anastomosis without making the patient seriously ill. It should be remembered, however, that anastomotic leakage and pelvic sepsis constitute potentially lethal complications that often require vigorous management.

3) *Sexual dysfunction* in the male may follow low anterior resection, especially in patients who have large tumors and require extensive dissection of the presacral space, the lateral ligaments, and the prostatic area.

References

Baker JW (1950) Low end to side recto-sigmoidal anastomosis. Arch Surg 61:143

Goligher JC et al. (1970) Anastomotic dehiscence after anterior resection of the rectum and sigmoid. Brit J Surg 57:109

Goligher JC (1975) Surgery of the anus, rectum and colon, 3rd edn. Bailliere, Tindall, London, p. 662

Goligher JC (1979) Use of circular stapling gun with peranal insertion of anorectal purse-string suture for construction of very low colorectal or colo-anal anastomoses. Brit J Surg 66:501

Parks AG, Thomson JPS (1977) Per-anal endorectal operative techniques. In: Rob C, Smith R (eds) Operative surgery, colon, rectum and anus, 3rd edn. Butterworth, London p. 157

Schrock TR et al. (1973) Factors contributing to leakage of colonic anastomoses. Ann Surg 177:513

Zollinger RM, Sheppard MH (1971) Carcinoma of the rectum and the rectosigmoid, a review of 729 cases. Arch Surg 102:335

31 Abdominoperineal Proctosigmoidectomy for Cancer

Indications

Adenocarcinoma of distal rectum

Carcinoid of lower rectum if invasive or over 1.8 cm in diameter

Squamous carcinoma of anus near dentate line if over 1 cm in diameter

Preoperative Preparation

Sigmoidoscopy and biopsy

Barium colon enema

Correction of anemia if necessary

Intravenous pyelogram

Bowel preparation as outlined in Chap. 25

Indwelling Foley catheter in bladder

Nasogastric tube

Perioperative antibiotics

Pitfalls and Danger Points

Hemorrhage

Presacral veins

Left iliac vein

Middle hemorrhoidal artery

Hypogastric arterial branches

Gastrointestinal

Rupture of rectum during dissection

Colostomy ischemia, producing postoperative necrosis

Colostomy under excessive tension, leading to postoperative retraction and peritonitis

Separation of pelvic peritoneal suture line, causing herniation and obstruction of small intestine; inadequate mobilization of pelvic peritoneum, resulting in failure of newly constructed pelvic floor to descend completely; resulting empty space, encouraging sepsis

Genitourinary

Ureteral trauma, especially during dissection in vicinity of lateral ligaments of rectum; inadvertent ureteral ligation, especially during reconstruction of pelvic floor

Urethral laceration during dissection of perineum in males

Operative Strategy

Abdominal Phase

Presacral Dissection: Prevention of Hemorrhage

Contrary to what apparently is a widely held perception, radical cancer surgery does *not* require stripping the presacral region down to the periosteum. The dissection of the perirectal tissues proximal to the carcinoma is necessary for the removal of *tumor emboli* within the lymph nodes and lymphatic channels. If tumor has invaded widely into the mesorectum and presacral tissues, the lesion is generally beyond cure by radical surgery.

There is a network of veins lying on the presacral periosteum that drain into the sacral foramina (see Fig. 30–6b). When these are torn by blunt dissection, clamping or ligation to control the hemorrhage that results often is impossible, since the torn vessel retracts into the foramen. The massive venous hemorrhage that can follow cannot be stemmed by ligating the hypogastric arteries. Most intraoperative fatalities during total proctectomy are caused by this type of presacral venous hemorrhage.

If the surgeon cannot very quickly control lacerated presacral veins with a hemostat or bone wax, the bleeding area should be covered with a sheet of Surgicel, over which a large gauze pack should be placed, filling the sacral hollow. This almost always controls the hemorrhage.

Unless the presacral vessels are directly invaded by a bulky tumor of the midrectum, massive presacral venous hemorrhage is entirely preventable. Blunt hand dissection of the presacral space is not a desirable technique. The surgeon's hand does not belong in this area until scissors dissection under direct vision has freed all the perirectal tissues from any posterior attachments to the sacrum. This should be done with a long Metzenbaum scissors, combined with gentle upward traction on the rectum. As the scissors are inserted on each side of the midline, the perirectal tissues can easily be lifted in an anterior direction *without removing the thin layer of endopelvic fascia that covers the presacral veins.* When the presacral dissection stays in the proper plane, the presacral veins are hidden from view by this layer of fascia, as Fig. 30–6a shows. Occasionally, branches of the middle sacral vessels enter the perirectal tissues from behind. These may be divided between Hemoclips.

This dissection is easily continued down to the area of the coccyx, where the fascia of Waldeyer becomes dense as it goes from the anterior surfaces of the coccyx and sacrum to attach to the lower rectum (see Fig. 31–8). Attempts to penetrate this fascia by blunt finger dissection may rupture the rectum rather than the fascia, which is strong. This layer must be incised sharply with a scissors or scalpel. When the posterior dissection has for the most part been completed, only *then* should the surgeon's hand enter the presacral space to sweep the dissection toward the lateral pelvic walls. This maneuver helps define the lateral ligaments. If this is done properly, the presacral veins will be covered by a thin layer of tissue and will not be visible. The dissection should be bloodless.

Other points of hemorrhage in the pelvic dissection may occur on the lateral walls. These can usually be readily identified and occluded by ligation or Hemoclips. Close attention should also be paid to the left iliac vein, which may be injured in the course of the dissection. As most serious bleeding in pelvic dissections is of venous origin, we do not ligate the hypogastric arteries routinely.

Presacral Dissection: Preservation of Hypogastric Nerves

As the rectum is elevated from the presacral space and the anterior surface of the aorta cleared of areolar and lymphovascular tissue, a varying number of preaortic sympathetic nerves of the superior hypogastric plexus can be identified. These are the contribution of the sympathetic nervous system to the bilateral inferior hypogastric (pelvic) plexuses. In males their preservation is necessary for normal ejaculation. After they cross the region of the aortic bifurcation and sacral promontory, they coalesce into two major nerve bundles, called the hypogastric nerves. Each nerve, which may have 1–3 strands, runs toward the posterolateral wall of the pelvis in the vicinity of the hypogastric artery (see Figs. 31–2c and 31–4). We agree with Goligher (1975) that in most malignancies of the distal rectum, these nerves can be preserved without compromising the patient's chances of cure.

After the inferior mesenteric artery and vein are divided and the lymphovascular tissues elevated from the bifurcation of the aorta by blunt dissection, the sympathetic nerves remain closely attached to the aorta and need not be damaged if the dissection is gently performed. At the promontory of the sacrum, if the rectum is dissected as described above, the right and left hypogastric nerves can be seen posterior to the plane of dissection and can be preserved—provided there is a sufficient distance separating them from the tumor. There also seems to be a diminution in the incidence of bladder dysfunction after nerve preservation.

Ureteral Dissection

To prevent damage to the ureters, these delicate structures must be identified and traced well down into the pelvis. The normal ureter crosses the common iliac artery at the point this structure bifurcates into its external and internal branches. Because the ureter and a leaf of incised peritoneum are often displaced during the course of dissection, if the ureter is not located in its usual position the undersurfaces of both the lateral and medial leaves of peritoneum should be inspected. The identity of the ureter can be confirmed if pinching or touching the structure with a forceps results in typical peristaltic waves. If doubt exists, the anesthesiologist may be instructed to inject indigo carmine dye intravenously; this stains the ureter blue, unless the patient is oliguric at the time of injection. The ureter should be traced into the pelvis beyond the point at which the lateral ligaments of the rectum are divided.

Inferior Mesenteric Artery Ligation and Preaortic Node Dissection

The highest point to which it is practical to extend the lymph node dissection in patients who have rectal cancer is the junction of the inferior mesenteric artery and the aorta. Ligation of the artery at this point, together with a preaortic lymph node dissection, has been recommended as a routine procedure. There is not yet sufficient data on postoperative survival to validate this level of ligation. The generally accepted apex point of the dissection (inferior mesenteric artery just distal to the takeoff of the left colic) (see Fig. 26–6) is located only about 4 cm from the aorta. Most of the lymphatic tissue in the intervening 3–4 cm can usually be swept downward with the specimen. On the other hand, if the surgeon notes that the lymph nodes near the aorta contain metastases in the proximal portion of the mesentery, then high ligation of the inferior mesenteric artery at the aorta may be performed (see Fig. 26–7).

Colostomy

The colostomy may be brought out through the left lower quadrant musculature, through the midline abdominal incision, or through the belly of the left rectus muscle. If the colostomy is brought out laterally, either the 3–5 cm gap between the colon and the lateral portion of the abdominal wall should be closed or a retroperitoneal colostomy should be performed. Otherwise the small bowel may become incarcerated in the lateral space. On the other hand, if the colostomy is brought out somewhere near the midline of the abdomen, there is no need to close this space, which becomes so large that movement of small bowel can take place freely without complication.

Goligher (1958) reported a method of bringing the colostomy through a retroperitoneal tunnel to the opening in the abdominal wall sited in the lateral third of the rectus muscle a few centimeters below the umbilicus. When the peritoneal pelvic floor is suitable for closure by suturing, this technique is another satisfactory method of creating the sigmoid colostomy (see Figs. 31–29 to 31–32). When the pelvic floor is not suitable for closure, we generally bring the colostomy through the midline incision.

To prevent necrosis of the colostomy, one must be certain there is adequate arterial blood flow to the distal portion of the exteriorized colon, just as would be required if an anastomosis were made at this point. Even in the presence of adequate arterial flow, ischemia of the colostomy may occur if an obese mesentery is constricted by a tight colostomy orifice.

Postoperative retraction of the colostomy may be brought on by abdominal distention that causes migration of the abdominal wall in an anterior direction. For this reason the limb of colon to be fashioned into a colostomy should protrude without tension for a distance of 5 cm beyond the level of the abdominal skin before any suturing takes place.

Immediate maturation of a colostomy, accomplished by inserting a mucocutaneous suture line between the colon and the subcuticular layer of the skin, has resulted in the virtual elimination of postoperative stricture and prolapse. If the maturation procedure is performed, retraction will not occur even though *no* additional sutures other than those attaching the colon to the subcuticular region are used.

Pelvic Floor

Because intestinal obstruction due to herniation of the ileum into a defect in the reconstructed pelvic floor is a serious complication, a number of surgeons now omit the step of resuturing the pelvic peritoneum. If no attempt is made to reperitonealize the pelvic floor, the small bowel will descend to the level of the sutured levators or subcutaneous layers of the perineum. Intestinal obstruction in the immediate postoperative period does not appear to be very common following this technique. However, if intestinal obstruction does occur at a later date, it becomes necessary to mobilize considerable small bowel, which is bound down by dense adhesions in the pelvis. This often results in extensive damage to the intestine, requiring resection and anastomosis to repair it. Thus it appears logical to attempt primary closure of the pelvic peritoneum to prevent this complication, provided enough tissue is available for closure without undue tension. The peritoneal floor should be *sufficiently lax to descend to the level of the reconstructed perineum.* This eliminates the dead space between the peritoneal floor and the other structures of the perineum. As total proctectomy is done primarily to remove lesions of the lower rectum, there is no need for a radical resection of the perirectal peritoneum. One should conserve as much of this layer as possible. If it appears that a proper closure will not be possible, it is preferable to leave the floor entirely open. Otherwise the dead space between the peritoneal diaphragm and the perineal floor often leads to disruption of the peritoneal suture line and to bowel herniation. The dead space also delays perineal healing and encourages sepsis.

Perineal Phase

Position

Turning the patient to a prone position provides the best exposure for the surgeon, but imposes a number of disadvantages upon the patient. First, circulatory equilibrium may be disturbed by turning the patient who is under anesthesia. Also, changing positions prolongs the operative procedure, as it is not possible to have one member of the surgical team close the abdominal incision while the perineal phase is in process. Similar objections can be raised about the lateral Sims position.

In recent years we have favored the position described by Lloyd-Davies, in which the patient lies supine, with the sacrum elevated on a folded sheet or sandbag and the lower extremities supported by Lloyd-Davies leg rests, causing the thighs to be widely abducted but flexed only slightly, while the legs are supported and moderately flexed. The mild flexion of the thighs does not interfere in any way with the abdominal procedure, and the second assistant can stand comfortably between the patient's legs while retracting the bladder (see Figs. 31–1a and 31–1b).

This position is identical with that used for the synchronous two-team method of performing a total proctectomy. Whether the abdominal and perineal phases are carried on synchronously by two operating teams or whether one team does the complete procedure, positioning the patient in this manner gives the surgeon the option of doing some portions of the procedure from below and then switching to the abdominal field in response to the exigencies of a particular step. This facilitates the safe lateral dissection of large tumors, as well as the achievement of complete hemostasis in the pelvis. Some vessels may be easier to control from below and some should be clamped from above. In addition, after the surgeon has completed suturing the pelvic peritoneum, suction can be applied from below to determine if there is a dead space between the pelvic floor and the perineal closure. After removing the specimen it is fairly simple to have closure of both the abdomen and perineum proceed simultaneously.

Closure of Perineum

Traditionally, after the perineal excision of the rectum the surgeon inserted a large gauze pack into the presacral space and closed the perineal skin loosely around the pack. The gauze was removed somewhere between the third and seventh postoperative day. This resulted in a huge open perineal wound, which required repeated irrigations, sitz baths, and a number of months for complete healing. Secondary infection of the large cavity was not uncommon.

If there has been no fecal spillage in the pelvis during the course of resection, and if good hemostasis has been accomplished, there is no need to leave the perineal wound open. Primary healing has been obtained in the vast majority of our patients operated upon for malignancy when the perineum is closed per primam with the insertion of two closed-suction drainage catheters. Kanamycin in a dose of 25 mg in 25 ml saline is injected into each of these catheters every 6 hours for the first 5 days. This serves the dual purpose of keeping the catheters open and instilling antibiotics into the retroperitoneal space. Suction applied to these catheters draws the reconstructed peritoneal pelvic floor downward to eliminate any empty space.

In patients who are experiencing major presacral hemorrhage, the area should be tamponaded with a sheet of Surgicel covered by a large gauze pack, which is brought out through the perineum. The gauze should be removed in the operating room on the first or second postoperative day.

In patients who have experienced contamination of the pelvis during the operation, the perineum should be closed only partially and drained with both latex and sump drains, followed by frequent postoperative irrigations with an antibiotic solution.

In female patients, management of the perineum depends on whether one has elected to remove the posterior vagina. For small anterior malignancies, the adjacent portion of the posterior vagina may be removed with the specimen, leaving sufficient vagina for primary closure of this organ with PG. When the entire posterior vaginal wall has been removed along with large anterior lesions, the perineum should be closed with sutures to the levator muscles, the subcutaneous fat, and the skin. This leaves a defect at the site of the vaginal excision, through which loose gauze packing should be inserted. If there is primary healing of the perineal floor, granulation will fill up this cavity and vaginal epithelium will regenerate in 1–3 months. Vaginal resection need not be done in cases of tumors confined to the posterior portion of the rectum.

Dissection of Perineum

The most serious pitfall in the perineal dissection is an inadvertent transection of the male urethra. This may be avoided if the anterior part of the dissection is delayed until the levator muscles have first been divided throughout the remainder of the circumference of the pelvis and the prostate identified. It is important not to divide the rectourethralis muscle at a point more cephalad than the plane of the posterior wall of the prostate (see Fig. 31–21). Alternatively, one should identify the transverse perineal muscles. If the dissection is kept on a plane posterior to these muscles, the urethra is out of harm's way.

Hemostasis

All bleeding during the perineal dissection can be controlled by the accurate application of electrocoagulation. Here, as elsewhere in abdominal surgery, if electrocoagulation is applied to a vessel that is well isolated from surrounding fat, ligature will not be necessary. Whether electrocoagulation is applied directly to a bleeding point or to a forceps or hemostat depends on the preference of the surgeon. With the cautery device it is possible to obtain complete control of bleeding in this area without undue loss of blood or time.

Operative Technique

Position

Place the patient in the supine position, with the sacrum elevated on several folded sheets or a sandbag and the thighs flexed only slightly but abducted sufficiently to allow adequate exposure of the perineum. The legs should be flexed slightly and the calves padded with foam rubber and supported in Lloyd-Davies leg rests (**Figs. 31–1a and 31–1b**). If the thighs are not flexed excessively, there will be no interference with the performance of the abdominal phase of the operation. The second assistant should stand between the patient's legs during the abdominal phase. Bring the indwelling Foley catheter over the patient's groin and attach it to a plastic tube for gravity drainage into a bag calibrated to facilitate measurement of hourly urine volume. In males fix the scrotum to the groin with a suture. Close the anal canal with a heavy purse-string suture.

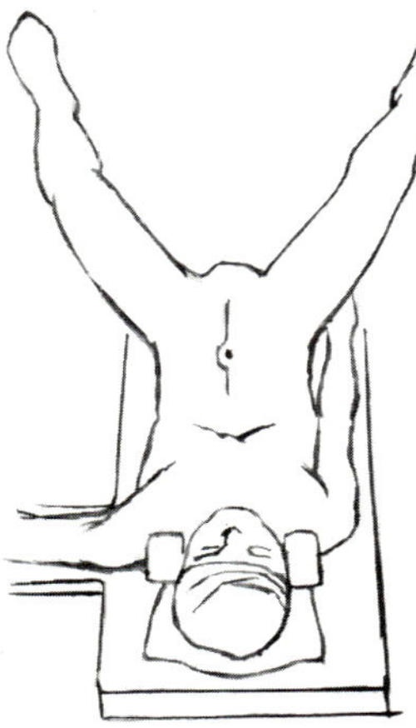

Fig. 31–1a

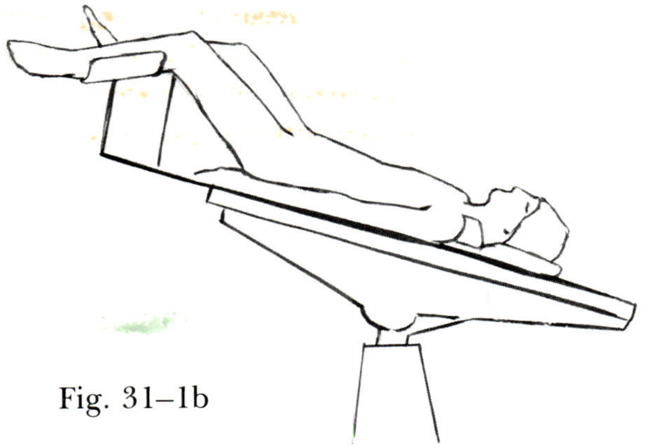

Fig. 31–1b

Carry out routine skin preparation of the abdomen, perineum, and buttocks. Drape the entire area with sterile sheets. After these steps have been completed, the operation can be performed either with two teams working synchronously or one team alternating between the abdomen and the perineum.

Incision and Exploration: Operability

Make a midline incision beginning at a point 8 cm above the umbilicus and continuing to the pubis (see Fig. 31–1a). Separate the pyramidalis muscles as the pubis is approached, for coming an extra 1–2 cm closer to the pubis improves the exposure significantly. Open the peritoneum and carry out general exploration. If one or two isolated liver metastases are identified and the patient has an otherwise resectable lesion, the solitary metastases should be individually excised, as the 5-year survival rate in cases of this type has been reported by Foster and Berman to approach 20%.

In most cases the resectability of a rectal carcinoma cannot generally be determined until a later step in the operation, when the presacral space is open. If the liver is heavily invaded by metastases, a proctectomy should not be performed. One exception to this rule is patients who are experiencing severe tenesmus or bleeding, as these symptoms are not usually relieved by colostomy alone. When there is advanced intra-abdominal metastasis, it would be desirable to destroy the rectal carcinoma by electrocoagulation. Unfortunately, in most cases of this type the rectal lesion is already almost circumferential, a finding that contraindicates fulguration. In circumferential lesions fulguration leads to fibrosis and obstruction. If the prognosis is that the patient will survive for more than 1 year, a proctectomy should be performed when it is anatomically feasible.

As for anatomical resectability, when a tumor invades the sacrum posteriorly or the prostate anteriorly, attempting to core out the rectum by forcing a plane through the tumor is a fruitless and sometimes dangerous endeavor. If much tumor is left behind in the presacral space, then the palliation attained is negligible, for if it should invade the presacral nerves it will produce the most distressing of all symptoms in this disease, extreme perineal pain. On the other hand, many tumors may be firmly adherent to the sacrum without actually having invaded it. These should be resected. Cases of borderline resectability may benefit from a course of radiation followed by reoperation.

Local invasion of the ureter does not contraindicate resection, as the divided ureter at this low level can be implanted into the bladder.

Mobilization of Sigmoid

With the patient in the Trendelenburg position, exteriorize the small intestine into a Vi-Drape intestinal bag. By drawing the sigmoid colon medially, several congenital attachments between the mesocolon and the posterolateral parietal peritoneum can be divided up to the mid-descending colon (**Fig. 31–2**). After doing

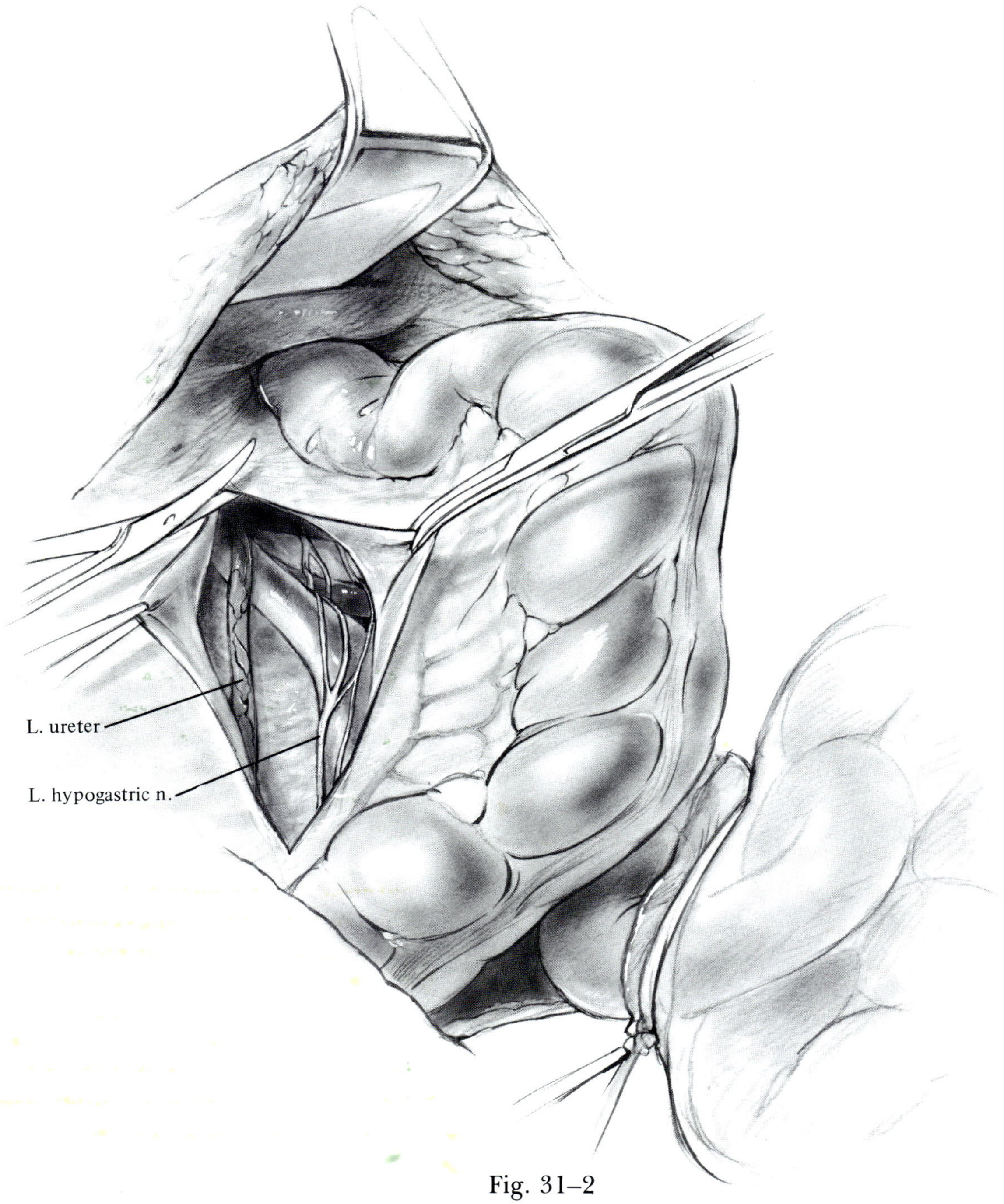

Fig. 31–2

so, identify the left ureter. If its course has not been altered by surgical dissection or pathological changes, the ureter crosses the common iliac artery at the point where the iliac artery bifurcates into its internal and external branches. Tag the ureter with a Vesseloop for later identification.

Use a scissors to continue the peritoneal incision along the left side of the rectum down to the rectovesical pouch (**Fig. 31–3**). Identify the course of the ureter well down into the pelvis. Most tumors that are managed by total proctectomy nowadays are located below the peritoneal reflection. In operating on them, the incision in the peritoneal floor of the pelvis should be designed to preserve as much peritoneum as possible.

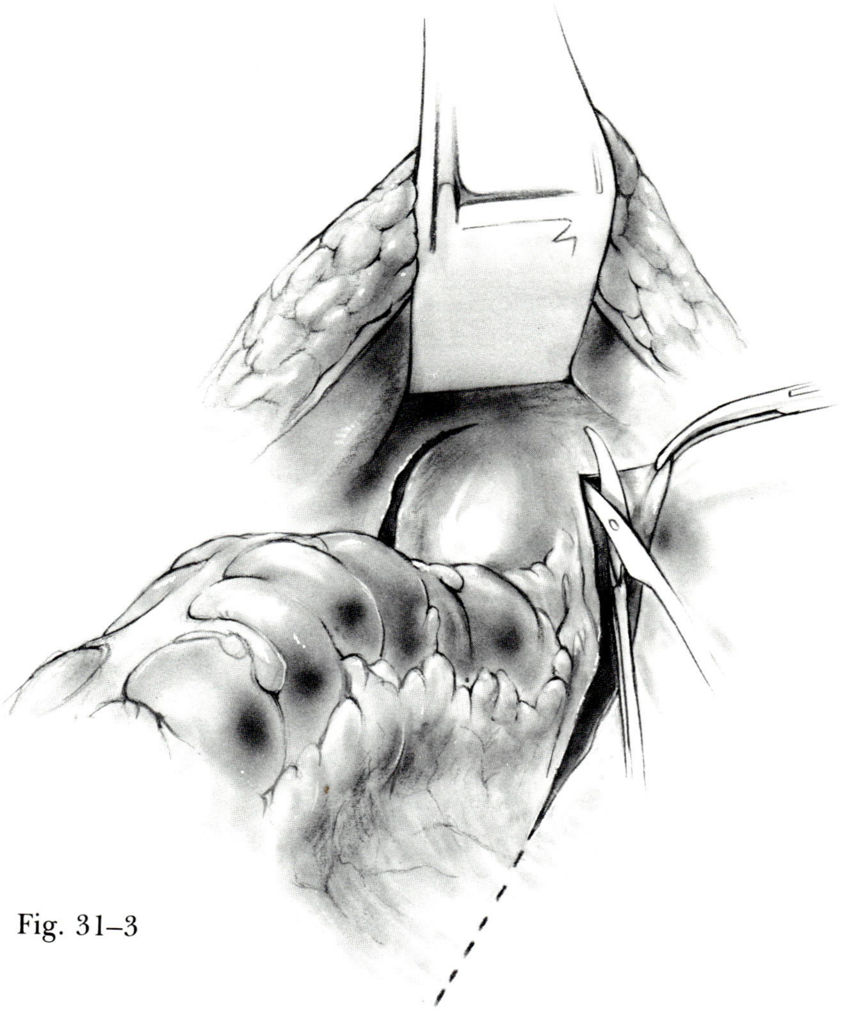

Fig. 31–3

Retract the sigmoid to the patient's left and make an incision on the right side of the sigmoid mesocolon. Begin at a point overlying the bifurcation of the aorta and continue in a caudal direction along the line where the mesosigmoid meets the right lateral leaf of peritoneum in the presacral space. Carry this incision down toward the rectovesical pouch after the right ureter has been identified (Fig. 31–3).

If exposure is convenient, incise the peritoneum of the rectovesical pouch, or rectouterine pouch in the female (**Fig. 31–4**). If exposure is not convenient, this step should be delayed until the presacral dissection has elevated the rectum sufficiently to bring the rectovesical pouch easily into the field of vision.

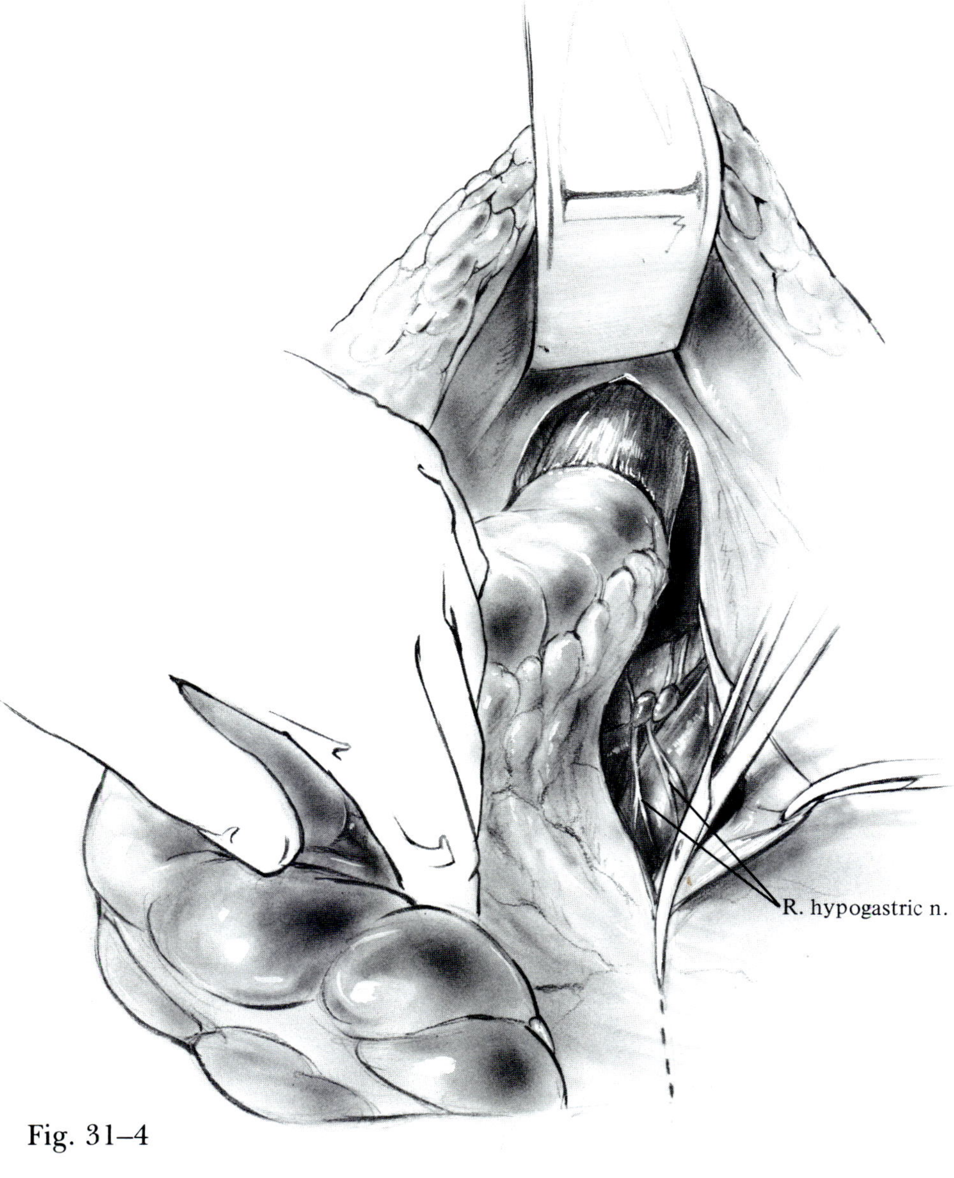

Fig. 31–4

Lymphovascular Dissection

Apply skyward traction to the colon, gently separate the gonadal vein from the lateral leaf of the mesocolon, and allow it to fall to the posterior. Insert an index finger between the deep margin of the mesosigmoid and the bifurcation of the aorta to feel the pulsation of the inferior mesenteric artery lying superficial to the finger. In patients who are markedly obese this vessel may be divided and ligated at the level of the aortic bifurcation without further dissection. In most patients, however, it is quite simple to incise the peritoneum overlying the origin of the inferior mesenteric artery, and to sweep the areolar and lymphatic tissue downward until one sees the point at which the inferior mesenteric artery gives off the left colic branch (Fig. 31–5).

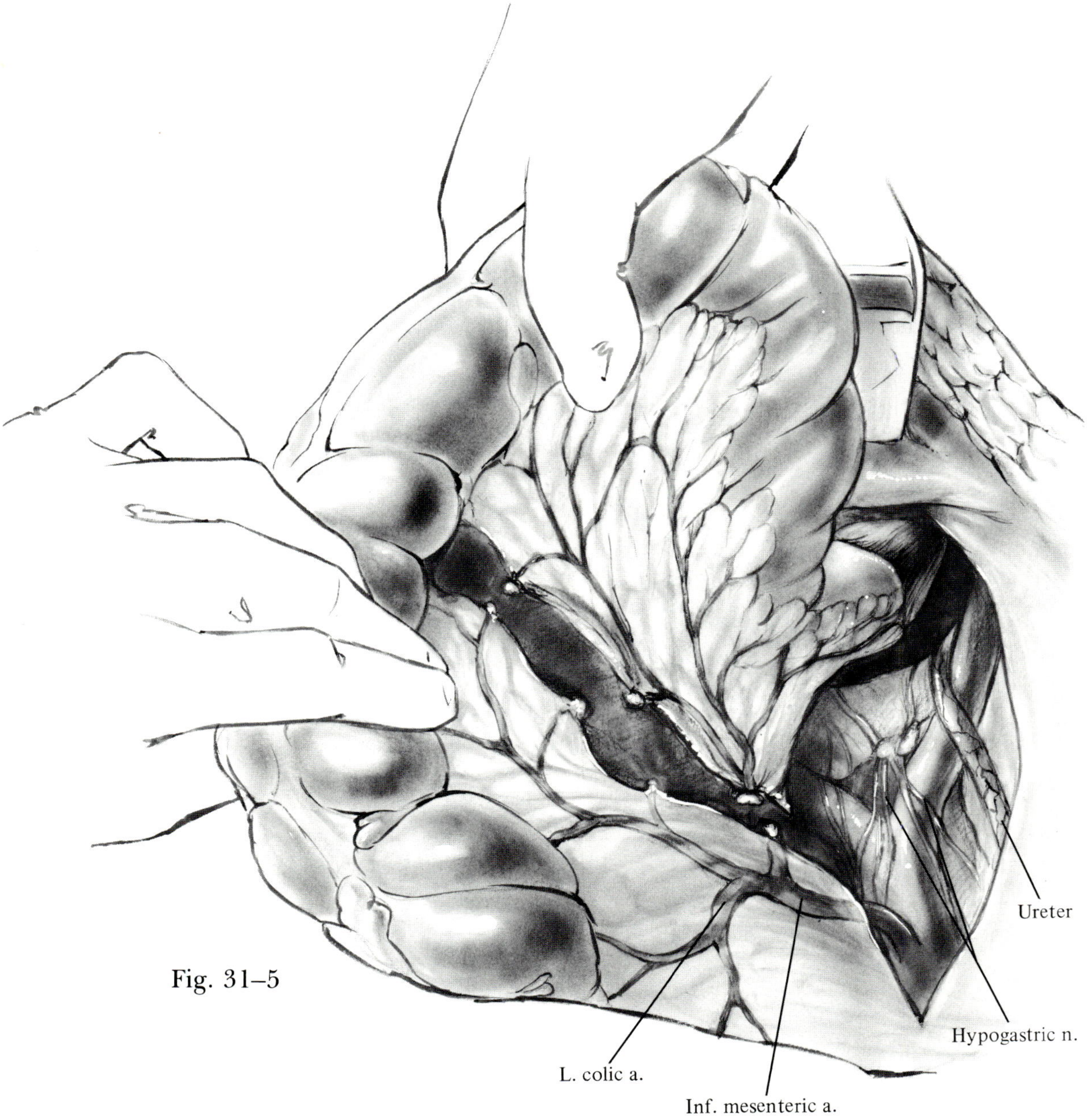

Fig. 31–5

In routine cases divide the inferior mesenteric vessels between 2–0 ligatures just distal to this junction. Then make a superficial scalpel incision along the surface of the mesosigmoid: begin at the point where the inferior mesenteric vessels were divided and continue to the wall of the sigmoid. Complete the division of the mesentery along this line by dividing it between serially applied Kelly hemostats and then ligating with 2–0 cotton or PG (**Fig. 31–5**). In nonobese patients it is feasible to incise the peritoneum up to the point where a vessel is visualized and then to apply hemostats directly to each vessel as it is encountered. With this technique, the surgeon will encounter only one or two vessels on the way to the marginal artery of the colon.

Sweep the mesosigmoid and the lymphovascular bundle (distal to the ligated inferior mesenteric vessels) off the anterior surfaces of the aorta and common iliac vessels by blunt dissection. Leave the preaortic sympathetic nerves intact. To minimize the time during which the patient's abdomen is exposed to possible fecal contamination, do not divide the sigmoid colon at this stage.

Presacral Dissection

With the lower sigmoid on steady upward retraction, it becomes evident that there is a band of tissue extending from the sacrum to the posterior rectum. On either side of this band there is only areolar tissue. Any tendency on the part of the surgeon to insert a hand into the presacral space at this stage should be stoutly resisted. Instead, a long, closed Metzenbaum scissors should be used as a blunt dissector (Fig. 31–6a). Insert it first to the right of the midline behind the rectum, and by gently elevating the mesorectum the proper presacral plane will be entered.

Repeat this maneuver identically on the left side of the midsacral line. Then direct attention to the remaining band of tissue, which contains branches of the middle sacral artery, and divide it with scissors after applying large Hemoclips (**Fig. 31–6a**).

At this time the surgeon will see a thin layer of fibroareolar tissue covering the sacrum. If a shiny layer of sacral periosteum, ligaments, or the naked presacral veins can be seen (**Fig. 31–6b**), the plane of dissection is *too deep,* presenting the danger of major venous hemorrhage. Elevate the *distal* rectum from the lower sacrum with gauze in a sponge holder. If the dissection has been completed properly, as described, note that the preaortic sympathetic nerves divide into two major trunks in the upper sacral area and then continue laterally to the right and left walls of the pelvis (Fig. 31–6a). Gently dissect these off the posterior wall of the specimen, unless the specimen has been invaded by tumor.

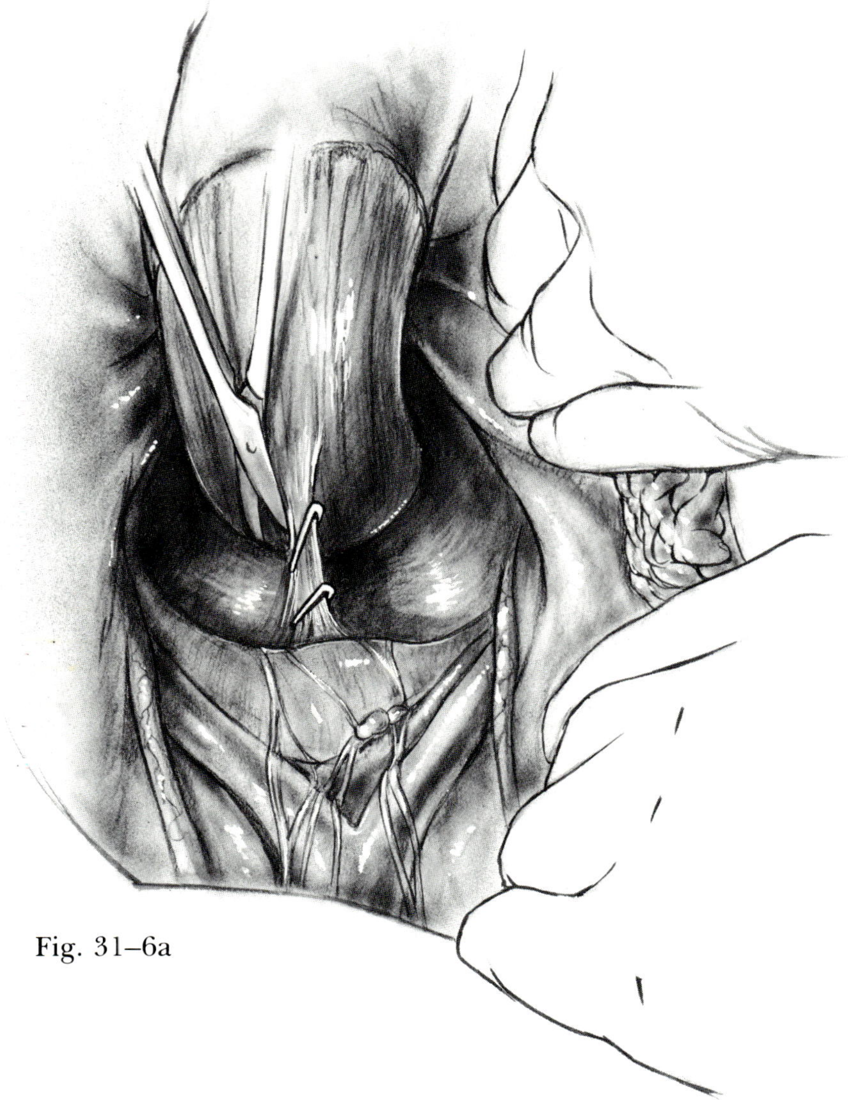

Fig. 31–6a

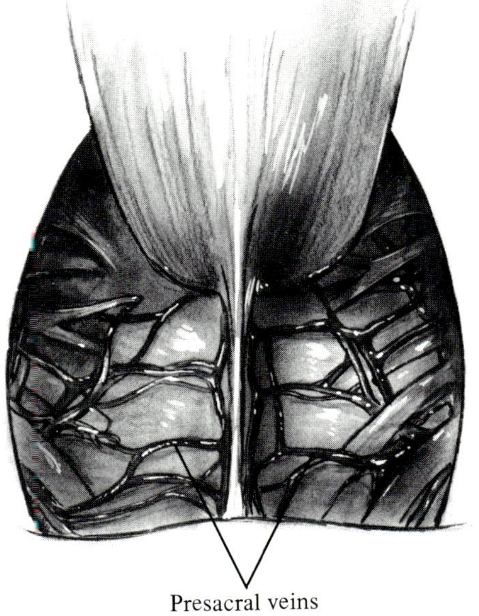

Fig. 31–6b

Now the surgeon may insert a hand into the presacral space, with the objective not of penetrating more deeply toward the coccyx, but rather of extending the presacral dissection laterally to the right and to the left, so that the posterior aspect of the specimen is elevated from the sacrum as far as the lateral ligament on each side. Place the lateral ligament on the left side on stretch by applying traction to the rectum toward the right. Apply large Hemoclips and divide the ligament between them (**Fig. 31–7**). In some cases the ligament may be 2 cm or more in width, so that additional pairs of Hemoclips may be needed.

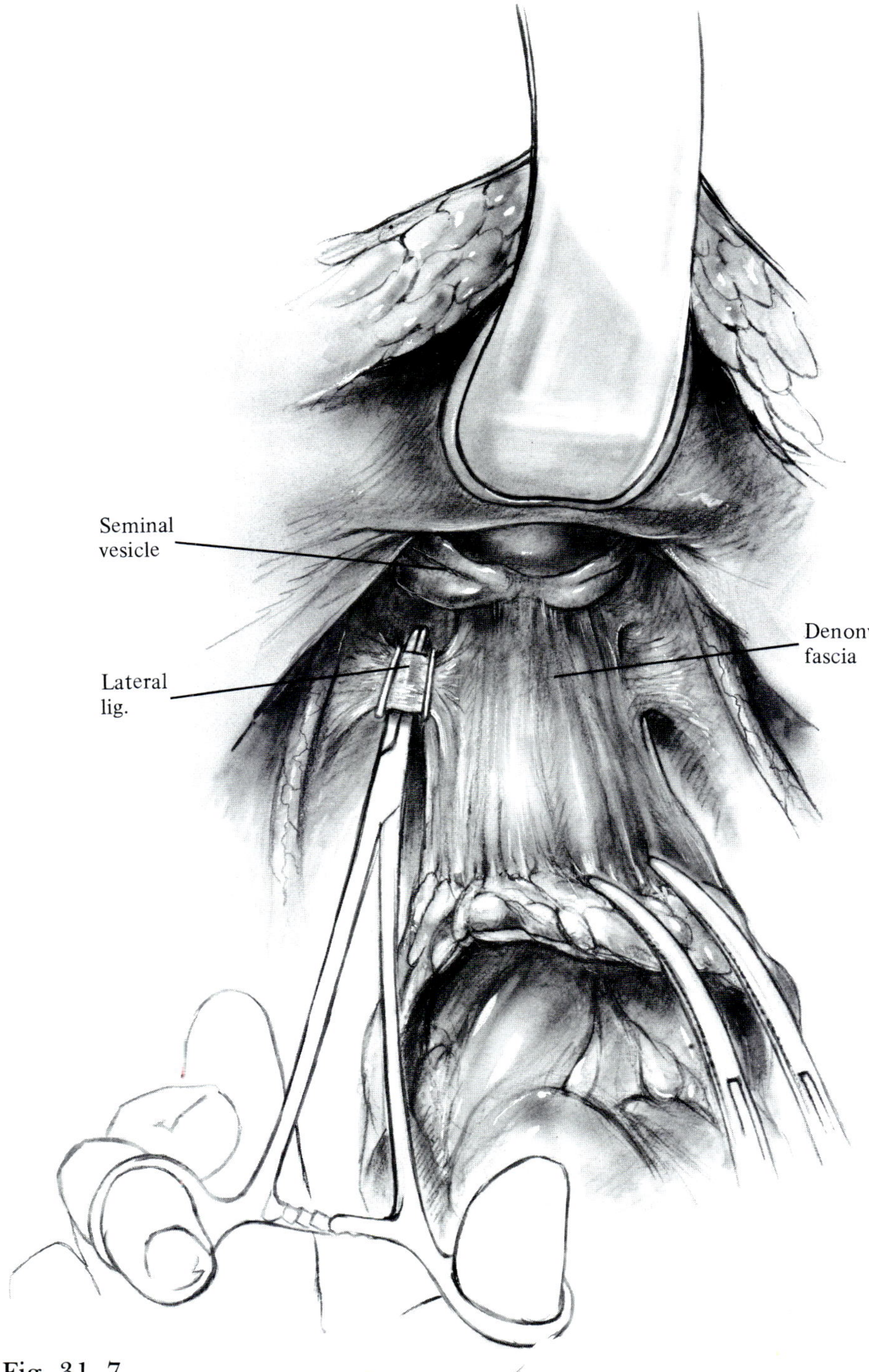

Fig. 31–7

Carry out a similar maneuver to divide the right lateral ligament. Before dividing each lateral ligament, recheck the position of the respective ureter and hypogastric nerve to be certain they lie lateral to the point of division. If for some reason difficulty is encountered in performing this step, division of the lateral ligaments may be delayed until perineal exposure has been achieved. This will permit clear identification of the ligaments by simultaneous visualization from above and from below.

The next step in exposing the levator diaphragm from above is to divide the fascia of Waldeyer, which extends from the coccyx to the posterior rectal wall (**Fig. 31–8**). This structure blocks the surgeon's hand from passing beyond the coccygeal area. Incise the fascia with a long Metzenbaum scissors. Do not injure the veins that run along the surface of the coccyx when incising this fascia.

Now direct attention to the anterior dissection. Use a Lloyd-Davies retractor to pull the bladder (in women, the uterus) in an anterior and caudal direction. If the peritoneum of the rectovesical pouch has not already been incised, perform this maneuver now, thereby connecting the incisions in the pelvic peritoneum previously made on the right and left sides of the rectum (see Fig. 31–4). Apply one or more

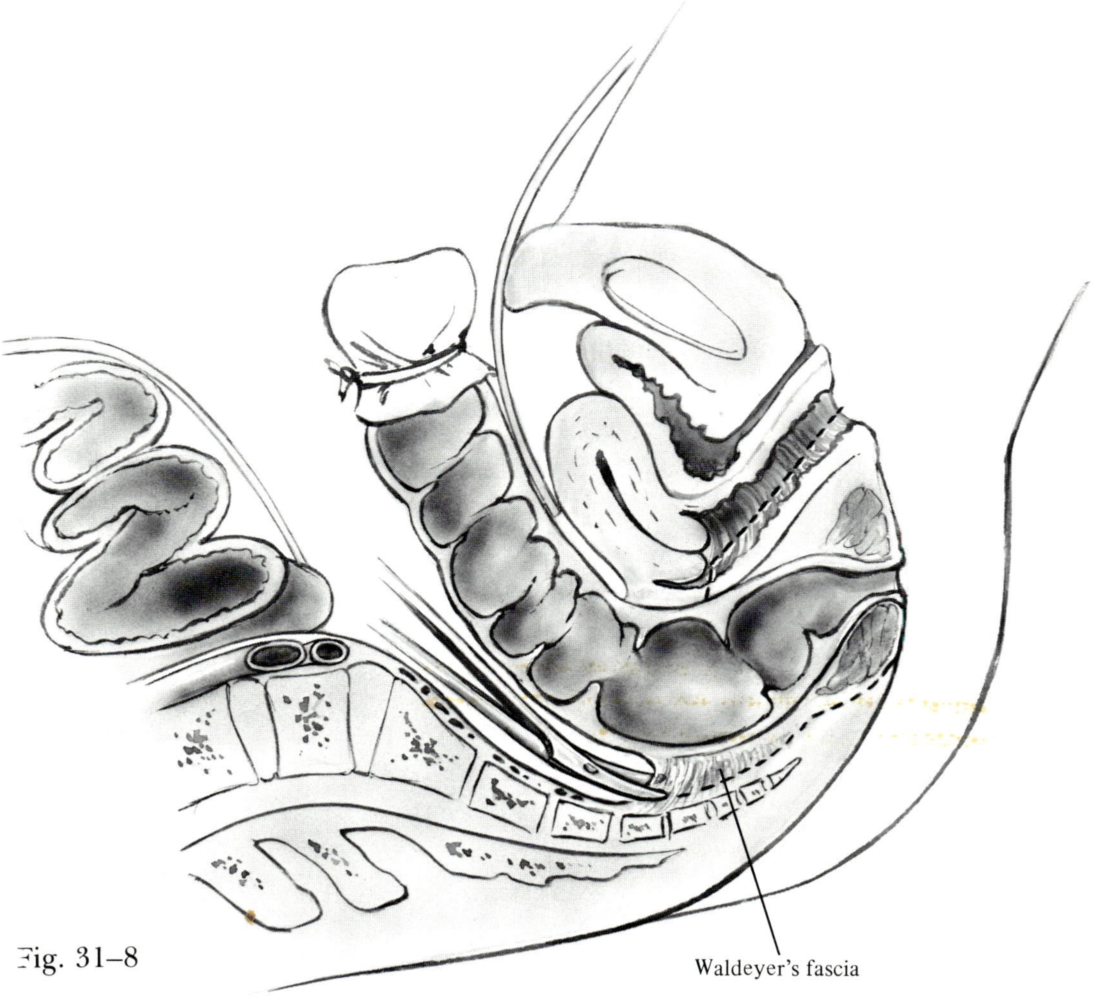

Fig. 31–8

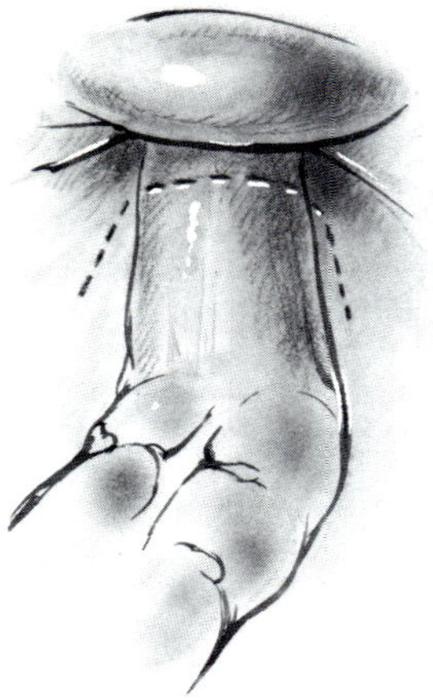

Fig. 31–9a

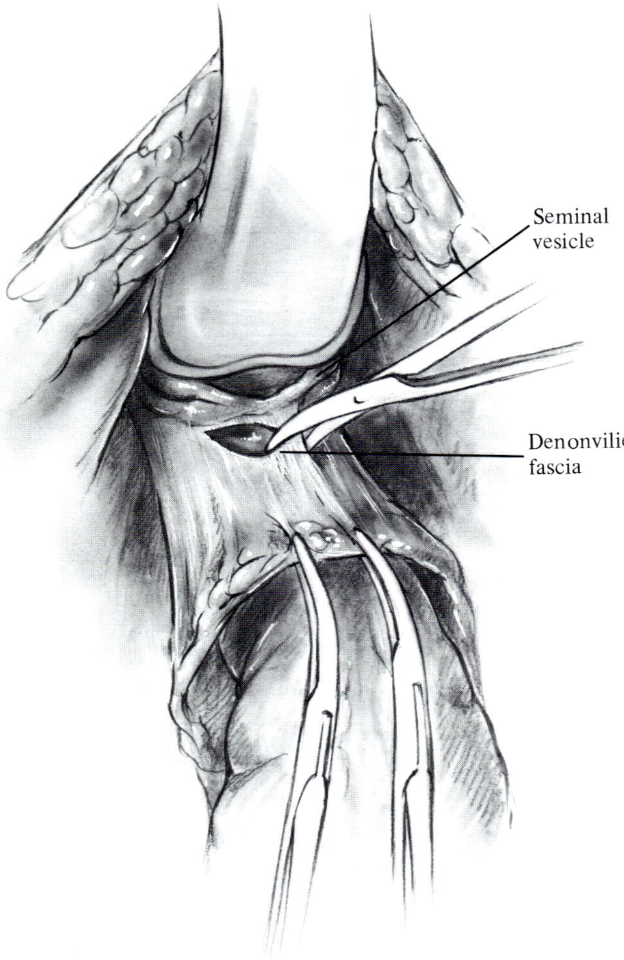

Fig. 31–9b

long hemostats or forceps to the posterior lip of the incised peritoneum of the rectovesical pouch. Place traction on these hemostats to draw the peritoneum and Denonvillier's fascia in a cephalad and posterior direction, and use Metzenbaum scissors dissection to dissect this layer from the seminal vesicles and prostate (**Figs. 31–9a and 31–9b**). Use blunt finger dissection to separate the rectum from the posterior wall of the prostate. Finally, secure hemostasis in this region by electrocoagulating multiple bleeding points.

In female patients the anterior dissection is somewhat simpler. With a Harrington retractor elevating the uterus, use scalpel dissection to initiate the plane of dissection elevating the peritoneum and fascia of Denonvillier from the posterior lip of the cervix until the proximal vagina has been exposed. If it is elected to remove the posterior wall of the vagina along with the specimen, this is more easily done during the perineal dissection. Some surgeons routinely perform bilateral salpingo-oophorectomy in women who have rectal and sigmoid cancer, because the ovaries are sometimes a site of metastatic deposit. Whether this step is of value has not been ascertained. We do not perform this maneuver in the absence of visible metastasis to the ovaries.

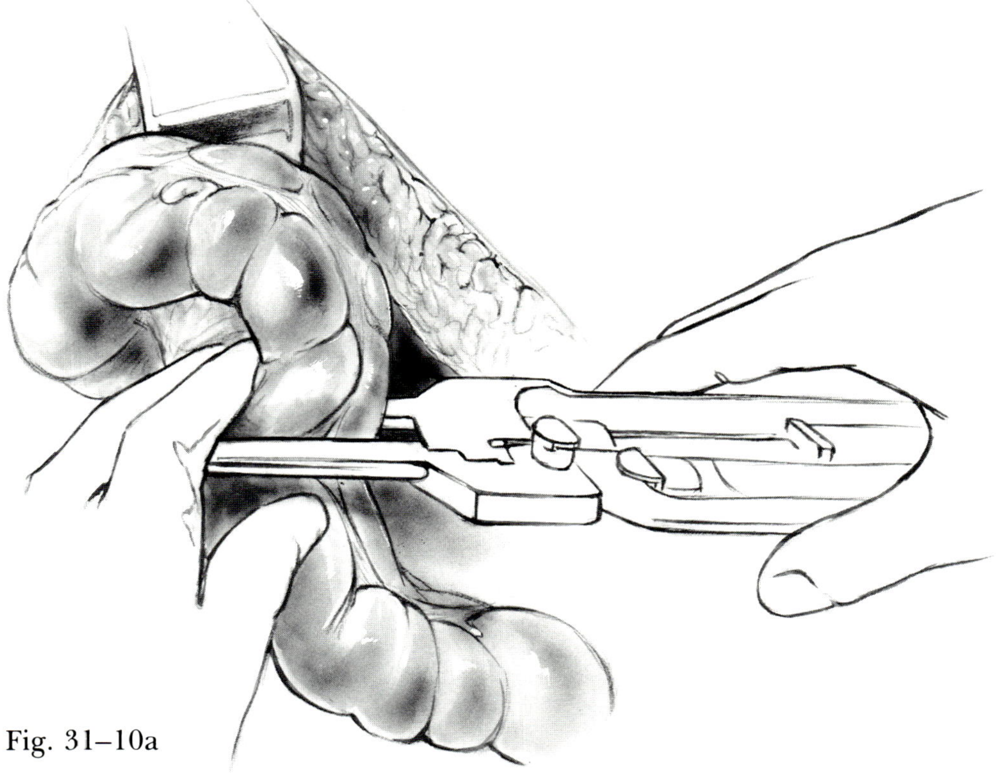

Fig. 31–10a

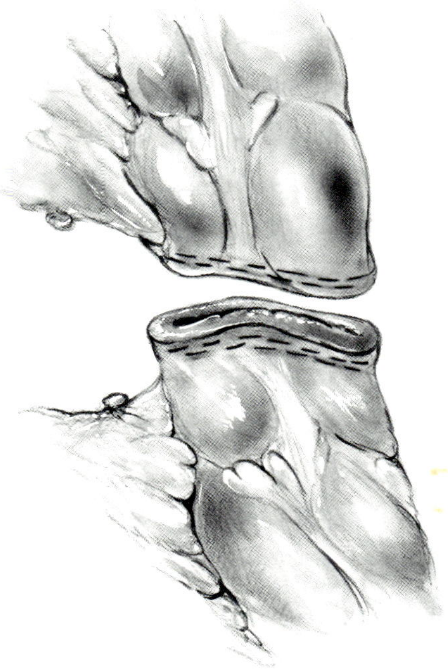

Fig. 31–10b

The last step in the abdominal portion of the procedure is to divide the sigmoid colon at a point that will permit the proximal colon to be brought out of the abdominal incision with at least 5 cm of slack. Use the GIA stapling device; it will simultaneously apply staples and divide the colon (**Figs. 31–10a and 31–10b**). Tie a rubber glove over the end of the distal sigmoid to preserve sterility (**Figs. 31–11a and 31–11b**). After this step abandon the abdominal dissection temporarily and initiate the perineal stage.

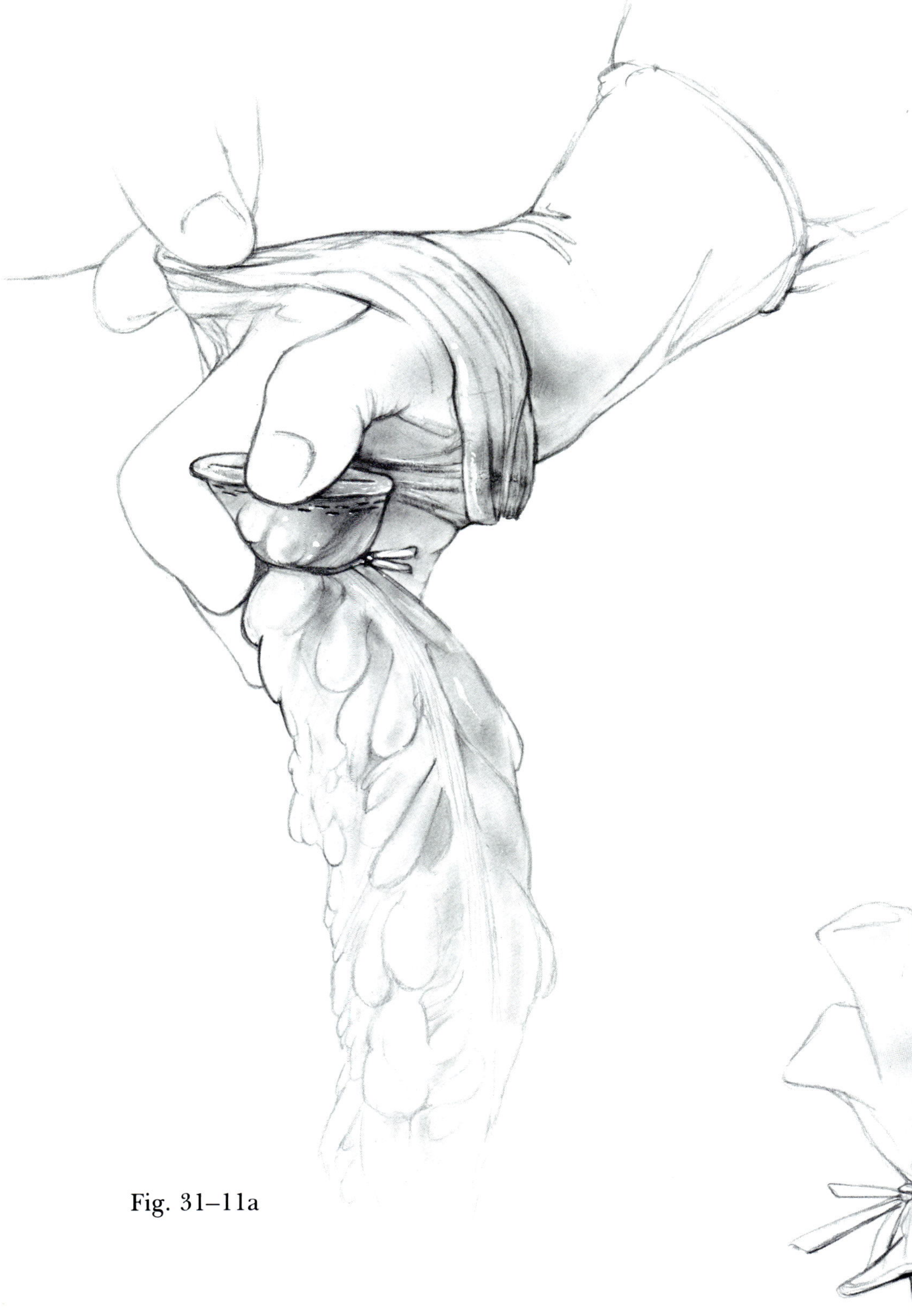

Fig. 31–11a

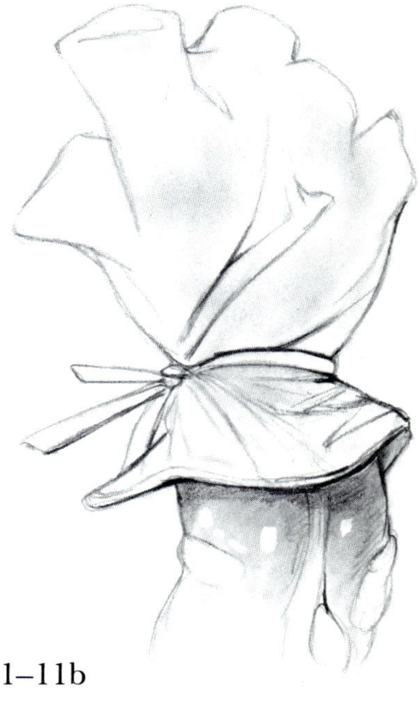

Fig. 31–11b

Pelvic Hemostasis

The entire pelvic dissection, if properly performed, should entail minimal blood loss. While Hemoclips may control clearly identified vessels along the lateral wall of the pelvis, they are rarely useful in the presacral area. Here the vessels consist of thin-walled veins, which are easily torn by metallic clips either in the act of application or during the act of sponging the area later. Except for a small, clearly defined bleeding point that can be held in a forceps, electrocoagulation may also be hazardous, as the coagulating tip may act as a scalpel and convert a small bleeding point into a major venous laceration. Here, a ball-tipped electrode is safer than those with sharp tips.

Almost invariably, presacral bleeding is the result of a tear in one of the veins that drain into the presacral foramina. If the hemorrhage cannot be controlled *promptly* with a hemostat, the area of bleeding should be covered by a sheet of Surgicel over which pressure should be applied with a large gauze pack. If the area of bleeding is only 1–2 cm in diameter, at a later stage in the operation an attempt may be made to remove the gauze pack, leaving the small piece of cellulose. This may result in complete hemostasis. If not, leave the gauze pack in the presacral space for 24–48 hours; then remove it under direct vision and under general anesthesia via the reopened perineal incision.

Perineal Dissection

The anus is already closed by a heavy, silk purse-string suture. In male patients make an elliptical incision in the skin beginning at a point 3–4 cm anterior to the anal orifice and terminating at the tip of the coccyx (**Fig. 31–12**). In females who have small posterior lesions make the incision from a point just behind the vaginal introitus to the tip of the coccyx. For anterior lesions in women, leave a patch of posterior vagina, including the posterior portion of the vaginal introitus, attached to the rectum in the region of the tumor (**Figs. 31–13 and 31–14**).

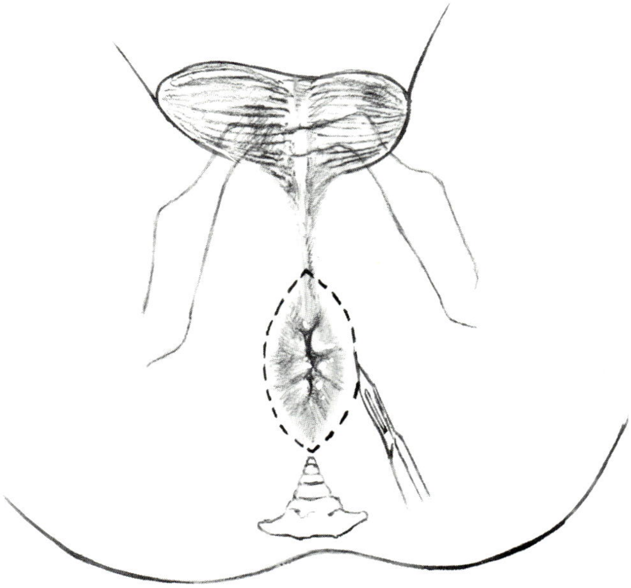

Fig. 31–12

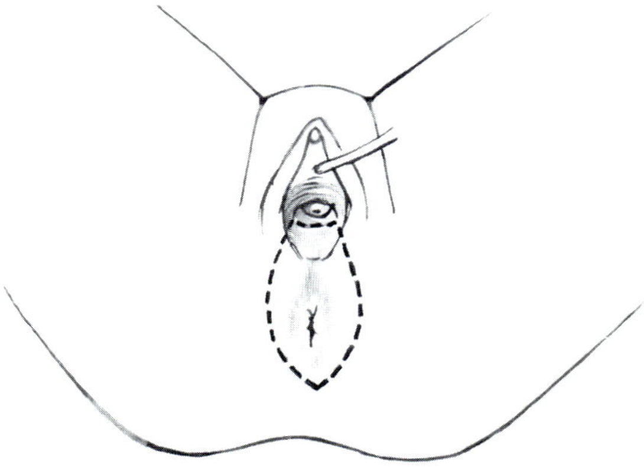

Fig. 31–13

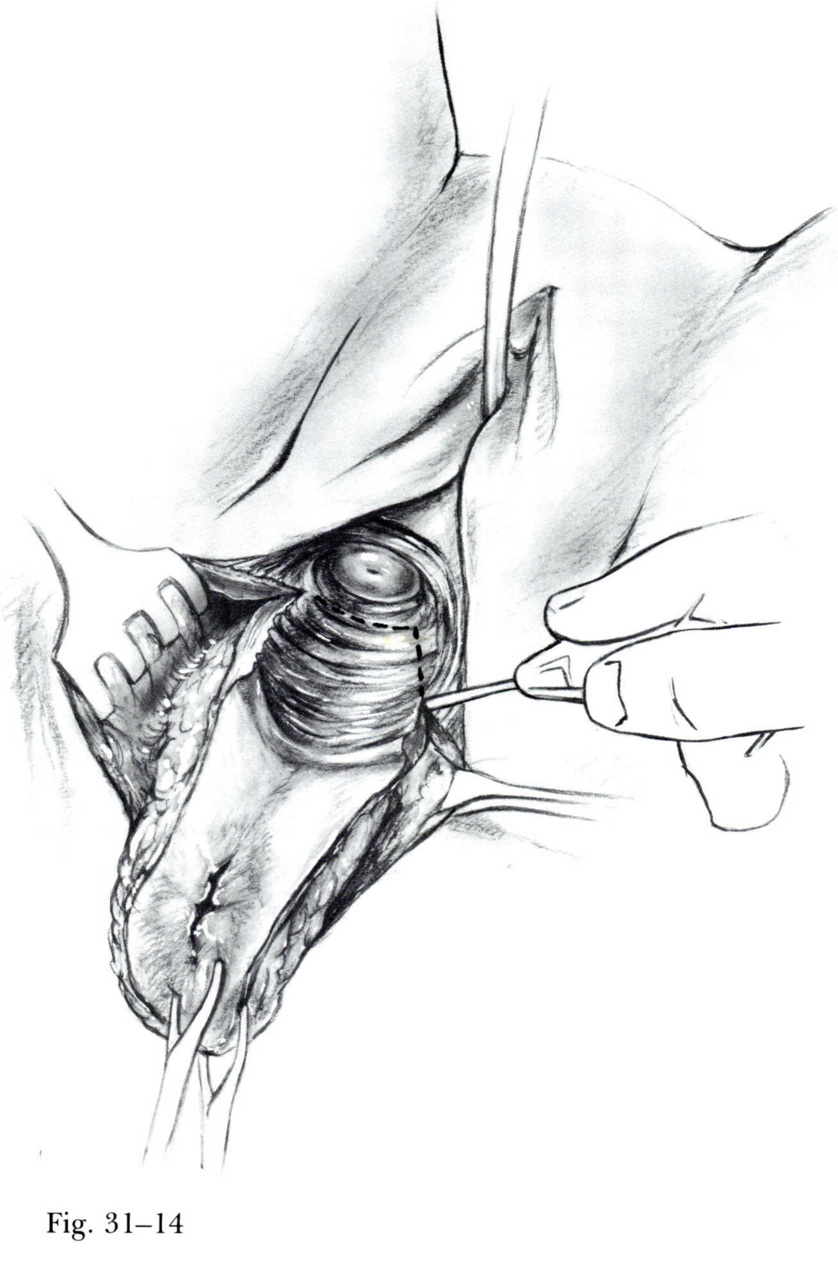

Fig. 31–14

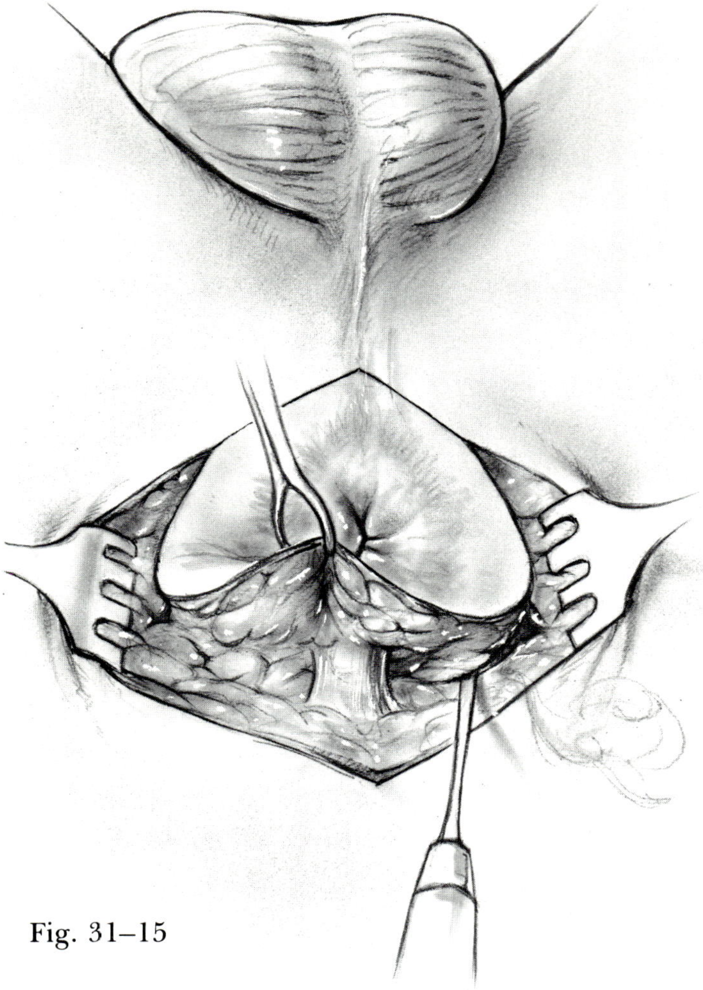

Fig. 31–15

In all cases carry the scalpel incision down into the perirectal fat and then grasp the ellipse of skin to be removed in three Allis clamps. While the anus is retracted to the patient's right, have the assistant insert a rake retractor to draw the skin of the perineum to the patient's left. Then incise the perirectal fat down to the levator diaphragm (**Fig. 31–15**). Generally, two branches of the inferior hemorrhoidal vessels will appear in the perirectal fat just superficial to the levators. Each may be occluded by electrocoagulation. Accomplish the identical procedure on the right side of the perineum.

After identifying the anococcygeal ligament at the tip of the coccyx, use the electrocoagulator to divide this ligament transversely from its attachment to the tip of the coccyx (**Figs. 31–16 and 31–17**). Note at this point that if the surgeon's index finger is inserted anterior to the tip of

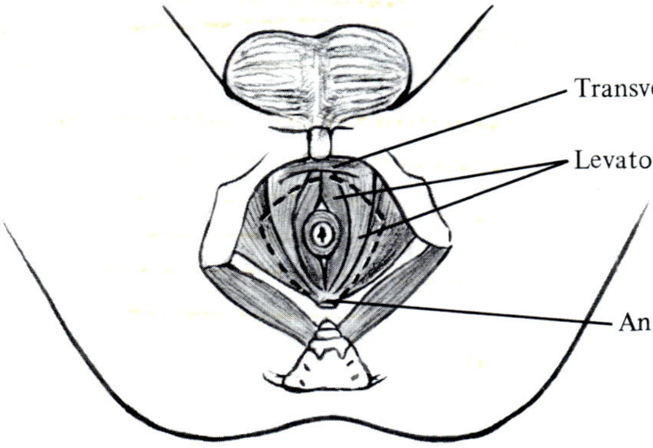

Fig. 31–16

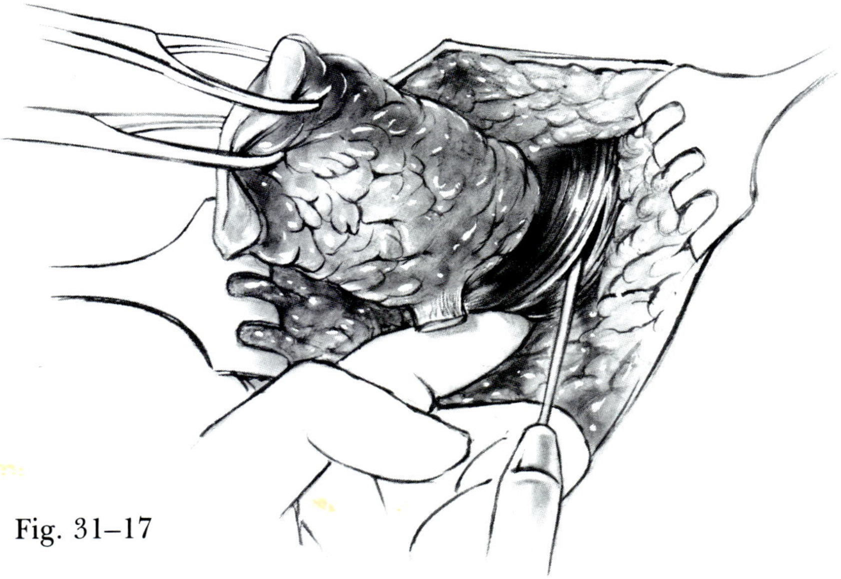

Fig. 31–17

the coccyx, it may be unable to enter the presacral space. A dense condensation of fascia (Waldeyer's fascia) attaches the posterior rectum to the presacral and precoccygeal area. If this fascia is torn off the sacrum by blunt technique, the presacral venous plexus may be entered, producing hemorrhage. Therefore, Waldeyer's fascia must be incised either at the termination of the abdominal portion of the presacral dissection or at the present stage in the perineal dissection. From the perineal aspect this is a simple maneuver, as it requires only sharp division of the fascia with a scalpel or electrocautery in the plane just deep to the anococcygeal ligament. As soon as this is accomplished it becomes evident that the abdominal and perineal phases of the dissection have joined.

The surgeon should then insert the left index finger beneath the left side of the levator diaphragm, and with the electrocoagulating current transect the levator muscles upward beginning from below, leaving a portion of the diaphragm attached to the specimen (**Fig. 31–17**). Continue this incision in the muscular diaphragm up to the region of the puborectalis sling on the anterior aspect of the perineum, but not through it.

Use the identical procedure to divide the right-hand portion of the levator diaphragm.

Because the greatest danger of the perineal dissection in males is the risk of traumatizing the urethra, the anterior portion of the dissection should be delayed until all the other landmarks in this area have been delineated. To facilitate this delineation, the transected rectosigmoid specimen may be delivered through the opening in the posterior perineum at this time (**Fig. 31–18**). Insert an index fin-

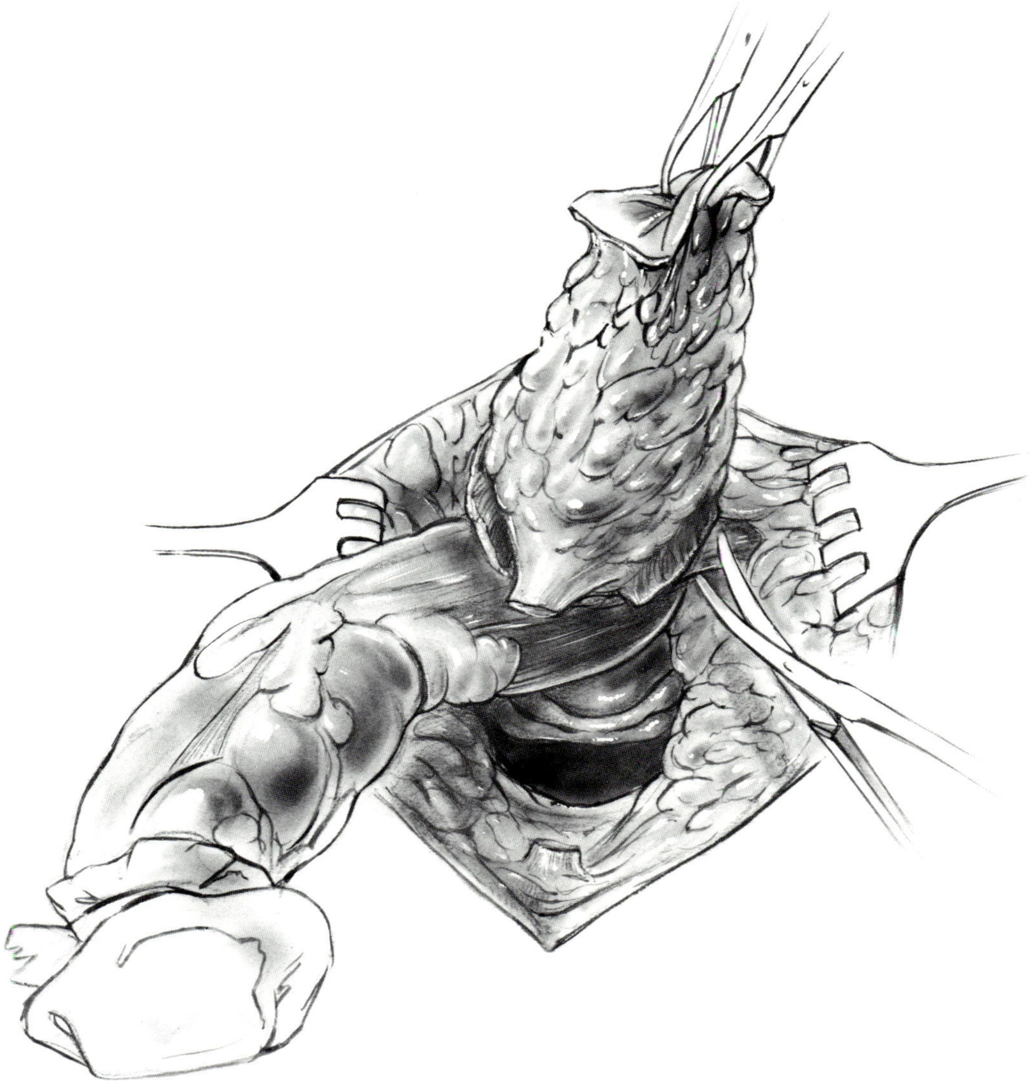

Fig. 31–18

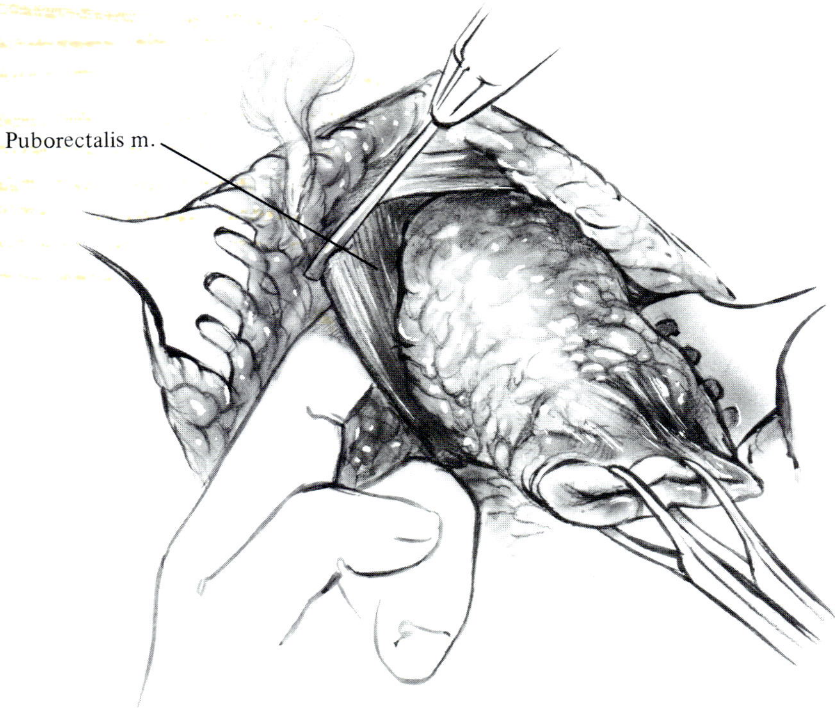

Fig. 31–19

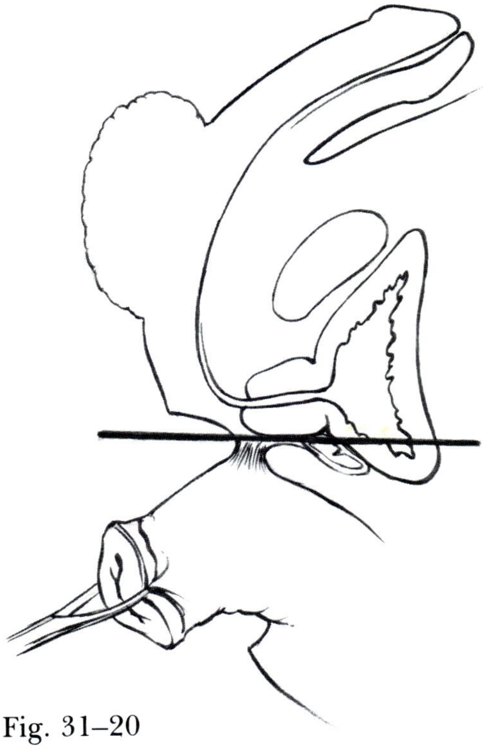

Fig. 31–20

ger beneath the puborectalis muscle and transect it with the electrocoagulator (**Figs. 31–18 and 31–19**). The prostate will have been exposed during the abdominal dissection; at this time palpate it and visualize it from below. Make a projection of the plane along the posterior aspect of the prostate gland (**Fig. 31–20**). Where this

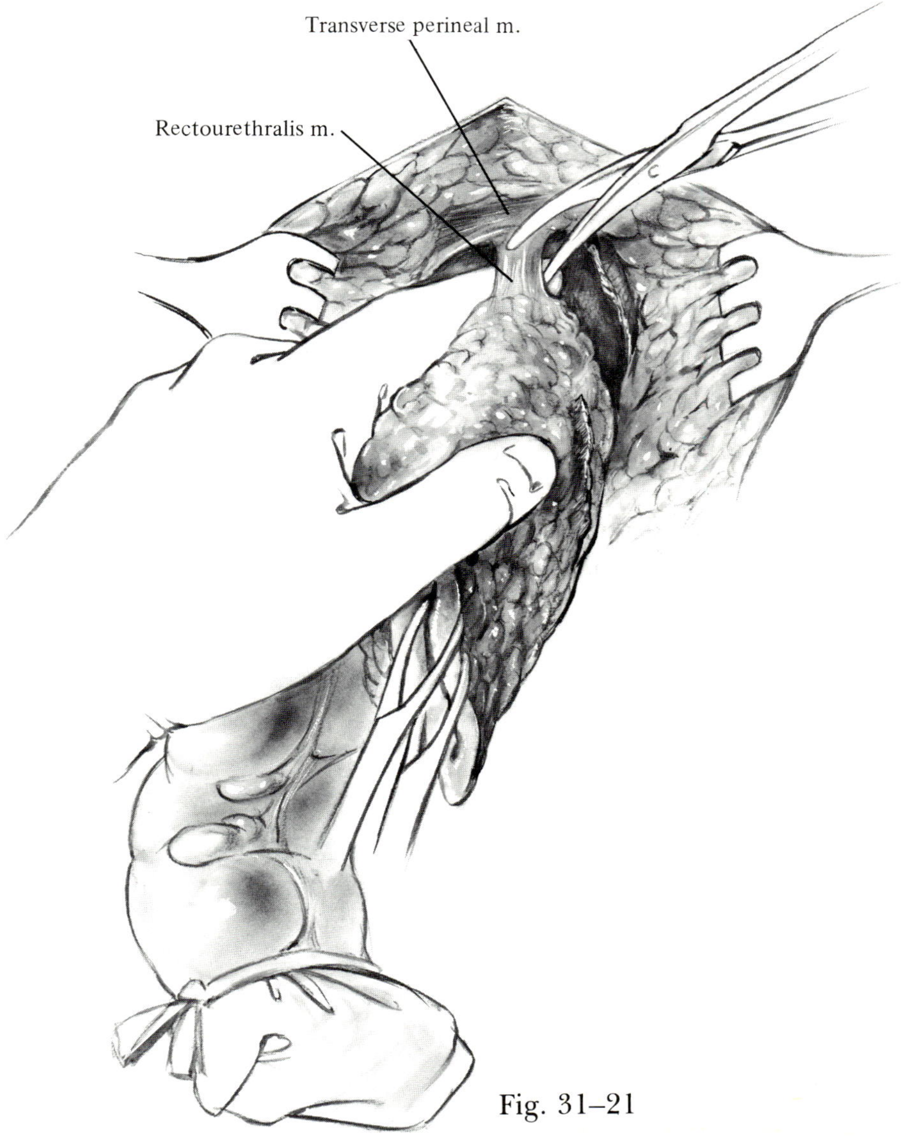

Fig. 31–21

plane crosses the rectourethralis muscle, the muscle may be transected safely and the specimen removed (**Fig. 31–21**). Another landmark, which is sometimes difficult to identify in obese patients, is the superficial transverse perineal muscles. The anterior plane of dissection should be posterior to these muscles. Finally, divide the remaining attachments to the prostate (**Fig. 31–22**) and remove the specimen.

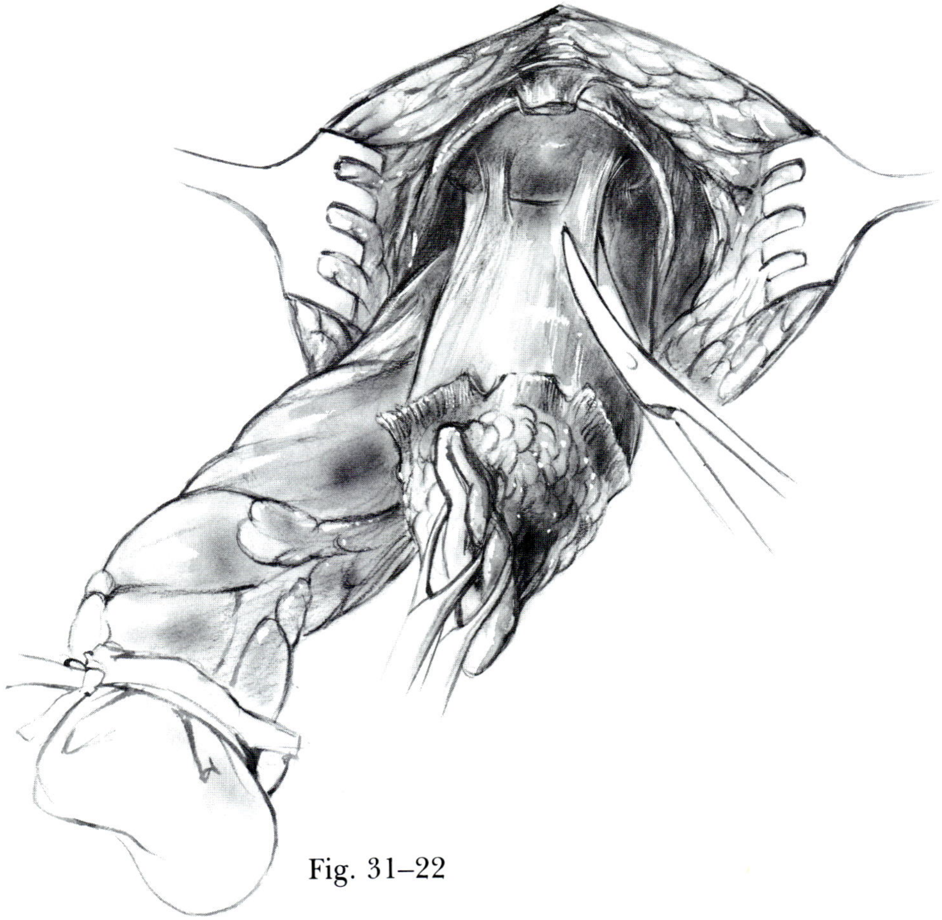

Fig. 31–22

In females the above precautions do not apply. If the vagina is to be preserved, the anterior dissection should follow a plane just posterior to the vagina. The wall of the vagina should not be traumatized or devascularized during this dissection, as this may well lead to perineovaginal fistula, which is difficult to manage. It is better to excise the posterior wall of the vagina than to partially devascularize it during the dissection. If the posterior wall of the vagina is to be removed, use the electrocautery to continue the perineal skin incision across the vaginal introitus (Fig. 31–14). When the vagina is incised by electrocoagulation, complete hemostasis is easily attained. Leave a patch of vagina of appropriate dimensions attached to the specimen.

Irrigate the presacral space with a dilute antibiotic solution. Hemostasis should be absolute and complete. This is easily accomplished using electrocoagulation and ligatures as one assistant works from above and the surgeon works from below.

Management of Pelvic Floor

In females whose posterior vaginal wall remains intact, and in all males, the perineum may be closed per primam if there has been no fecal contamination and if hemostasis is excellent. First, accomplish

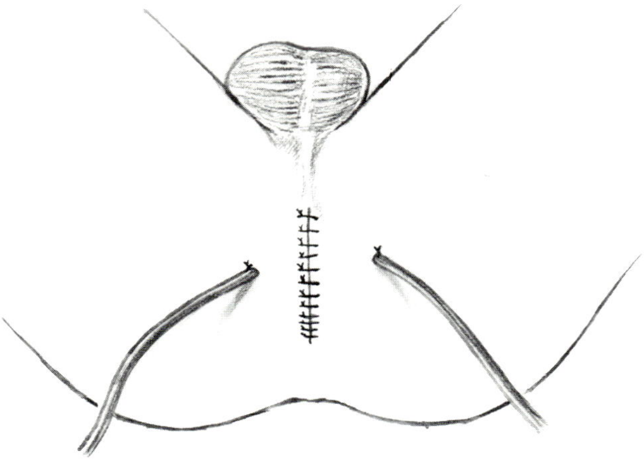

Fig. 31–23

presacral drainage by inserting two closed-suction drainage catheters, each 6 mm in diameter. Introduce one catheter through a puncture wound of the skin in the posterior portion of the perineum about 4 cm to the left of the coccyx, and a second through a similar point at the right. Suture each catheter to the skin surrounding its exit wound (**Fig. 31–23**). Place the tips of the catheters in the presacral space. In some cases the posterior levator diaphragm may be partially reconstructed, using 2–0 PG sutures. Accomplish the remainder of the perineal closure with one or two layers of interrupted PG to the subcutaneous fat and a subcuticular suture of 4–0 PG to close the skin. As soon as the abdominal surgeon has closed the pelvic peritoneum, apply continuous suction to the two drainage catheters in order to draw the peritoneum down to the newly reconstructed pelvic floor. The surgeon's aim must be to *eliminate any possible dead space* between the peritoneal closure and the pelvic floor.

When the posterior vaginal wall and the specimen have been excised, attempt to fabricate a substitute posterior wall with interrupted PG sutures to the perineal fat and to the residual levator muscle (**Fig. 31–24**). If this can be accomplished, within a few months after the operation the vaginal mucosa will grow over this newly constructed pelvic floor, restoring the vaginal tube. Pack the posterior defect loosely with sterile gauze. This should be brought out through the newly reconstructed vaginal introitus after the remainder of the perineal fat and skin have been closed, as described above (**Fig. 31–25**). If it is deemed desirable, a sump catheter can be brought out from the presacral space through the same defect, but this is not a routine procedure.

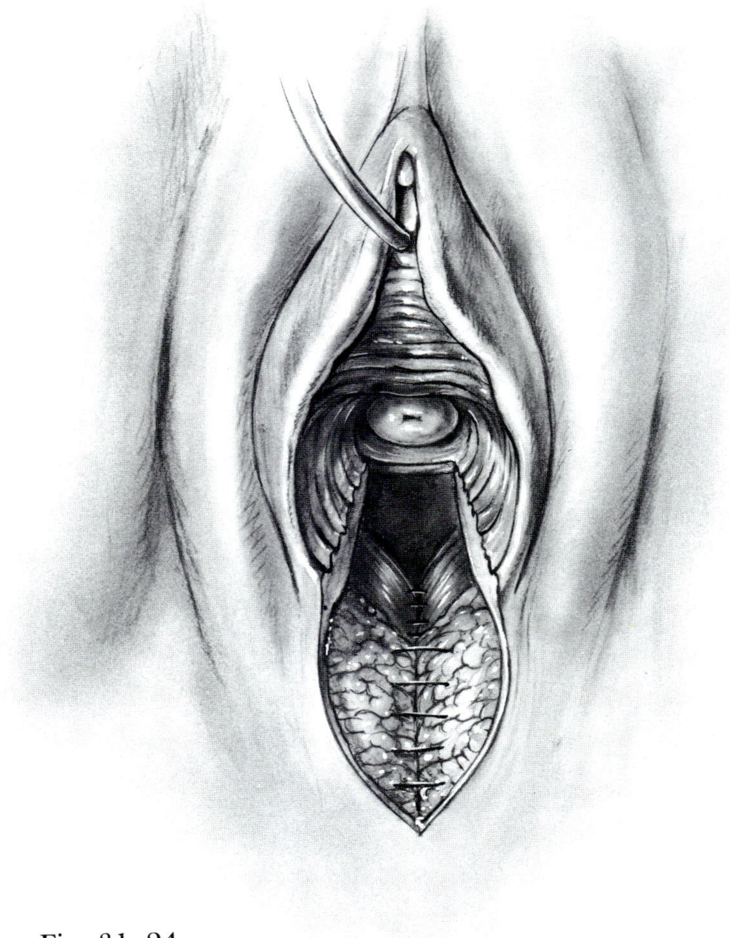

Fig. 31–24

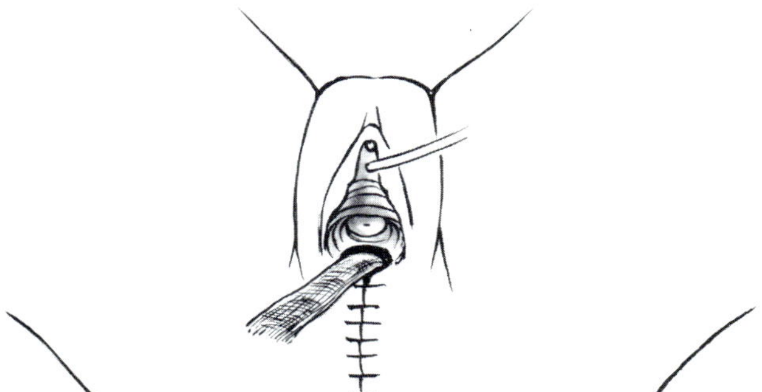

Fig. 31–25

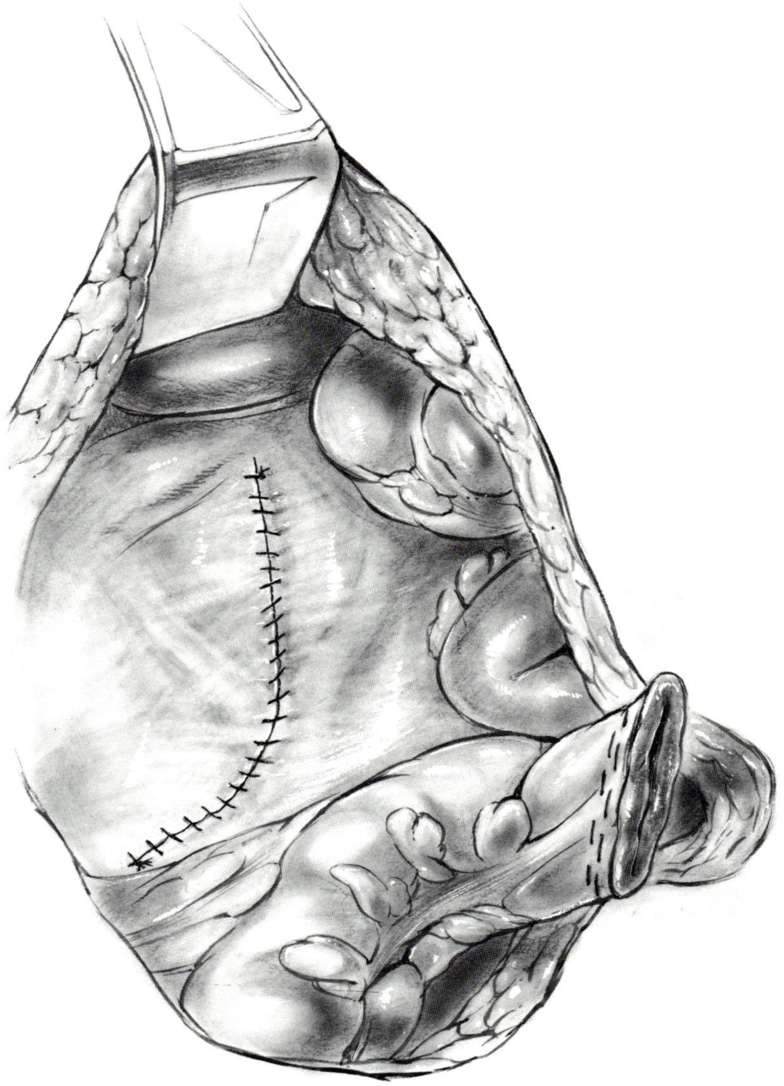

Fig. 31–26

While the assistant is closing the perineum, the surgeon should return to the abdominal approach to dissect the pelvic peritoneum free from its surrounding attachments to the lateral pelvic walls and bladder. This enables the peritoneum to be closed without tension (**Fig. 31–26**). Use a continuous atraumatic suture of 2–0 PG. If there is insufficient peritoneum to permit the peritoneal diaphragm to descend to the level of the newly constructed perineal floor, leave the peritoneum completely unsutured.

Colostomy

The colostomy may be brought out through the upper portion of the midline incision, in which case it is not necessary to close the intraperitoneal gap lateral to the colostomy. Through the midline incision, at a point where 5 cm will protrude from the anterior abdominal skin surface without tension, bring out the segment of colon previously selected for formation of the colostomy. If this point is near the umbilicus, excise the umbilicus for greater postoperative cleanliness. Close the abdominal wall with one layer of monofilament 2–0 stainless steel wire; an index finger should fit without tension between the colostomy and the next adjoining wire suture. Close the skin above and below the colostomy with a continuous subcuticular suture of 4–0 PG. Before closing the skin, insert a small plastic catheter with many perforations through a puncture wound in the skin of the suprapubic region and bring it up along the anterior rectus fascia almost to the level of the colostomy. This provides closed-suction drainage for 4 days, as well as an avenue for the intermittent subcutaneous administration of antibiotics (see Chap. 2).

After all these steps have been completed, excise the line of staples previously used to occlude the colon. Immediately mature the colostomy, using interrupted or continuous sutures of 4–0 PG to attach the full thickness of the colon to the subcuticular plane of the skin (**Figs. 31–27 and 31–28**). No additional sutures are necessary to attach the colon to the fascia or to any other layer of the abdominal wall.

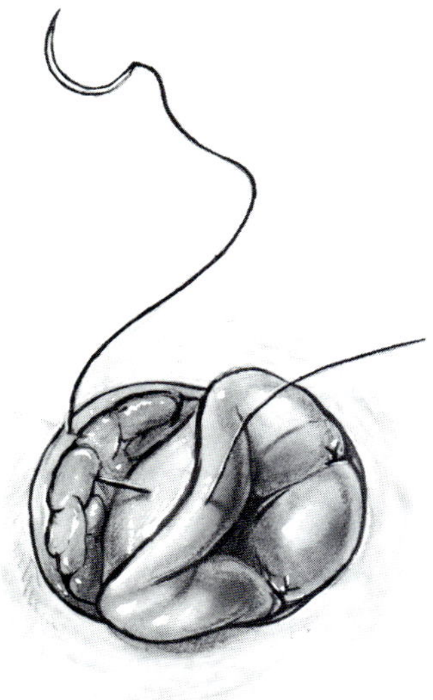

Fig. 31–27

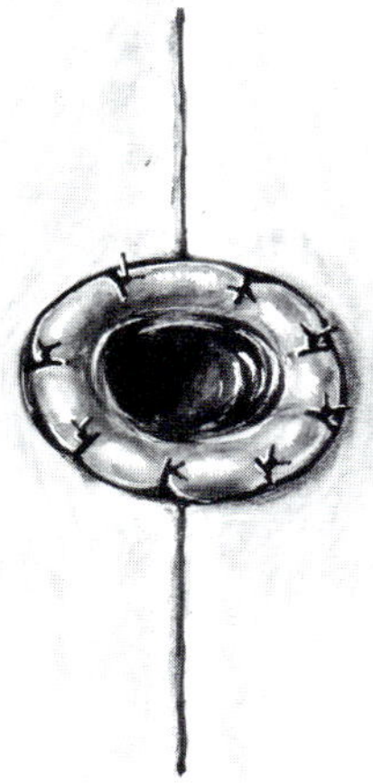

Fig. 31–28

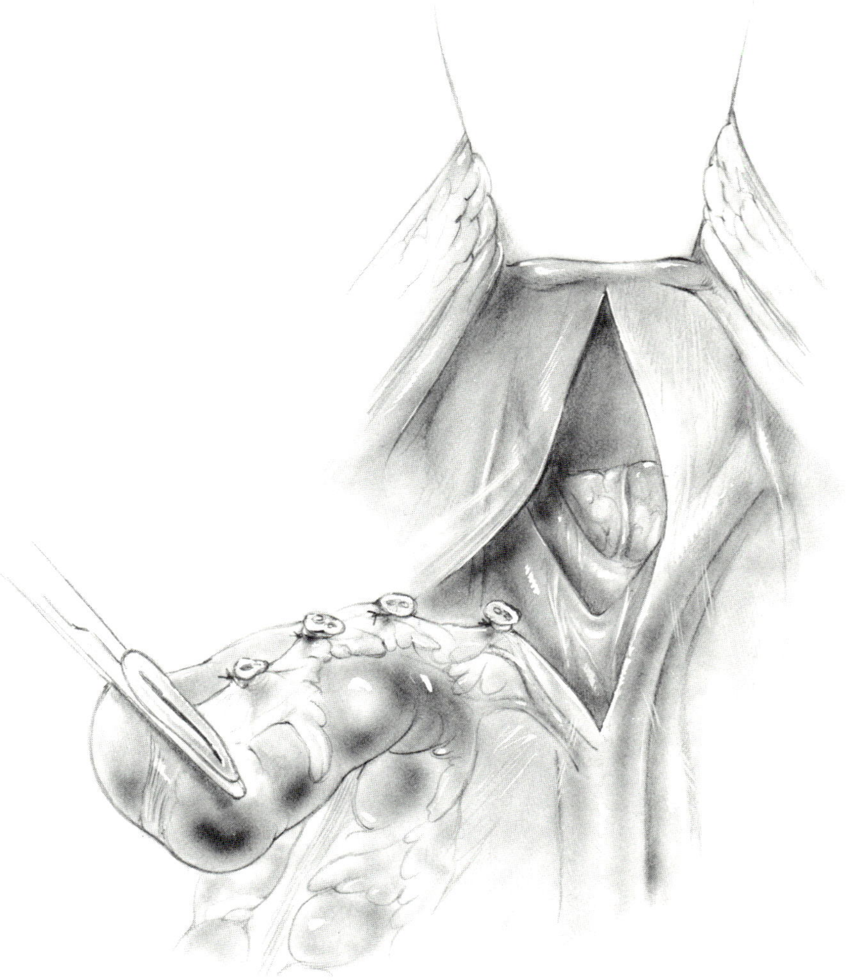

Fig. 31–29

When the peritoneal pelvic floor is suitable for reconstruction by suturing, the retroperitoneal type of colostomy may be performed. Elevate the previously incised peritoneum of the left paracolic gutter from the lateral abdominal wall by finger dissection. Continue until a hand is freely admitted up to the point in the lateral portion of the rectus muscle that has been previously selected for the colostomy (**Figs. 31–29 and 31–30**). This is generally about 4–5 cm below the level of the umbilicus.

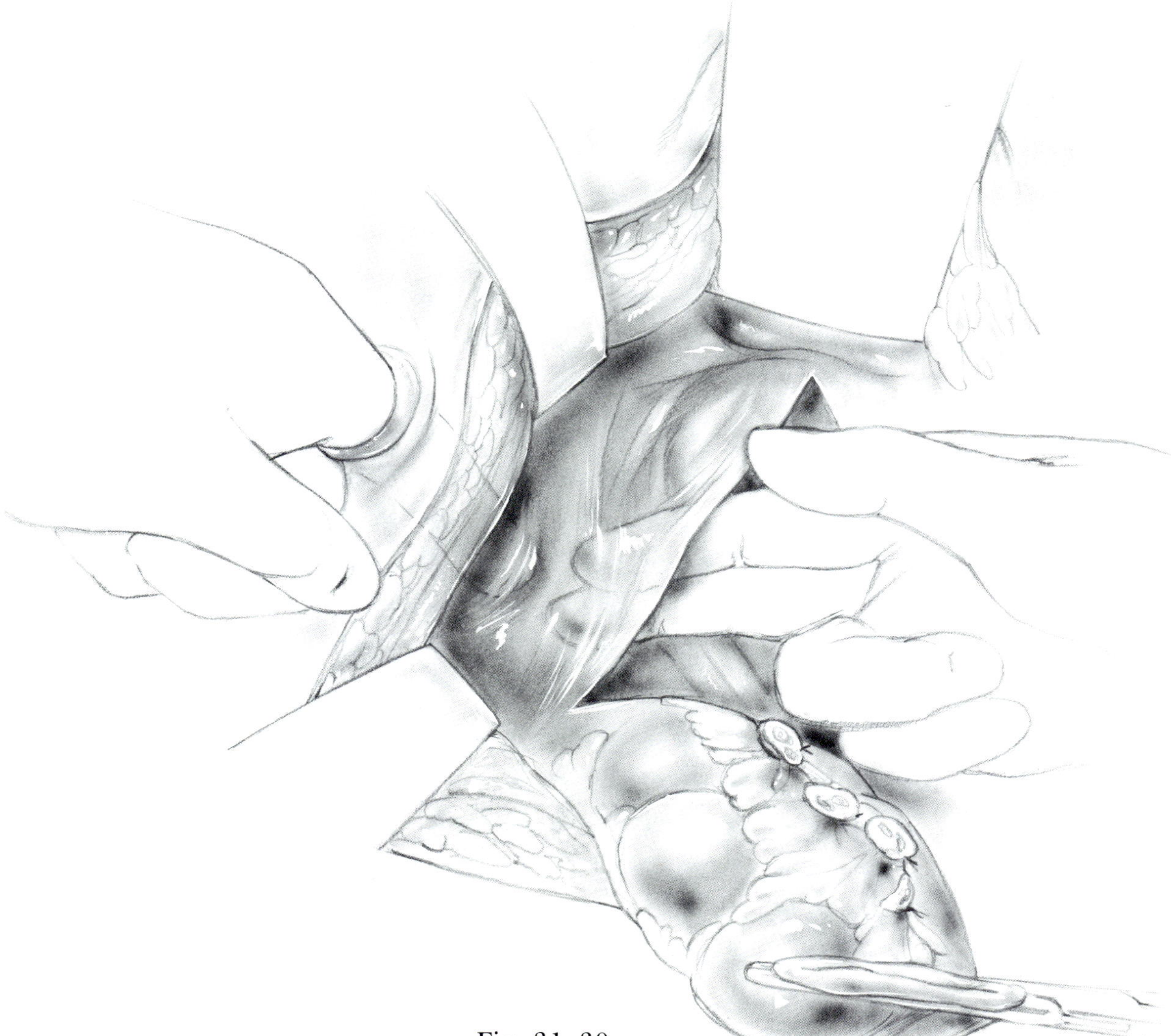

Fig. 31–30

Excise a circle of skin about the size of a nickel and expose the fascia of the left rectus muscle. Make cruciate incisions in the anterior rectus fascia, separate the rectus muscle fibers bluntly, and incise the underlying posterior rectus sheath and peritoneum. The aperture in the abdominal wall should be large enough to admit two fingers.

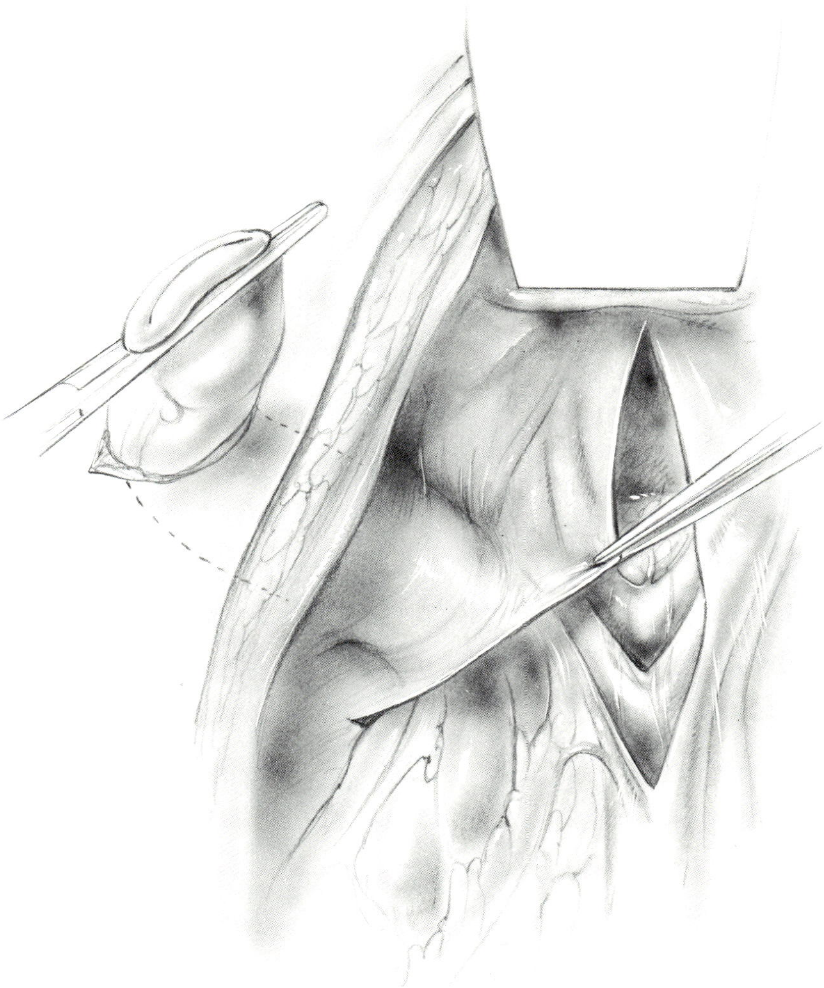

Fig. 31–31

Bring the colon through the retroperitoneal tunnel and out the opening made for the colostomy (**Fig. 31–31**). Begin the suture line closing the pelvic peritoneum near the bladder. Continue this suture of 2–0 atraumatic PG in a cephalad direction, closing the entire defect by suturing the free edge of the peritoneum to the anterior seromuscular wall of the sigmoid colon as it enters the retroperitoneal tunnel to become a colostomy (**Fig. 31–32**).

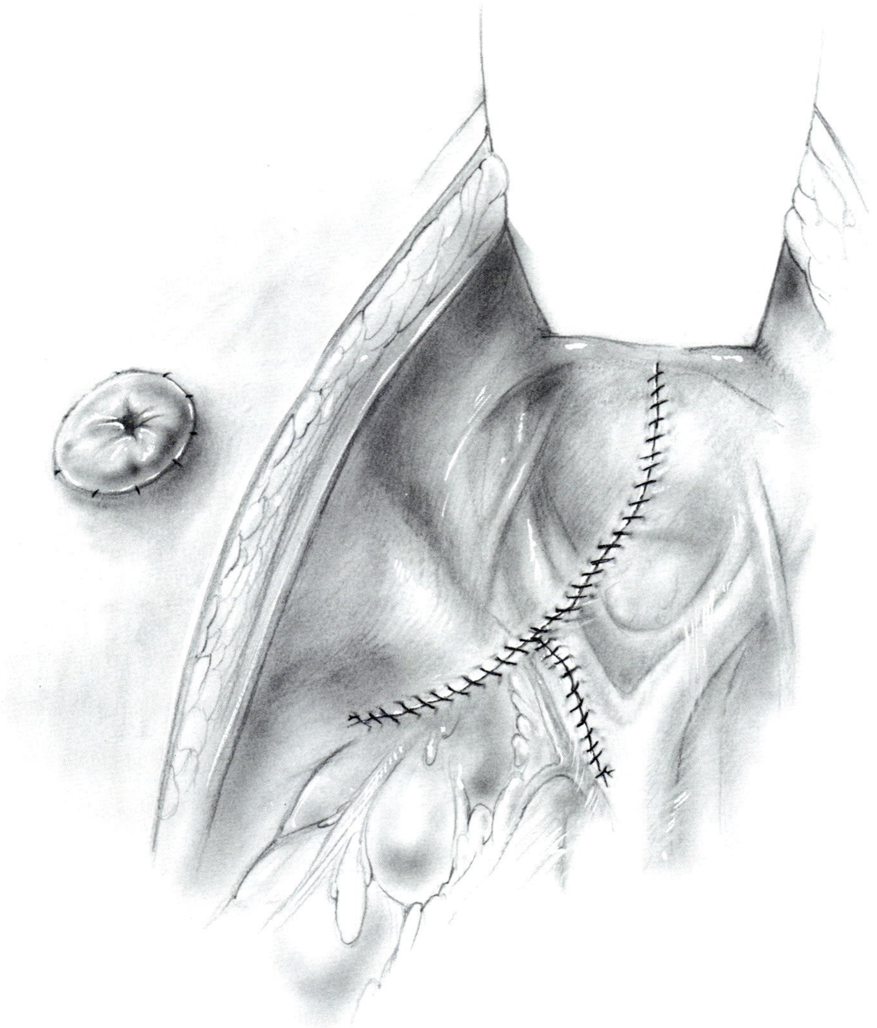

Fig. 31–32

Then close the abdominal incision. Mature the colostomy by a mucocutaneous suture as described above. Attach a temporary colostomy bag to the abdominal wall at the conclusion of the operation. We prefer the bags manufactured by the Hollister Co., which can remain in use until the patient learns proper colostomy irrigation.

Postoperative Care

Antibiotics

Continue perioperative antibiotic therapy, which had been initiated 1–2 hours before the start of operation, for 24–48 hours.

Nasogastric Suction

Continue nasogastric suction until the patient expels flatus or stool into the colostomy bag. This may take 4–7 days.

Bladder Drainage

The Foley catheter in the bladder should generally remain until the seventh postoperative day. At that time, inject sterile saline into the bladder through the catheter until the patient feels slightly uncomfortable. Then remove the catheter. If the patient cannot void within 1–2 hours, promptly replace the catheter for an additional period of 3 days, giving the patient 15 mg bethanechol chloride three times daily to stimulate bladder tone.

Perineal Care

Patients who have undergone excision of the posterior vagina have a small amount of gauze packing inserted into the perineum through the residual vaginal defect. This gauze should be removed on the third day, followed by daily saline irrigation of the area. As soon as the patient can sit comfortably, initiate sitz baths daily and discontinue irrigation.

Those patients who have had large gauze packs inserted in the presacral region to control hemorrhage should be brought back to the operating room on the first or second postoperative day so that the pack can be removed under general anesthesia. The sheet of oxidized cellulose, which had been applied to the sacrum, is left undisturbed. The patient should be observed briefly to ascertain that the hemorrhage is under complete control. If the abdominal contents descend to occupy the cavity in the presacral space that had been created by the gauze packing, then the perineal floor can be closed tightly around two closed-suction drains, as described above. If a large dead space remains, insert a sump and several latex drains and close the pelvic floor loosely around them. Administer postoperative irrigations with 0.1% kanamycin solution through the sump catheter every 6 hours.

Most of our patients leave the operating room with the perineum closed per primam. Every 6 hours, 25 ml of 0.1% kanamycin solution should be injected into each of the two closed-suction catheters that exit from puncture wounds in the perineal skin. Except for 20 minutes following each injection, the catheters should be subjected to constant suction. After perineal drainage ceases, generally on the fifth postoperative day, remove the catheters. Administer sitz baths twice daily to provide symptomatic relief of perineal soreness.

Chronic perineal sinus may occur, especially following a proctectomy for colitis. The etiology of this complication, which may persist for years, is not clear, but chronic sepsis and inadequate drainage are the probable causes. Local treatment by curettage, irrigations with a pulsating water jet as noted by Sohn and Weinstein, and perineal hygiene will remedy most chronic sinuses. Frequent shaving is necessary to prevent loose hair from entering deep into the sinus and producing a foreign-body granuloma.

Colostomy Care

Observe the colostomy daily through the transparent bag to detect signs of possible necrosis. That the colostomy does not function during the first 6–7 days following the operation need not be a cause for concern, if the patient does not develop abdominal distention or cramps. If there is no function beyond this date, abdominal X rays must be performed to rule out an obstruction of the small bowel.

The patient should begin receiving instructions in daily colostomy irrigations during the second week of hospitalization. No patient should leave the hospital before acquiring the skills necessary to perform the irrigations effectively.

It is important to understand that the aim of colostomy irrigation is not simply to wash out the distal few inches of colon. Patients sometimes insert a catheter a few inches into the colon, and when the water runs into the colon they permit it promptly to run out alongside the catheter. This is ineffective. Water is instilled into the distal colon for the purpose of dilating the area sufficiently to produce a reflex peristaltic contraction that evacuates the entire distal colon. For many patients this may require the injection of over a liter of water before they begin to feel "crampy" discomfort. At this point the catheter should be removed and the patient encouraged to keep the colostomy orifice occluded for a few more minutes, until peristalsis is well underway.

Some patients use a cone-shaped device, through which the fluid channel passes, to occlude the lumen. In other cases, the patient may be able to occlude the lumen by lightly grasping and manually compressing the abdominal wall around the inflow catheter or cone. There are many variations in devices and techniques in colostomy management; when any of them fails, however, it usually is because the patient has not retained the injected fluid long enough for distention of the distal colon to occur. Without this distention there can be no reflex peristaltic contraction.

All patients must be urged to exercise extreme caution in passing the catheter or any other irrigating device, so as to avoid the possibility of perforating the colon. This complication may occur even in patients who have had 15–20 years of experience in irrigating their colostomy. It is generally heralded promptly by the onset of severe abdominal pain during the irrigation. The patient should be urged to report *immediately* for examination if pain occurs at any time during irrigation.

Postoperative Complications

Acute Intestinal Obstruction

The small intestine may become obstructed either by adhesion to the pelvic suture line or herniation through a defect in the pelvic floor. Adhesions elsewhere in the abdomen which may occur after any abdominal procedure, can also cause obstruction. If colostomy function has not begun by the sixth or seventh postoperative day, X rays of the abdomen should be taken. If small bowel obstruction appears to have occurred, and there is no evidence of strangulation, a *brief* trial of a long intestinal tube may be initiated. If this is not promptly successful (3–4 days), secondary laparotomy for the relief of the obstruction is indicated.

Hemorrhage

Hemorrhage should be extremely rare in properly managed cases. If there is evidence of significant bleeding, either by vital signs and laboratory tests or by visible bleeding from the perineal drains, prompt reoperation is preferable to expectant management.

Sepsis

Sepsis that occurs following primary closure of the perineal wound is generally not difficult to detect. It is accompanied by fever, local pain, and purulent drainage through the suction catheters. Under these conditions the perineal incision should be opened sufficiently to insert two fingers, a sump, and several latex or Penrose drains. Intermittent or continuous irrigations with an antibiotic solution should be instituted promptly. If this is not successful in relieving the infection quickly, the entire wound may be reopened and a gauze pack inserted. The gauze should be changed at least once daily.

Bladder Obstruction

Because many men who undergo proctocolectomy for carcinoma are at an age when prostatic hypertrophy is common, this factor, combined with the loss of bladder support in the absence of the rectum, as well as some degree of nerve injury, leads to a high incidence of urinary tract obstruction. If the obstruction cannot be managed by conservative means, urological consultation and prostatectomy may be necessary.

Sexual Impotence

Some studies have indicated that virtually all operations for the radical removal of malignancies in the middle and lower rectum of males have been followed by sexual impotence, although Goligher's findings were not so bleak. This complication has been rare after operations for benign disease when special precautions are observed (see Chap. 36).

Colostomy Complications

Postoperative pericolostomy sepsis has been rare following immediate maturation of the colostomy. This technique has virtually eliminated the late complications of stricture formation and prolapse.

Chronic Perineal Sinus

Although a persistent perineal sinus is rare after a properly managed resection for carcinoma, it appears to be common following operations for inflammatory bowel disease. If all the local measures fail and the sinus persists for several years, Silen recommends a saucerization procedure consisting of excision of the coccyx and the chronically infected wall of the sinus down to its apex. After saucerization is done, persistent attention to encouraging healing from the bottom has proved successful. Another technique, suggested by Turnbull, is the insertion of a perforated split-thickness skin graft following local debridement and cleansing.

References

Anderson R, Turnbull RB Jr (1976) Grafting the unhealed perineal wound after coloproctectomy for Crohn's disease. Arch Surg 111:335

Foster JH, Berman MM (1977) Solid liver tumors. Saunders, Philadelphia, p. 225

Goligher JC (1958) Extraperitoneal colostomy or ileostomy. Br J Surg 46:97

Goligher JC (1975) Surgery of the anus, rectum and colon, 3rd edn. Baillière, Tindall, London, p. 760

Silen W, Glotzer DJ (1974) The prevention and treatment of the persistent perineal sinus. Surgery 75:535

Sohn N, Weinstein MA (1977) Unhealed perineal wound: lavage with a pulsating water jet. Am J Surg 134:426

32 Subtotal Colectomy with Ileoproctostomy or Ileostomy and Sigmoid Mucous Fistula

Indications

- Familial polyposis
- Chronic ulcerative colitis
- Toxic megacolon, unresponsive to 48 hours of medical management
- Intractable systemic complications such as arthritis, pyoderma gangrenosum, or liver disease
- Threat of carcinoma, especially after 10 years of pancolitis
- Intractable symptoms
- Crohn's colitis
- Perforation
- Obstruction
- Inflammatory mass unresponsive to conservative management
- Intractable colonic fistulas to skin, small intestine, bladder, perineum
- Massive hemorrhage

Concept: Choice of Operation

In the management of the above conditions the surgeon must choose among total colectomy with proctectomy, subtotal colectomy with ileoproctostomy, or subtotal colectomy with ileostomy and mucous fistula. Occasional cases of localized Crohn's colitis will respond, at least temporarily, to a segmental resection of the colon.

Familial polyposis is most frequently treated by subtotal colectomy and ileoproctostomy, followed by lifelong observation and electrocoagulation of the residual polyps in the rectum. If there is a likelihood that periodic postoperative observation of the rectum will not be faithfully carried out, it is safer to perform immediate total proctectomy, as there is a high probability that the untreated rectum of patients who suffer from familial polyposis will develop carcinoma.

In inflammatory bowel disease the condition of the rectum is the main determinant in selecting the proper operation. For advanced disease of the rectal mucosa or in cases of multiple perineal fistulas, total proctocolectomy in one stage is advisable. Immediate ileoproctostomy may be performed when the rectum is relatively healthy; at least half the patients have the prospect of a satisfactory result. When patients who suffer from ulcerative colitis have mild to moderate disease in the rectum, subtotal colectomy, ileostomy, and rectosigmoid mucous fistula offer an opportunity for continued observation of the rectum while the patient makes a complete nutritional recovery from the disease. In a year, especially if the ileostomy content becomes thick rather than watery in consistency, a secondary ileorectal anastomosis may be offered to the patient, with the proviso that the result is uncertain. Results in this category of ulcerative colitis patients have been quite variable. Eventually proctectomy may be necessary because the inflammatory disease has become aggravated or rectal carcinoma has developed. Continued observation is necessary. Many surgeons believe that ileoproctostomy is *rarely* indicated in ulcerative colitis.

If an emergency operation is required for severe toxic megacolon, Turnbull has recommended a diverting loop ileostomy and a colostomy instead of a colon resection in order to avoid the hazard of accidentally rupturing the colon during the operation. Colectomy, says Turnbull, should be performed at a later date. At present, however, the data reported by other surgeons is not adequate to evaluate this procedure.

Total colectomy, including proctectomy by the Soave technique, leaving intact the serosa of the rectum and the external sphincter muscle, followed by an ileoanal anastomosis, has been revived. Martin et al. and Ravitch and Sabiston have reported that the preserved sphincter mechanism produces fairly satisfactory results in these cases. This procedure must still be considered experimental, though.

Kock has described an ileostomy pouch which does not require that the patient wear a bag to contain the ileal excretions. As this operation produces many complications that require reoperation, the Kock ileostomy cannot yet be recommended for general use.

Preoperative Preparation

The preoperative care of patients who undergo *elective* surgery is the same as that used when the colon is resected for malignancy, except that colitis patients who have cachexia should receive preoperative intravenous hyperalimentation. For *emergency* colectomy, restitution with blood and electrolytes should be accomplished. Colitis cases complicated by toxic megacolon or perforation require appropriate antibiotic therapy.

Pitfalls and Danger Points

Operative contamination of the peritoneal cavity with colonic contents, leading to sepsis (in toxic megacolon)

Improper construction of ileostomy

Operative Strategy

Sepsis is not uncommon following an emergency colectomy for inflammatory bowel disease and its complications. In Crohn's disease one often finds a fistula to the adjacent bowel or to the skin. In some cases paracolic abscesses are encountered, making gross contamination of the peritoneal cavity inevitable. In operations for fistula, abscess, or toxic megacolon, intensive preoperative treatment with systemic antibiotics (aminoglycoside, ampicillin, and clindamycin) as well as frequent intraoperative irrigations with an antibiotic solution are indicated. When performing a resection for toxic megacolon, the surgeon should be aware that the colon, especially the distal transverse colon and splenic flexure, may have the consistency of wet tissue paper and may be ruptured by even minimal manipulation. This will cause massive and sometimes fatal contamination of the abdominal cavity. It must be avoided. No attempt should be made to dissect the omentum off the transverse colon, as this may unseal a perforation. Elevation of the left costal margin by a "chain" retractor will generally provide good exposure of the splenic flexure.

Another precaution to take to help prevent perforating the colon during the operation is to pass a 40F catheter through a purse-string suture in the ileum. Pass the tube into the ascending colon and, by gravity, drain the semiliquid contents of the colon out into a plastic bag away from the operative field.

Accomplish technical simplification of the colectomy by dividing the mesentery at a point of convenience nearer to the colon than would be the case in resections for carcinoma. Extensive mesenteric excision is not necessary.

Postoperative ileostomy complications have been reduced remarkably since the advent of the immediate maturation technique, which uses the mucocutaneous suture. Stricture and prolapse are rare after primary healing of this suture line has been accomplished. Peristomal skin erosions and other difficulties with ileostomy appliances can be minimized if the surgeon constructs an ileostomy that protrudes permanently from the abdominal wall, like a cervix, for 2 cm. This helps prevent the contents of the small bowel from leaking between the appliance and the peristomal skin. It also greatly simplifies the patient's task of placing the appliance accurately. Finally, the gap between the cut edge of ileal mesentery and the lateral abdominal wall must be closed to avoid internal herniation.

Operative Technique

Placement of Ileostomy

On the day before the operation the surgeon should obtain a face plate from an ileostomy appliance, or some facsimile, and apply it tentatively to the patient's abdominal wall. Test proper placement with the patient sitting erect. In some patients, if the appliance is not properly placed, the rim may strike the costal margin or the anterior spine of the ilium. Generally, the proper location is somewhere near the outer margin of the right rectus muscle, about 5 cm lateral to the midline and 4 cm below the umbilicus. In this position the face plate does not impinge upon the midline scar, the umbilicus, the anterior superior spine, or the costal margin no matter what position the patient assumes. The stoma should also be sited so that the patient can see it when he or she is erect.

Operative Position

If there is a possibility that both colectomy and total proctectomy will be performed in one stage, position the patient in Lloyd-Davies leg rests (see Figs. 31–1a and 31–1b). Otherwise, the usual supine position is satisfactory.

Incision

We prefer a midline incision because it does not interfere with the ileostomy appliance. It also leaves the entire left lower quadrant free of scar, in case, in the future, ileostomy revision and reimplantation may become necessary. On the other hand, many surgeons use a left paramedian incision to permit a wider margin between the ileostomy and the scar. The incision should extend from the upper epigastrium down to the pubis (**Fig. 32–1**). Since the splenic flexure is foreshortened in many cases of ulcerative colitis and toxic megacolon, exposure for this area is often good, with the "chain" retractor applied to the left costal margin. If it is not, make a T extension from the midline incision transversely across the left rectus muscle to improve the exposure of the splenic flexure.

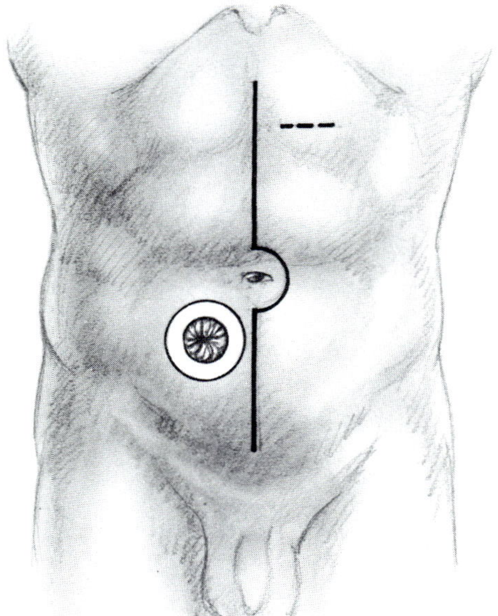

Fig. 32–1

Evacuation of Stool

For patients undergoing an operation for acute toxic megacolon, insert a heavy purse-string suture on the anterior surface of the terminal ileum. After applying a Wound Protector ring-drape to the abdominal wall, incise the ileum and insert a large 40F multiperforated tube through the purse-string suture into the ascending colon. Permit the semiliquid content of the distended colon to drain by gravity into a bag away from the operative field. After the colon has been adequately decompressed, remove the tube and tie the purse-string suture.

Dissection of Right Colon and Omentum

Make an incision in the right paracolic peritoneum lateral to the cecum and insert the left index finger to elevate the avascular peritoneum, which should be

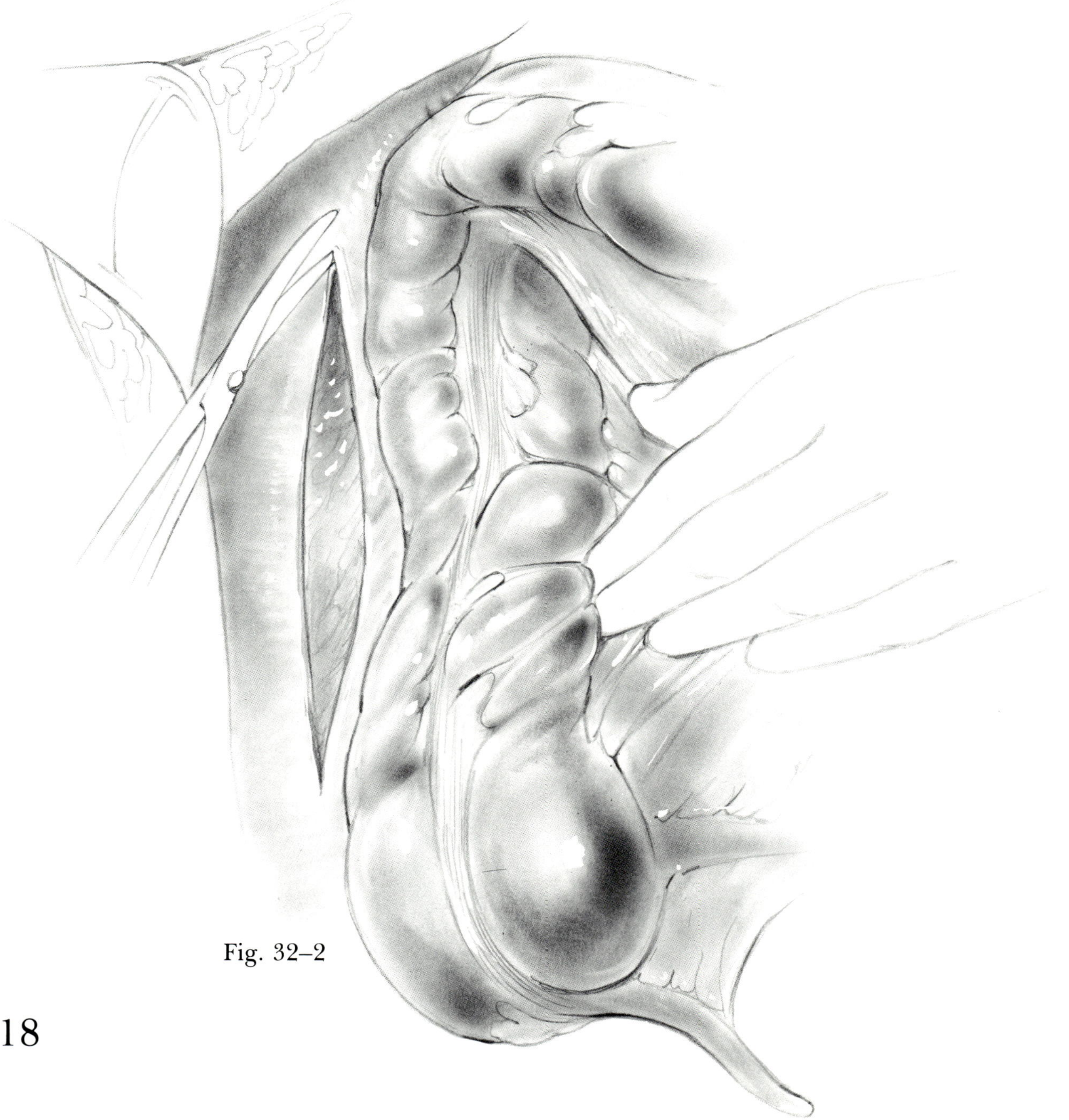

Fig. 32–2

divided by scissors in a cephalad direction (**Fig. 32–2**). If local inflammation has produced increased vascularity in this layer, use the electrocoagulator to carry out the division. Throughout the dissection, keep manipulation of the colon to a minimum. Continue the paracolic incision around the hepatic flexure, exposing the anterior wall of the duodenum.

In emergency operations for toxic megacolon, divide the omentum between Kelly hemostats 5 cm above its line of attachment to the transverse colon. In some cases, if the omentum is fused to the transverse mesocolon it may be divided simultaneously with the mesocolon, in one layer. In most elective operations, the omentum can be dissected off the transverse colon through the usual avascular plane (**Fig. 32–3**).

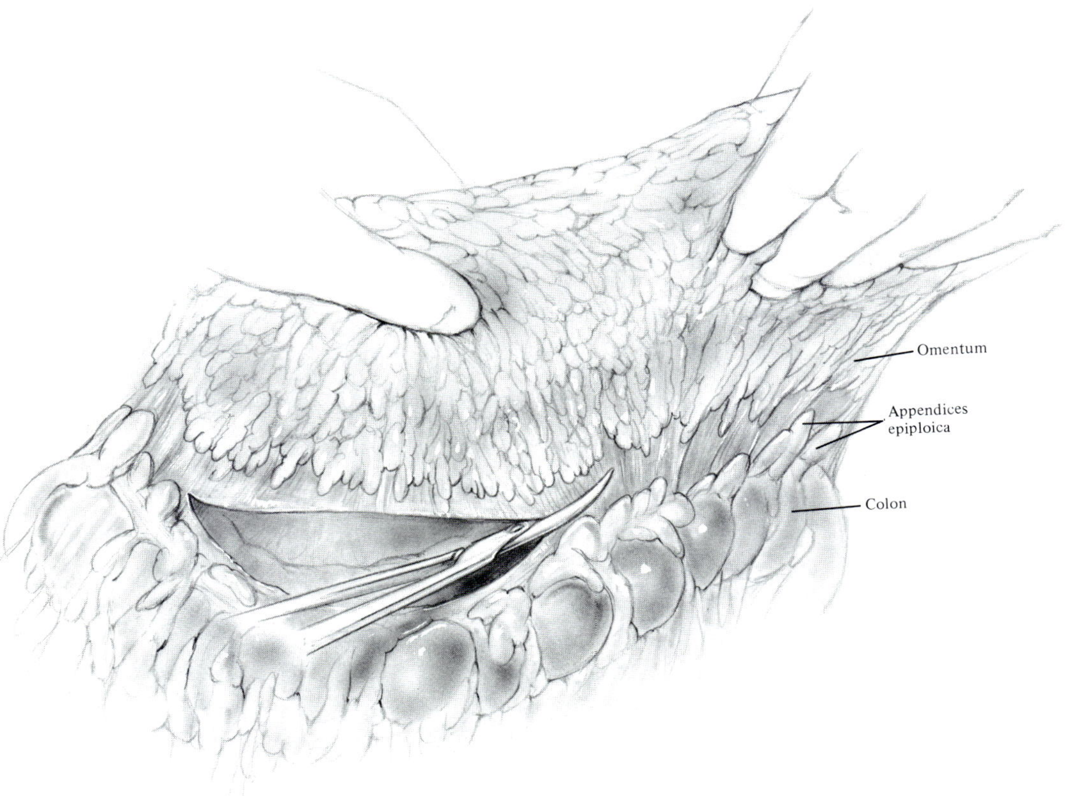

Fig. 32–3

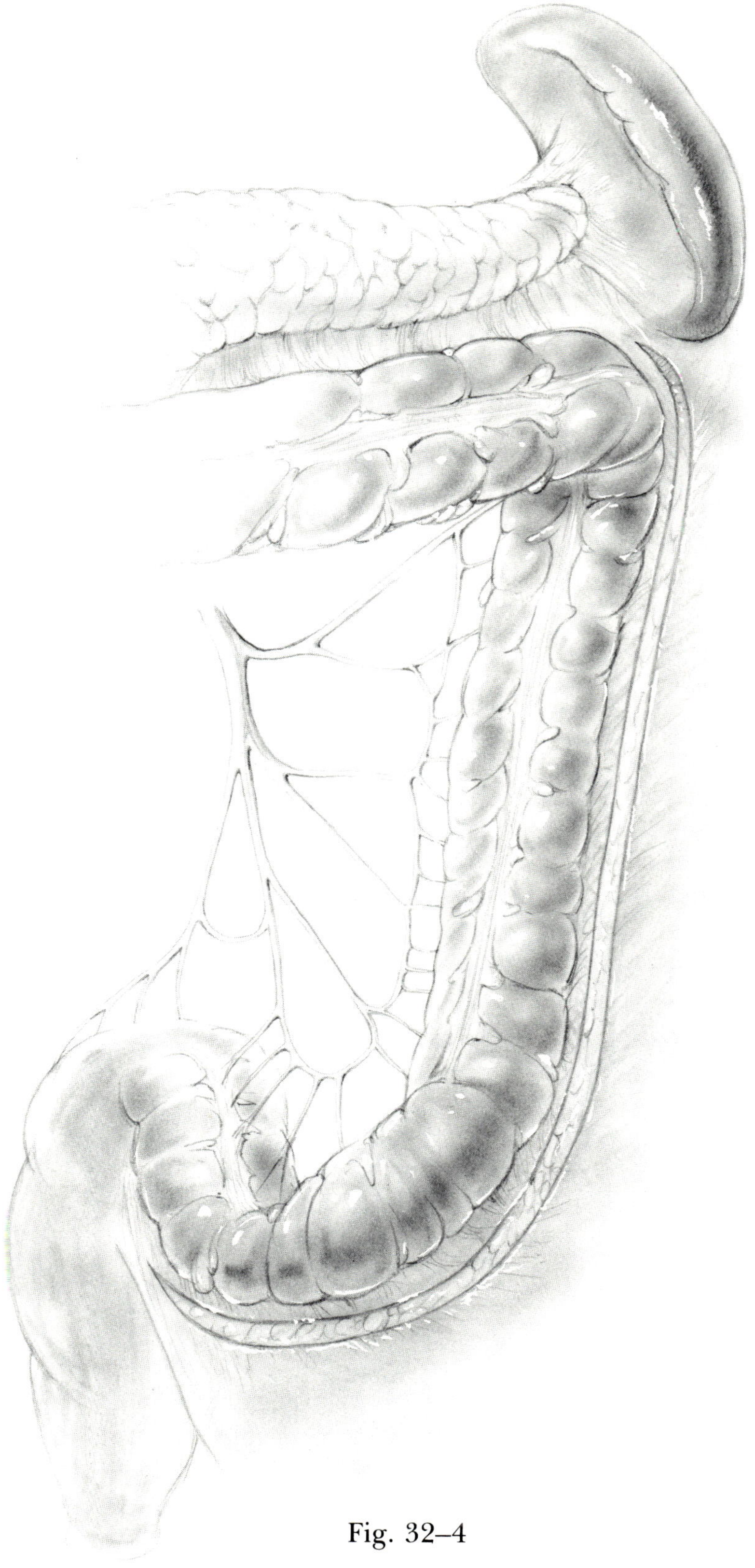

Fig. 32–4

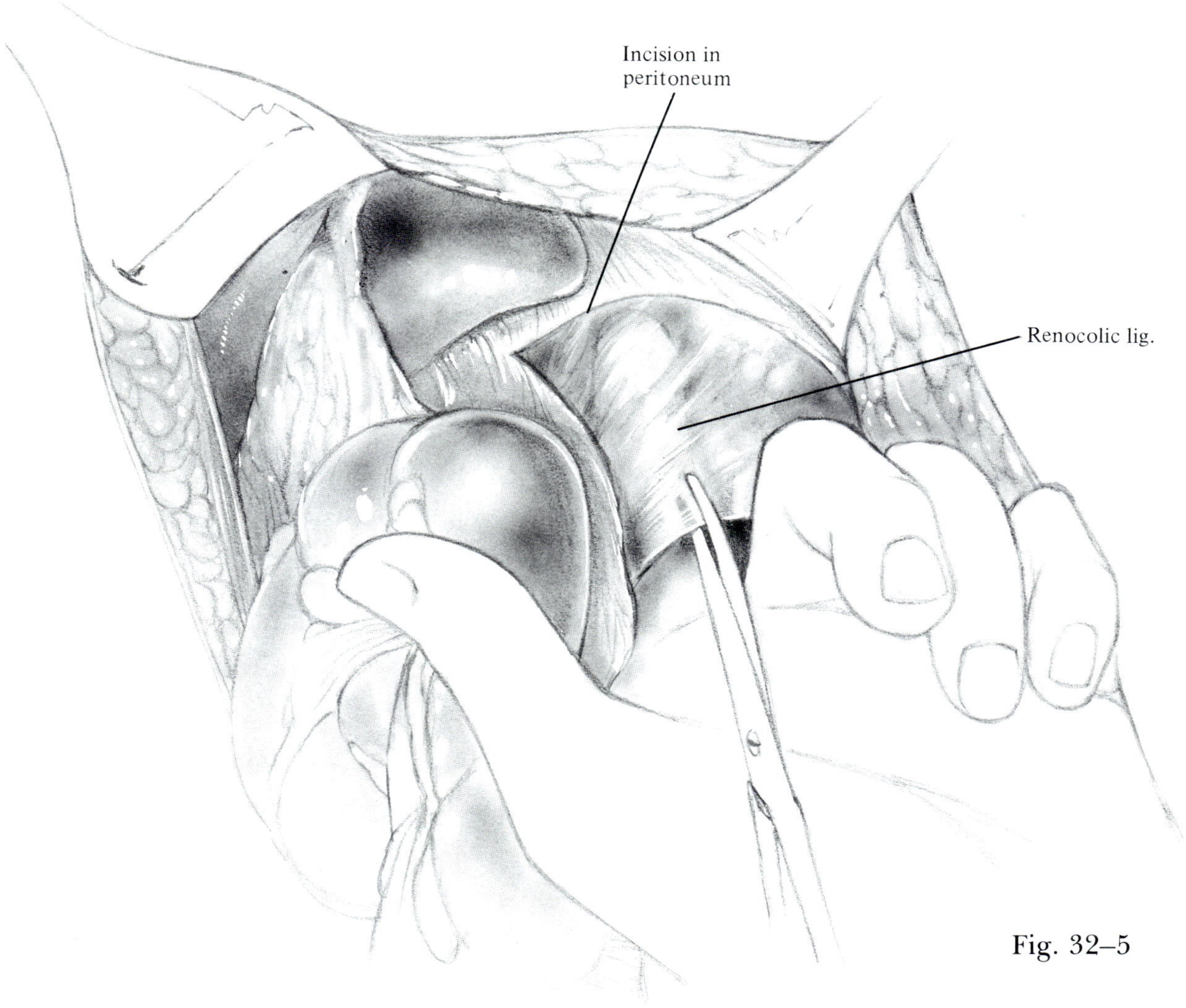

Fig. 32–5

Dissection of Left Colon

Remain at the patient's right side and make an incision in the peritoneum of the left paracolic gutter in the line of Toldt, beginning at the sigmoid. With the aid of the left hand elevate the avascular peritoneum and divide it in a cephalad direction with a Metzenbaum scissors. Carry this incision up to and around the splenic flexure (**Fig. 32–4**).

After the peritoneal attachments of the splenic flexure have been divided, divide the renocolic ligament (**Fig. 32–5**), which stretches between Gerota's fascia and the undersurface of the mesocolon.

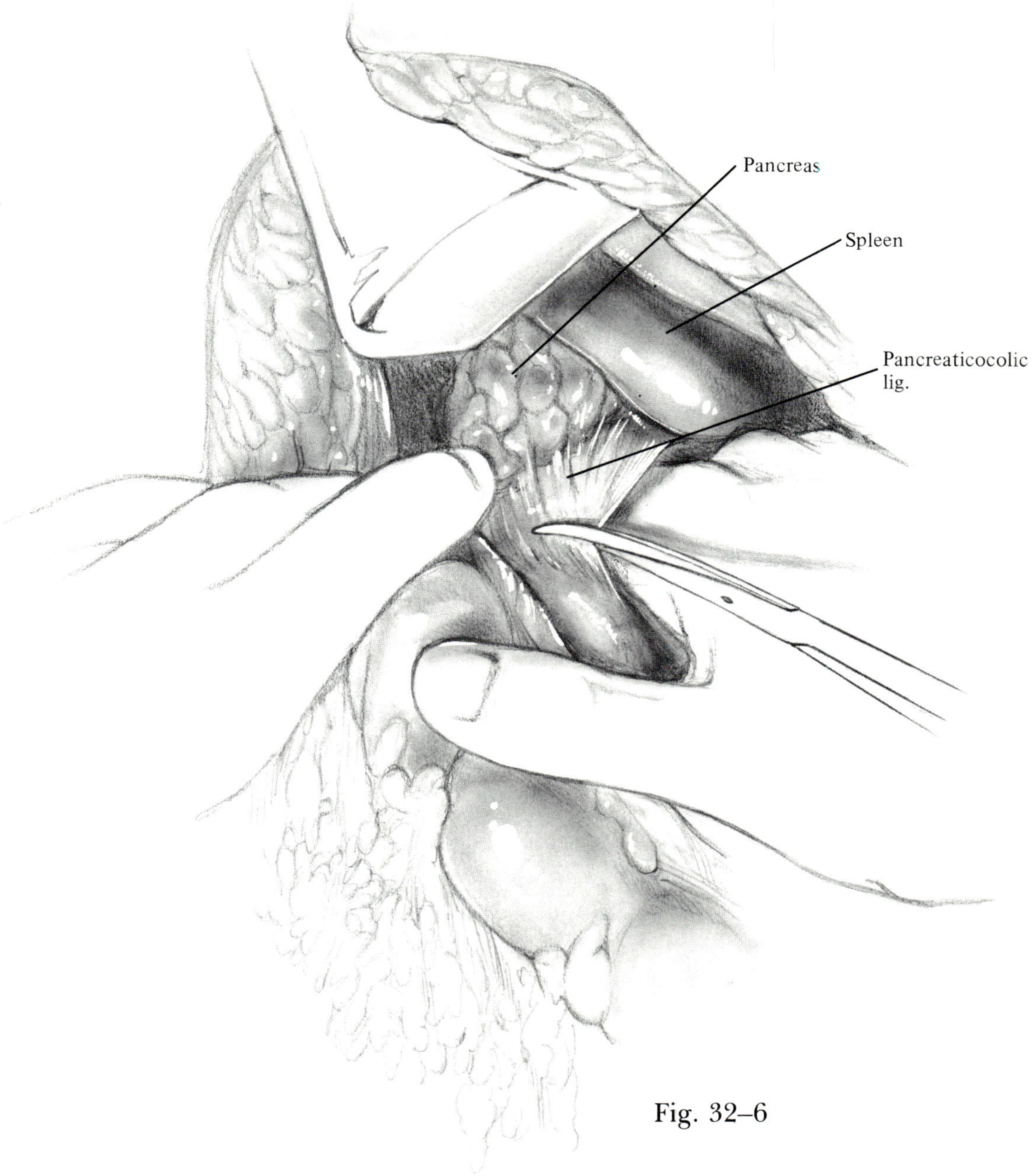

Fig. 32–6

Divide in a cephalad direction until the avascular ligament between the tail of the pancreas and the left transverse colon is encountered (**Fig. 32–6**). Transect this "pancreatico-colic ligament," leaving the mesocolon as the only attachment the colon has to the patient. In patients who suffer from toxic megacolon, this dissection should be done with extreme caution, so as not to perforate the colon.

Division of Mesocolon

Turn now to the ileocecal region. If the terminal ileum is not involved in the disease process, its blood supply should be preserved and the point of transection should be close to the ileocecal valve. Divide the mesocolon along a line indicated in **Fig. 32–7**. Since most patients who require this operation are thin, each vessel can be visualized, doubly clamped, and divided accurately. Ligate each vessel with 2–0 PG or cotton ligatures and divide the

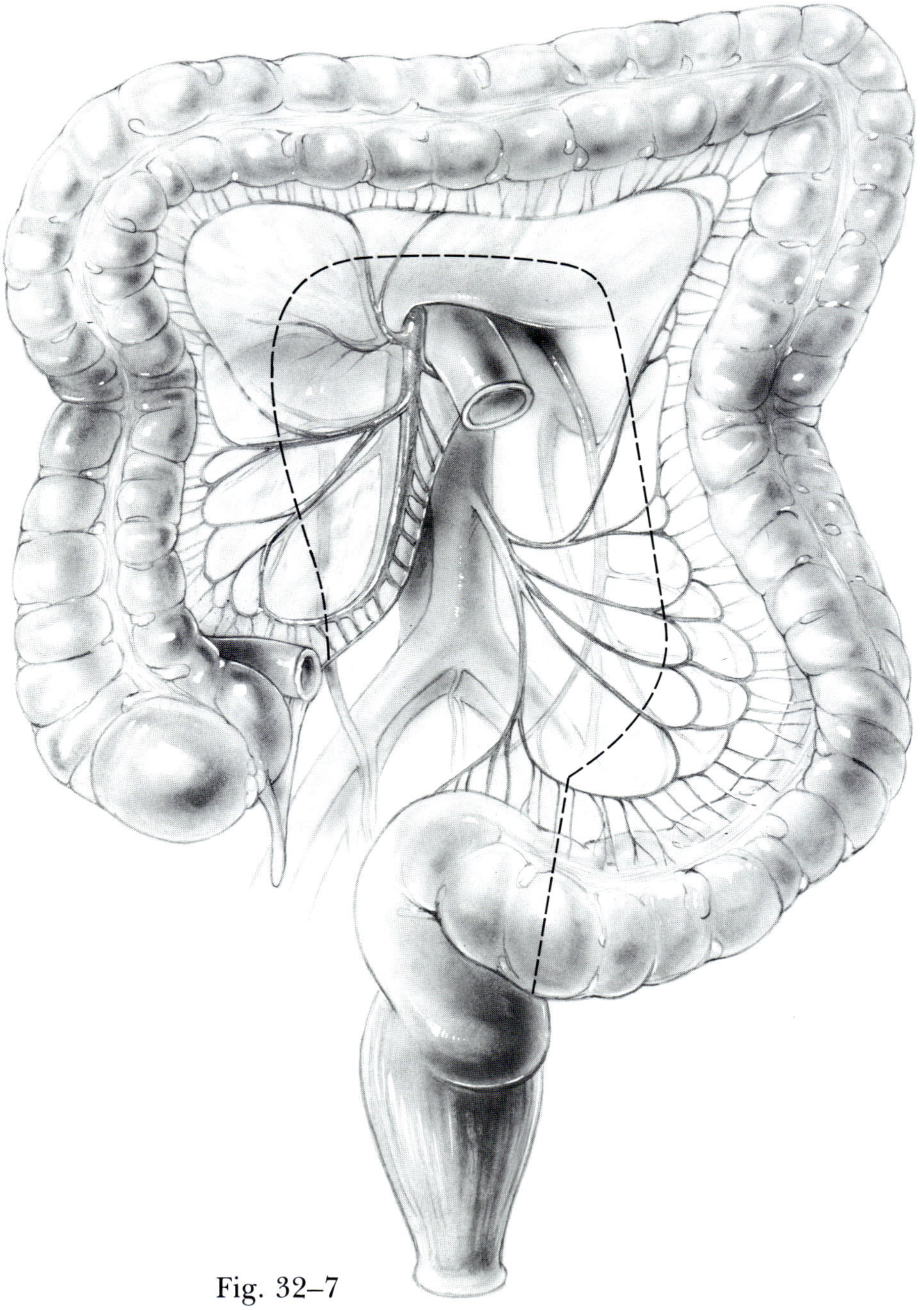

Fig. 32–7

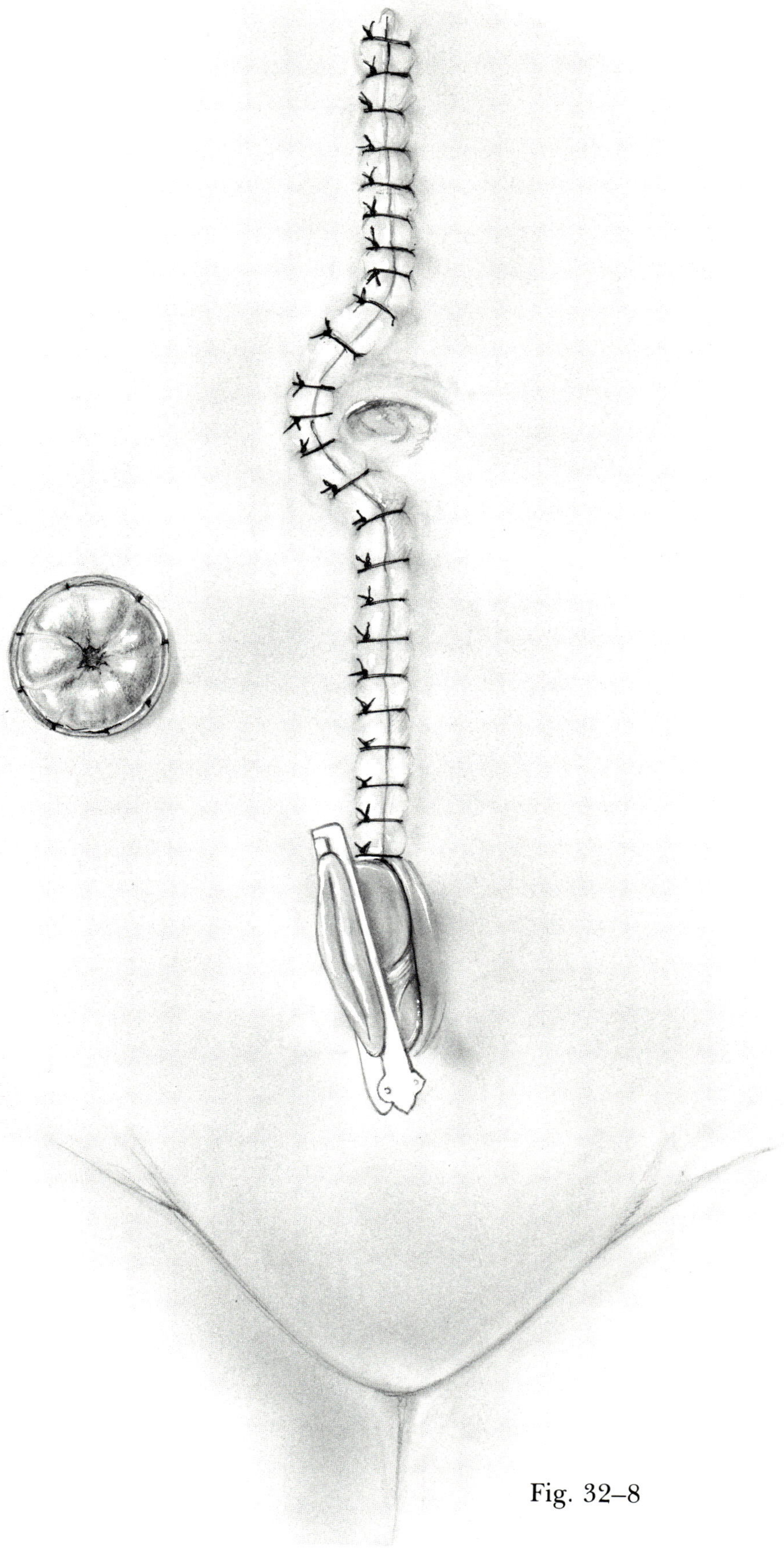

Fig. 32–8

intervening avascular mesentery with a Metzenbaum scissors. In the same way, divide and ligate sequentially the ileocolic branches, the right colic, the middle colic, the two branches of the left colic, and each of the sigmoidal arteries.

Ileostomy and Sigmoid Mucous Fistula

The technique of fashioning a permanent ileostomy, including suturing the cut edge of the ileal mesentery to the right abdominal wall, is depicted in Figs. 34–1 through 34–9.

After the sigmoid mesentery has been divided up to a suitable point on the wall of the distal sigmoid, apply DeMartel clamps. Divide the colon and remove the specimen. Remove the Wound Protector drape. Bring out the stump of the rectosigmoid, its orifice closed by the DeMartel clamp, through the lower pole of the incision (**Fig. 32–8**). Fix the rectosigmoid stump to the lower pole with a few 3–0 PG sutures, approximating the mesocolon and the appendices epiploica to the anterior rectus fascia. Close the abdominal incision around the mucous fistula.

Ileoproctostomy

When an ileorectal anastomosis is elected, we prefer the side-to-end technique, which is the same as that described by Baker (see Figs. 30–10 through 30–21) for the colorectal anastomosis. After the mesentery has been cleared at the point selected for the transection of the ileum, apply transversely and fire a TA–55 stapler using 3.5 mm staples. Apply an Allen clamp to the specimen side of the ileum and with a scalpel transect the ileum flush with the stapler. Lightly electrocoagulate the everted mucosa and remove the stapling device. Inspect the staple line to assure that proper B formation of the staples has occurred.

Divide the mesentery of the rectosigmoid up to the point on the upper rectum that has been selected for transection. This is generally opposite the sacral promontory. Apply a right-angle kidney clamp to the colon to exclude colonic contents from the field. Dissect fat and mesentery off the serosa of the rectum at the site to be anastomosed. Make a linear scratch mark on the antimesenteric border of the ileum beginning at a point 1 cm proximal to the staple line and continuing in a cephalad direction for a distance equal to the diameter of the rectum, usually 4–5 cm.

The first layer should consist of interrupted 4–0 cotton seromuscular Cushing sutures inserted by the technique of successive bisection. After the sutures are tied, cut all the tails except for the two end sutures, to which small hemostats should be attached. Then make an incision on the antimesenteric border of the ileum. Also incise the back wall of rectum (**Fig. 32–9**). Initiate the closure of the posterior mucosal layer by inserting a double-armed 4–0 PG suture in the middle point of the posterior layer and tying it. With one needle insert a continuous locked suture to approximate all the coats of the posterior layer, going from the midpoint to the right corner of the anastomosis. Use the

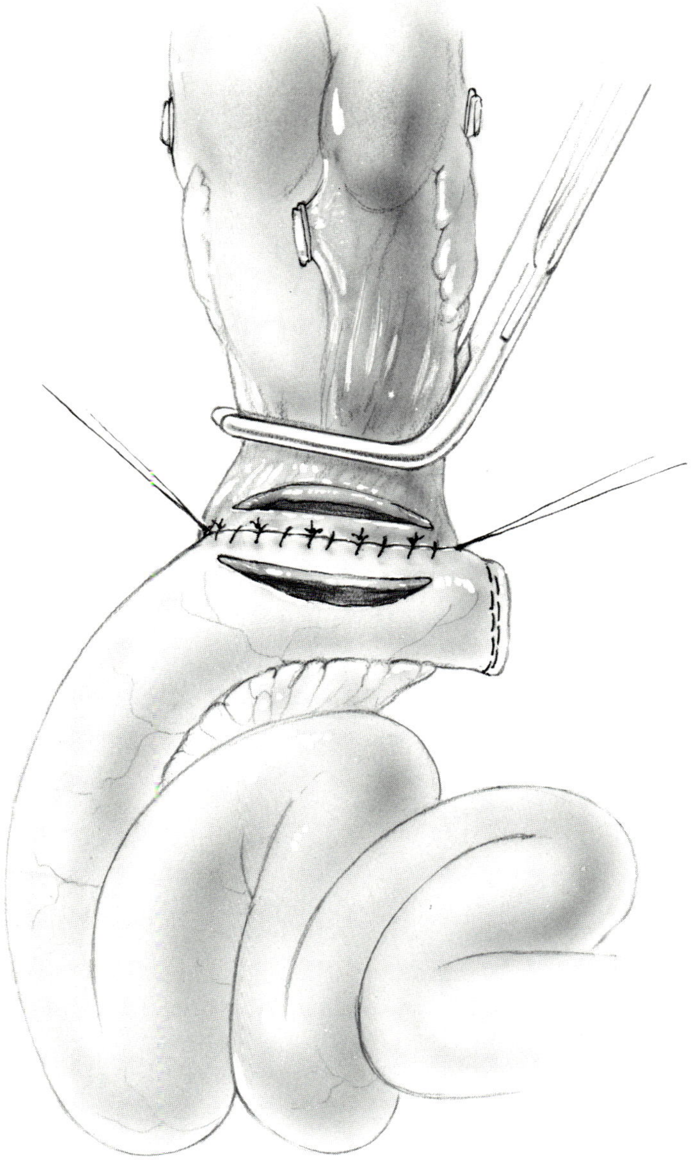

Fig. 32–9

other needle to perform the same maneuver going from the midpoint to the left (**Fig. 32–10**). Use a continuous Cushing, Connell, or seromucosal suture to approximate the anterior mucosal layer, terminating the suture line at the midpoint of the anterior layer. Close the final anterior seromuscular layer with interrupted 4–0 cotton Cushing sutures (**Fig. 32–11**). If possible, cover the anastomosis with omentum.

Approximate the cut edge of the ileal mesentery to the cut edge of the right lateral paracolic peritoneum with a continuous 2–0 atraumatic PG suture. Do not close the left paracolic gutter. Irrigate the abdominal cavity with an antibiotic solution. Remove the Wound Protector ring drape.

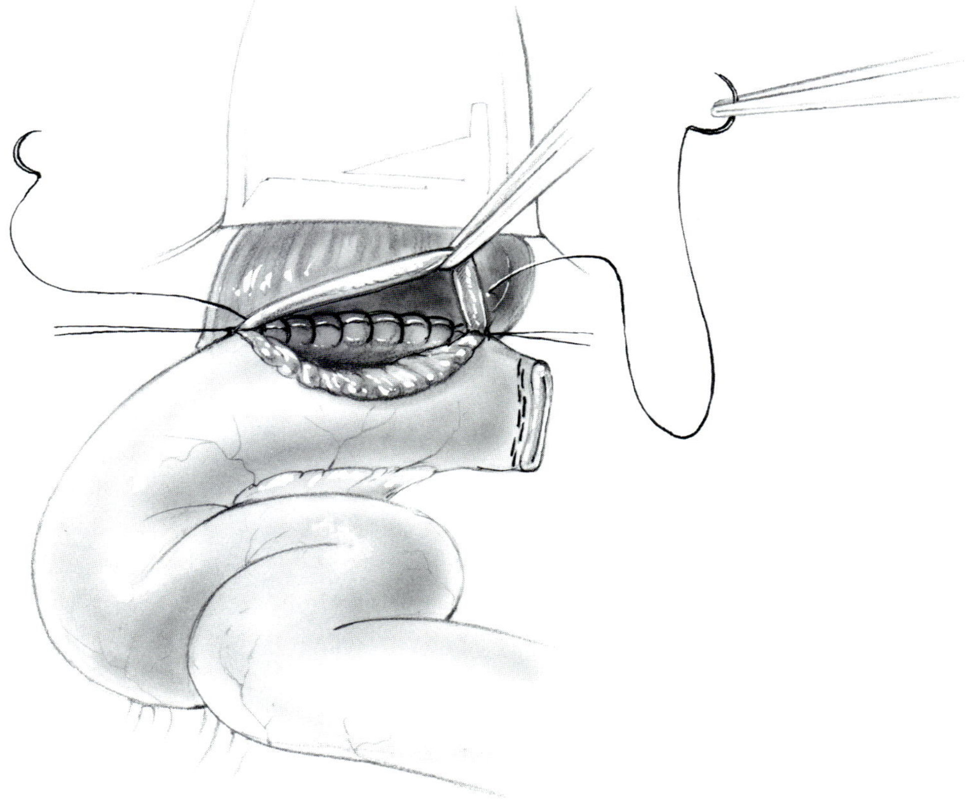

Fig. 32–10

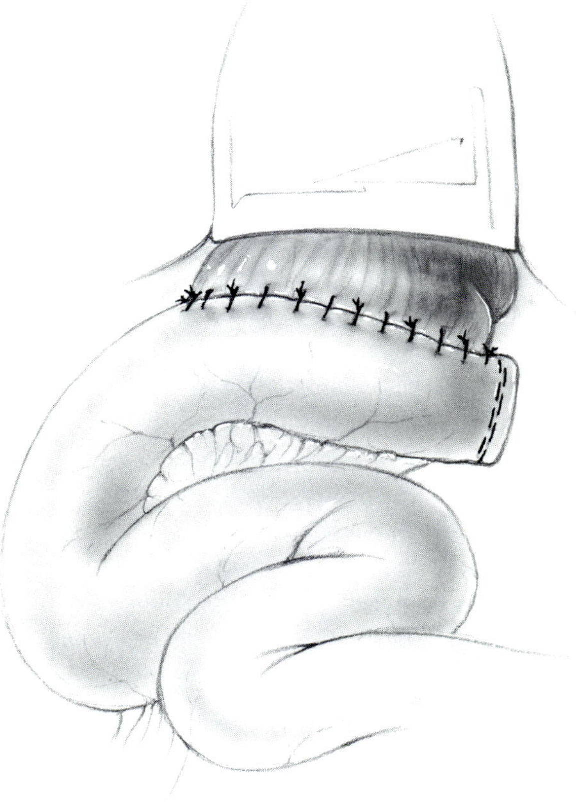

Fig. 32–11

Subtotal Colectomy Combined with Immediate Total Proctectomy

When a proctectomy is performed at the same stage as a subtotal colectomy, occlude the rectosigmoid by a layer of TA–55 staples. Apply an Allen clamp to the specimen side of the colon, which should be transected with the removal of the specimen. Construct the ileostomy as depicted in Figs. 34–1 through 34–9. Then accomplish the abdominoperineal proctectomy by the technique described under "Total Proctectomy for Benign Disease" in Chap. 36.

Closure of the Abdominal Incision

Irrigate the abdominal cavity with a dilute antibiotic solution and close the abdominal wall in routine fashion (see Chap. 5). Insert a long subcutaneous plastic catheter throughout the length of the abdominal incision in the subcutaneous layer. Bring it out through a puncture wound near the upper pole of the incision, so it can be used for closed-suction drainage and the intermittent injection of antibiotics. Then close the skin with a continuous subcuticular suture of 4–0 PG or with interrupted 4–0 nylon stitches.

Postoperative Care

Continue nasogastric suction and intravenous fluids until there is good ileostomy function or, in the case of ileoproctostomy, for at least 7 days.

If there is no operative contamination, discontinue the perioperative antibiotics within 24 hours. Otherwise, order them when they are indicated by the operative findings and the postoperative course.

In the operating room apply a Stomahesive disc to the ileostomy after cutting a properly sized opening. Over the disc place a temporary ileostomy bag. Instruct the patient in the details of ileostomy management and encourage him or her to join one of the organizations of ileostomates, where considerable emotional support can be derived by meeting patients who have been successfully rehabilitated.

Complications

1) *Intra-abdominal abscess* is more common after colon resection for inflammatory bowel disease than for other conditions. When signs of intra-abdominal infection appear, prompt, laparotomy for evacuation of the abscess is indicated.

2) *Intestinal obstruction* due to adhesions is not rare following this group of operations, because of the extensive dissection. If treatment by a long intestinal suction tube does not bring a prompt response, laparotomy for enterolysis will be necessary.

3) Leakage of the anastomosis may follow ileoproctostomy. In case of a major leak, immediate laparotomy for a diverting loop ileostomy (see Chap. 35), followed by pelvic drainage, is mandatory. Alternatively, the anastomosis may be dismantled and the ileum brought out as a terminal ileostomy.

References

Kock N et al. (1977) Ileostomy. Curr Probl Surg 14:1

Martin LW et al. (1977) Total colectomy and mucosal proctectomy with preservation of continence in ulcerative colitis. Ann Surg 186:477

Ravitch MM, Sabiston DC (1947) Anal ileostomy with preservation of the sphincter: a proposed operation in patients requiring total colectomy for benign lesions. Surg Gynecol Obstet 84:1095

Turnbull R, Weakley FL (1971) Surgical treatment of toxic megacolon: ileostomy and colostomy to prepare patients for colectomy. Am J Surg 122:325

33 Subtotal Colectomy for Massive Colonic Hemorrhage

Indications

Angiodysplasia
Diverticulosis

Concept

In many patients (especially the elderly) the etiology of colon hemorrhage is an *angiodysplasia,* usually located in the right colon. When this has been identified by arteriography, resection of the right colon, rather than subtotal colectomy, is indicated. While well tolerated by most patients, subtotal colectomy does produce disabling diarrhea in some. Ottinger reported that 16% of the patients studied were disabled by six or more bowel movements a day, after subtotal colectomy had been performed for noninflammatory conditions of the colon.

In the majority of cases, bleeding from *diverticulosis* does not exceed 1500 ml. Occasionally, especially in patients whose diverticulosis extends from the cecum to the rectosigmoid, major life-threatening hemorrhage of the colon does take place. In these cases the source of bleeding is more commonly located in the right colon than the left. Sometimes, there is more than one bleeding point. For these reasons, Drapanas et al. have recommended emergency subtotal colectomy for these patients. On the other hand, Boley et al. have found that if the location of a bleeding diverticulum has been identified by arteriography, *partial* colectomy is followed by recurrent bleeding in less than 20% of the cases. When a bleeding point has been demonstrated angiographically, we generally do a segmental rather than subtotal colectomy, especially in elderly patients.

Occasionally, the bleeding can be stopped by an intra-arterial infusion of vasopressin, and an emergency operation will be unnecessary.

Preoperative Preparation

In most cases of hemorrhage, an operation is performed as an emergency procedure and the routine bowel preparation cannot be carried out. After blood loss has been replaced, insert a nasogastric tube and Foley catheter, initiate perioperative systemic antibiotics, and schedule an operation immediately.

Operative Strategy

The colon is rarely inflamed in cases of major hemorrhage, which makes the operation technically simple. The major blood supply to the colon may be transected just proximal to the marginal artery, where the right colic, the middle colic, and left colic branches are ligated easily. In the lower left colon, the sigmoidal vessels are ligated, rather than the inferior mesenteric. A side-to-end anastomosis is constructed between the ileum and the upper rectosigmoid. No dissection is necessary in the presacral space in most cases.

It is hoped that the severity of postoperative diarrhea may be reduced if the terminal ileum is preserved. This is accomplished by avoiding ligation of the ileocolic trunk. Rather, the blood supply to the terminal ileum is preserved and the ileum divided close to the ileocecal valve in order to preserve, as much as possible, its water-absorbing capability.

In agreement with Drapanas et al. we perform a side-to-end (Baker) anastomosis because it is technically simpler and safer than is an end-to-end ileocolonic suture line, which would require an extensive Cheatle slit of the ileum. The incision on the antimesenteric border of the ileum for this anastomosis should begin no more than one centimeter from the end of the ileum, which we generally close with staples.

Operative Technique

(See Chap. 32.)

References

Boley SJ et al. (1979) Lower intestinal bleeding in the elderly. Am J Surg 137:57

Drapanas T et al. (1973) Emergency subtotal colectomy: preferred approach to management of massively bleeding diverticular disease. Ann Surg 177:519

Ottinger LW (1978) Frequency of bowel movements after colectomy with ileorectal anastomosis. Arch Surg 113:1048

34 Ileostomy, End

Indications

An end ileostomy is generally done in conjunction with a subtotal or total colectomy for inflammatory bowel disease. Occasionally a temporary end ileostomy and mucous fistula of the distal end of the bowel is constructed after the resection of a gangrenous segment of intestine or a perforated cecal lesion, when primary anastomosis is contraindicated.

Pitfalls and Danger Points

Devascularization of an excessive amount of terminal ileum, with resultant necrosis and stricture formation

Ileocutaneous fistula resulting from too deep a stitch in the seromuscular layer of the ileum when fashioning the ileostomy

Operative Strategy

Immediate maturation of the ileostomy by mucocutaneous suture, which prevents the occurrence of the serositis that is uniformly present when the serosa is exposed outside the body, has virtually eliminated a host of ileostomy complications, such as prolapse, obstruction, and excessive secretion.

The prevention of peristomal skin excoriation, which results from the escape of small bowel contents underneath the face plate of the ileostomy appliance, requires the formation of a permanently protruding ileostomy. Properly performed, the ileostomy should resemble the cervix of the uterus. A permanent protrusion of 2.0–2.5 cm is desirable. This allows for the likelihood that an underweight patient will accumulate a subcutaneous layer of fat following successful surgery for colitis.

To prevent herniation of small bowel, the gap between the cut edge of the ileum and the lateral abdominal wall should be closed in the formation of a permanent ileostomy.

Operative Technique

Preoperative Selection of Ileostomy Site

Apply the face plate of an ileostomy appliance tentatively to various positions in the right lower quadrant of the patient, to make sure it does not come into contact with the costal margin or the anterior superior spine when the patient is in a sitting position. The face plate should not extend beyond the midrectus line or the umbilicus.

In emergency operations, when an ileostomy has not been contemplated, the site for the ileostomy may be placed approximately 5 cm to the right of the midline and about 4 cm below the umbilicus.

Incision

Since ileostomy generally is not the main part of the contemplated operation, a midline incision will have already been made. Now make a circular incision in the previously selected site in the right lower quadrant and excise a circle of skin the diameter of a nickel (2 cm) (**Fig. 34–1**). The incision will then spontaneously stretch to the proper diameter. It is not necessary to excise a core of subcutaneous fat. Make a linear incision down to the anterior rectus fascia and insert retractors to expose the fascia. Make a longitudinal 2 cm incision in the fascia, exposing the rectus muscle (**Fig. 34–2**). Separate the muscle fibers with a Kelly hemostat (**Fig. 34–3**), and make a longitudinal incision in the peritoneum. Then dilate the opening in the abdominal wall by inserting two fingers (**Fig. 34–4**).

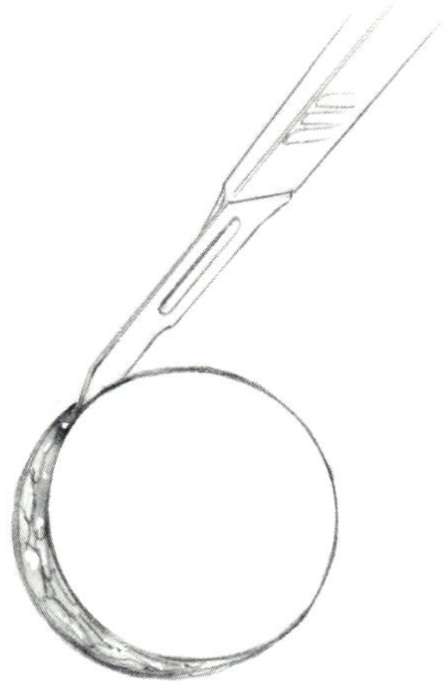

Fig. 34–1

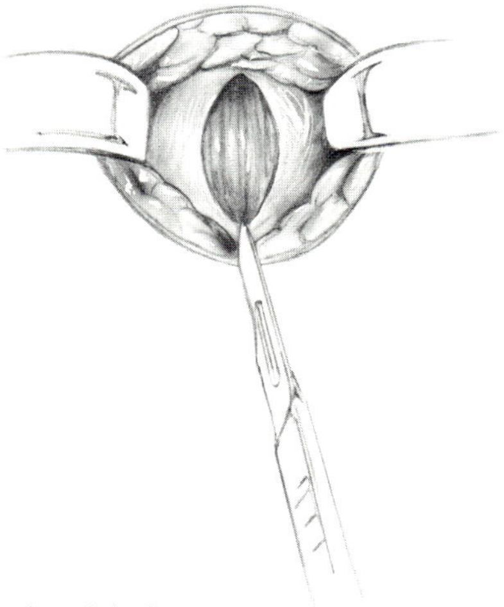

Fig. 34–2

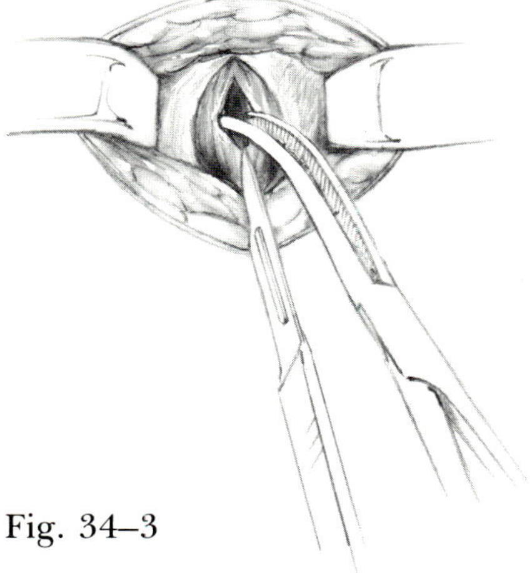

Fig. 34–3

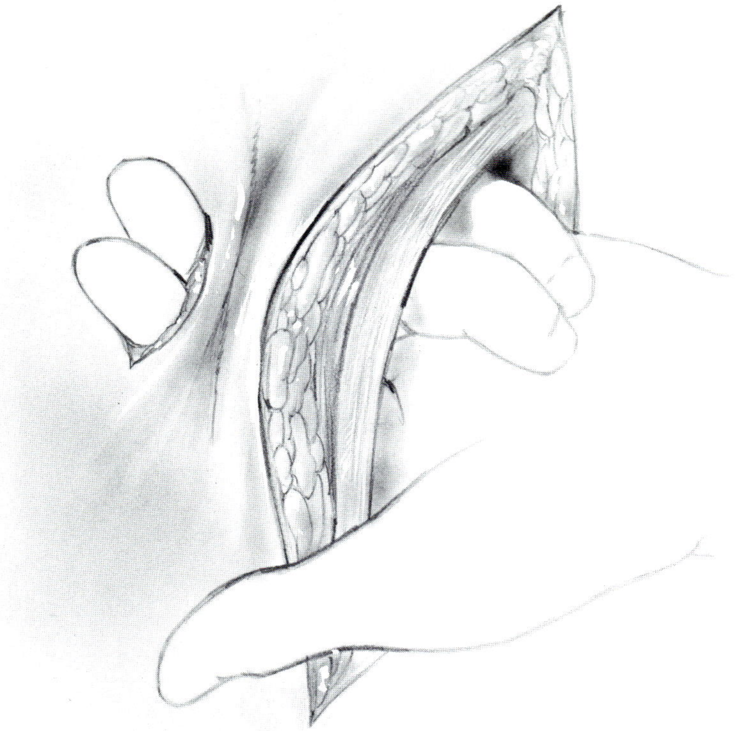

Fig. 34–4

Fashioning the Ileal Mesentery

A 6–7 cm length of ileum is required beyond the point at which the ileum meets the peritoneum if a proper ileostomy of the protruding type is to be made. If the entire mesentery is removed from this length of ileum, necrosis of the distal ileal mucosa will take place in many patients. Consequently, the portion of the ileum that passes through the abdominal wall must retain a sufficient width of mesentery to assure vascularity. The "marginal" artery can be visualized in the mesentery within 2 cm of the ileal wall. Preserve this segment of vasculature while carefully dividing the mesentery. Complete removal of the mesentery is well tolerated by the distal 2–3 cm of the ileum.

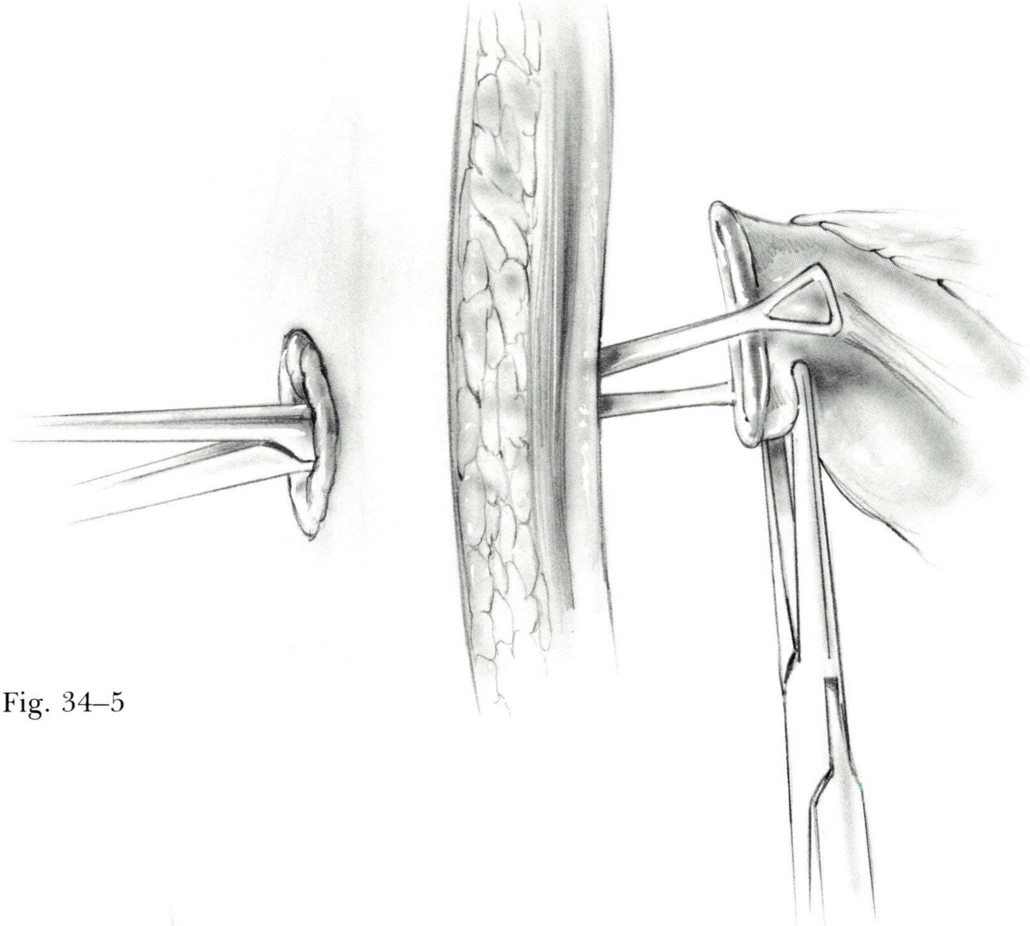

Fig. 34–5

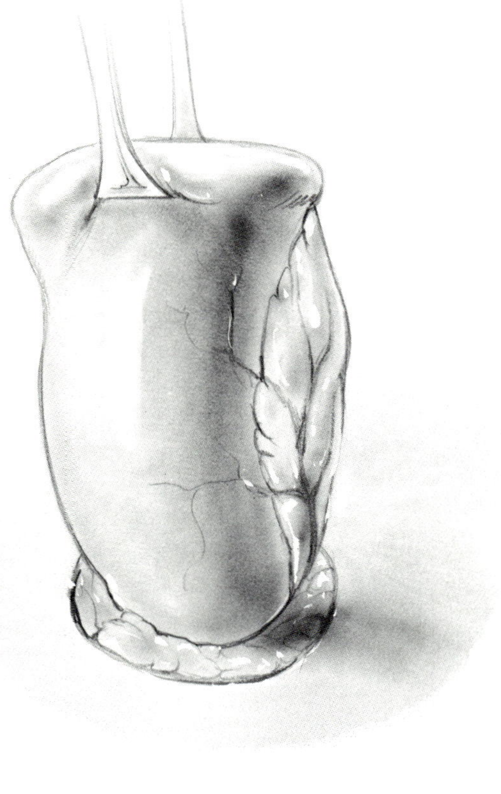

Closure of Mesenteric Gap

Insert a Babcock clamp into the abdominal cavity through the opening made for the ileostomy. Grasp the terminal ileum with the clamp and gently bring it through this opening, with the mesentery placed in a cephalad direction (**Fig. 34–5**). Place no sutures between the ileum and the peritoneum or the rectus fascia (**Fig. 34–6**).

Fig. 34–6

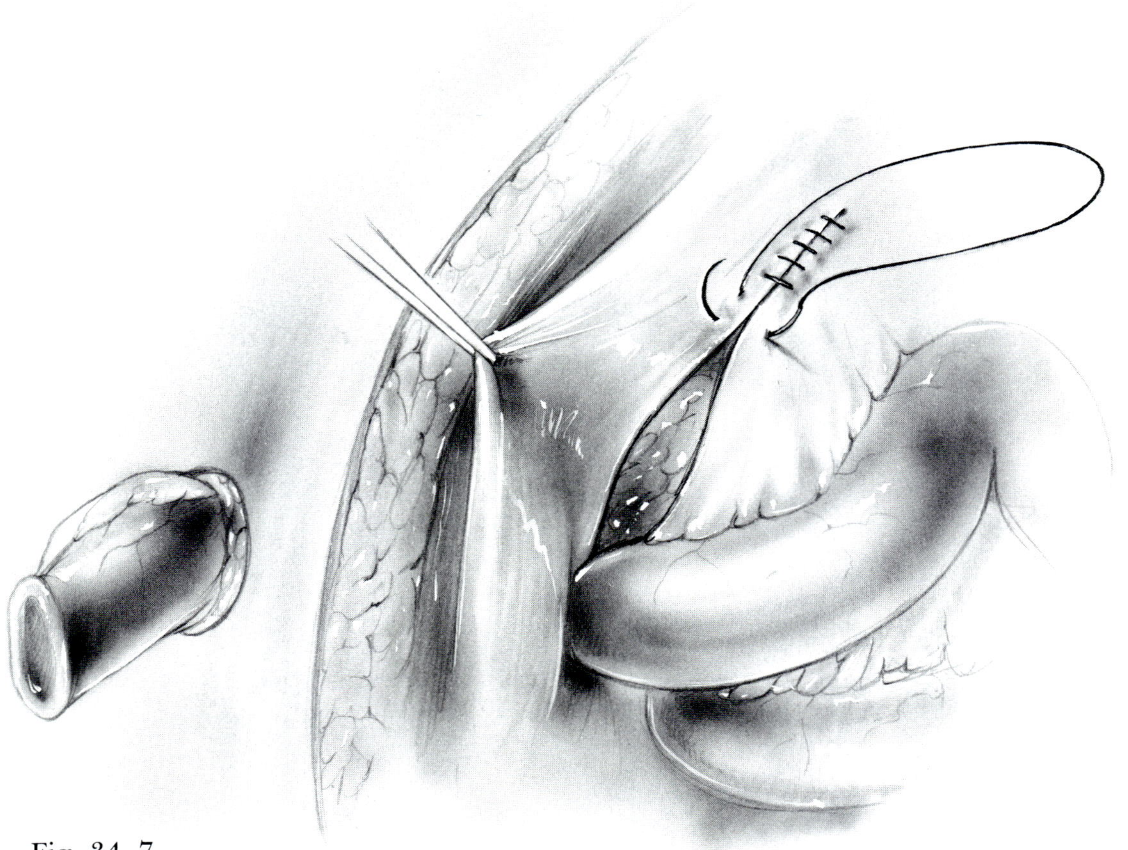

Fig. 34–7

Using a continuous 2–0 PG suture, suture the cut edge of the ileal mesentery to the cut edge of the paracolic peritoneum. This will completely obliterate the mesenteric defect (**Fig. 34–7**).

Mucocutaneous Fixation of Ileostomy

Construct a "cervix" by inserting interrupted 4–0 PG sutures through the full thickness of the terminal ileum and then using the same needle to take a shallow seromuscular bite of the lateral wall of the ileum, which is situated opposite the level

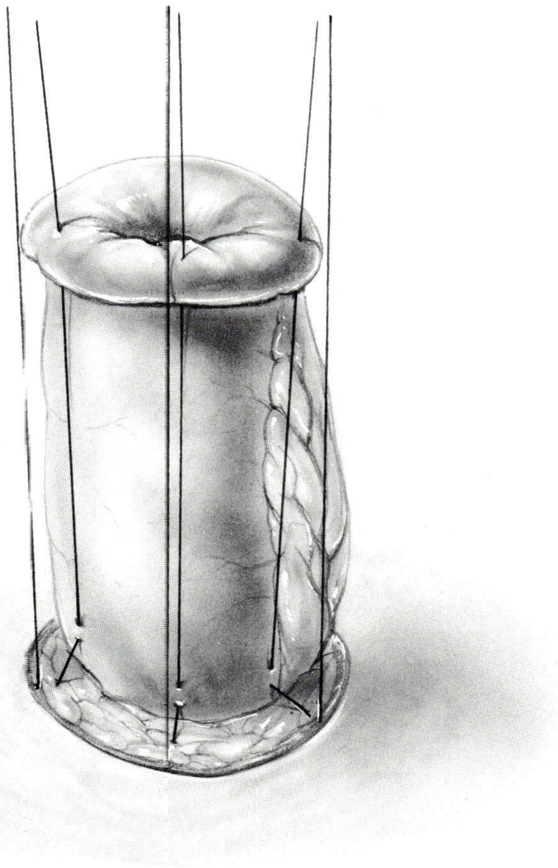

Fig. 34–8

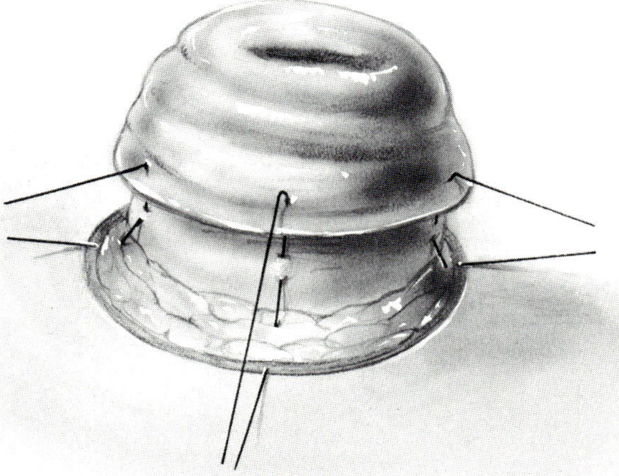

Fig. 34–9

of the skin. Complete the suture by taking a bite of the subcuticular layer of skin (**Fig. 34–8**).

Temporarily hold the stitch in a hemostat and place identical stitches in each of the other quadrants of the ileostomy. After all the sutures have been inserted, gently tightening them will evert the ileum (**Fig. 34–9**). Then tie the sutures. Place one additional suture of the same type between each of the four quadrant sutures, completing the mucocutaneous fixation.

Postoperative Care

Nasogastric suction until ileostomy function begins

Perioperative antibiotics

Apply Stomahesive disc to the ileostomy in the operating room; place an ileostomy bag over disc

Instruct patient in ileostomy care

Complications

Early

Although rare when good technique is used, occasional cases of slough of distal ileum have been observed

Peristomal infection or fistula

Late

Prolapse of ileostomy

Stricture of ileostomy

Obstruction of ileostomy due to food fiber

Peristomal skin ulceration

35 Ileostomy, Loop

Indications

Temporary ileostomy is used on rare occasions as the first stage of a subtotal colectomy for inflammatory bowel disease. It has been advocated by Turnbull and Weakley for use in combination with a skin-sutured transverse colostomy in emergency operations for toxic megacolon.

It is also a temporary method of diverting the fecal stream in patients who undergo ileoproctostomy following subtotal colectomy.

Pitfalls and Danger Points

If the ileum is not transected at the proper point, so as to make the proximal stoma the dominant one, total fecal diversion will not be accomplished.

Operative Strategy

Properly performed, this technique is a good method of achieving, temporarily, the total diversion of the intestinal contents. It can be used as the first stage of a subtotal colectomy. At the second stage, the distal ileum is detached inside the abdomen and the ileostomy need not be taken down.

Operative Technique

If a loop ileostomy is being performed as a primary procedure, a midline incision beginning at the umbilicus and going caudal for 8–10 cm is adequate. Identify the distal ileum and identify the segment selected for ileostomy by applying a single marking suture to that segment of the ileum that will form the *proximal* limb of the loop ileostomy.

Select the proper site in the right lower quadrant (see Chap. 34) and excise a nickel-size circle of skin. Expose the anterior rectus fascia and make a 2 cm longitudinal incision in it (see Fig. 34–1). Separate the rectus fibers with a large hemostat and make a similar vertical incision in the peritoneum (see Figs. 34–2 and 34–3). Then stretch the ileostomy orifice by inserting two fingers (see Fig. 34–4).

After this has been accomplished, insert a Babcock clamp through the aperture into the abdominal cavity. Arrange the ileum so that the proximal segment will emerge on the *caudal* side of the ileostomy. Then have the Babcock clamp grasp the ileum just distal to the marking suture. With the aid of digital manipulation from inside the abdomen, deliver the loop of ileum into the aperture made in the right lower quadrant. The proximal limb with the marking suture should be on the *inferior* surface of the ileostomy.

Use a hemostat to pierce the mesentery of the ileum close to its posterior wall. Pass a narrow, short glass rod into this opening in the mesentery behind the ileum after the hemostat has been removed.

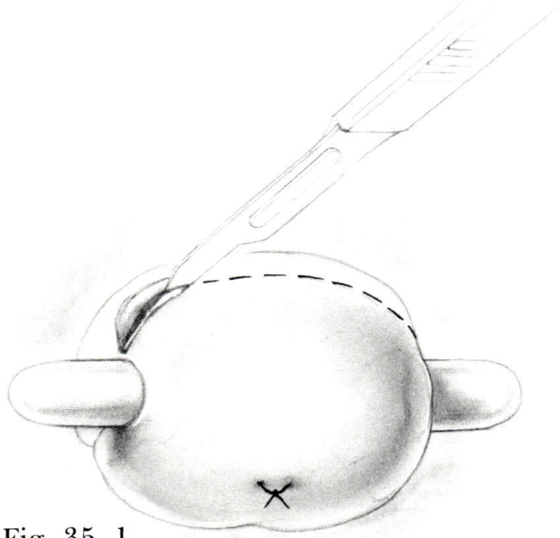

Fig. 35–1

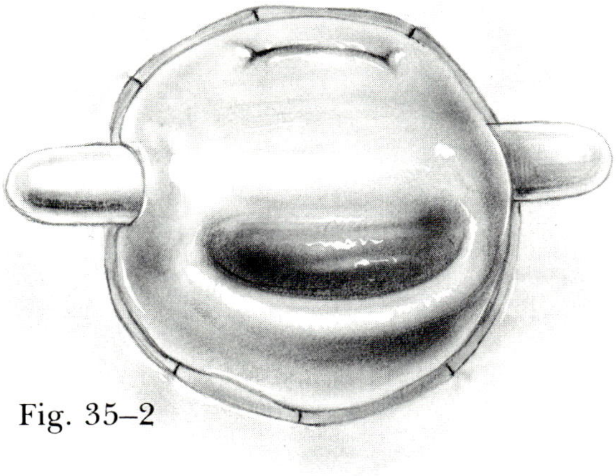

Fig. 35–2

Transect the anterior wall of the ileum at a point about 2 cm distal to the marking suture (**Fig. 35–1**). This will appear on the cephalad aspect of the apex of the ileostomy. Because the incision is placed away from the apex of the ileostomy, the proximal and distal stomas are not equal in size. The proximal stoma is much larger and, therefore, dominates the ileostomy; this assures complete diversion of the fecal stream. Fig. 35–1 shows how the incision encompasses slightly more than 50% of the circumference of the ileum to accomplish this end.

Mature the cut ends of the ileostomy by interrupted mucocutaneous sutures of 4–0 atraumatic PG. The sutures should penetrate the full thickness of the ileum and attach it to the subcuticular layer of skin (**Fig. 35–2**). The glass rod should remain in place for about 5 days. This does not interfere with the application of an ileostomy appliance.

Postoperative Care

(See Chap. 34.)

Complications

(See Chap. 34.)

Reference

Turnbull R, Weakley FL (1971) Surgical treatment of toxic megacolon: ileostomy and colostomy to prepare patients for colectomy. Am J Surg 122:325

36 Abdominoperineal Proctectomy for Benign Disease

Indications

Inflammatory bowel disease, including ulcerative colitis and Crohn's colitis with intractable rectal involvement

Familial polyposis (a controversial indication)

Preoperative Preparation

(See Chap. 31.)

Pitfalls and Danger Points

Operative damage to or interruption of pelvic autonomic nerves in male patients, leading to sexual impotency or failure of ejaculation

Pelvic sepsis, especially in patients who have perineal fistulas

Inadequate management of perineal wound, resulting in chronic perineal draining sinus

Operative Strategy

The failure of normal ejaculation is caused by the transection of the hypogastric sympathetic nerve trunks that cross over the anterior aorta. Beyond the aortic bifurcation these nerves diverge into two bundles going toward the region of the right and left hypogastric arteries, where they join the inferior hypogastric plexus on each side. According to Lee et al. the *parasympathetic* sacral autonomic outflow will be interrupted if the lateral ligaments are divided too far lateral to the rectum or if the nerve plexus between the rectum and prostate is damaged. Parasympathetic nerve damage results in the failure of erection. Proper strategy requires that the mesentery in the region of the rectosigmoid be divided along a line just adjacent to the colon, leaving considerable fat and mesentery in the presacral space to protect the hypogastric nerves. The remainder of the pelvic dissection should be carried out as close to the rectum as possible, *especially in the region of the lateral ligaments and prostate.*

As long as there are not multiple perineal fistulas, it is generally possible to achieve primary healing of the perineum *if dead space between the closed levators and the peritoneal pelvic floor is eliminated.* Because there is no need for radical excision of the pelvic peritoneum, as much of this as possible should be preserved. Additional pelvic peritoneum should be mobilized from the lateral walls of the pelvis and the bladder. If there is sufficient peritoneum to permit the pelvic peritoneal suture line to come down easily into contact with the reconstructed levator diaphragm, then the pelvic peritoneum should be closed. Otherwise it is much better to leave the pelvic peritoneum entirely unsutured to permit the small bowel to fill this space and rest on the levator diaphragm. To aid in preventing perineal sinus formation due to chronic low-grade sepsis, insert closed-suction catheters into the presacral space and instill an antibiotic solution postoperatively.

In operations done for inflammatory bowel disease, Lyttle and Parks advocate the preservation of the external sphincter muscles in proctectomy. They begin the perineal dissection with an incision near the dentate line of the anal canal and continue the dissection in the intersphincteric space between the internal and external sphincters of the anal canal. Thus the rectum is cored out of the anal canal, leaving the entire levator diaphragm and external sphincters intact. This, say Lyttle and Parks, results in less operative trauma and further minimizes dead space. We have not used this technique. It promises to reduce the incidence of damage to the prerectal nerve plexus. The results reported by Parks do not indicate that this technique has consistently achieved the goal of primary healing in the perineal wound.

Operative Technique: Abdominal

Incision and Position

With the patient positioned on Lloyd-Davies leg rests, thighs abducted and slightly flexed, make a midline incision from the midepigastrium to the pubis (see Fig. 31–1a). If the patient has previously undergone subtotal colectomy with ileostomy and mucous fistula, free the mucous fistula from its attachments to the abdominal wall. Ligate the lumen with umbilical tape and cover it with a sterile rubber glove.

Mesenteric Dissection

Divide the mesentery between sequentially applied Kelly clamps along a line *close to the posterior wall* of the rectosigmoid. Continue the line of dissection well into the presacral space. This leaves a considerable amount of fat and mesentery behind to cover the bifurcation of the aorta and sacrum (**Fig. 36–1**). The fat and mesentery prevent injury to the hypogastric nerve bundles, which travel from the preaortic area down the promontory of the sacrum toward the hypogastric vessels on each side to join the hypogastric plexuses on each side (see Fig. 31–2 and 31–4).

Rectal Dissection

Incise the pelvic peritoneum along the line where the peritoneum joins the rectum, preserving as much peritoneum as possible. Accomplish this first on the right and then on the left side (see Fig. 31–3). Note the location of each ureter (see Fig. 31–4). Divide the posterior mesentery to the midsacral level. The posterior wall of rectum can now be seen, for at this point the blood supply of the rectum comes from the lateral wall of the pelvis. Elevate the rectum from the distal sacrum by blunt dissection, and with a Metzenbaum scissors incise Waldeyer's fascia close to the rectum. Draw the rectum in a cephalad direction, and place the peritoneum of the rectovesical or rectouterine pouch on stretch. This perito-

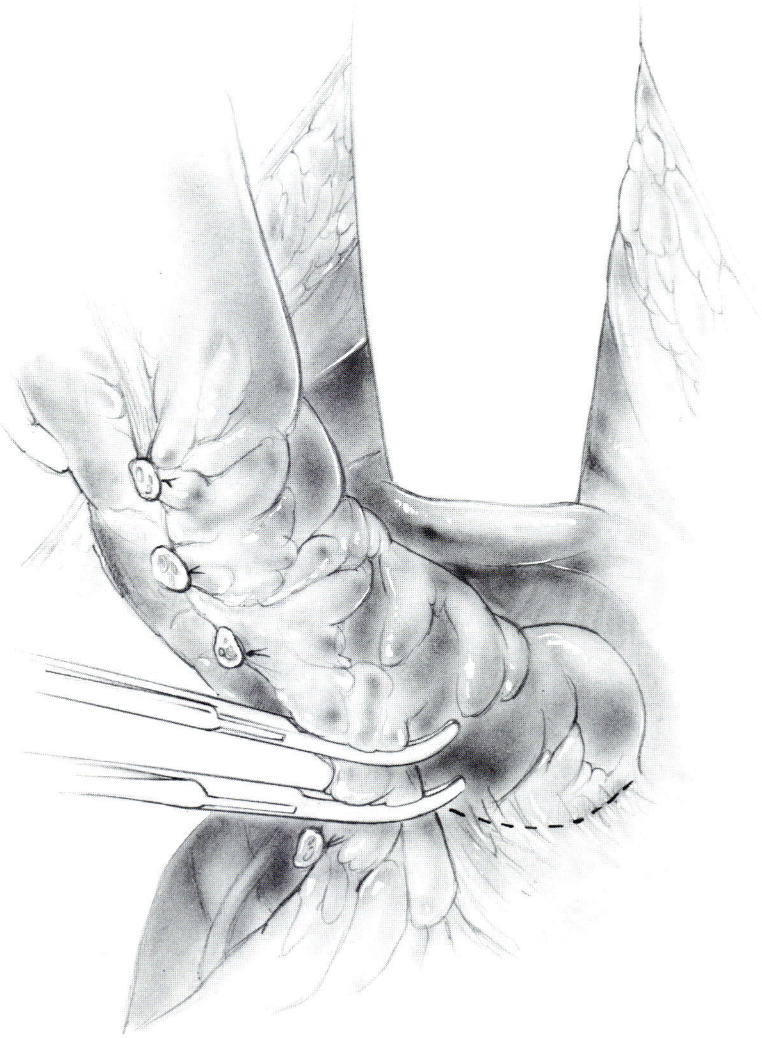

Fig. 36–1

neum can now be divided easily with a Metzenbaum scissors. Occlude the lateral ligament on each side with a large Hemoclip (see Fig. 31–7) and divide them *close* to the rectum. This maneuver often has to be repeated, as the lateral ligament may extend for several centimeters on each side. With cephalad traction on the rectum and a Lloyd-Davies retractor holding the bladder forward, divide Denonvillier's fascia at the level of the proximal portion of the prostate (see Fig. 31–9b). Keep the dissection *close to the anterior rectal wall,* which should be bluntly separated from the body of the prostate. (In females, the dissection would separate the rectum from the vagina.) When the dissection has continued beyond the tip of the coccyx posteriorly and the prostate anteriorly, initiate the perineal dissection.

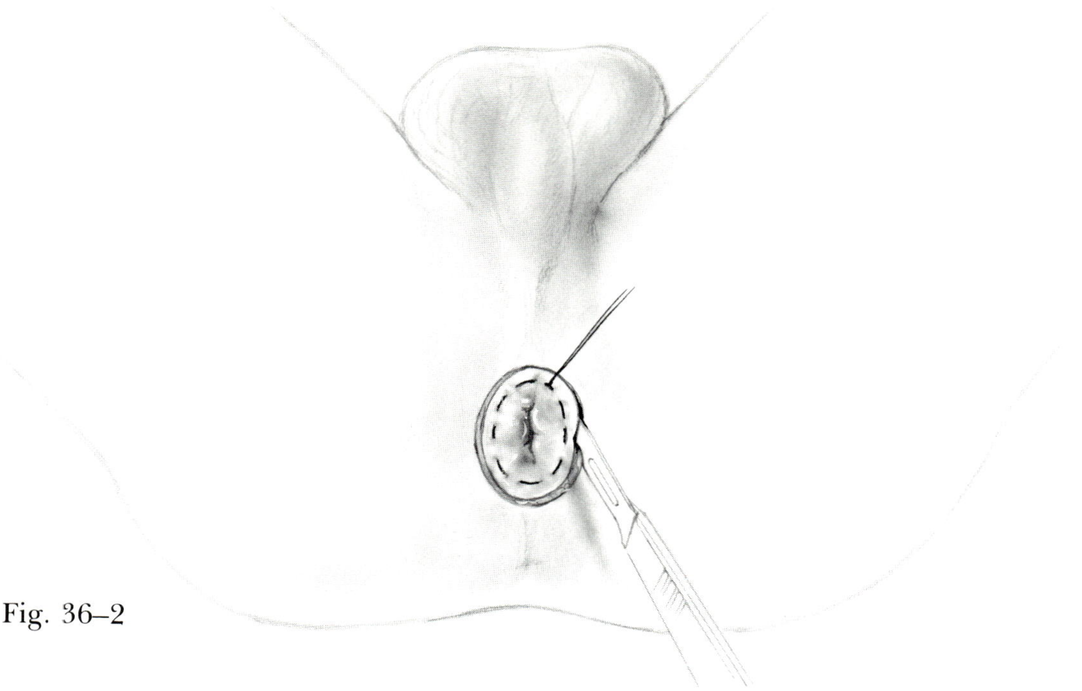

Fig. 36–2

Operative Technique: Perineal

Incision

Close the skin of the anal canal with a heavy purse-string suture (**Fig. 36–2**). Then make an incision circumferentially in the skin just outside the sphincter muscles of the anus. Carry down the dissection *close* to the sphincters to the levator muscles (**Fig. 36–3**). The inferior hemorrhoidal vessels will be encountered running toward the rectum overlying the levator muscles. Occlude these vessels by electrocoagulation. After the incision has been deepened to the levators on both sides, expose the tip of the coccyx. Transect the anococcygeal ligament by electrocautery and enter the presacral space posteriorly. The fascia of Waldeyer, which attaches to the anterior surfaces of the lower sacrum and coccyx and to the posterior rectum, forms a barrier blocking entrance into the presacral space from below even after the anococcygeal ligament has been divided.

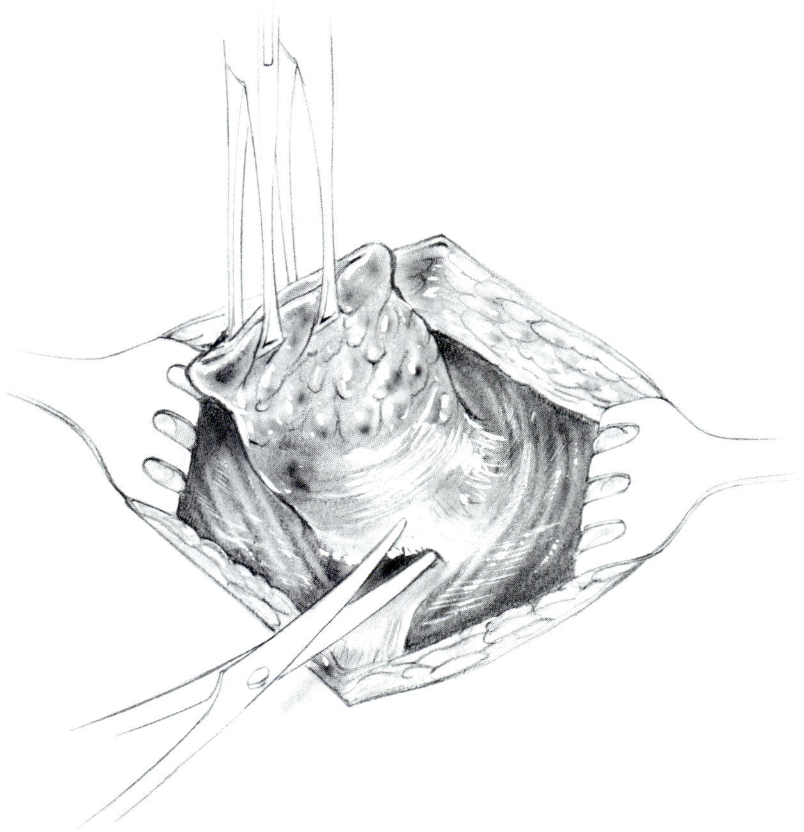

Fig. 36–3

If this fascia is elevated from the sacral periosteum by forceful blunt dissection in the perineum, venous bleeding and damage to the sacral neural components of the nervi erigentes may occur. Consequently, the fascia of Waldeyer should be divided with a long scissors or scalpel, taking the abdominal approach (see Fig. 31–8), or by *sharp* dissection from below, before an attempt is made to enter the presacral space from below.

Division of Levator Diaphragm

From the perineal approach, insert the left index finger into the opening into the presacral space and place it in the groove between the rectum and the levator muscles. Use the electrocoagulator to divide the levators close to the rectum on either side. Then deliver the specimen from the presacral space down through the posterior perineum, so that the anal canal is attached only anteriorly. Visualize the prostate gland. Using the electrocautery, transect the puborectalis and rectourethralis muscles close to the anterior rectal wall. Carry down this dissection to the level of the prostate and remove the specimen.

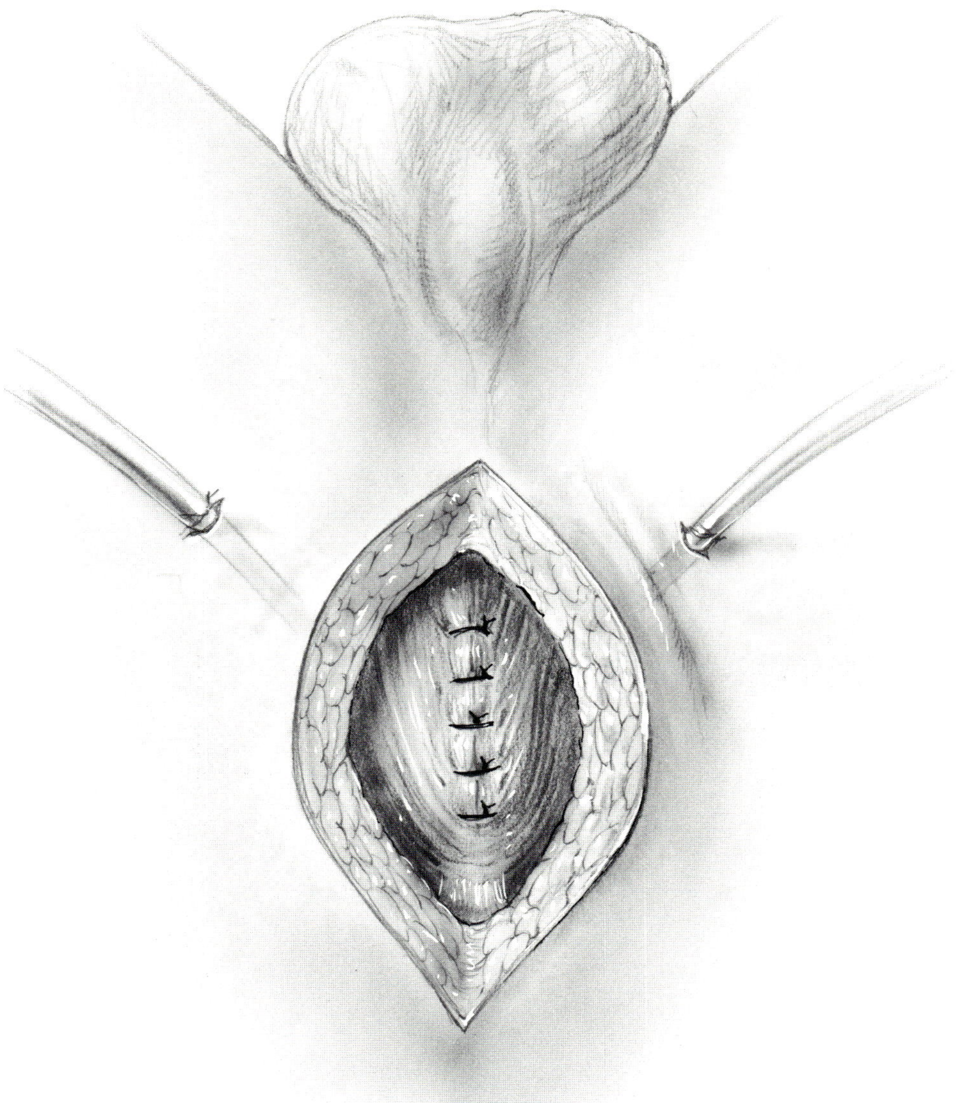

Fig. 36–4

Closure of Pelvic Floor

Insert large (6 mm) plastic catheters through the skin of the perineum and the levator muscles into the presacral space, one on each side of the midline, for closed-suction drainage.

Close the defect in the levator diaphragm, using interrupted sutures of 2–0 PG, after thoroughly irrigating the pelvis with an antibiotic solution and achieving perfect hemostasis (**Fig. 36–4**). Close the skin with subcuticular sutures of 4–0 PG. Attach the catheters to suction for the remainder of the procedure while an assistant closes the peritoneum of the pelvic floor with continuous 2–0 PG using the abdominal approach.

Abdominal Closure

After checking the integrity of the peritoneal pelvic suture line and making certain that it is contiguous with the pelvic floor, irrigate the abdominal cavity and pelvis with antibiotic solution. Approximate the abdominal wall with interrupted sutures using the modified Smead-Jones technique. Perform a routine skin closure over a long, subcutaneous closed-suction catheter, which should be brought out through a puncture wound alongside the lower pole of the incision.

Postoperative Care

(See Chap. 31.)

Complications

(See Chap. 31.)

References

Lee JF et al. (1973) Anatomic relations of pelvic autonomic nerves to pelvic operations. Arch Surg 107:324

Lyttle JA, Parks AG (1977) Intersphincteric excision of the rectum. Br J Surg 64:413

37 Operations for Colon Obstruction

Concept: Primary Resection and Anastomosis versus Staged Procedures

Many authorities report that it is safe to perform a primary resection with ileocolonic anastomosis for a mechanical obstruction of the *right* colon. Anastomosis of the obstructed small intestine is much safer than a similar anastomosis of the obstructed colon. If there is a large amount of stool in the transverse or left colon, however, primary anastomosis should be avoided. Anastomosis should also be deferred in patients who undergo emergency resection in the presence of advanced peritonitis. Such cases should be managed by resection accompanied by ileostomy and by exteriorization of the distal cut end of colon as a mucous fistula. Do not by any means perform a primary resection and anastomosis to treat obstructing lesions of the left colon. This operation has a much higher mortality rate than if preliminary colostomy were performed and followed by colon resection ten days later. The colostomy should be closed at a third operation. For perforated obstructing lesions of the left colon, perform an immediate resection with end colostomy and a mucous fistula.

Concept: Cecostomy or Colostomy?

While considerable heated debate has in the past attended discussions of the relative merits of cecostomy and colostomy for obstructions of the left colon, a rational analysis reveals clear indications for each procedure. Patients who have marked distention of the cecum may develop patches of ischemic necrosis. Performance of a transverse colostomy in such cases will not prevent perforation and subsequent peritonitis in this necrotic area. Consequently, when the preoperative X ray of the abdomen discloses a cecal diameter in excess of 12–15 cm, or if there is right lower quadrant tenderness, a cecostomy is the proper decompressive operation. This permits direct inspection of the cecum. A surgeon who wishes to perform a transverse colostomy in a patient whose cecum is markedly distended is obligated, at the very least, to make a laparotomy incision of sufficient length to permit careful exploration of the cecum in order to check for impending perforation or gangrene.

In the past two decades, cecostomy has deservedly lost popularity as a definitive treatment for the usual case of left colon obstruction. This is because the traditional *tube* cecostomy provides inadequate decompression. Even when catheters of large caliber are used, removal of fecal matter from an obstructed colon requires hourly irrigation of the catheter for many days. Since nursing personnel to accomplish this successfully is often lacking, the results of the tube cecostomy leave much to be desired. Its only attractive feature is the ease, after the cecostomy is no longer needed, of withdrawing the tube and permitting the cecal fistula to close spontaneously.

A skin-sutured cecostomy, as described below, can on the other hand prove quite effective in decompressing and cleansing the obstructed colon. When there is no indication for exposing the cecum, a transverse colostomy is more efficient in accomplishing decompression and cleansing.

Some surgeons have suggested that a colostomy situated in the left colon, proximal to a colon obstruction, would permit more effective cleansing. It also would have the advantage, they say, of eliminating the colostomy at the time of colon resection. Unfortunately, the anatomy of the colon is such that performing a colostomy in the *descending* colon is often not possible without liberating the splenic flexure, for there is no redundancy of colon in this location. Using the sigmoid colon would place the colostomy too close to the tumor unless the lesion were situated at or below the rectosigmoid. Consequently, this concept does not have wide applicability.

38 Cecostomy

Indications

A cecostomy is indicated when there is impending perforation of the cecum secondary to a colon obstruction or colonic ileus.

Concept

In left colon obstruction, when the diameter of the cecum is over 12–15 cm, as measured on abdominal X rays, an impending rupture of the cecum must be suspected. If the X-ray finding is accompanied by tenderness in the right lower quadrant, it is mandatory to explore the area of the cecum, as patches of pressure-caused necrosis may be present. If a transverse colostomy is done in this situation, the necrotic patch may nevertheless perforate, producing fatal peritonitis. Sometimes, in left colon obstruction, serosal tears can be noted. Whether the findings are large diameter and tenderness or serosal tears, it is safer to perform a skin-sutured cecostomy than a transverse colostomy, as the former permits inspection of the cecum, excision of possible necrotic patches, and immediate decompression.

If free perforation of the cecum has already occurred, an immediate resection of the perforated segment with ileostomy and mucous fistula is safer than cecostomy in most cases.

The skin-sutured cecostomy is a satisfactory method of decompressing obstructions of the left colon, but the use of a tube cecostomy for this purpose is not effective, as the tube will frequently become obstructed with particles of stool.

Tube cecostomy is, however, effective in cases of colonic ileus or a pseudo-obstruction of the type seen following Caesarian section. In these cases the problem is not one of removing stool, but simply of preventing the accumulated gas from perforating the cecum. It is a self-limiting condition; spontaneous remission occurs after 4–7 days. The tube cecostomy heals following the removal of the tube; the major disadvantage of the skin-sutured cecostomy is that a formal operation for closure is necessary later.

Preoperative Preparation

- Perioperative antibiotics
- Nasogastric suction
- Fluid resuscitation
- Preoperative barium colon enema X ray

Pitfalls and Danger Points

A cecostomy introduces the danger that fecal matter may spill into the peritoneal cavity.

Operative Strategy

In the attempt to avoid fecal contamination of the abdominal cavity during this operation, the cecum may be sutured to the external oblique aponeurosis before being incised for the mucocutaneous suture.

Operative Technique

Skin-sutured Cecostomy

Incision

Make a transverse incision about 4–5 cm long over McBurney's point and carry it in the same line through the skin, external oblique aponeurosis, internal oblique, and transversus muscles, as well as through the peritoneum. Do not attempt to split the muscles along the line of their fibers.

Exploration of Cecum

Rule out patches of necrosis in areas beyond the line of incision by carefully exploring the cecum. To accomplish this without the danger of rupturing the cecum, insert a 16-gauge needle attached to an empty 50-cc syringe, which will release some of the pressure. After this has been accomplished, close the puncture wound with a fine suture. Elevate the abdominal wall with a retractor to expose the anterior and lateral walls of the cecum. If the exposure is inadequate, make a larger incision. If a necrotic patch of cecum can be identified, this is the area that should be selected for the cecostomy, for it enables the surgeon to excise the necrotic patch during the procedure.

Cecal Fixation

Suture the wall of the cecum to the external oblique aponeurosis with a continuous 4–0 PG suture on a fine needle, so as to prevent any fecal spillage from reaching the peritoneal cavity (**Fig. 38–1**).

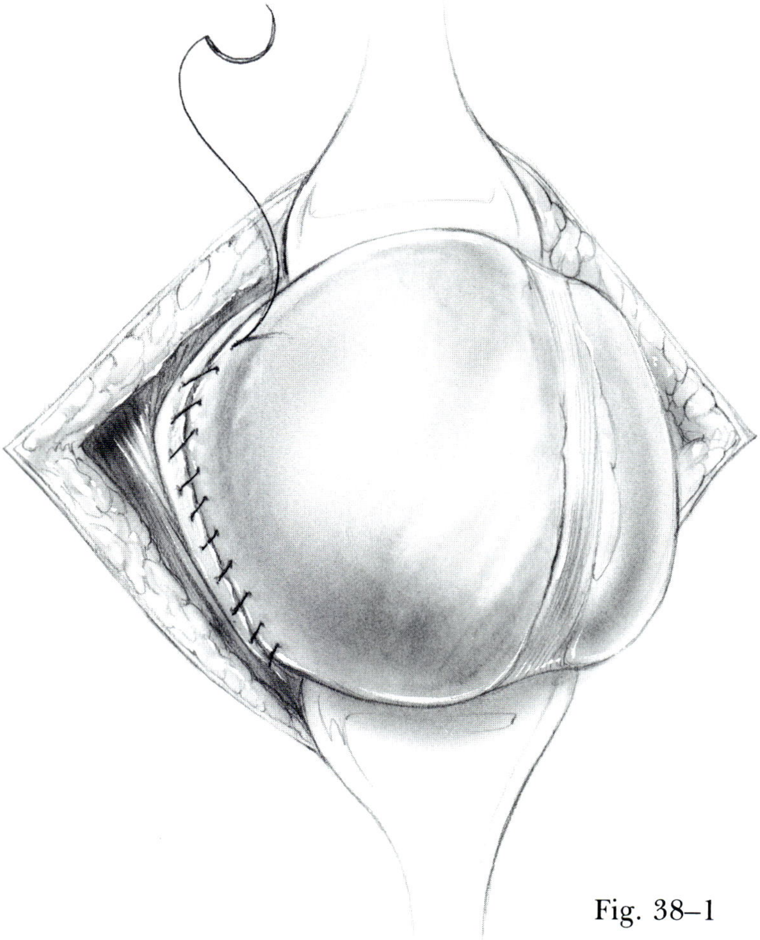

Fig. 38–1

If the incision in the external oblique aponeurosis is longer than 4–5 cm, narrow it with several PG sutures. Narrow the skin incision also to the same length with several fine PG subcuticular sutures.

Mucocutaneous Suture

Make a transverse incision in the anterior wall of the cecum 4 cm long (**Fig. 38–2**) and aspirate liquid stool and gas. Then suture the full thickness of the cecal wall to the subcuticular layer of the skin with a continuous or interrupted suture of 4–0 chromic catgut on an atraumatic needle (**Fig. 38–3**). Place a properly fitted ileostomy bag over the cecostomy at the conclusion of the operation.

Tube Cecostomy

The abdominal incision and the exploration of the cecum for a tube cecostomy are identical to those done for a skin-sutured cecostomy. Insert a purse-string suture in a circular fashion on the anterior wall of the cecum, using 3–0 atraumatic PG. The diameter of the circle should be 1.5 cm. Insert a second purse-string outside the first, using the same suture material. Then make a stab wound in the

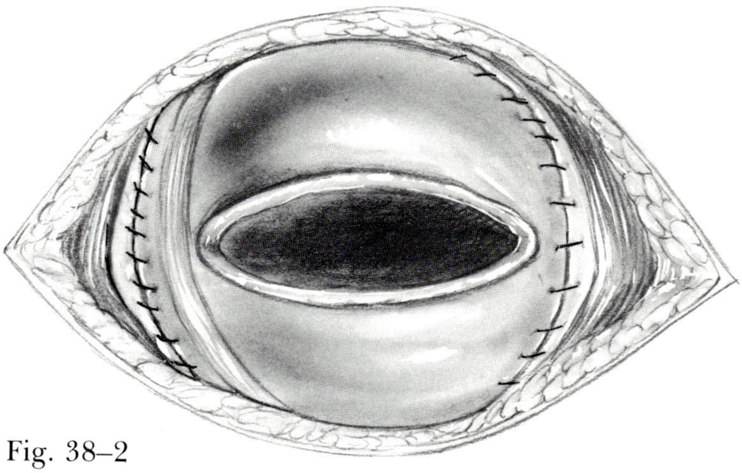

Fig. 38–2

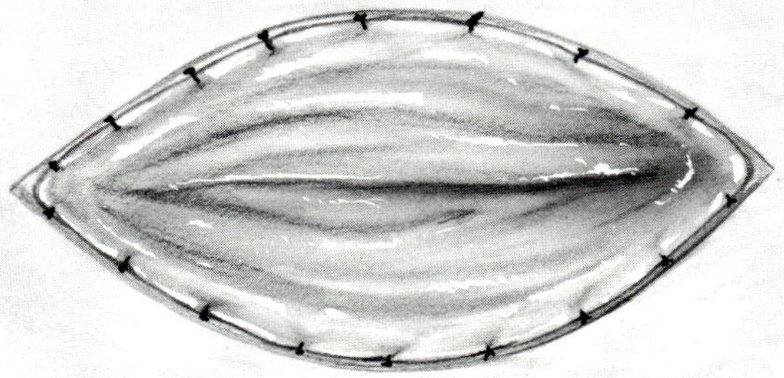

Fig. 38–3

middle of the purse-string; insert a 36F soft-rubber tube into the purse-string and for about 5 or 6 cm into the ascending colon. Tie the first purse-string around the rubber tube; then tie the second purse-string so as to invert the first. It is helpful if several large side holes have been cut first in the distal 3–4 cm of the rubber tube.

Select a site about 3 cm above the incision for a stab wound. Bring out the rubber tube through this stab wound and suture the cecum to the peritoneum close to the stab wound. Use four interrupted 3–0 PG atraumatic sutures to keep the peritoneal cavity free of any fecal matter that may leak around the tube.

Close the abdominal incision in a single layer by the modified Smead-Jones technique, using interrupted 3–0 monofilament stainless steel wire or 0 PG sutures. Do not close the skin wound; insert several 4–0 nylon interrupted skin sutures, which will be tied 6–8 days after operation.

Postoperative Care

Manage the skin-sutured cecostomy in the operating room by applying an adhesive-backed ileostomy-type disposable plastic appliance to it.

The tube cecostomy requires repeated irrigation with saline to prevent it from being plugged by fecal particles. It may be removed after the tenth postoperative day if it is no longer needed.

Complications

The major postoperative complication of this procedure is peristomal sepsis, for the possibility of bacterial contamination of the abdominal incision cannot be completely eliminated. Nevertheless, peristomal sepsis is much less common than one would anticipate in an operation of this type.

39 Transverse Colostomy

Indications

Relief of obstruction due to lesions of left colon

Diversion of fecal stream

Complementary to left colon anastomosis

Preoperative Preparation

Before performing a colostomy for colon obstruction, do a barium colon enema X ray to confirm the diagnosis and rule out such causes of obstruction as fecal impaction; use preoperative flat X ray of abdomen to identify position of transverse colon relative to a fixed point, such as a coin placed over the umbilicus

Fluid restitution

Nasogastric tube

Perioperative antibiotics

Pitfalls and Danger Points

Performing colostomy in error for diagnoses such as fecal impaction

Be certain the "ostomy" is, in fact, being constructed in transverse colon (we are aware of cases in which procedure was performed erroneously in sigmoid colon and, in one instance, in gastric antrum!)

In advanced colon obstruction, be aware of possibility of impending rupture of cecum, for which transverse colostomy is an inadequate operation

Operative Strategy

Impending Rupture of Cecum

In routine cases of left colon obstruction, with the diagnosis confirmed by barium enema X ray, the colon may be approached through a small transverse incision in the right rectus muscle. This incision should be made for the colostomy alone; the rest of the abdominal cavity does not have to be explored. Exceptions to this policy should be made for patients who suffer a sigmoid volvulus, who are suspected of having ischemic colitis or perforation, and in whom an advanced obstruction threatens an impending rupture of the cecum. Impending rupture should be suspected when the diameter of the cecum, measured on the flat abdominal X ray, is in the 12–15 cm range, and especially when the patient demonstrates right lower quadrant tenderness. In such cases, direct inspection of the cecum is mandatory. This may be accomplished with a midline laparotomy incision or a transverse right lower quadrant incision made over the cecum. If tears of the serosa can be seen, cecostomy should be performed. If there is an area of impending necrosis, this should be excised and the defect in the cecum converted to a skin-sutured cutaneous cecostomy (see Chap. 38). This provides satisfactory decompression of the obstructed colon while it eliminates the possibility of cecal rupture.

Importance of Immediate Maturation of Colostomy

With the discovery in 1951–52 by Patey and Brooke that fixing the bowel mucosa in apposition to the dermal epithelium eliminates serositis, the traditional loop colostomy over a glass rod became an obsolete operation. It became obsolete for a number of reasons:

1) *Exteriorization* of the posterior wall of the transverse colon over a glass rod requires more dissection as well as a longer incision than does a matured colostomy.

2) *Exposure* of the outer surface of the bowel outside the body results in marked serositis, manifested by much edema and inflammation.

3) *Closure* of the colostomy has to be delayed for at least 4–6 weeks to permit the serositis and edema to subside. When the colostomy is eventually closed, the fibrosis, which follows the serositis, often mandates a formal resection of the colostomy, including anastomosis. A colostomy that has been immediately matured by skin sutures, however, may be closed at any time. The need for resection and anastomosis following the latter technique is rare.

4) The *bulky nature* of the loop colostomy over a glass rod makes it difficult to manage. Application of a colostomy bag is often followed by leakage. On the other hand, the matured colostomy is fitted with an appliance in the operating room, making postoperative management far simpler.

Though it would appear that contamination of the subcutaneous tissues by fecal spillage during the act of suturing the mucosa to the skin would invariably lead to subcutaneous abscess, this has rarely occurred. Since 1961 we have been quite satisfied using the mucocutaneous suture technique for all colostomies.

Diversion of Fecal Stream

Contrary to widespread medical opinion, it is not necessary to construct a double-barreled colostomy, including complete transection of the colon, in order to divert the stool from entering the left colon. We agree with Turnbull and Weakley that if a 5 cm longitudinal incision is made on the antimesenteric wall of the transverse colon and is followed by immediate maturation, fecal diversion is accomplished even in the absence of a supporting glass rod. Fecal diversion is accomplished with this operation because the long incision in the colon permits the posterior wall to prolapse. This in effect results functionally in separate distal and proximal stomas.

It should be remembered, however, that in the presence of spreading peritonitis from perforated sigmoid diverticulitis, no type of transverse colostomy can prevent the column of stool situated between the colostomy and the sigmoid perforation from passing through the point of leakage and perpetuating sepsis. In cases such as these, immediate resection with end colostomy and mucous fistula is the only operation that will prevent further fecal leakage.

Operative Technique

Incision

Make a transverse incision over the middle and lateral thirds of the upper right rectus muscle (**Fig. 39–1**). The length of the skin incision, ideally, would equal the length of the longitudinal incision to be made in the colon (5–6 cm). To accomplish this, it is necessary to identify the

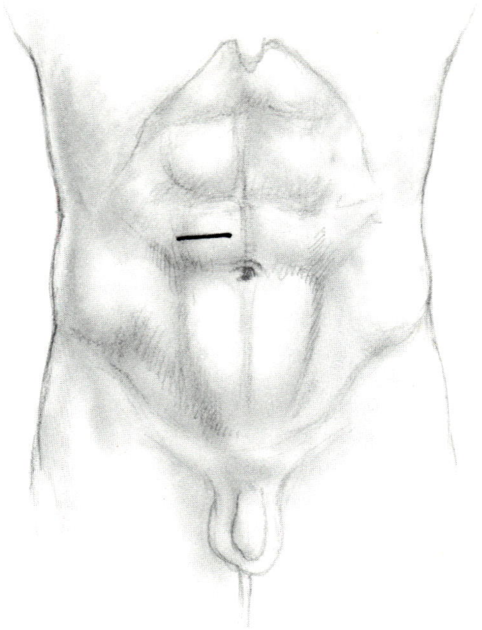

Fig. 39–1

level at which the transverse colon crosses the path of the right rectus muscle. This may be done by a preoperative flat X ray of the abdomen, followed by confirmation by percussion of the upper abdomen in the operating room. Make the transverse incision sufficiently long to accomplish accurate identification of the transverse colon. The incision should be partially closed subsequently, leaving a 5 cm gap to accommodate the colostomy.

When the transverse colostomy is to precede a subsequent laparotomy for the removal of colon pathology, begin the transverse incision 2 cm to the right of the midline and extend it laterally. If this is done, the colostomy will not prevent the surgeon from using a long midline incision for the second stage of the operation.

After the skin incision is made, incise the anterior rectus fascia with a scalpel. Insert a Kelly hemostat between the muscle belly and the posterior rectus sheath. Incise the rectus muscle transversely over the hemostat with the coagulating electrocautery for a distance of 6 cm. Then enter the abdomen in the usual manner by incising the posterior rectus sheath and peritoneum.

Identification of Transverse Colon

Even though the transverse colon is covered by omentum, in the average patient the omentum is thin enough so that the colon can be seen through it. Positive identification can be made by observing the taenia. The omentum should be divided for 6–7 cm over the colon. If colon is not clearly visible, extend the length of the incision.

Exteriorize the omentum and draw it in a cephalad direction; its undersurface will lead to its junction with the transverse colon. At this point make a window in the overlying omentum so that the transverse colon may protrude through the incision. Then replace the omentum into the abdomen.

Immediate Maturation of Colostomy

In patients who undergo operations for colon obstruction, the transverse colon is often so tensely distended that it is difficult to extract the anterior wall of the colon from the abdominal cavity without causing damage. To solve this problem, apply two Babcock clamps 2 cm apart to the anterior wall of the transverse colon. Insert a No. 16 needle, attached either to a low-pressure suction line or to a 50-cc syringe from which the barrel has been removed, into the colon between the Babcock clamps (**Fig. 39–2**). After the gas has been allowed to escape through the needle, the colon can be exteriorized easily.

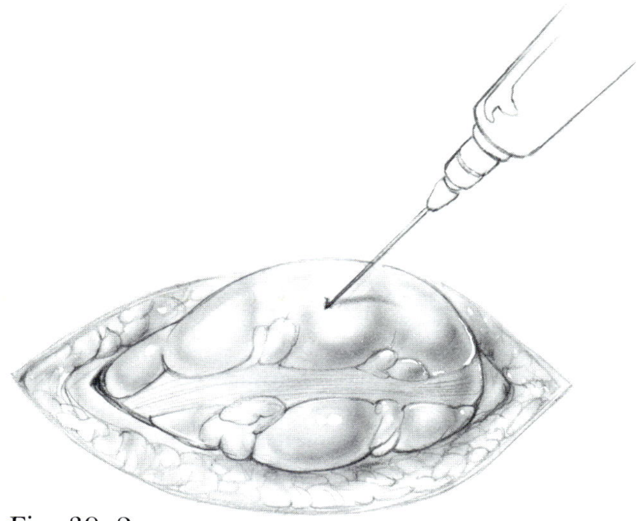

Fig. 39–2

At this point, Turnbull and Weakley insert a layer of chromic catgut sutures between the serosa of the colon and either the anterior rectus sheath or the deep subcutaneous fascia. We have omitted this step and have not discerned any ill effect from the omission.

The incision in the abdominal wall should be about 6 cm long. If it is longer than 6 cm, then close the lateral portion with interrupted No. 1 PG sutures of the Smead-Jones type. Use interrupted 4–0 nylon skin sutures to shorten the skin incision appropriately.

Immediate maturation can be accomplished by making an incision, 5–6 cm long, longitudinally along the anterior wall of the colon, preferably in the taenia (**Fig. 39–3**). Aspirate the bowel content. Irrigate

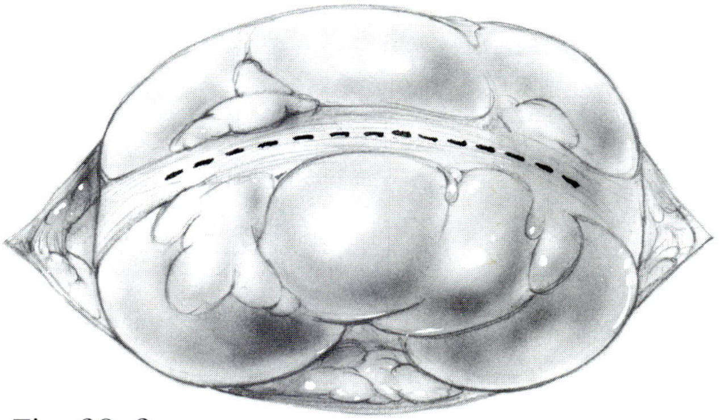

Fig. 39–3

the operative field with 0.1% kanamycin solution. Then suture the full thickness of the colon wall to the *subcuticular* layer of the skin with 4–0 chromic catgut or PG sutures, either interrupted or continuous (**Fig. 39–4**). Attach a disposable ileostomy or colostomy bag to the colostomy.

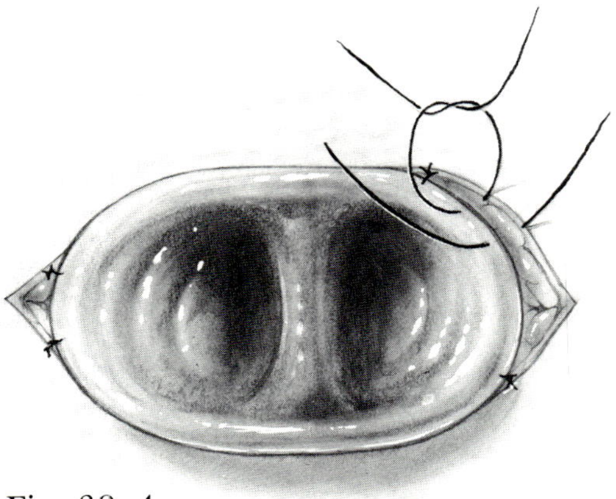
Fig. 39–4

Modification of Technique Using Glass Rod

We prefer not to interrupt the suture line between the colon and skin by the use of a glass rod. In markedly obese patients who have a short mesentery, a modified glass rod technique may be used to prevent retraction while it keeps the colocutaneous suture line intact. This may be accomplished by the technique of Turnbull and Weakley. Make a stab wound through the skin at a point about 4 cm caudal to the midpoint of the proposed colostomy. By blunt dissection pass a glass or plastic rod between the subcutaneous fat and the anterior rectus fascia, going in a cephalad direction. Pass the rod deep to the colon and have it emerge from a second stab wound 4 cm cephalad to the colostomy (**Fig. 39–5**). This technique permits the subcutaneous fat to be protected from postoperative contamination by stool. It also simplifies the application of the colostomy bag.

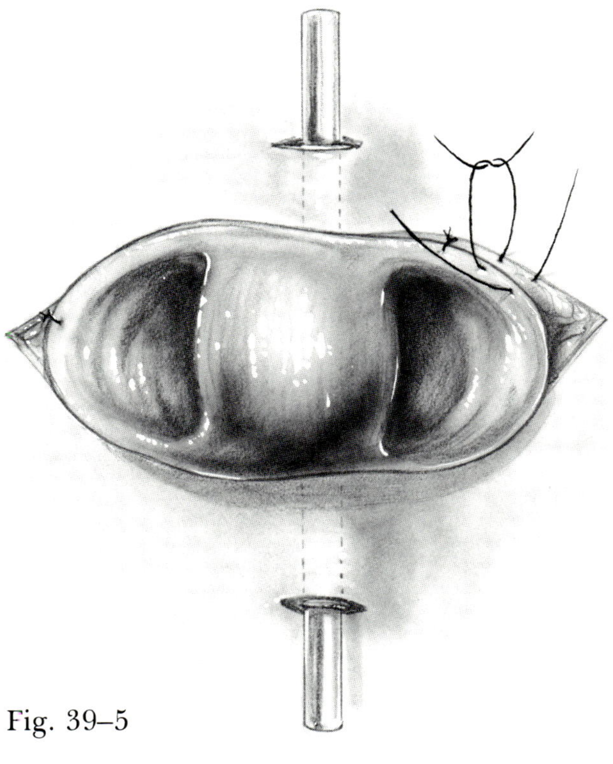
Fig. 39–5

One alternative to the solid rod is a Silastic tube, 6 mm in diameter. We prefer this because it produces minimal inflammatory tissue response. However, since the Silastic tube is soft, it has to be fixed to the skin of the two stab wounds with nylon sutures.

Postoperative Care

- In the operating room apply a plastic disposable adhesive-type colostomy bag, with a karaya gum facing or Stomahesive disc to the colostomy
- Nasogastric suction until colostomy functions

Complications

Peristomal sepsis is surprisingly uncommon. Treatment requires local incision and drainage. Massive sepsis would require moving the colostomy to another site.

References

Brooke BN (1952) The management of ileostomy including its complications. Lancet 2:102

Patey, DH (1951) Primary epithelial apposition in colostomy. Proc R Soc Med 44:423

Turnbull RB Jr, Weakley FL (1967) Atlas of intestinal stomas. Mosby, St Louis

40 Closure of Temporary Colostomy

Concept: When to Close a Colostomy

There are reports in the surgical literature—Wheeler and Barker, Knox et al., and Yaiko et al. among them—describing many complications and even mortality following operations for closure of a colostomy. In many instances it is emphasized that the complications are more numerous when a colostomy is closed before 30–90 days have passed after the formation of the colostomy. On the other hand, we have had excellent results even when colostomies were closed 2–3 weeks after the initial operation. The discrepancy exists because all of our colostomies were immediately matured by mucocutaneous suture. Most of the authors who report complications from colostomy closure and who require the passage of 30–90 days to make closure safer do a loop colostomy over a glass rod. If immediate mucocutaneous suture is not done, several weeks must elapse before granulation and contraction results in spontaneous maturation of the colostomy. Because this type of colostomy often is accompanied by considerable fibrosis and inflammation, the surgeon should indeed wait 60–90 days before attempting closure. Turnbull and Weakley agree that when the colostomy has been matured by mucocutaneous suture at the initial operation, the colostomy closure may take place whenever indicated by the patient's condition. Also, in our experience the matured colostomy can generally be closed without the need to resect and anastomose a segment of colon.

The absence of distal obstruction in the colon is another requirement for safe closure of a colostomy. This should be confirmed by a barium colon enema X ray before colostomy closure.

Preoperative Preparation

Barium colon enema X ray to demonstrate patency of distal colon

Nasogastric tube

Routine mechanical and antibiotic bowel preparation (see Chap. 25); in addition, carry out saline irrigations of inactivated left colon segment

Perioperative systemic antibiotics

Pitfalls and Danger Points

Suture-line leak

Intra-abdominal abscess

Wound abscess

Operative Strategy

Suture-line leakage can follow when traumatized or devascularized colon tissue is used in the closure. Another common cause of leakage is tension on the suture line due to inadequate lysis of the adhesions between the transverse colon and surrounding structures. To avoid these complications a sufficient segment of transverse colon must be freed of all surrounding adhesions. If necessary, the incision in the abdominal wall should be enlarged to provide exposure. If the tissue in the vicinity of the colostomy has been devascularized by operative trauma, do not hesitate to resect a segment of bowel and perform an end-to-end anastomosis instead of a local reconstruction. Proper suturing or stapling of healthy colon tissue—minimizing fecal contamination—combined with local antibiotic irrigation helps prevent formation of abscesses.

Infection of the operative incision is rather common following colostomy closure. This is in part the result of failure to minimize the bacterial inoculum into the wound. Another phenomenon that contributes to wound infection is the retraction of subcutaneous fat that occurs around the colostomy. This can produce a gap between the fascia and the epidermis when the skin is sutured closed. If the fat does retract, the skin should be left open at the conclusion of the operation.

Operative Technique

Incision

Occlude the colostomy by inserting a small gauze packing moistened with providone-iodine solution. Make an incision in the skin around the colostomy 3–4 mm from the mucocutaneous junction (**Fig. 40–1**). Continue this incision parallel to the mucocutaneous junction until the entire colostomy has been encircled. (Applying three Allis clamps to the lips of the defect in the colon expedites this dissec-

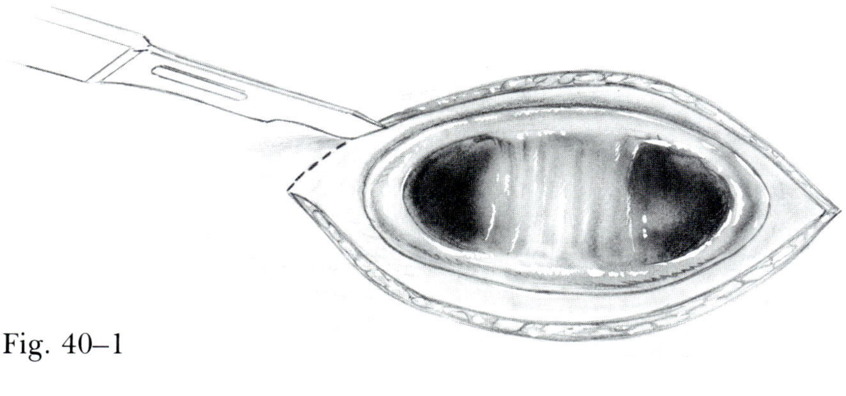

Fig. 40–1

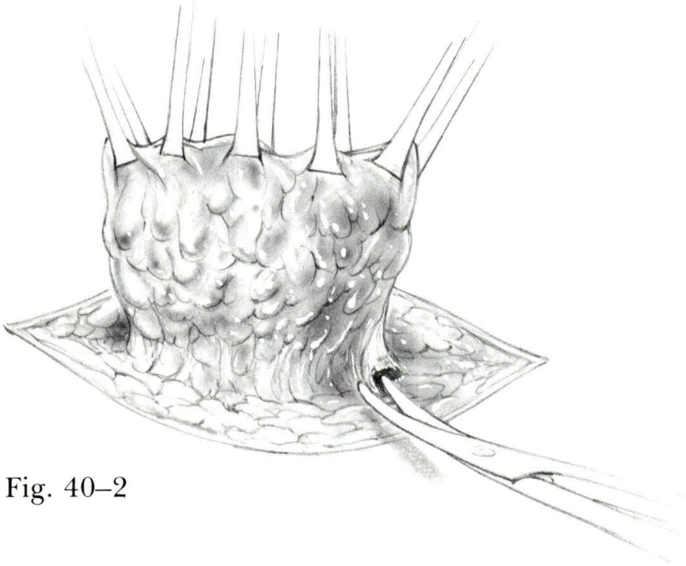

Fig. 40–2

tion and helps prevent contamination.) Deepen the incision by scalpel dissection until the seromuscular coat of colon can be identified. Then separate the serosa and surrounding subcutaneous fat by Metzenbaum-scissors dissection (**Fig. 40–2**). This dissection should be carried out with meticulous care in order to avoid trauma to the colon wall. Carry down the dissection to the point where the colon meets the anterior rectus fascia.

Fascial Dissection

Identify the fascial ring and use a scalpel to dissect the subcutaneous fat off the anterior wall of the fascia for a width of 1–2 cm, until a clean rim of fascia is visible all around the colostomy. Then dissect the colon away from the fascial ring until the peritoneal cavity is entered.

Peritoneal Dissection

Once the peritoneal cavity has been identified, it is often possible to insert the index finger and gently dissect the transverse colon away from the adjoining peritoneal attachments. Under the guidance of the index finger, separate the remainder of the colon from its attachments to the anterior abdominal wall. This can often be accomplished without appreciably enlarging the defect in the abdominal wall. However, if any difficulty whatever is encountered in freeing the adhesions between the colon and peritoneum, extend the incision laterally by dividing the remainder of the rectus muscle with the electrocautery for a distance adequate to accomplish the dissection safely.

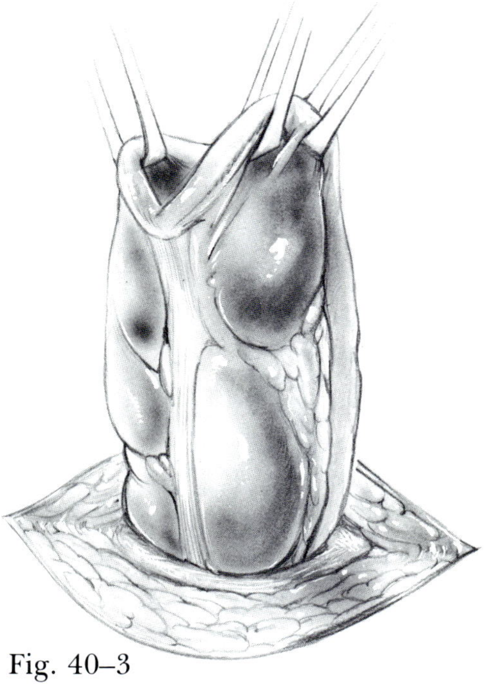
Fig. 40–3

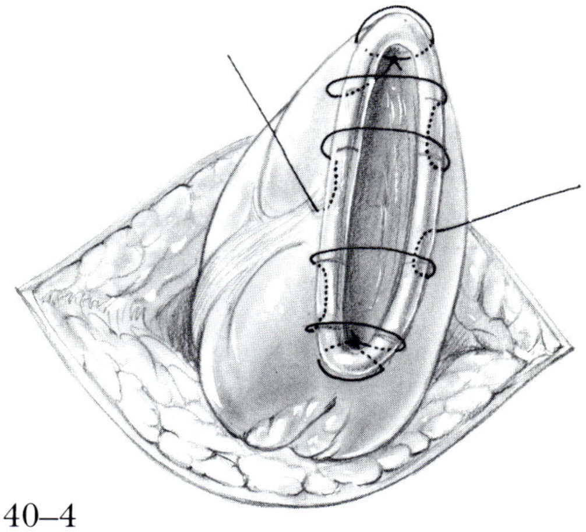
Fig. 40–4

Closure of Colon Defect by Suture

After the colostomy has been freed from all attachments for a distance of 5–6 cm (**Fig. 40–3**), detach the rim of skin from the colon. Carefully inspect the wall of the colon for injury. A few small superficial patches of serosal damage are of no significance as long as they are not accompanied by devascularization. In most cases, merely freshening the edge of the colostomy by excising a rim of 3–4 mm of scarred colon tissue will reveal healthy tissue.

The colon wall should now be of relatively normal thickness. In these cases, the colostomy defect, which resulted from a longitudinal incision in the transverse colon at the initial operation, should be closed in a transverse direction. Initiate an inverting stitch of 4–0 PG on an atraumatic curved needle at the caudal margin of the colonic defect and pursue it as a continuous Connell or continuous Cushing suture to the midpoint of the defect (**Fig. 40–4**). Then initiate a second suture of the same material on the cephalad margin of the defect and continue it also to the midpoint. Terminate the suture line here (Fig. 40–4). Then invert this layer with another layer of interrupted 4–0 cotton atraumatic seromuscular Lembert sutures (**Fig. 40–5**). Because of the transverse direction of the suture line, the lumen of the colon is quite commodious at the conclusion of the closure. There should be no tension whatever on this suture line. Finally, irrigate with a dilute antibiotic solution and reduce the colon into the abdominal cavity.

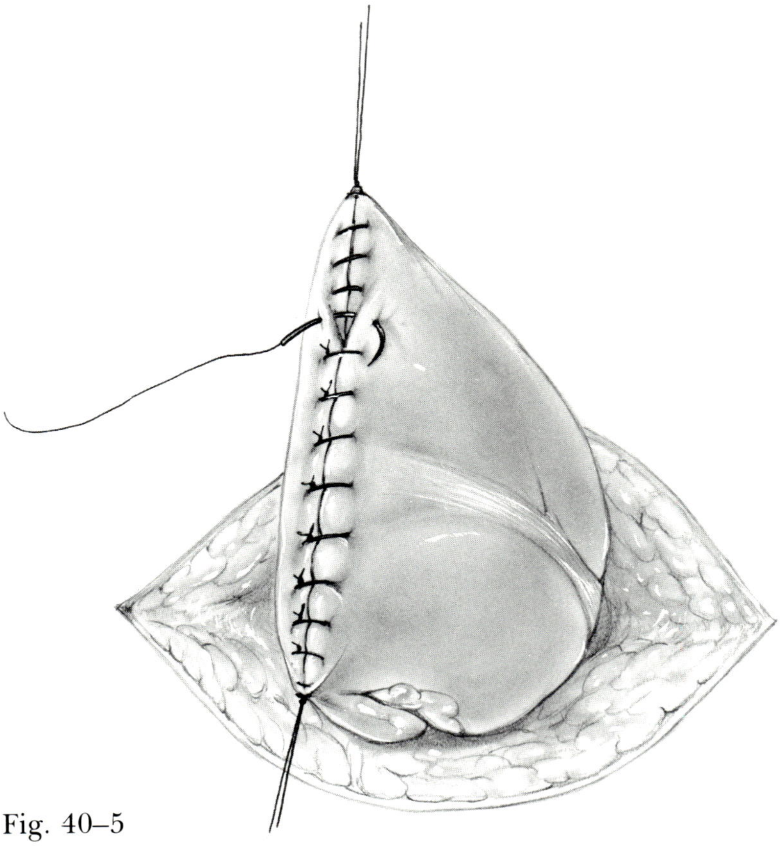

Fig. 40–5

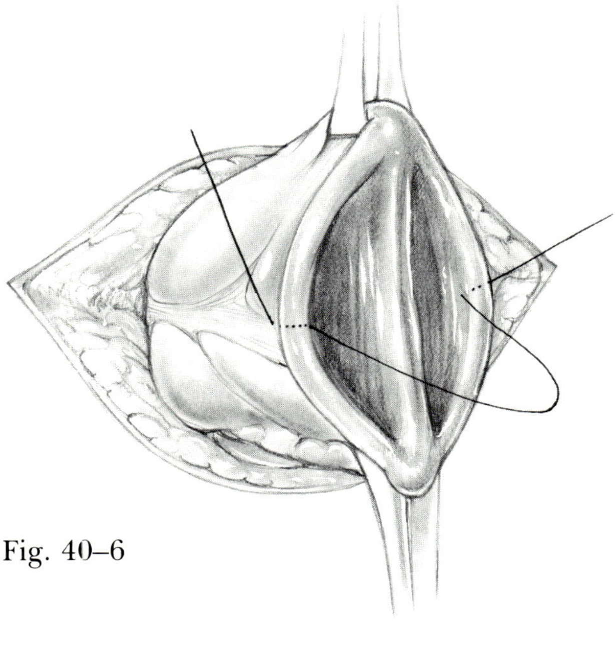

Fig. 40–6

Closure of Colonic Defect by Staples

If the colon wall is not so thick that compressing it to 2 mm will produce necrosis, stapling is an excellent method of closing the colon defect. Align the defect so that the closure can take place in a transverse direction. Place a single guy suture to mark the midpoint of the transverse closure (**Fig. 40–6**) and apply Allis clamps to approximate the colon staple line with the bowel wall in eversion.

Carry out stapling by triangulation with two applications of the TA–55 device. First, in the TA–55 device grasp the everted mucosa supported by the Allis clamps on the caudal aspect of the defect and the guy suture. Drive home the alignment pin of the TA–55 and tighten the device so the vernier marks coincide. Fire the staples and use a Mayo scissors to excise the redundant everted mucosa flush with the stapler. Leave the guy suture at the midpoint of the closure intact.

Make the final application of the TA–55 as the device is positioned deep to the Allis clamps on the cephalad portion of the defect (**Fig. 40–7**). It is important to position the guy suture so as to include the previous staple line in this second line of staples, assuring that no gap will exist between the two staple lines. Then drive home the alignment pin, tighten the stapler so that the vernier marks overlap, and

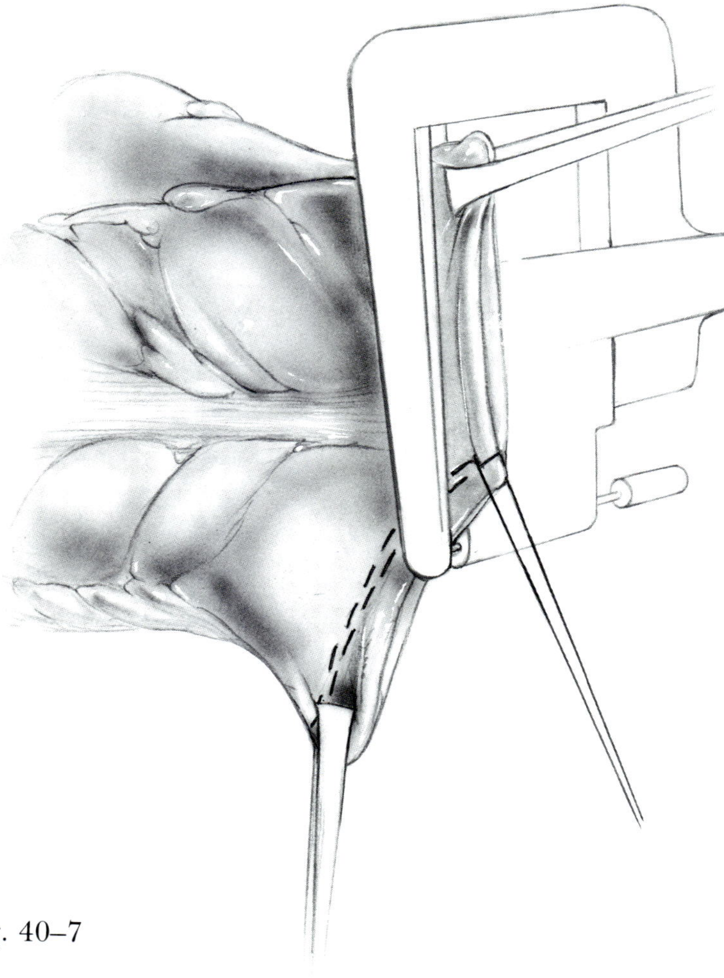

Fig. 40–7

fire the staples. Remove any redundant mucosa by excising it with Mayo scissors flush with the stapler. Lightly electrocoagulate the everted mucosa. Carefully inspect the integrity of the staple line to insure that proper B formation has taken place. It is important, especially with stapling, to ascertain that no tension is exerted on the closure.

Resection and Anastomosis of Colostomy

Whenever the tissue is of inadequate quality for closing, the incision in the abdominal wall must be enlarged and resection of a segment of colon carried out. A sufficient section of the right transverse colon must also be mobilized. Occasionally, the hepatic flexure will have to be freed from the abdominal wall too. Dissect the omentum off the transverse colon both proximal and distal to the defect. After the proximal and distal segments of the colon have been sufficiently mobilized and the traumatized tissue excised, end-to-end anastomosis can be constructed by the usual two-layer technique (see Figs. 28–16 through 28–24). Alternatively, a functional end-to-end colocolonic anastomosis may be constructed by the stapling technique (see Figs. 28–33 through 28–36).

Closure of Abdominal Wall

Irrigate the area with a dilute antibiotic solution and apply a Kocher clamp to the midpoint of the abdominal wall on the caudal and cephalad aspects of the wound. Then close the incision by the modified Smead-Jones technique (see Chap. 5).

Management of Skin Wound

Frequently the colostomy can be closed without enlarging the skin incision, which was no longer than 5–6 cm. In such cases we simply insert a loose packing of gauze into the subcutaneous space, which we allow to heal by granulation and contraction. If desired, several interrupted vertical mattress sutures of nylon may be inserted; but do not tie them until the eighth or tenth postoperative day. The subcutaneous tissue should be kept separated with moist gauze packing. There is a high incidence of wound infection following primary closure of the skin. To avoid it, the surgeon must eliminate bacterial contamination or leave the skin open.

Postoperative Care

Nasogastric suction until gastrointestinal function resumes

Systemic antibiotics are not continued beyond the perioperative period unless there was a serious degree of wound contamination during surgery

Complications

Wound infection

Abdominal abscess

Colocutaneous fistula

References

Knox AJS et al. (1971) Closure of colostomy. Br J Surg 58:669

Turnbull RB Jr, Weakley FL (1967) Atlas of intestinal stomas. Mosby, St. Louis

Wheeler MH, Barker J (1977) Closure of colostomy—a safe procedure? Dis Col Rectum 20:29

Yaiko RD et al. (1976) Morbidity of colostomy closure. Am J Surg 132:304

41 Operations for Colonic Diverticulitis

Indications

Elective

Recurrent diverticulitis

Colovesical fistula

Urgent

Diverticular abscess or phlegmon, unresponsive to medical management

Complete colon obstruction

Suspicion of coexistent carcinoma

Emergent

Spreading or generalized peritonitis

Massive colonic hemorrhage

Concept: Selection of Operation

Management of Typical Acute Diverticulitis

The typical case of acute sigmoid diverticulitis appears with fever, leukocytosis, and pain and tenderness in the left lower quadrant. The patient may or may not have a palpable mass in the lower abdomen or in the pelvis. Initial therapy depends upon intravenous antibiotics and nasogastric suction. After 2–3 days the patient is much improved. Tenderness and fever will diminish. By the end of a week the pelvic or abdominal mass may no longer be palpable. During the second week, if improvement continues, a barium or diatrizoate sodium colon enema radiographic study may be performed *with caution.* If this is the patient's first attack, surgery is not generally indicated unless the X ray shows an extravasation of contrast material outside the lumen of the colon.

On the other hand, if the patient's toxicity and physical findings advance despite 2 days of intensive therapy, urgent surgery is indicated. In such a case, at laparotomy one finds a leaking pericolonic abscess, sometimes with advancing peritonitis. Occasionally, instead of peritonitis, one finds a retromesenteric abscess and phlegmon.

It should be emphasized that in the vast majority of cases acute diverticulitis is caused by intramural and pericolonic cellulitis (phlegmon) rather than a collection of pus (abscess). For this reason many cases of severe acute diverticulitis respond to conservative therapy. In many patients, not only does conservative therapy avoid the need for surgery, it enables the surgeon to perform a *one-stage* resection at a time of election instead of the traditional three-stage procedure.

In those patients for whom conservative therapy has failed, performance of a proximal colostomy and local drainage may prove inadequate for the control of *spreading sepsis*, according to Alexander-Williams and Eng et al. Because of the column of stool in the left colon situated between the colostomy and the perforation, the progression of sepsis is likely if there is a continuing leak. Also, the surgeon may fail to identify a retro or intermesenteric abscess. In these patients the preferred operation is either a Hartmann or a sigmoid resection with exteriorization of the proximal segment as an end colostomy and the distal segment as a mucous fistula.

Obviously, when acute diverticulitis presents initially, with signs of extensive or generalized peritonitis, an operation should be performed on an emergency basis immediately following the administration of antibiotics and fluids.

Elective Left Colon Resection with Anastomosis, One Stage

Patients who have recovered from an attack of acute diverticulitis may undergo primary resection as early as 2–3 weeks following the attack, provided all the signs of local inflammation have receded rapidly. Many surgeons prefer to delay the operation for 3 months. Delay for a period of time longer than 3 months appears to be of no incremental value, as the operation does not become technically easier with the passage of additional time.

If a reading of the X rays raises the suspicion of carcinoma, either the operation should be done within 3 weeks following the attack or an attempt should be made by colonoscopy to rule out carcinoma.

Transverse Colostomy for Complete Colon Obstruction

A few patients who have diverticulitis present with signs of a complete obstruction. In the absence of localized tenderness, fever, and leukocytosis, these patients can be treated the same way as those having an obstruction due to carcinoma: a simple transverse colostomy can be performed on them as the first stage of a three-stage operation. If on physical examination there are local findings of acute inflammation, a midline incision should be made and the sigmoid colon explored and evaluated.

If preoperative abdominal X rays disclose evidence of small bowel obstruction, laparotomy should be performed to mobilize the segment of the small bowel adherent to the diverticular mass.

Emergent Operation for Massive Colonic Hemorrhage

Massive colonic hemorrhage is an uncommon complication of diverticulosis. Many cases of massive colonic hemorrhage, previously attributed to diverticulosis, have proved on arteriography to be due to angiodysplasia in the cecum. Arteriography may also identify the point of bleeding in cases of diffuse diverticulosis. In such cases the intra-arterial administration of vasopressin often controls bleeding and avoids the need for emergency surgery.

For uncontrolled colonic hemorrhage immediate subtotal colectomy is indicated, with a side-to-end anastomosis between the terminal ileum and rectosigmoid (see Chap. 33).

Colovesical Fistula

When a colovesical fistula develops as the result of sigmoid diverticulitis having eroded into the bladder, if proper preoperative preparation is carried out it is generally possible to perform a primary resection of the diseased sigmoid, including immediate anastomosis. The fibrotic area in the bladder is generally small in diameter and may be excised and repaired by a primary closure of the bladder accompanied by constant bladder drainage with a large Foley catheter.

Summary

At present the indications for a diverting transverse colostomy and simple drainage of acute diverticulitis are limited in number. Many of the patients who in previous years underwent the three-stage operation are now treated conservatively. This permits a primary resection and anastomosis 2–3 weeks later.

Patients who have generalized or advancing peritonitis are best treated by a resection of the diseased sigmoid, which eliminates the feeding focus of the sepsis. This should be accompanied by a colostomy and a mucous fistula or a Hartmann pouch. This operation often is indicated also for those patients who have failed to respond to conservative management. In these patients, routinely thrusting a drain in the left lower quadrant and making a diverting colostomy may cause the surgeon to overlook a retromesenteric abscess and fail to control the source of infection. When this possibility can be eliminated by careful exploration at laparotomy, the three-stage resection is an acceptable alternative method of therapy.

Preoperative Preparation

(See Chap. 25.)

Primary Resection and Anastomosis

Operative Strategy

The operative technique for the resection of the left colon and for the anastomosis is similar to that described for left colectomy for carcinoma—but with a number of important exceptions.

Because there is no need to perform a high lymphovascular dissection in the absence of cancer, the mesentery may be divided at a point much closer to the bowel, unless the mesentery is so inflamed and edematous that it cannot hold ligatures.

In most cases it is not necessary to elevate the rectum from the presacral space, as this area is rarely the site of more than an occasional diverticulum. The anastomosis can be done a few centimeters proximal to the promontory of the sacrum.

Though it is important to remove the greatest concentration of diverticulae, in an elderly patient it is not necessary to do an extensive colectomy just because there are some innocent diverticulae in the ascending or transverse colon. At the site selected for anastomosis, however, there should be no diverticulae or any gross muscle hypertrophy.

Primary anastomosis should be performed only if the proximal and distal bowel segments selected for anastomosis are free of cellulitis and of marked muscle hypertrophy. Also, if an abscess has been encountered in the pelvis, so that the anastomosis will lie on the wall of an evacated abscess cavity, it is wiser to delay the anastomosis for a second-stage operation.

Operative Technique

Incision

Make a midline incision from the upper epigastrium to the pubis.

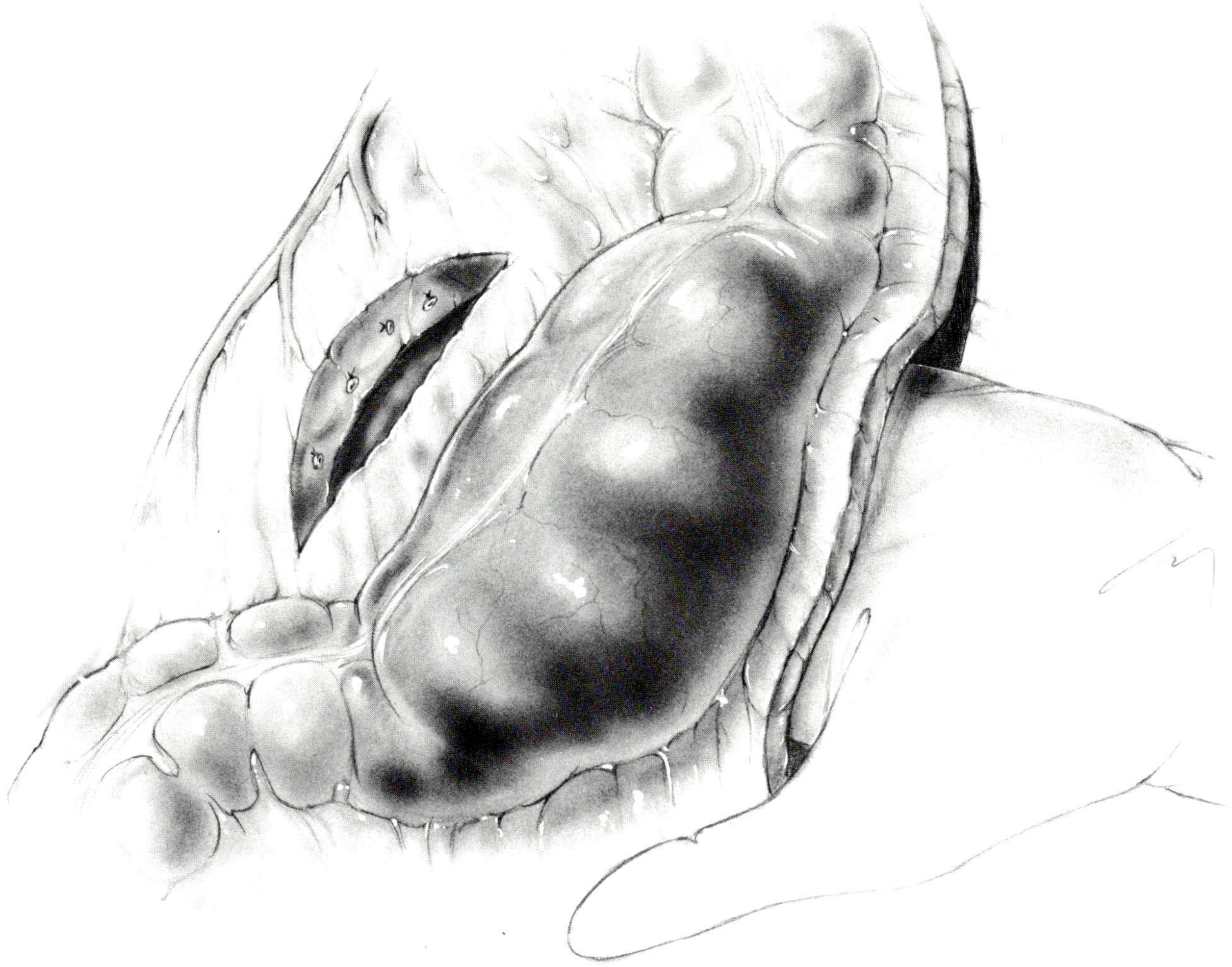

Fig. 41–1

Liberation of Sigmoid and Left Colon

Initiate the dissection in the region of the upper descending colon by incising the peritoneum in the paracolic gutter. Then insert the left hand behind the colon (**Fig. 41–1**), in an area above the diverticulitis, to elevate the mesocolon. Continue the incision in the paracolic peritoneum down to the descending colon and sigmoid to the brim of the pelvis.

At this point, to safeguard the left ureter from damage, it is essential to locate it in the upper portion of the dissection, where the absence of inflammation simplifies its identification. Then trace the ureter down into the pelvis. It may have to be dissected off an area of fibrosis in the sigmoid. When this dissection has been completed, the sigmoid is free down to the promontory of the sacrum.

Division of Mesocolon

In the elective case the mesentery generally may be divided serially between Kelly hemostats at a point no more than 4–6 cm from the bowel wall (Fig. 41–1). Initiate the line of division at a point on the left colon that is free of pathology. This sometimes requires the liberation of the splenic flexure and distal transverse colon. Continue the dissection to the rectosigmoid. Remove the specimen after applying Allen clamps.

Anastomosis

Perform an open type of anastomosis, either in one layer or two layers, or by stapling as described in Chap. 28 (Figs. 28–10 through 28–36). In a rare case it may be necessary to make the anastomosis at a lower level, where the ampulla of the rectum is significantly larger in diameter than the proximal colon. In that case a side-to-end Baker anastomosis is preferable, as described in Chap. 30 (see Figs. 30–10 through 30–20).

At frequent intervals during the above dissection and during the anastomosis, irrigate the abdominal and pelvic cavities with an antibiotic solution.

Abdominal Closure

In the absence of any intra-abdominal or pelvic abscesses, close the abdomen in the usual fashion (see Chap. 5), using no intraperitoneal drains. Manage the skin incision as a contaminated wound (see Chap. 2).

Primary Resection, End Colostomy with Mucous Fistula

Operative Strategy and Technique

After the sigmoid colon has been liberated, but before complete division of the mesentery, it is important to decide whether or not to perform an immediate anastomosis. If a residual abscess has been encountered in the pelvis, where the anastomosis is to be made, then anastomosis should be delayed until a second-stage operation is performed. A small collection of pus behind the colon is not a contraindication to primary anastomosis, provided that the proximal and distal bowel are normal and that the anastomosis will not be situated adjacent to the wall of a pelvic abscess. The vicinity of the anastomosis should be essentially clean.

If it is decided to delay the anastomosis for a second stage, then it is not necessary to excise every bit of inflamed bowel, as this frequently requires a Hartmann pouch at the site of the rectosigmoid transection and makes the second stage more difficult than if a mucous fistula can be constructed. In almost every case, proper planning of the operation will permit the exteriorization of the distal sigmoid as a mucous fistula, which can be brought out through the lower margin of the midline incision after a De Martel or other clamp is applied (**Fig. 41–2**). Divide the mesocolon so as to preserve the vascularity of the mucous fistula. Then bring out an uninflamed area of the descending colon as an end colostomy through a separate incision in the lateral portion of the left rectus muscle and excise the intervening diseased colon. The second stage of this operation, with removal of the colostomy and mucous fistula and anastomosis of the descending colon to the rectosigmoid, may be carried out after a delay of several weeks.

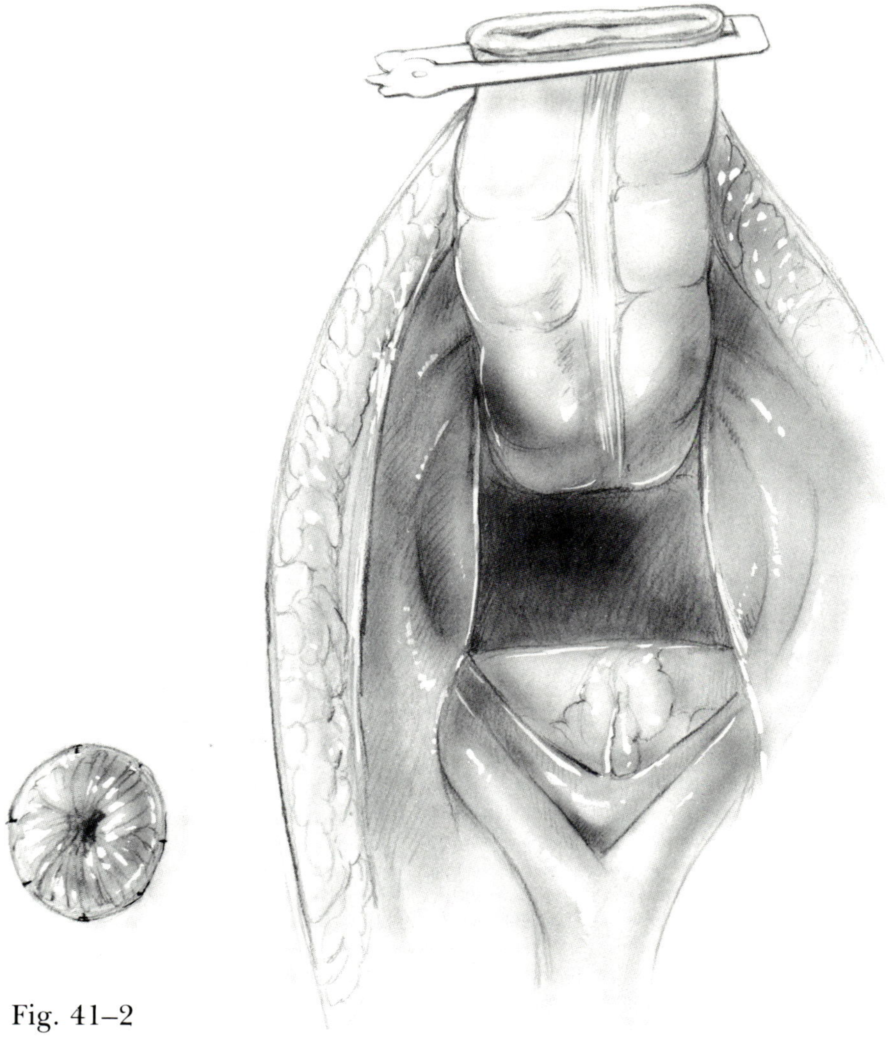

Fig. 41–2

Emergency Sigmoid Colectomy with End Colostomy and Hartmann's Pouch

Indications

For patients suffering generalized or spreading peritonitis secondary to perforated sigmoid diverticulitis, a conservative approach, with diverting transverse colostomy and local drainage, carries a mortality of more than 50%. Immediate excision of the perforated bowel is necessary to remove the focus of sepsis. Following this excision the preferred procedure is a mucous fistula and end colostomy. However, if excising the perforated portion of the sigmoid leaves an insufficient amount of distal bowel with which to form a mucous fistula, then Hartmann's operation is indicated. It is not wise to attempt to make a mucous fistula by extensive presacral dissection, in the hope of lengthening the distal segment, as this only opens new planes to potential sepsis.

Preoperative Preparation

Preoperative preparation primarily involves rapid resuscitative measures using intravenous fluids, blood, and antibiotics, as some patients are admitted to the hospital in septic shock. Colon preparation is not possible. Nasogastric suction and bladder drainage with a Foley catheter should be instituted.

Operative Technique

Incision and Liberation of Left Colon

The steps for the incision and the liberation of the left colon are identical to those described on p. 467 above. It is essential to find the proper retromesenteric plane by initiating the dissection above the area of maximal inflammation. Once this has been achieved, with the left hand elevate the sigmoid colon and the diseased mesocolon—which is generally the site of a phlegmon—so that the left paracolic peritoneum may be incised safely (see Fig. 41–1). Again, it is essential to identify the left ureter in the upper abdomen in order to safeguard it from damage. There sometimes is a considerable amount of blood oozing from the retroperitoneal dissection, but this can often be controlled by moist gauze packs while the dissection continues. After the left colon has been liberated, divide the mesentery serially between hemostats, as above.

Hartmann's Pouch

Often in acute diverticulitis the rectosigmoid is not involved to a great extent in the inflammatory process. Mesenteric dissection should be terminated at this point. If the thickness of the rectosigmoid is not excessive, occlude it by an application of the TA–55 stapler. In the presence of mild or moderate thickening, use the 4.8 mm staples. Place an Allen clamp on the specimen side of the sigmoid and divide the bowel flush with the stapler. After the stapling device is removed there should be slight oozing of blood through the staples, which is evidence that excessively thickened tissue has not been necrotized by using the stapling technique on it (**Fig. 41–3**).

If the tissue is so thick that compression to 2 mm by the stapling device will result in necrosis, then the technique is contraindicated and the rectal stump should be closed by a continuous layer of locked sutures of 3–0 PG. Invert this layer with a second layer of continuous 3–0 PG Lembert sutures. Suture the apex of the Hartmann pouch to the pelvic fascia near, or if possible, higher than the promontory of the sacrum, in order to prevent retraction low into the pelvis which would make a secondary anastomosis more difficult.

End Colostomy

Use an uninflamed area of the left colon as an end colostomy. In a patient who is desperately ill, the colostomy may be brought out through the upper portion of the midline incision if this will save time. Otherwise, bring it out through a transverse incision over the lateral portion of left rectus muscle. The incision should admit two fingers. Bring out the cut end of the colon and immediately suture it with 4–0 chromic catgut, either interrupted or continuous, to the subcuticular layer of the skin incision.

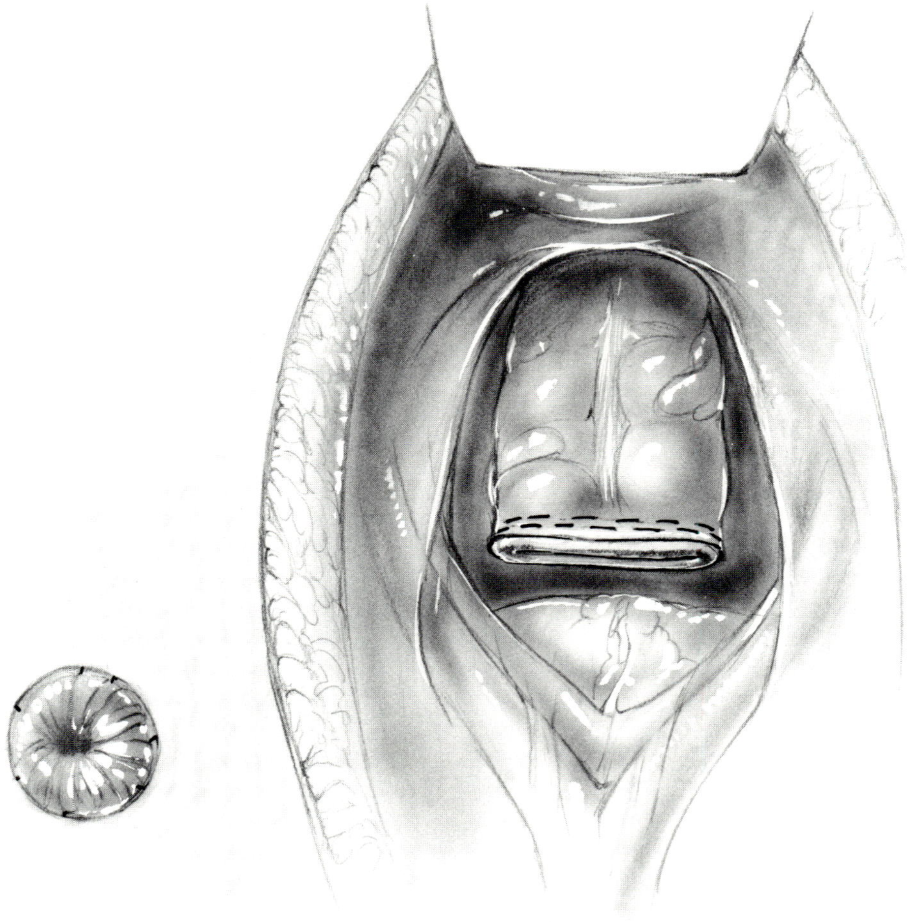

Fig. 41–3

Wound Closure

Any rigid abscess cavities that cannot be excised should be managed by the insertion of sump drains for antibiotic irrigation and suction. If no rigid abscess walls have been left behind, then the abdomen, which has been irrigated with antibiotic solution at intervals during the operation, should be closed in the usual fashion without drainage. The skin can be managed either by delayed primary closure or by McIlrath's method (see Chap. 2).

References

Alexander-Williams J (1976) Management of acute complications of diverticular disease—the dangers of colostomy. Dis Colon Rectum 19:289

Eng K et al. (1977) Resection of the perforated segment—a significant advance in the treatment of diverticulitis with free perforation of abscess. Am J Surg 133:67

42 Operation for Rectal Prolapse (Ripstein)

Indications

This operation is indicated for the management of a complete prolapse of the rectum.

Preoperative Preparation

- Routine bowel preparation (see Chap. 25)
- Sigmoidoscopy
- Barium colon enema
- Foley catheter in bladder
- Nasogastric tube

Concept: Selection of Operation

For many years it was believed that massive rectal prolapse resulted from the weakness of the levator diaphragm anterior to the rectum. This hypothesis explained prolapse as a sliding hernia of the rectum through the defect in the anterior part of this diaphragm. Ripstein in 1965 emphasized that the normal rectum curves posteriorly and follows the contour of the sacrum, to which it is closely attached. Only when the rectum reaches the puborectalis sling does it change sharply to an inferior direction at the anal canal. In the normal individual, straining tends to force the rectum in a posterior direction against the hollow of the sacrum. Radiological observation of barium in the rectum of patients who have rectal prolapse demonstrates that when they increase their intraabdominal pressure, the rectum assumes a straight-line position from the lumbar region to the anal canal. This permits intussusception of the rectal wall through the anal musculature. It is likely that the weakness of the levator diaphragm is secondary to many years of constipation and prolapse, rather than the cause of prolapse. This explains how prolapse can occur in young patients who have strong levator musculature.

The concept underlying the operation is the application of a permanent polypropylene mesh that fixes the anterior three-quarters of the circumference of the rectum to the presacral fascia. This restores the normal posterior curve of the rectum and eliminates intussusception and prolapse. Although an abdominal approach is used, Gordon and Hoexter have found the mortality in over 1000 cases to be less than 0.5%, and the recurrence rate 2%–3%.

In extremely poor-risk patients, a Thiersch operation is often performed. This consists of inserting a silver wire around the anal musculature, thereby constricting the anal canal to the diameter of about one finger. In the experience of most surgeons, this operation lasts no more than 1–2 years, as the wire either breaks or perforates.

Low anterior resection has also been advocated for this condition. Whatever efficacy this operation possesses probably results from the scar tissue that attaches the anastomosis and rectal stump to the presacral fascia. However, a low colorectal anastomosis carries with it a mortality higher than that of the Ripstein operation and seems to have a somewhat higher recurrence rate.

Another procedure advocated for this condition is amputation of the prolapsed segment, with colorectal anastomosis performed outside the anal canal. This too carries a higher mortality rate than the Ripstein procedure.

Pitfalls and Danger Points

Excessive constriction of rectum by the mesh, which may result in partial obstruction or, on rare occasions, erosion of mesh into lumen of rectum

Disruption of suture line between mesh and presacral space

Presacral hemorrhage

Operative Strategy

To prevent undue constriction of the rectum when the mesh is placed around it, there should be sufficient room left for the surgeon to pass two fingers behind the rectum after the mesh has been fixed in place.

The success of the Ripstein operation is *not predicated upon any degree of constriction* of the rectum. It will suffice if the mesh simply prevents the rectum from advancing in an anterior direction away from the hollow of the sacrum.

The site on the rectum selected for the placement of the mesh is important. The upper level of the mesh should be 5 cm below the promontory of the sacrum. This requires opening the rectovesical or rectouterine peritoneum. In most cases the lateral ligaments of the rectum need not be divided.

Damage to the hypogastric nerves in the presacral area should be avoided, especially in males, in whom transection interferes with sexual function.

Operative Technique

Incision

A midline incision between the umbilicus and pubis provides excellent exposure in most patients. In young women, the operation is accompanied by improved cosmetic results if it is performed through a Pfannenstiel incision. Place the Pfannenstiel incision just inside the pubic hairline, in the crease that goes from one anterior superior iliac spine to the other (**Fig. 42–1**). It should be 12–15 cm long. With the scalpel, divide the subcutaneous fat down to the anterior rectus sheath and the external oblique aponeurosis. Divide the anterior rectus sheath in the line of the incision about 2 cm above the pubis (**Fig. 42–2**). Extend the incision in the rectus sheath laterally in both directions into the external oblique aponeurosis. Apply Allis clamps to the cephalad portion of this fascial layer and bluntly dissect it off the underlying rectus muscles almost to the level

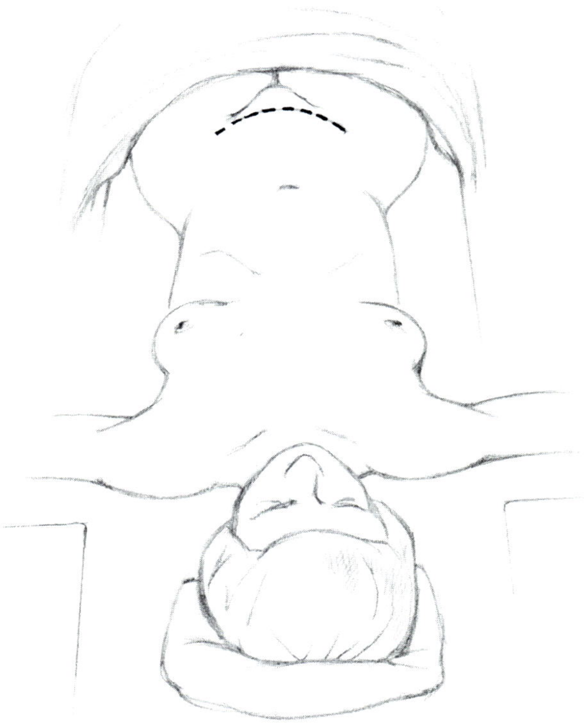

Fig. 42–1

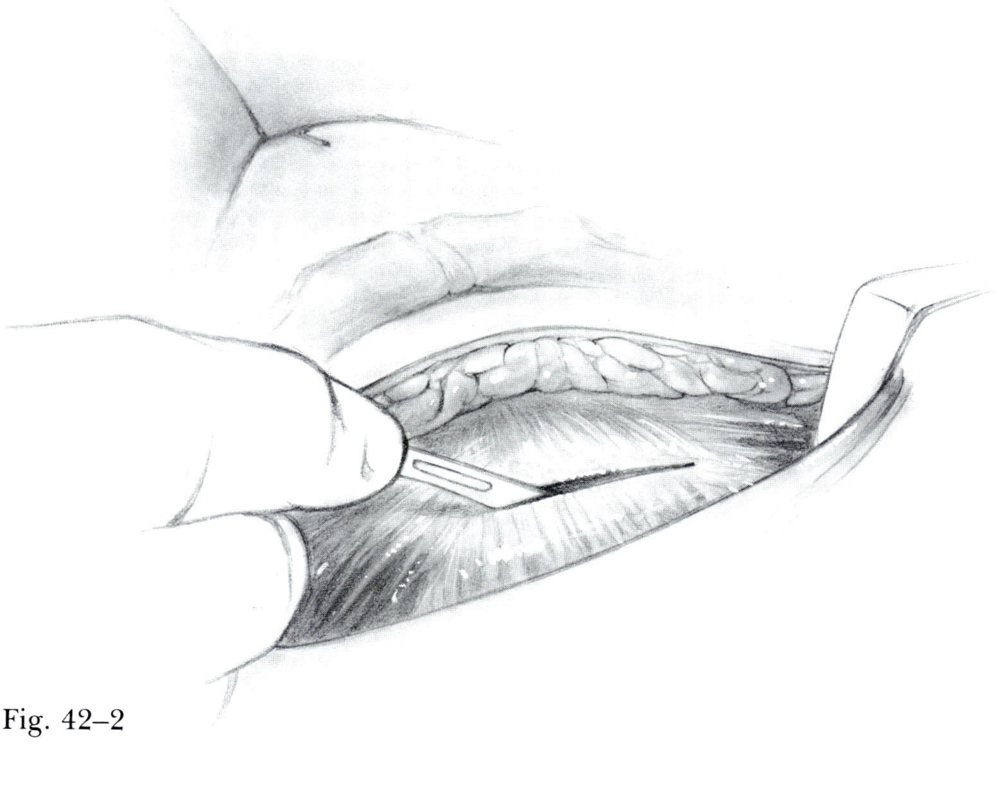

Fig. 42–2

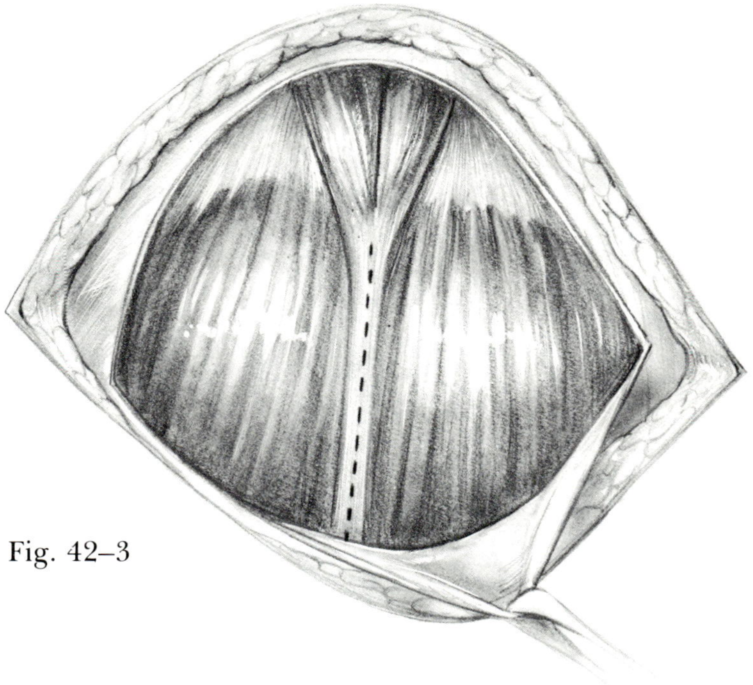

Fig. 42–3

of the umbilicus (**Fig. 42–3**). Separate the rectus muscles in the midline, exposing the preperitoneal fat and peritoneum. Grasp these in an area sufficiently cephalad to the bladder so as not to endanger that organ. Incise the peritoneum, open the abdominal cavity, and explore it for coincidental pathology. A moderate Trendelenburg position is helpful.

Incision of Pelvic Peritoneum

Retract the small intestine in a cephalad direction. Make an incision in the pelvic peritoneum beginning at the promontory of the sacrum and go along the left side of the mesorectum down as far as the cul de sac. Identify the left ureter.

Make a second incision in the peritoneum on the right side of the mesorectum, where the mesorectum meets the pelvic peritoneum. Extend this incision down to the cul de sac too and identify and preserve the right ureter. Join these two incisions by dividing the peritoneum at the depth of the rectovesical or rectouterine pouch, using a Metzenbaum scissors (see Figs. 31–2 through 31–4). Frequently, the cul de sac is quite deep in patients with rectal prolapse. Further dissection between the rectum and the prostate or the vagina is generally not necessary.

Presacral Dissection

In cases of rectal prolapse the rectum can be elevated with ease from the hollow of the sacrum. Enter the presacral space via a Metzenbaum dissection, a method similar to that described for anterior resection (see Chap. 30). Take the usual precautions to avoid damage to the presacral veins. Inspect the presacral area for hemostasis, which should be perfect before the procedure is continued.

Application of Mesh

Fit a section of Prolene mesh measuring 5 cm × 10 cm or 5 cm × 12 cm into place overlying the lower rectum. The upper margin of the mesh should lie over the rectum at a point 4–5 cm below the sacral promontory. Using a small Mayo

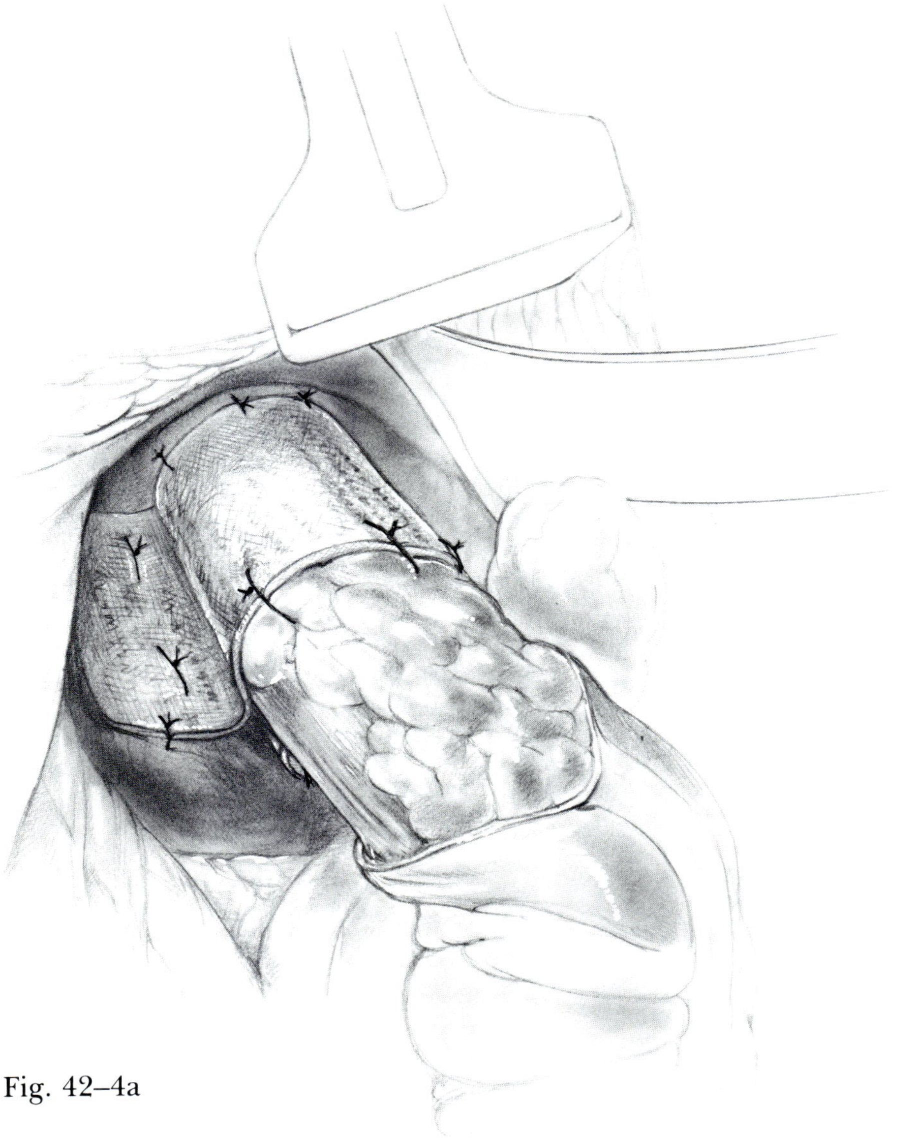

Fig. 42–4a

needle, insert three interrupted sutures of 2–0 Prolene or Tevdek into the right margin of the mesh and attach the mesh to the sacral periosteum along a line about 1–2 cm to the right of the midsacral line. Use the same technique to insert three interrupted sutures in the left lateral margin of the mesh and through the sacral fascia and periosteum (**Fig. 42–4a**). Tie none of these sutures yet, but apply a hemostat to each of them temporarily. After all six sutures have been inserted, have the assistants draw them taut. Then insert two fingers between the rectum and sacrum in

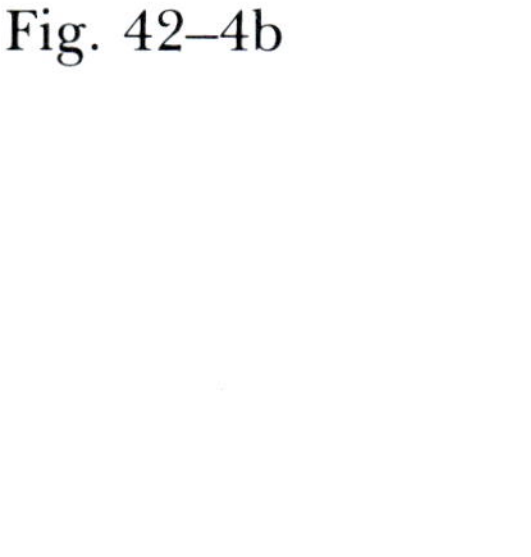

Fig. 42–4b

order to check the tension of the mesh, so as to ensure against excessive constriction (**Fig. 42–4b**). Now tie all six sutures. Use additional sutures of 3–0 atraumatic Prolene or Tevdek to attach both the proximal and distal margins of the mesh to the underlying rectum so that there will be no possibility of the rectum sliding forward beneath the mesh.

Closure of Pelvic Peritoneum

Irrigate the pelvic cavity with an antibiotic solution. Close the incision in the pelvic peritoneum with a continuous suture of 2–0 atraumatic PG (**Fig. 42–5**).

Wound Closure

For closure of the Pfannenstiel incision, grasp the peritoneum with hemostats and approximate it with a continuous 2–0 atraumatic PG suture. Use several sutures of the same material loosely to approximate the rectus muscle in the midline.

Close the transverse incision in the rectus sheath and external oblique aponeurosis with interrupted sutures of atraumatic 2–0 PG. Close the skin with a continuous 4–0 PG subcuticular suture.

Generally, no pelvic drains are necessary. If hemostasis is not perfect, bring a 6 mm Silastic catheter out from the presacral space through a puncture wound in the lower abdomen and attach it to a closed-suction device (Fig. 42–5).

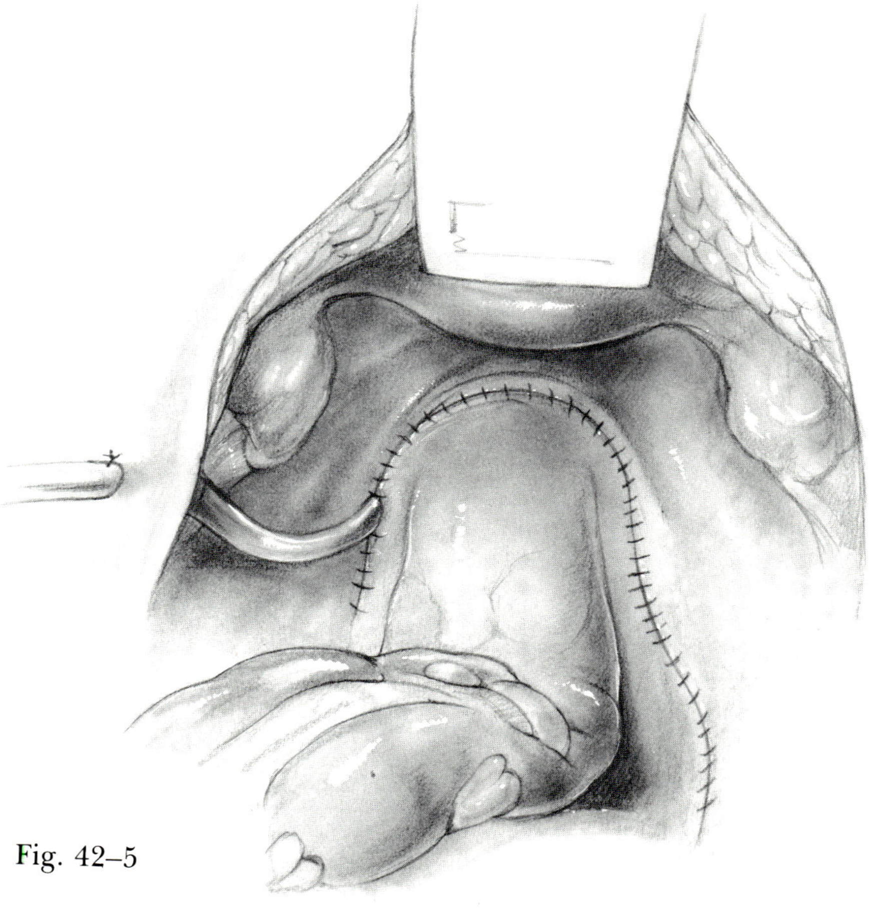

Fig. 42–5

Postoperative Care and Complications

Continue nasogastric suction only until the patient begins to pass flatus, then initiate feeding. Antibiotics should not be prescribed routinely.

Most patients who have a complete prolapse have suffered from years of constipation. The colon may require continued use of laxative medications for this condition, although in some cases there is a definite improvement in the patient's bowel function following the operation.

Fecal incontinence, as a result of many years of dilatation of the anal sphincters by repeated prolapse, is also common among these patients. Correction of the prolapse will not automatically eliminate incontinence. This condition may improve if the patient is encouraged to persist in exercises aimed at strengthening the sphincter mechanism.

References

Gordon PH, Hoexter B (1978) Complications of the Ripstein procedure. Dis Colon Rectum 21:277

Ripstein CB (1965) Surgical care of massive rectal prolapse. Dis Colon Rectum 8:34

Appendixes

A Some Mechanical Basics of Operative Technique

Rare is the novice who has the inborn talent to accomplish all the mechanical manipulations in surgery with no more thought or analysis than the natural athlete gives to hitting a ball. Most surgeons in training can gain a great deal from analyzing such basics of surgery as foot position, hand and arm motion, and the efficient use of instruments.

In considering the mechanics discussed here, remember that underlying all aspects of surgical technique are the fundamental principles articulated by Halsted, who emphasized that the surgeon must minimize trauma to tissues by using gentle technique. Halsted also stressed the importance of maintaining hemostasis and asepsis.

Bear in mind that this text has been written from the vantage point of the right-handed surgeon. Left-handed surgeons should of course reverse the instructions where appropriate.

Importance of Surgeon's Foot and Body Position

For every activity involving the use of hands and arms, there is a body stance that allows the greatest efficiency of execution. For example, the right-handed professional who uses a baseball bat, a tennis racket, a wood chisel, or a golf club places the left foot forward, the right foot 30–50 cm to the rear, and directs the right arm and hand motion toward the left foot. And for the greatest efficiency in sewing, the surgeon assumes a body position such that the point of the needle is aimed toward the left foot. This stance allows the shoulder, arm, and wrist to occupy positions that are free of strain. It permits the surgeon to perceive proprioceptive sensations as the needle moves through the tissues. Only in this way can the surgeon "feel" the depth of the suture bite. Combining this proprioceptive sense with visual monitoring of the depth of the needle bite is the best way to assure consistency in suturing. Because accuracy in grasping submucosa with the suture is one of the most important factors in the proper construction of an intestinal anastomosis, the surgeon must make every effort to perfect this skill.

Fig. A–1 illustrates the proper foot position of the surgeon who is inserting Lembert sutures in the construction of an anastomosis situated at right angles to the long axis of the body. If the surgeon were to insert sutures of the Halsted type instead, they would require one forehand pass with a needle holder, followed by a second pass with the same strand of suture material, using a backhand motion; there should be no alteration of foot position. To insert sutures backhand, the needle should be directed toward the surgeon's right foot. Similarly, cutting by scalpel is properly performed with a backhand motion directed toward the surgeon's right foot (**Fig. A–2**). In using scissors, however, the point of the scissors should be directed toward the surgeon's *left* foot.

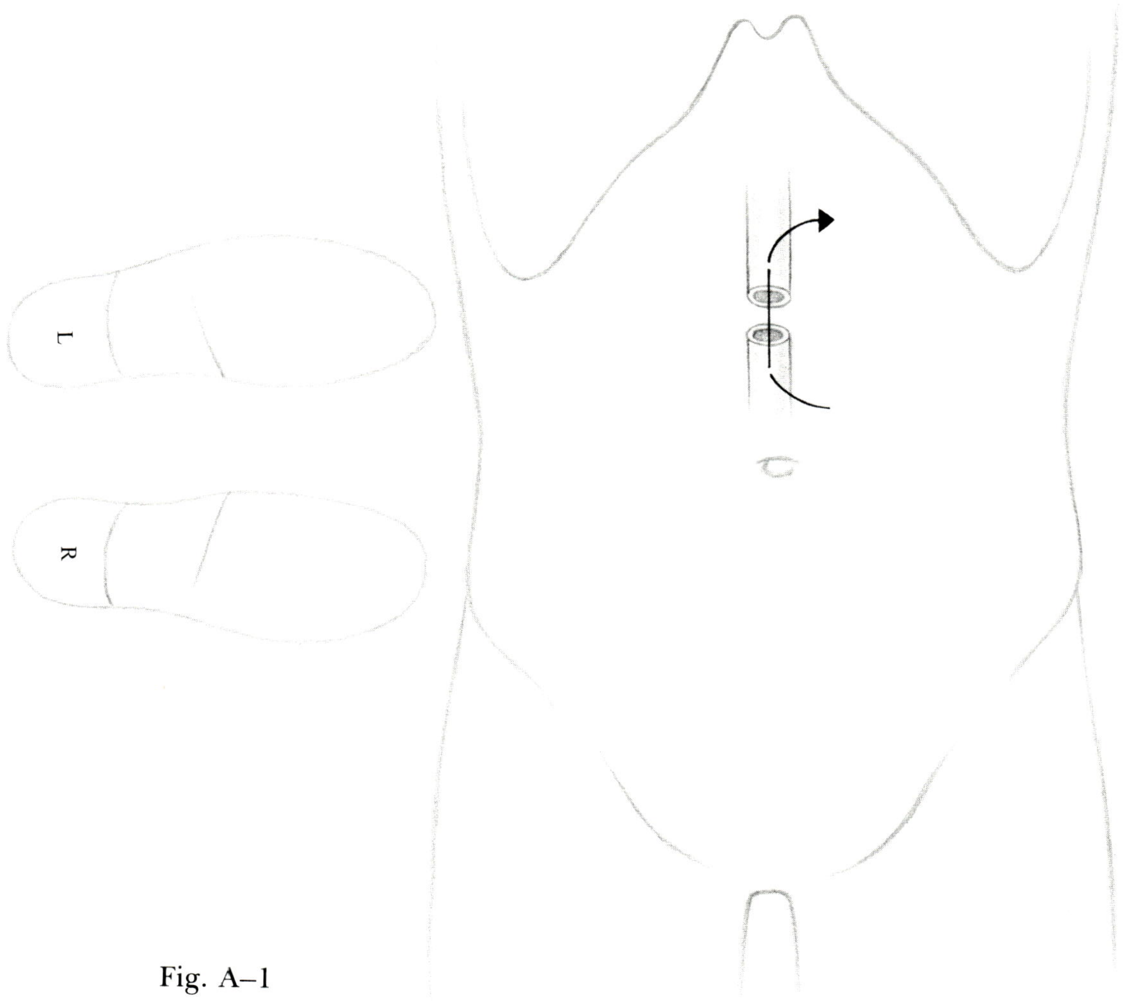

Fig. A–1

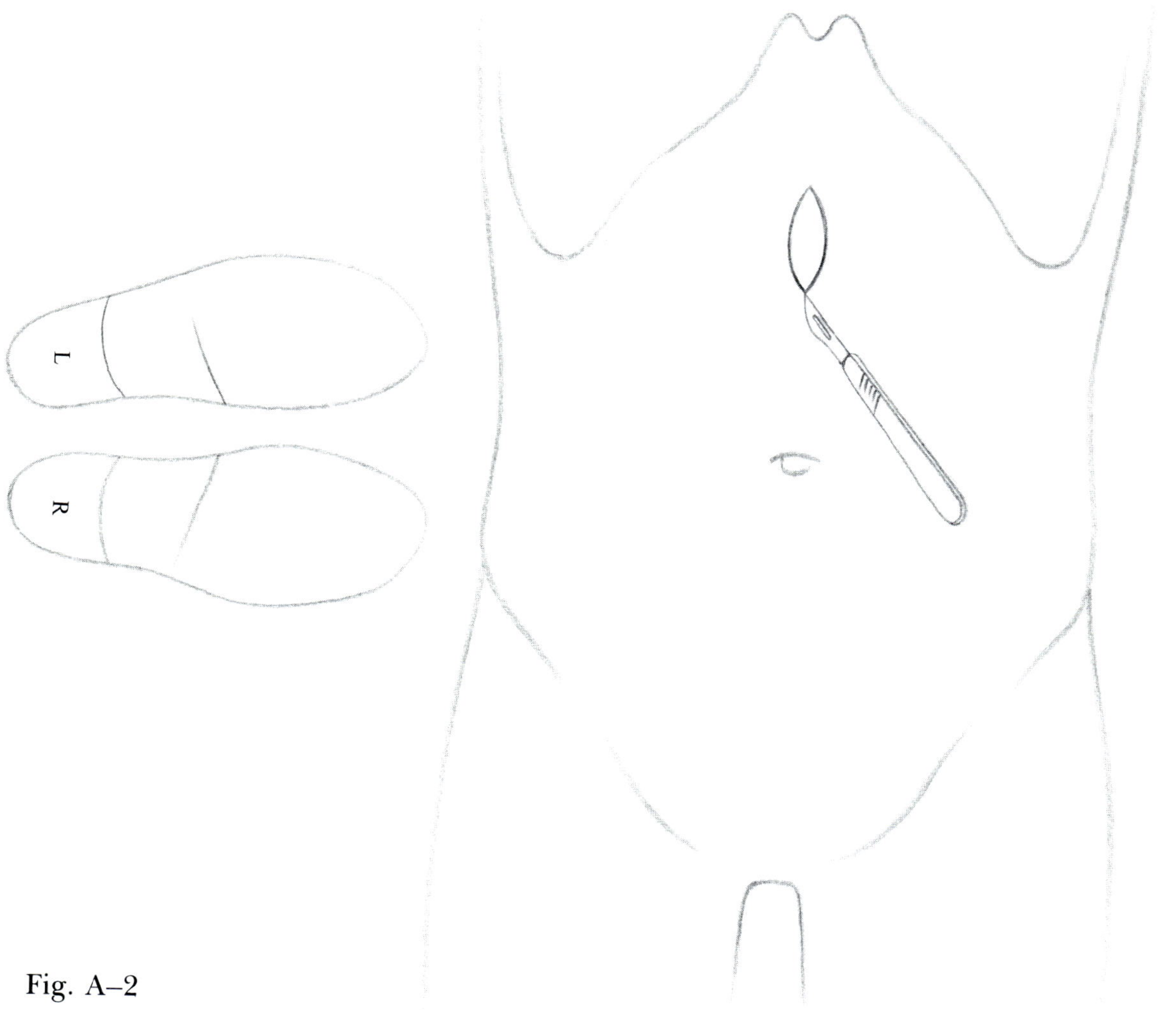

Fig. A–2

The proper foot position for inserting Lembert sutures in an anastomosis oriented in a line parallel to the long axis of the body is shown in **Fig. A–3.**

Some surgeons do not have a highly developed proprioceptive sense when they use the backhand suture. Therefore, whenever it is feasible they should avoid this maneuver in seromuscular suturing. This is almost always possible if the surgeon rearranges the direction of the anastomosis or assumes a body stance that permits optimal forehand suturing.

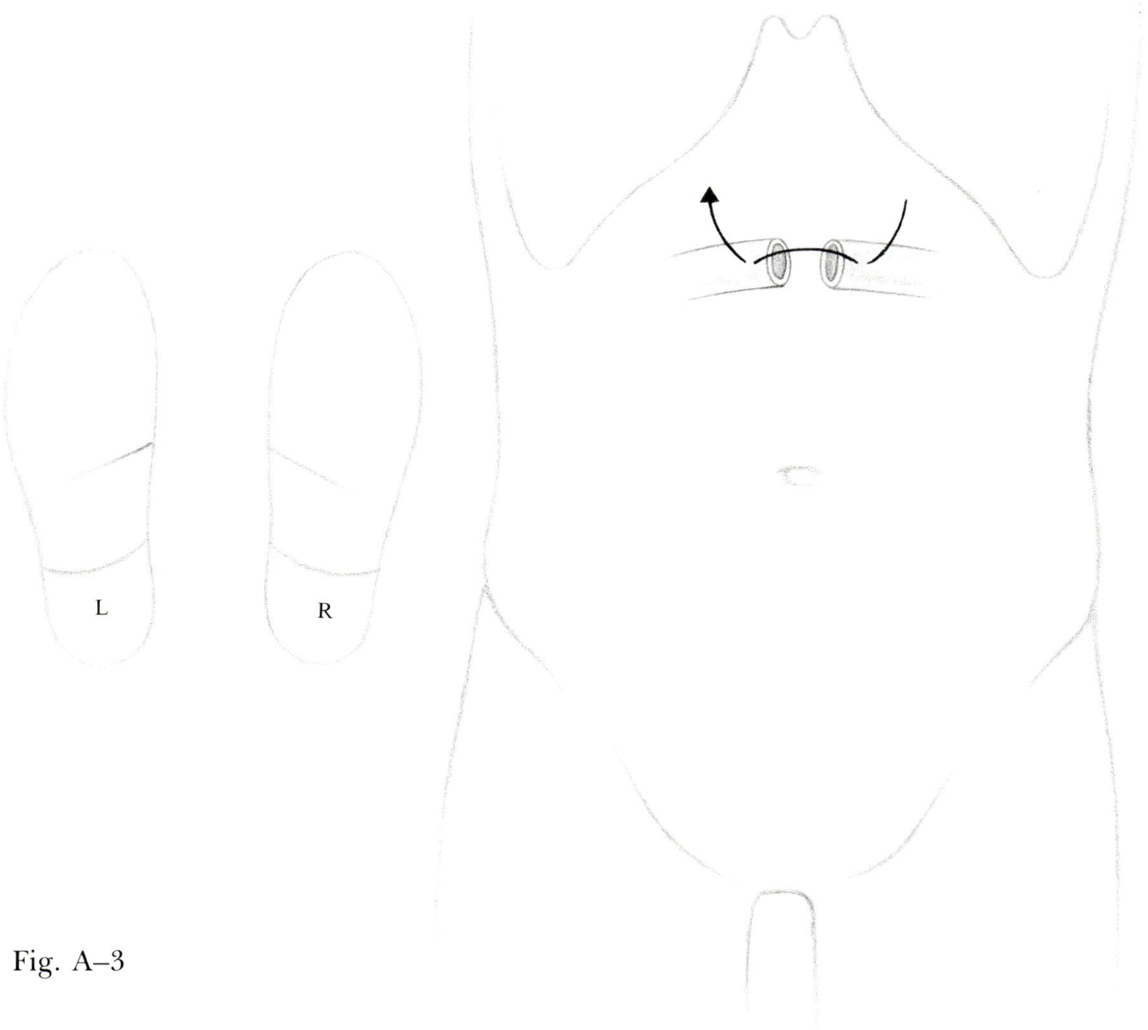

Fig. A–3

The method of changing body position so that all sutures can be placed with a forehand motion is illustrated in **Fig. A–4.** It shows Cushing sutures being inserted into an esophagogastric anastomosis, with the surgeon standing on the left side of the patient. When the needle is passed through the gastric wall from the patient's left to right, the surgeon's left foot is planted close to the operating table along the *left* side of the patient's abdomen.

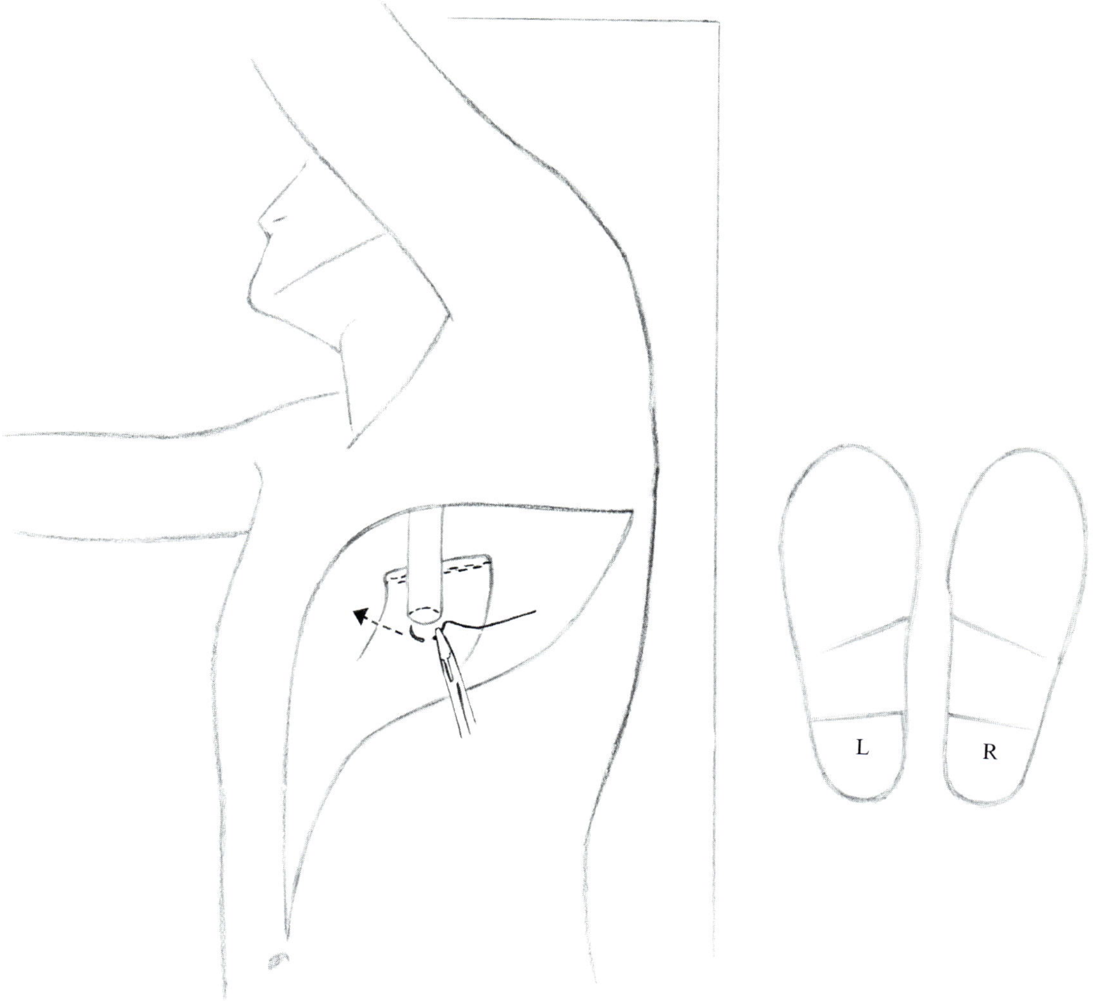

Fig. A–4

The surgeon's right foot is placed more laterally. When the suture is passed from the patient's right to left, on the posterior aspect of the esophageal wall, the surgeon's right foot is placed alongside the operating table. The surgeon's body faces toward the patient's feet and the surgeon's left foot is somewhat lateral to the right foot (**Fig. A–5**). Generally, this directs the point of the needle toward the surgeon's left foot at all times.

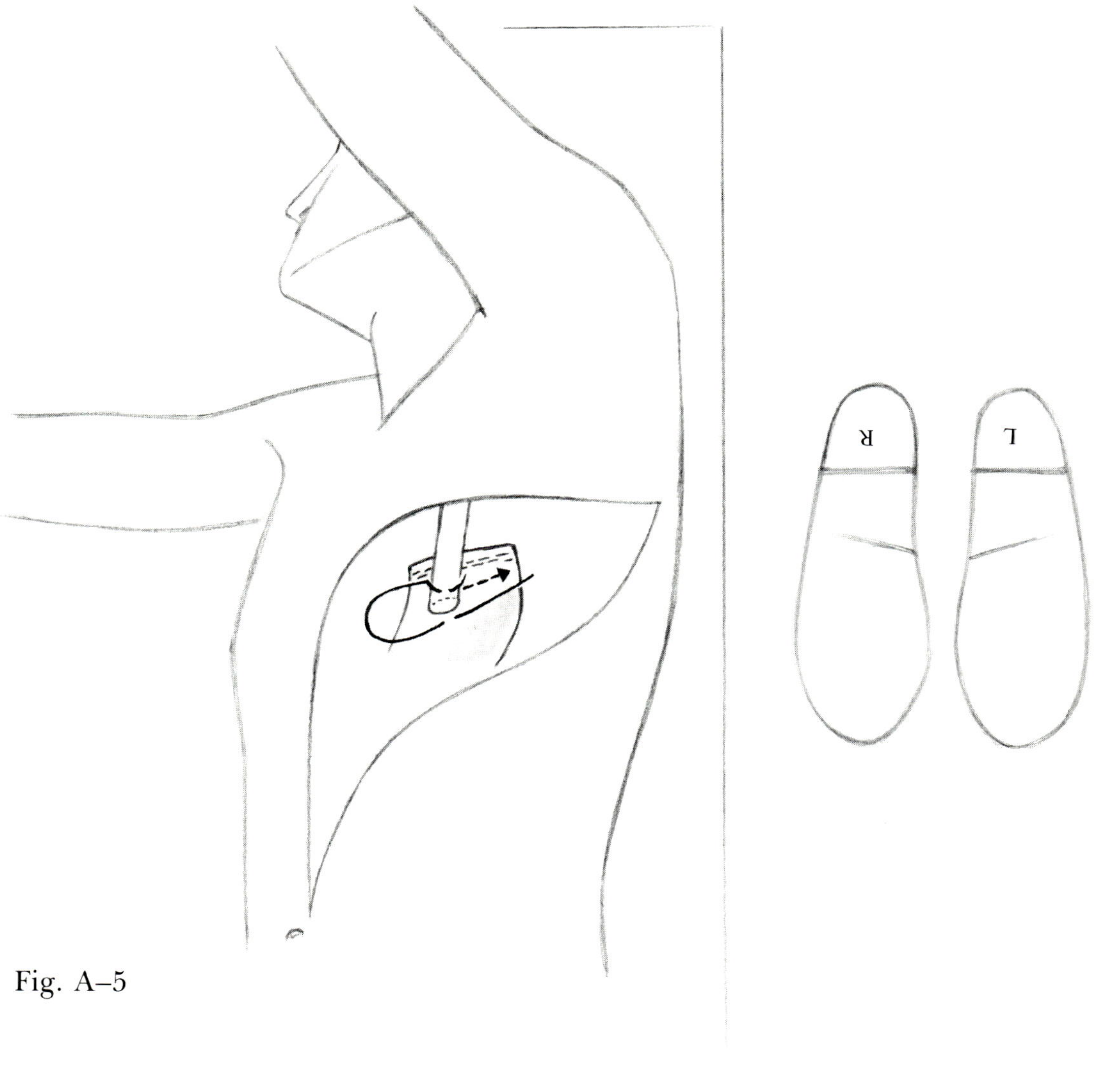

Fig. A–5

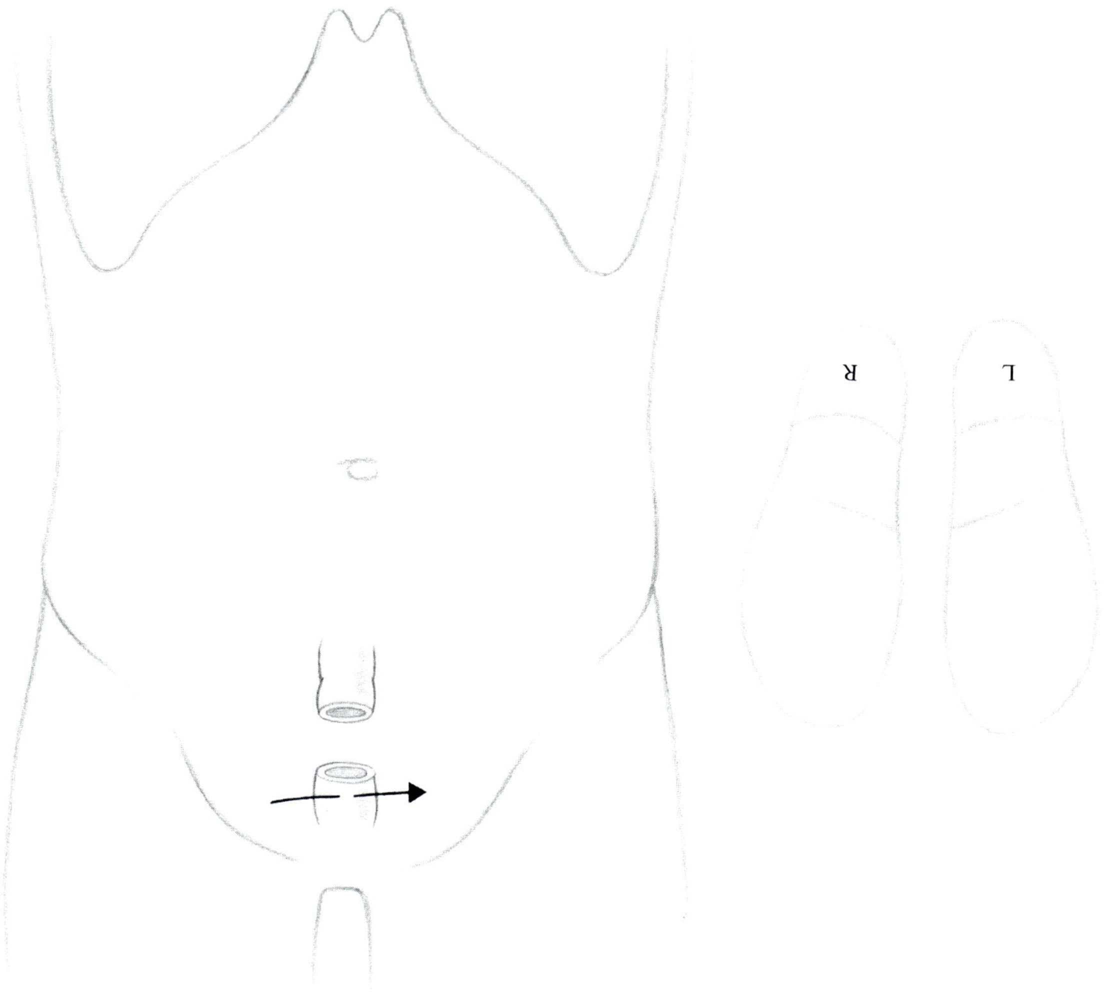

Fig. A–6

A similar change in body stance is illustrated in **Figs. A–6 and A–7**, where Cushing sutures are being inserted into a low-lying colorectal anastomosis. Of course, if the surgeon chose to use the Lembert-type suture in either an esophagogastrostomy or coloproctostomy, a single stance would be efficient for the entire anastomosis.

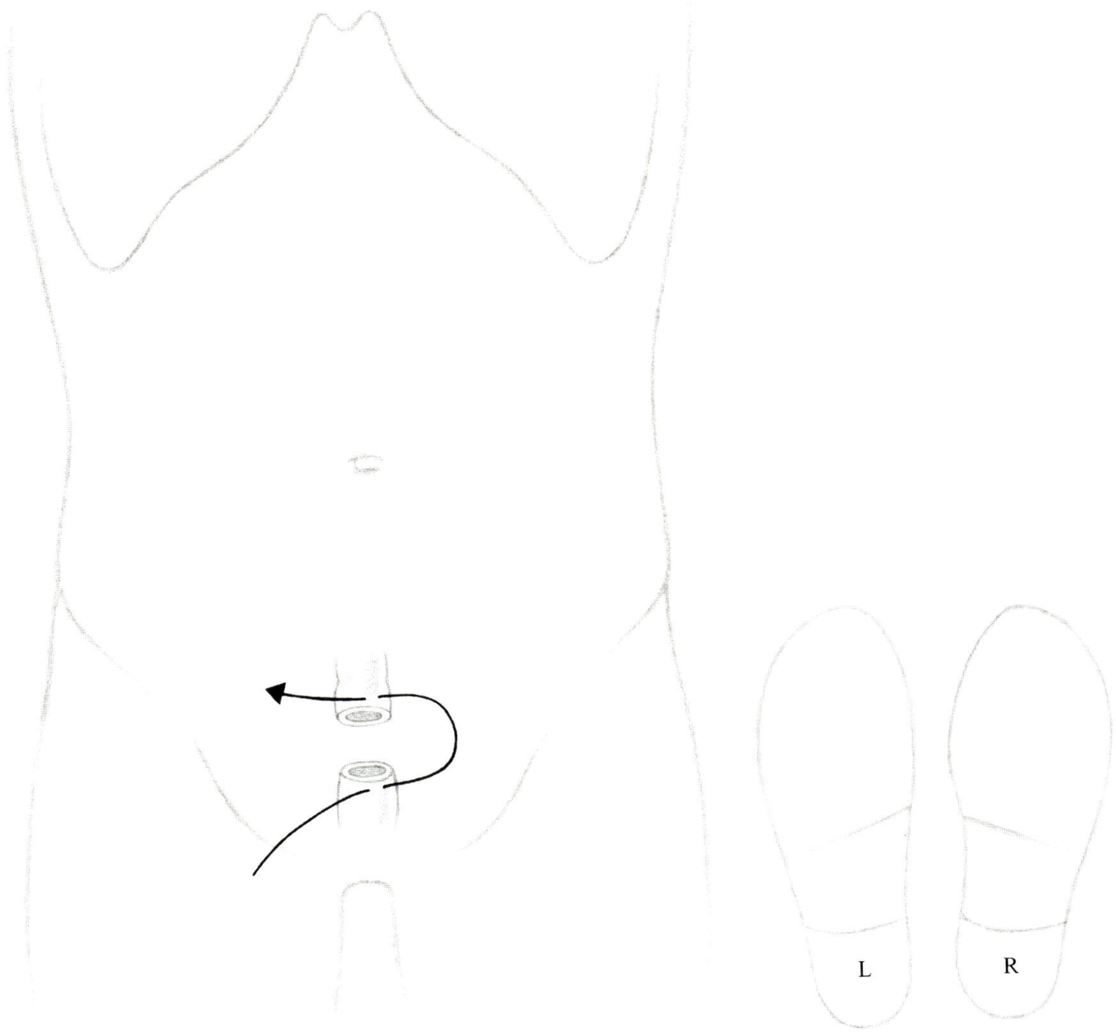

Fig. A–7

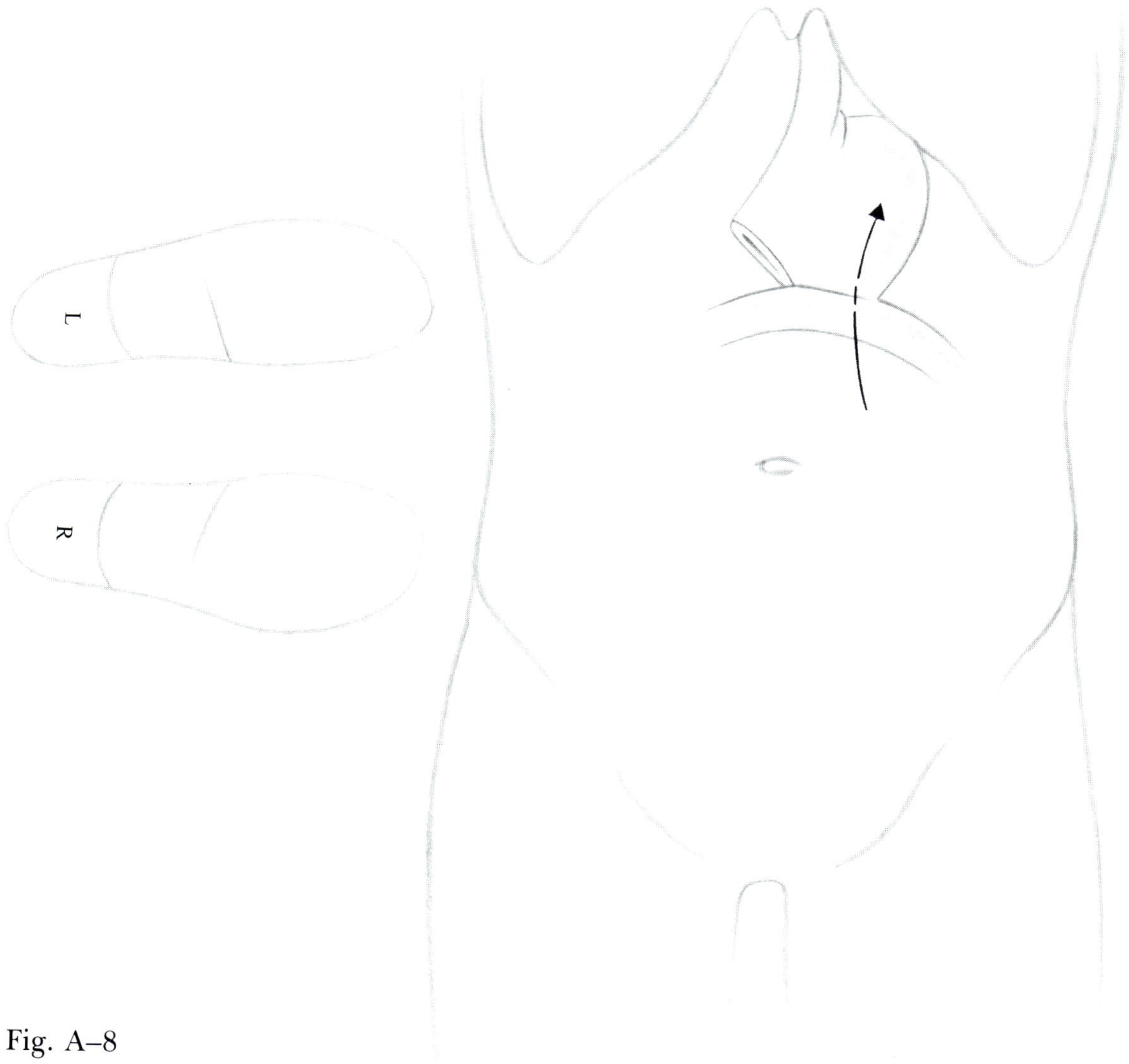

Fig. A–8

Figs. A–8 and A–9 illustrate the insertion of Lembert sutures for the final layer of a gastrojejunal anastomosis, showing the foot position of the surgeon who is standing on the patient's right side as compared with a position on the patient's left.

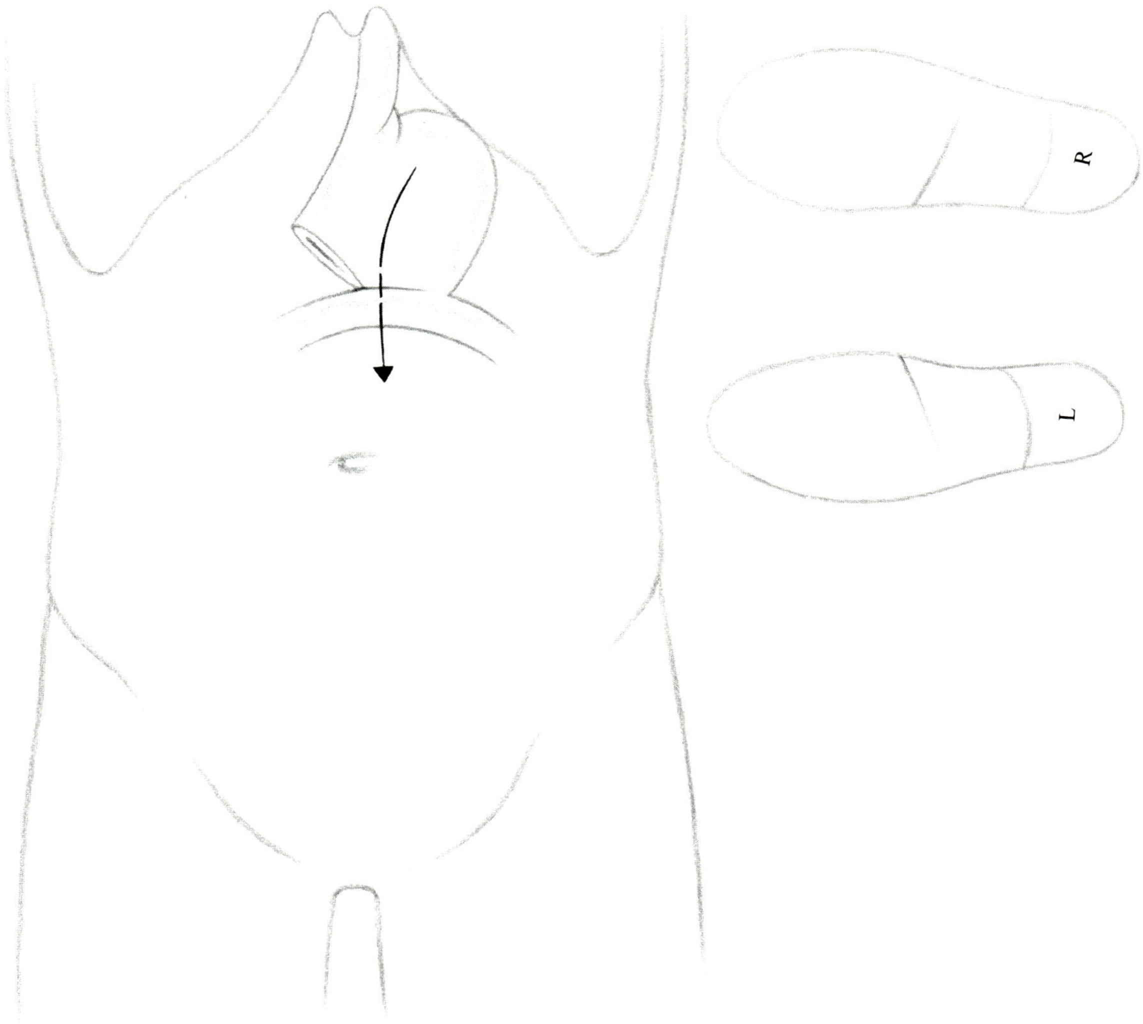

Fig. A–9

Fig. A–10 illustrates closure of an upper vertical midline abdominal incision. **Fig. A–11** shows a lower midline incision with the surgeon standing at the patient's right side.

Though it is true that some surgeons are able to accomplish effective suturing in spite of awkward or strained body and hand positions, it must be emphasized that in surgery, as in athletics, good form is an essential ingredient in producing consistently superior performance.

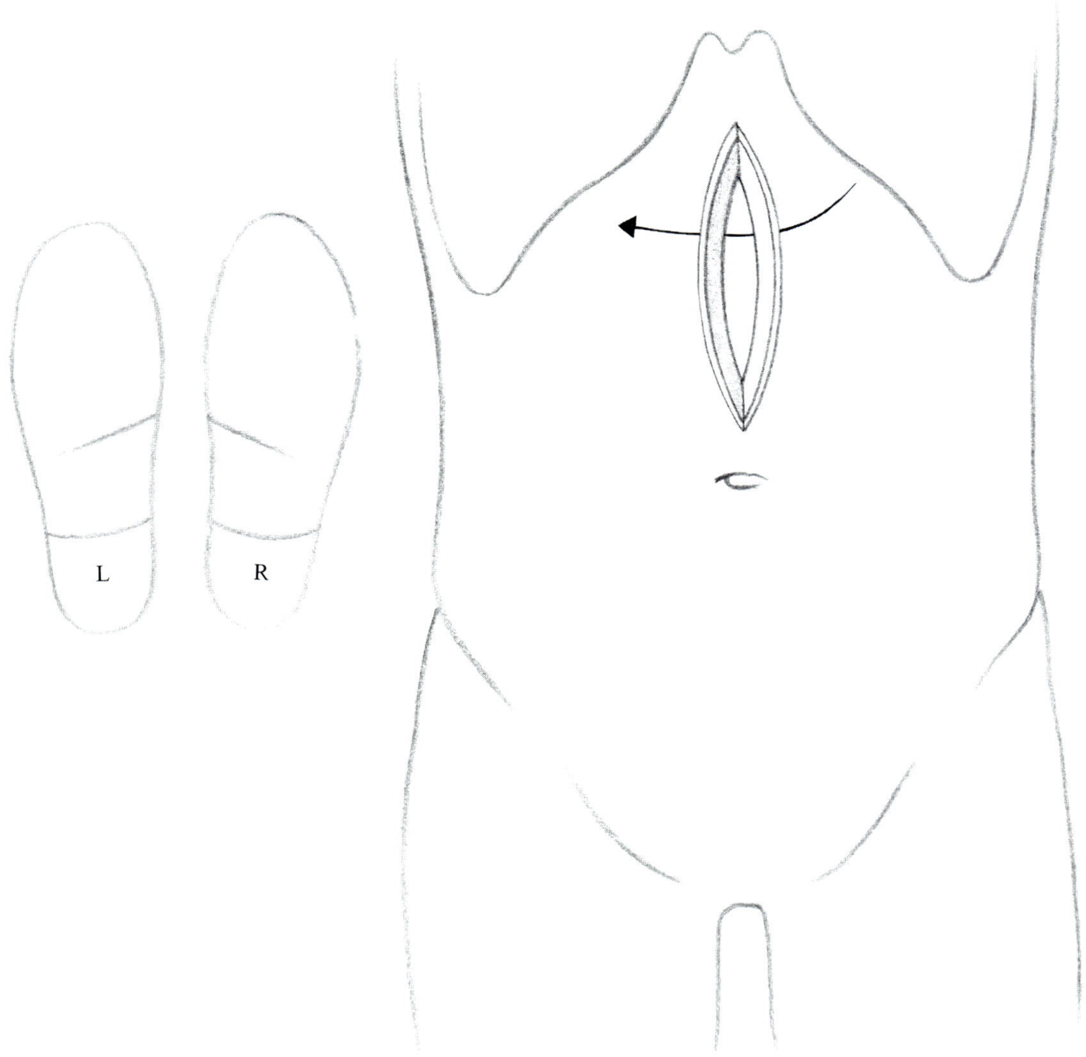

Fig. A–10

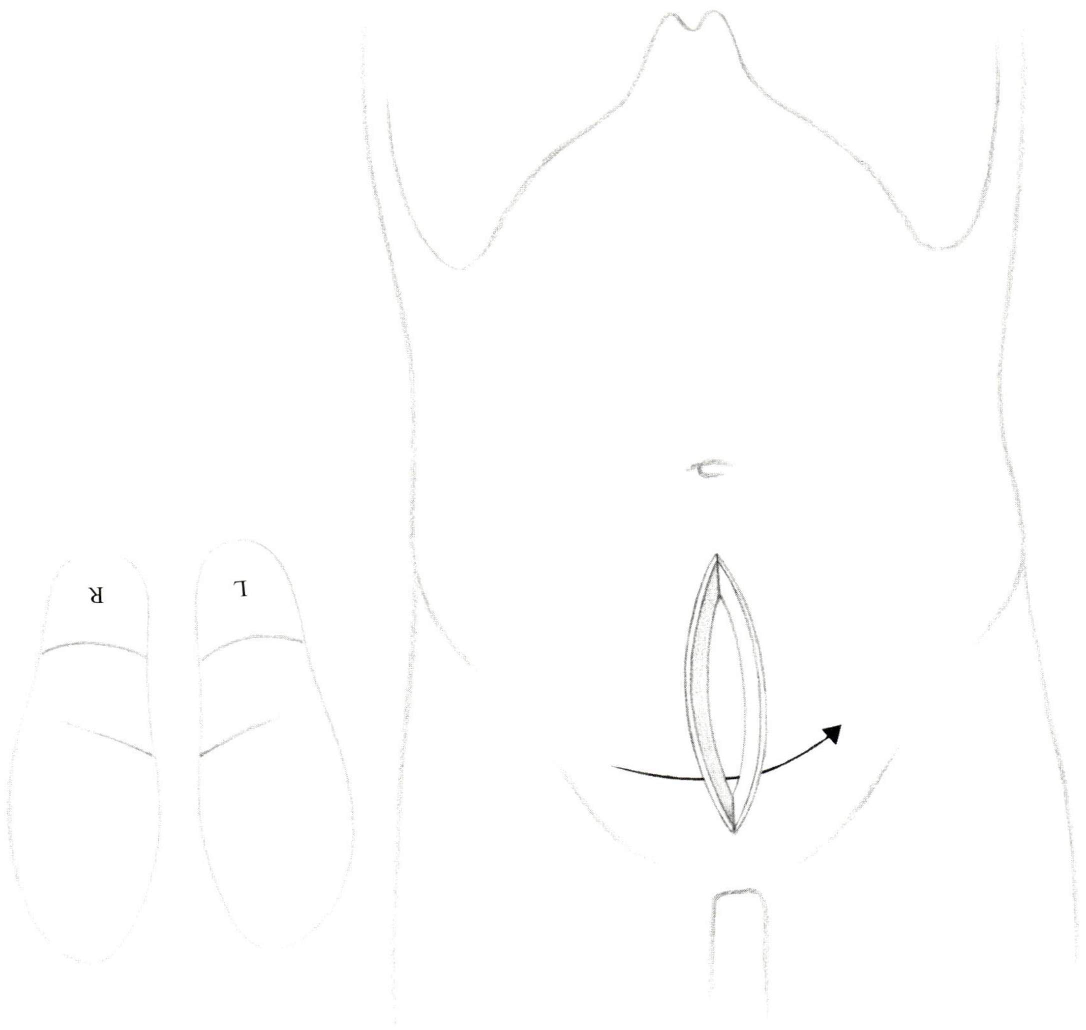

Fig. A–11

Use of Instruments

With rare exceptions, all surgical instruments used in soft tissue dissection should be held with fingertip pressure; they should not be held in a tight vise-like grip. The loose grip is essential if the surgeon is to perceive proprioceptive sensations as the instrument is applied to the tissue. This requirement applies whether the instrument used is a scalpel, forceps, needle-holder, or scissors.

Scalpel

When making the initial scalpel incision in the skin, the surgeon can minimize tissue trauma by the use of a bold stroke through the skin and subcutaneous fat. This does indeed require a firm grip. In most other situations, however, the scalpel should be held gently between the thumb on one side of the handle and the other fingers on the opposite side. Long, deliberate strokes with the scalpel are preferred. Generally, cutting is best done with the belly of the scalpel blade. This enables the surgeon to control the depth of the incision by feel as well as by eye. The scalpel is a particularly effective instrument when broad surface areas are to be dissected, as in radical mastectomy or inguinal lymphadenectomy.

In situations such as an attempt to define the fascial ring surrounding an incisional hernia, the surgeon can clear overlying adherent fat rapidly from broad areas of fascia by using a scalpel. The efficiency of knife dissection is greatly enhanced when the tissues being incised are kept in a state of tension; this can be brought about by traction between the surgeon's left hand and countertraction by the first assistant.

The surgeon must always be alert to observe the nuances of anatomy revealed by each scalpel stroke, especially if a structure appears in an unexpected location. This is not possible if the surgeon is in the habit of making rapid little chopstrokes with the scalpel, like a woodpecker. Rapid, frenzied motions do not afford sufficient time for the surgeon's brain to register and analyze the observations made during the dissection. Nor do they allow sufficient time for feedback to control the hand motions. Slow, definitive, long sweeping strokes with the scalpel make the most rapid progress and allow enough time to permit the activation of cerebral control mechanisms and prevent unnecessary damage.

Metzenbaum Scissors

The round-tipped Metzenbaum scissors is a valuable instrument because it serves a number of essential functions. The closed Metzenbaum is an excellent tool for dissection. It may be inserted behind adhesions or ligaments to elevate and delineate planes of dissection before dividing them. Properly held, with the ring finger and thumb in the two orifices and the index finger and middle finger extended along the handle, *this instrument serves as an extension of the hand in detecting sensations* and in providing the surgeon with information concerning the density, pliability, and thickness of the tissue being dissected. As with other instruments, this proprioceptive function is enhanced if the hand grasps the instrument gently.

The Electrocautery as a Cutting Device

Some surgeons prefer to use the electrocautery, set for the "cutting" current, for such maneuvers as elevating the skin flaps during mastectomy or incising subcutaneous fat. Transecting fat with a cutting current makes hemostasis only partially effective, but tissue trauma is minimal. If the current is set for "coagulation," considerable heat is generated, causing the fat to boil. The trauma produced is excessive for the amount of hemostasis gained and Madden et al. and Cruse and Foord have observed that the incidence of wound infections is doubled. On the other hand, the transection of muscle bellies, as for instance in the subcostal or thoracic incision, may be accomplished efficiently when the electrocoagulator is set for "coagulation" or "blend" current. This provides good hemostasis and appears not to injure the patient significantly. Occasionally, the peritoneum and ligaments in the paracolic gutters become somewhat vascular secondary to inflammation. The electrocoagulator can be used to divide these structures.

In many areas, such as the neck, breast, and abdominal wall, it is feasible to cut with the electrocautery set for "cutting." To divide a small blood vessel, change the switch from "cutting" to "coagulation" and occlude the isolated blood vessel by electrocautery. Carefully performed, this sequence of dissection seems not to be damaging. If the incidence of wound infections, hematoma, or local edema is increased by using this technique, the surgeon is overcoagulating the tissues and not isolating the blood vessels effectively.

Forceps

Care must be taken to avoid unnecessary trauma when applying forceps to body tissues. As with other instruments, hold the forceps gently. It is surprising how little force need be applied when holding the bowel with a pair of forceps while inserting a suture. If the imprint of the forceps appears upon the wall of the bowel after the forceps have been removed, this is a clear warning that excessive force has been applied in grasping the tissue.

With the goal of avoiding unnecessary trauma, in selecting forceps recognize immediately that the "smooth" as well as the "mouse-toothed" forceps are contraindicated when handling delicate tissue. Applied to the bowel, the smooth forceps requires excessive compression to avoid slipping. In this situation a DeBakey-type forceps does not require excessive compression to prevent the tissue from slipping from the jaws of the forceps. For more delicate dissection, the Brown-Adson type forceps is even more suitable. This instrument contains many tiny interdigitating teeth, which allow the surgeon to hold delicate tissues with *minimal* force.

Needle-holder

It should be obvious that when a curved needle is used it must be inserted with a circular motion to avoid a tear at the site of the needle's point of entry into the tissue. What is required is a rotatory motion of the surgeon's wrist which, in turn, is aided by proper body stance and a relaxed shoulder and elbow position. Stability is enhanced if the elbow can be kept close to the body. Many novices tend to ignore the need for this rotatory wrist motion, especially when the suture line is in a poorly accessible anatomical location. They tend to insert a curved needle with a purely horizontal motion of the needle-holder, thus causing excessive injury at the entrance hole.

Using the same hand grip throughout the suturing sequence enhances the surgeon's capacity to detect proprioceptive impulses from the needle-holder. It is difficult to sense the depth of the needle bite accurately if some of the time the surgeon's fingers are in the orifices of the instrument's handle and at other times are not. For gastrointestinal suturing, where proprioception is of great importance, we prefer a grip with the thumb in one orifice and the ring finger in the other, steadying the handle with the extended index and middle fingers.

While most suturing is accomplished using a needle-holder with a straight shaft, some situations require a needle-holder whose shaft is angled or curved. This is so, for example, in the low colorectal and in some esophago-gastric anastomoses. In both instances inserting the suture with a smooth rotatory motion may not be possible unless a curved needle-holder like the Stratte or Finochietto is used (see Fig. D–15).

Hemostat

Ideally, the hemostat should be applied to a vessel just behind the point of bleeding, and the bite of tissue should be no larger than the diameter of the vessel. Obtaining hemostasis may *seem* to take less time if large bites of tissue are grasped by large hemostats than if small, accurate bites are taken. On the other hand, with small bites *many* bleeding points can be rapidly controlled by electrocoagulation rather than ligature, a technique that is especially helpful in operations such as those for radical mastectomy.

Whenever possible, small Halsted or Crile hemostats should be employed. The choice between straight- and curve-tipped hemostats is a matter of personal preference, as either may be applied with equal accuracy. For deeper vessels, such as the cystic artery, Adson clamps provide greater length of handle combined with delicate jaws.

Occasionally it is more efficient to use a single, large Kelly hemostat to grasp a large pedicle containing a number of vascular branches than to cause additional bleeding by dissecting each small branch away from the pedicle. An example is the ligation of the left gastric artery–coronary vein pedicle along the lesser curvature of the stomach during gastric resection. A right-angled Mixter clamp is useful for obtaining hemostasis in the thoracic cavity and when dividing the vascular tissue around the lower rectum during the course of anterior resection.

In all cases the preferred hand grip for holding hemostats is identical with that for holding the needle-holder and scissors. When the hemostat has a curved tip, the instrument should be held so that the tip curves in the same direction in which the surgeon's fingers flex.

References

Cruse PJ, Foord R (1973) A five-year prospective study of 23,649 surgical wounds. Arch Surg 107:206

Madden JE et al. (1970) Studies in the management of the contaminated wound, IV. Resistance to infection of surgical wounds made by knife, electrosurgery, and laser. Am J Surg 119:222

B Dissecting and Sewing

The Art of Dissecting Planes

Of all the skills involved in the craft of surgery, perhaps the single most important is the discovery, delineation, and separation of anatomical planes. When this is skillfully accomplished, there is scant blood loss and tissue trauma is minimal. The delicacy and speed with which dissection is accomplished can mark the difference between the master surgeon and the tyro.

Of all the instruments available to expedite the discovery and delineation of tissue planes, none is better than the surgeon's *left index finger*. (References here are again to right-handed surgeons). This digit gets insinuated behind the lateral duodenal ligament in the performance of the Kocher maneuver, behind the renocolic ligament during colon resection, and behind the gastrophrenic ligament in the performance of a gastric fundoplication. These structures can then be divided very rapidly, for the underlying left index finger is visible through the transparent tissue. Dissection of all these structures by other techniques is not only more time consuming, it is frequently more traumatic and produces more blood loss.

In identifying adhesions between the bowel and peritoneum, the left index finger can often be passed behind the adhesion. This maneuver can produce gentle traction on the tissue to be incised. If the finger is visible through the adhesion it can aid dissection.

If there is insufficient space for the insertion of the surgeon's left index finger, often the *Metzenbaum scissors*, with the blades closed, can serve the same function when inserted underneath an adhesion for delineation and division. This maneuver is also useful in incising the adventitia of the axillary vein during radical mastectomy. To do this, the closed Metzenbaum scissors is inserted between the adventitia and the vein itself; then it is withdrawn, the blades are opened, and one blade is inserted beneath the adventitia; finally, the jaws of the scissors are closed and the tissue divided. This maneuver gets repeated until the entire adventitia anterior to the vein has been divided.

In many situations a closed blunt-tip right-angle *Mixter clamp* may be used the same way as a Metzenbaum scissors for the dissection and delineation of anatomical structures. Identification and skeletonization of the inferior mesenteric artery or the cystic artery and delineation of the circular muscle of the esophagus during cardiomyotomy are just some of the uses to which this instrument can be put.

The *scalpel* is the instrument of choice when developing a plane that is not a natural one, such as in elevating skin flaps over the breast. When the scalpel is held at a 45° angle to the direction of the incision (**Fig. B–1**), it is also quite useful in clearing fascia of overlying fat.

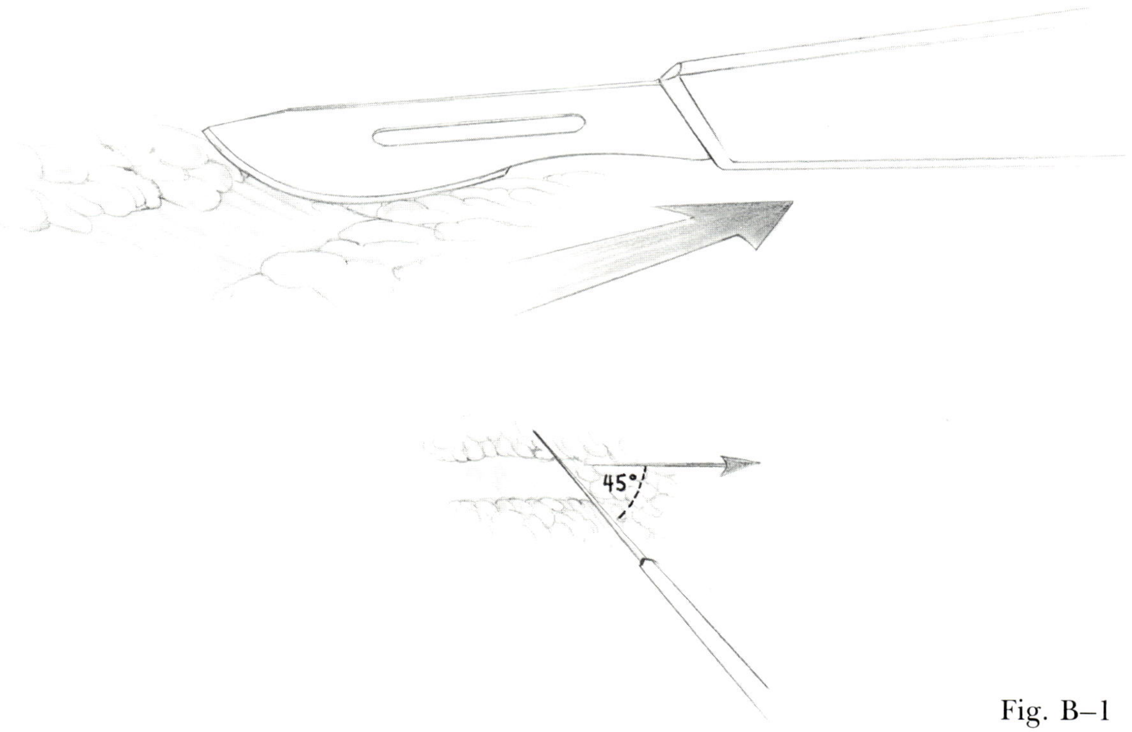

Fig. B–1

More important, when the surgeon must cope with advanced pathological changes involving dense scar tissue, such as may exist when elevating the posterior wall of the duodenum in the vicinity of a penetrating duodenal ulcer, the scalpel is the only instrument that will divide the dense scar accurately until the natural plane of cleavage between the duodenum and pancreas is reached, beyond the diseased tissue.

The *peanut sponge* (Kutner dissector), a small, 1.5 cm gauze sponge grasped in a long hemostat, is an appropriate device to separate fat and areolar tissue from anatomical structures. It should not be used to tear tissues while making a plane. After the peritoneum overlying the cystic duct and artery has been incised, the peanut sponge can separate peritoneum and fat from the underlying duct and artery. It is useful for the elevation of a thyroid lobe from its capsule. After sharp dissection has exposed the major arteries during the course of a colon resection, the peanut sponge is able to skeletonize the vessels and sweep the lymphatic and areolar tissue toward the specimen.

A folded 10 cm × 10 cm *gauze square* grasped in a sponge holder has occasional application in sweeping perirenal fat from the posterior aspect of the peritoneum in lumbar sympathectomy. It is useful also in separating the posterior wall of the stomach from peripancreatic filmy peritoneal attachments. Because the use of a large sponge does not permit anatomical precision, small veins may be torn in this type of gross dissection; therefore the sponge's applicability should be limited to avascular planes.

The surgeon who wants to perform accurate dissections is greatly aided by a *talent for quickly recognizing tissues and structures* as they are revealed by the scalpel or scissors. A truly alert surgeon can make a prompt evaluation of the structural characteristics of a nerve, blood vessel, ureter, or common bile duct, so that each is identifiable at a glance, even before the structure is thoroughly exposed. This requires an intimate knowledge of anatomy, so that the surgeon knows *exactly where each structure will appear*, even before it has been revealed by dissection.

Sewing Technique

Use of Needle-holder

Smooth rotatory wrist action and the surgeon's awareness of what it feels like when a needle penetrates the submucosa of the bowel are important when suturing with a typical half-circle needle on a needle-holder. (Also see Appendix A.)

Selection of Needle: Straight or Curved?

Most surgeons prefer to place seromuscular sutures into the gastrointestinal tract with a fine half-curved needle in a needle-holder. However, for those who wish to learn the technique it is possible to accomplish the same seromuscular bite with a straight needle held between thumb and fingers. This is done by first angling the needle toward the lumen of the bowel at a 45° angle. After penetrating the submucosa the needle direction is abruptly changed to an outward direction away from the lumen.

It is in the insertion of the mucosal layer of sutures that the straight needle demonstrates its distinct superiority. The needle should be directed at a right angle to the long axis of the bowel and passed directly through the entire wall in a single thrusting motion. The first assistant should then grasp the tip of the needle with a straight hemostat, pull it through, and hand it back to the surgeon, who will then be prepared to insert the next stitch in the continuous layer. Considerable time can be saved by avoiding the need to reposition the needle in a needle-holder at each step.

The needle selected for any use should have the least possible thickness commensurate with adequate strength to achieve its purpose.

Size of Bite

The width of the tissue enclosed in the typical seromuscular suture will vary between 4 and 6 mm, depending on the thickness and consistency of the tissue involved. Hypertrophied gastric wall requires a larger bite than the normally thin colon. When closing the abdominal wall by our version of the Smead-Jones closure, a bite of abdominal wall 3 cm wide is appropriate, as this stitch serves as a buried "retention" suture and must resist considerable muscle pull without tearing out.

Distance between Sutures

The distance between bites in the typical approximation of the seromuscular layer with interrupted Lembert sutures is 5 mm. When continuous mucosal or other sutures are used, the width of the bites and the distance apart should be approximately the same as those specified for interrupted stitches.

After one layer of sutures has been inserted, the surgeon should use the forceps in order tentatively to test the optimal degree of inversion that will permit the second layer to be inserted without tension (see Figs. 15–26a and 15–26b).

Size of Suture Material

As there must never be any tension on an anastomosis in the gastrointestinal tract, it is not necessary to use suture material heavier than 4–0. Failure of healing is often due to tearing of a stitch through the tissue and almost never to a broken suture. When two layers of sutures are used for an anastomosis in the GI tract, the inner layer should be 4–0 chromic catgut. This layer provides immediate and accurate approximation of the mucosa and, in some instances, hemostasis. Therefore, this layer of suture material need not persist more than 4–6 days before it is absorbed. In esophagogastric anastomoses, interrupted 4–0 PG should be used for the inner layer, which has the additional function of contributing strength to the anastomosis. For this purpose, slower absorption is desirable.

When taking large bites of tissue that has considerable tensile strength, such as in the Smead-Jones closure of the abdominal wall, heavier suture material is indicated. Here, 2–0 monofilament stainless steel wire or No. 1 PG is suitable. Obviously, the size of the suture material must be proportional to the strength of the tissues into which it is inserted and to the strain it has to sustain.

Continuous versus Interrupted Sutures

An end-to-end anastomosis of the GI tract should always be done with interrupted seromuscular sutures in order to avoid the possibility that the purse-string effect of the continuous stitch will narrow the lumen. A continuous suture of 4–0 catgut is often permissible in the mucosal layer if it is inserted with care to avoid narrowing. Rapid absorption of the catgut will help avoid permanent stomal constriction. However, if the lumens of the two segments of intestine to be anastomosed seem narrow, *both* the seromuscular and mucosal layers should be interrupted. When an anastomosis is large, as in gastrojejunostomy, the use of two continuous layers of PG appears to be quite safe.

In performing inguinal hernia repair by the Shouldice technique, we have found multiple layers of continuous 3–0 Tevdek to be satisfactory.

How Tight the Knot?

If the knot on a suture approximating the seromuscular coats of two segments of intestine is tied so tightly as to cause ischemic necrosis, an anastomotic leak may follow. This is especially likely if the stitch has been placed erroneously through the entire wall of the bowel into the lumen. Since considerable edema follows the construction of an anastomosis, knots should be tied with only sufficient tension to provide apposition of the two seromuscular coats. Caution must be exercised when tying suture material such as silk or Prolene, which are slippery enough so that each knot may have the effect of a noose that is repeatedly tightened with the tying of each additional knot. One advantage of cotton is its high coefficient of friction, which minimizes the tendency that the second knot will cause further constriction. Nylon sutures evidence excessive slippage; even when the first knot has been applied with proper tension, each succeeding knot often produces further constriction. When nylon sutures in the skin have been tied with too much tension, marked edema, redness, and cross-hatching can be seen at the site of each stitch. The same ill effects occur when intestinal sutures are made too tight, but the result is of course not visible to the surgeon.

Catching Both Walls of Intestine with One Pass of the Needle-holder

Most surgeons who insert seromuscular sutures to approximate two segments of intestine were taught to insert the Lembert suture through the intestine on one side of the anastomosis. Then they pick up the needle with the needle-holder to take another Lembert stitch in the opposite wall of the bowel. Occasionally, under ideal conditions, it is possible to pass a needle of proper length through one side of the intestine and then, without removing the needle-holder, pass the needle through the opposite wall before pulling the thread through.

The danger in performing this shortcut is that one may traumatize the entrance wound made on the side of the intestine through which the needle was first inserted. This can happen as the surgeon moves the needle and the intestinal wall in a lateral direction to bring it closer to the opposing intestine, thus making a small tear at the entrance hole (**Fig. B–2**).

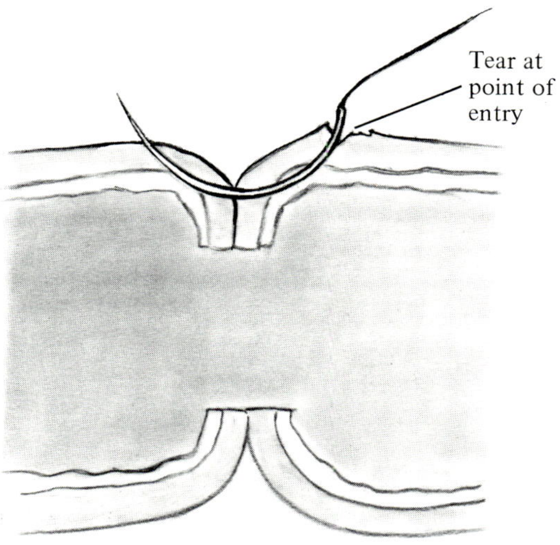

Fig. B–2

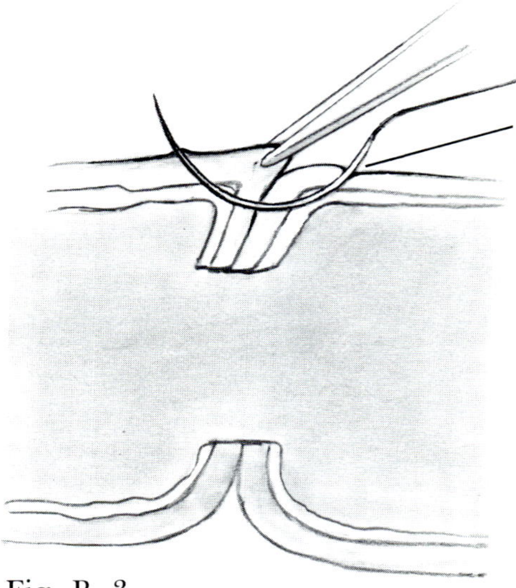

Fig. B–3

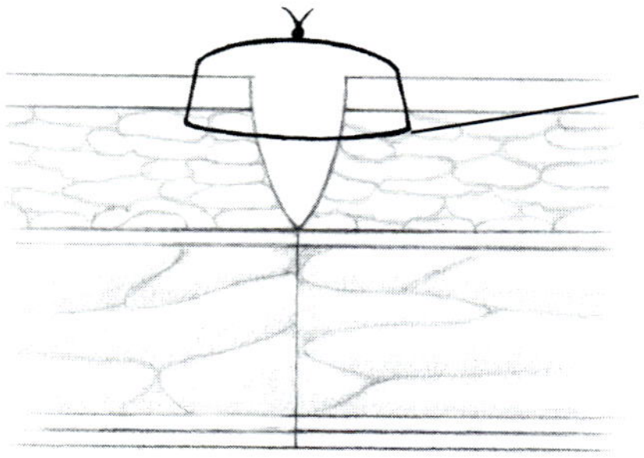

Fig. B–4

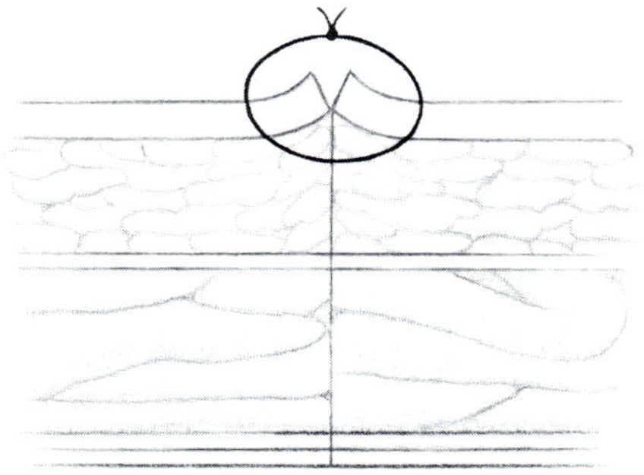

Fig. B–5

With proper technique this shortcut can be accomplished without undue trauma. After the needle has been passed through the first segment of intestine, the surgeon should avoid any *lateral* movement of the needle-holder. Instead, the surgeon should *gently* pick up the opposing segment of intestine with a forceps and bring this bowel to the needle. Then, with a purely *rotatory* motion of the wrist, the surgeon should allow the needle to penetrate the second side (**Fig. B–3**). If the surgeon remains conscious of the need to avoid trauma and uses a rotatory maneuver, there are situations in which this technique is acceptable and efficient.

Types of Stitches

Simple Everting Skin Stitch

In closing skin, eversion of the edges is desired. Consequently, the wrist should be pronated and the needle inserted so that the deeper portion of the bite will be slightly wider than the superficial portion (**Fig. B–4**). When this stitch is tied, the edges will be everted (**Fig. B–5**).

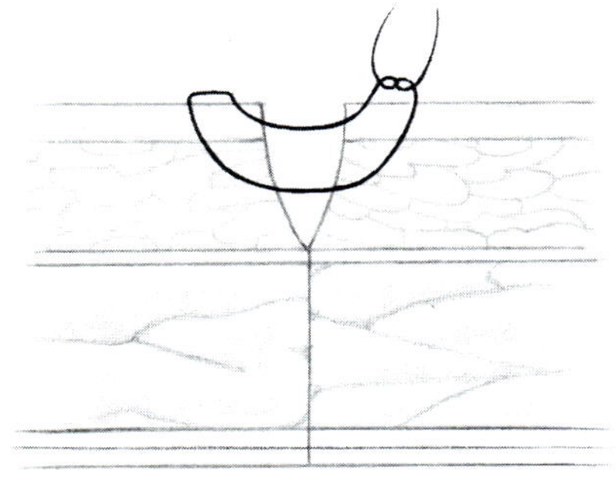

Fig. B–6

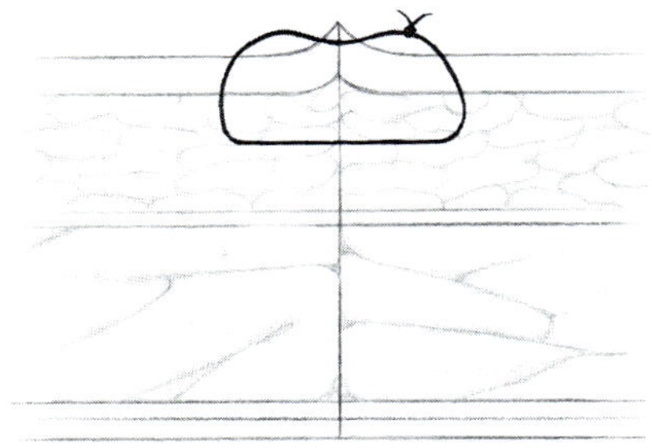

Fig. B–7

Vertical Mattress (Stewart) Stitch

In the classic, Stewart method of skin suturing, eversion is guaranteed by the nature of the vertical mattress stitch (**Figs. B–6 and B–7**). Neither of these two types of skin sutures should be tied with excessive tension if cross-hatching is to be avoided.

Continuous Subcuticular Stitch

In the continuous subcuticular stitch 4–0 PG may be employed on an atraumatic, curved, or straight cutting needle. With practice the surgeon may insert it rapidly and get a good cosmetic result (**Fig. B–8**). Because it is absorbable there are no sutures to be removed postoperatively. If preferred, continuous 3–0 nylon may be used, with lead shot fixing the stitch at its points of origin and termination. This stitch should not be removed for 10–14 days following the operation. If the nylon stitch is longer than 7–8 cm, it may break during the attempt at its removal.

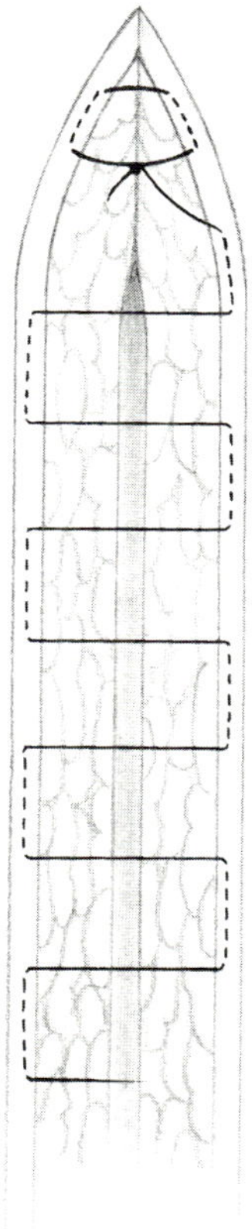

Fig. B–8

Skin Staples

The new stapling devices developed by the U.S. Surgical and the Ethicon companies have made the Michel clips obsolete. The new staples can be applied with force just sufficient to achieve approximation without producing cross-hatching of the skin. They also obtain good cosmetic results. Depending upon the thickness of the skin and the underlying structures, staples may be placed 5–10 mm apart (**Fig. B–9**).

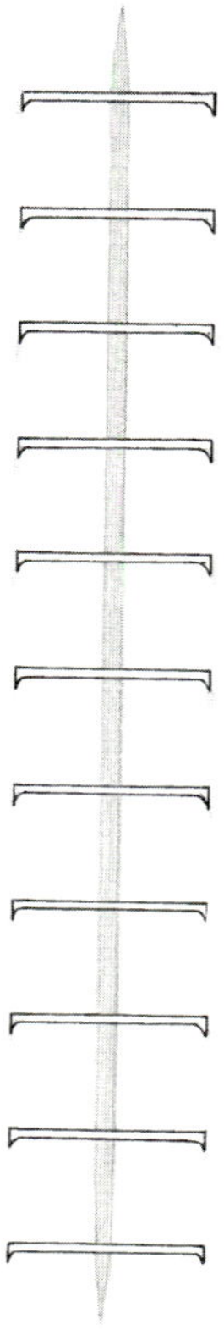

Fig. B–9

Simple Interrupted Fascial Stitch

In the traditional abdominal closure, the fascia is closed by interrupted simple stitches, which catch 8–10 mm of tissue with each bite, as shown in **Fig. B–10**. Except for its use in the McBurney and Pfannenstiel incisions, this type of abdominal wall closure should be considered obsolete (see Chap. 5).

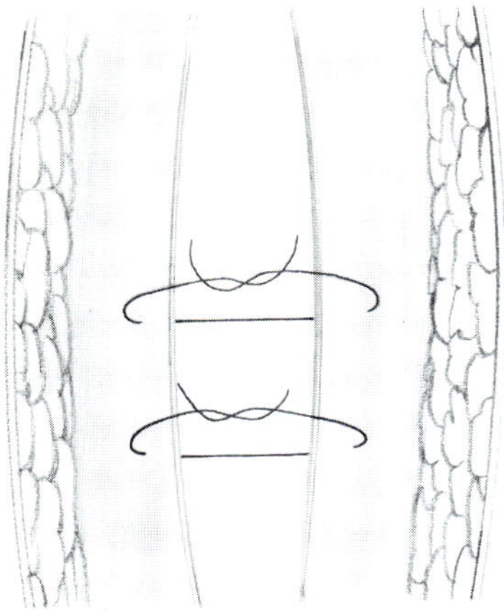

Fig. B–10

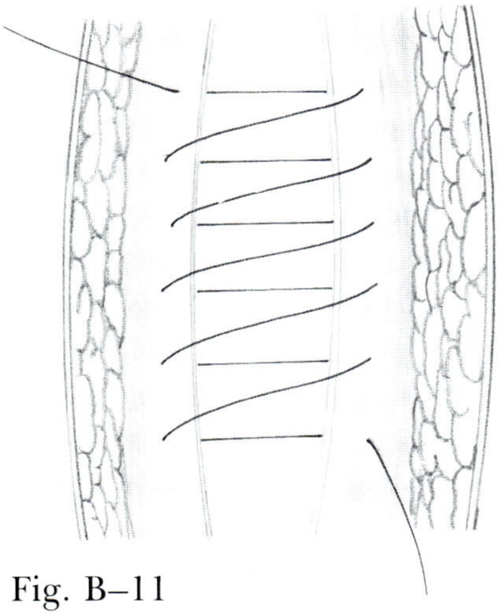

Fig. B–11

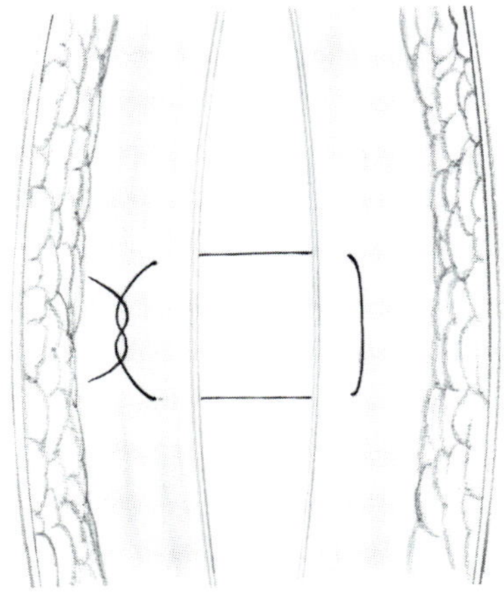

Fig. B–12

Continuous Simple Over-and-Over Stitch

Fig. B–11 illustrates the simple over-and-over continuous stitch which frequently is used for closure of the peritoneum and is sometimes applied to the mucosal layer of bowel anastomoses.

Horizontal Mattress Stitch

The mattress suture is used to close fascia and, sometimes, for ventral hernia repair (**Fig. B–12**). It can also serve as a hemostatic stitch.

Smead-Jones Stitch

The Smead-Jones stitch is well suited for the closure of major abdominal incisions. It is, in essence, a buried "retention" suture, for it encompasses all the layers of the abdominal wall, except the skin, in its large loop. The large loop is followed by a small loop, which catches only 4–5 mm of linea alba on each side (**Fig. B–13**). The purpose of this small loop is

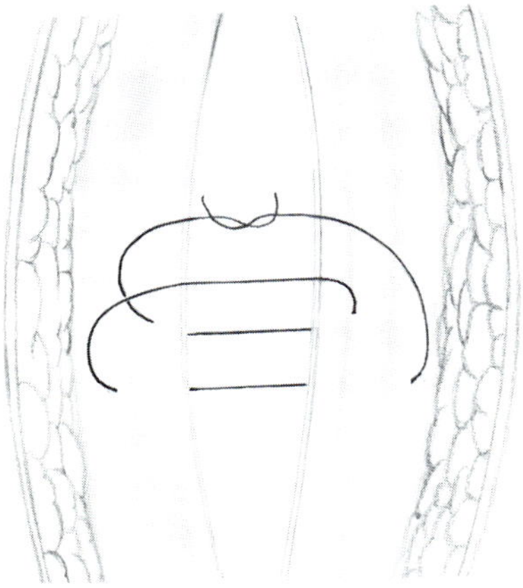

Fig. B–13

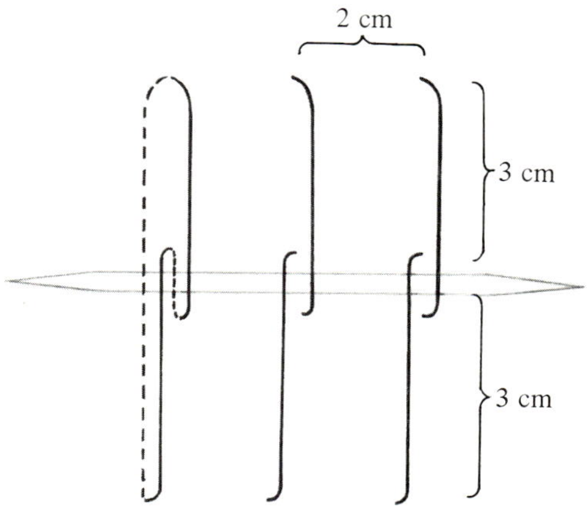

Fig. B–14

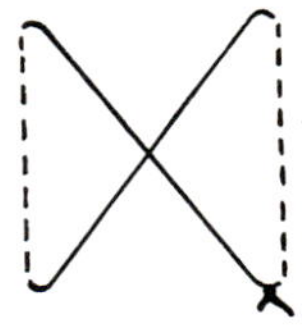
Fig. B–15

to orient the abdominal wall in perfect apposition. It is described in detail in Chap. 5. Its dimensions are diagrammed in **Fig. B–14**.

Hemostatic Figure-of-Eight Stitch

The classic hemostatic stitch, the figure-of-eight, for the occlusion of a bleeding vessel that has retracted into muscle or similar tissue is illustrated in **Fig. B–15**.

Seromucosal Bowel Stitch

In recent years bowel anastomoses that employ one layer of sutures have become acceptable. An effective method of accomplishing both inversion and approximation simultaneously is by the use of what we have called the seromucosal stitch (**Fig. B–16**). This is an inverting stitch that catches the seromuscular and submucosal layer as well as a small amount of mucosa. When properly applied, it produces a slight inversion of the mucosal layer as well as approximation. It is not necessary to pass this stitch deeper than the submucosal layer.

If this stitch is passed into the lumen before emerging from the mucosal layer, it is identical with that described by Gambee, whose technique was at one time applied to the one-layer closure of the Heinecke-Mikulicz pyloroplasty. Used either in an interrupted or in continuous fashion, it is an excellent alternative to the Connell stitch for the inversion of the anterior mucosal layer of a two-layer bowel anastomosis. When used for the construction of a single-layer intestinal anastomosis, it should, of course, be done only in interrupted fashion.

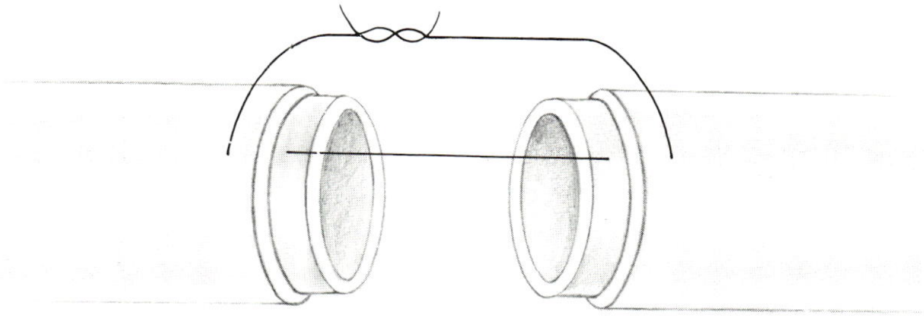
Fig. B–16

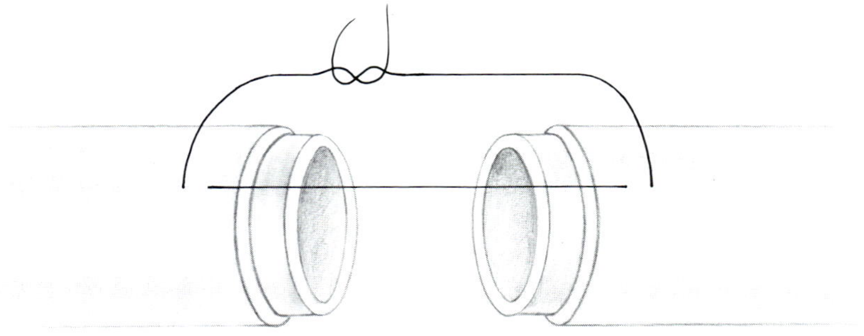

Fig. B–17

Lembert Stitch

Perhaps the most widely used technique for the approximation of the seromuscular layer of a bowel or gastric anastomosis is the Lembert stitch (**Fig. B–17**). This catches about 5 mm of tissue, including a bite of submucosa, and emerges 1–2 mm proximal to the cut edge of the serosa. This stitch also has been used for one-layer intestinal anastomoses. Under proper circumstances, it may be applied in a continuous fashion.

Cushing Stitch

The Cushing stitch is similar to the Lembert stitch, except that it is inserted parallel to the cut edge of the bowel, 2–4 mm from the cut edge. It should catch about 5 mm of the bowel, including the submucosa. It is especially applicable for seromuscular approximation in anastomoses in poorly accessible locations, such as the low colorectal anastomosis. The interrupted Cushing technique is illustrated in **Fig. B–18a**. When used as a continuous stitch (**Fig. B–18b**), the Cushing is a good alternative to the Connell stitch for inverting the anterior mucosal layer of an anastomosis. The main

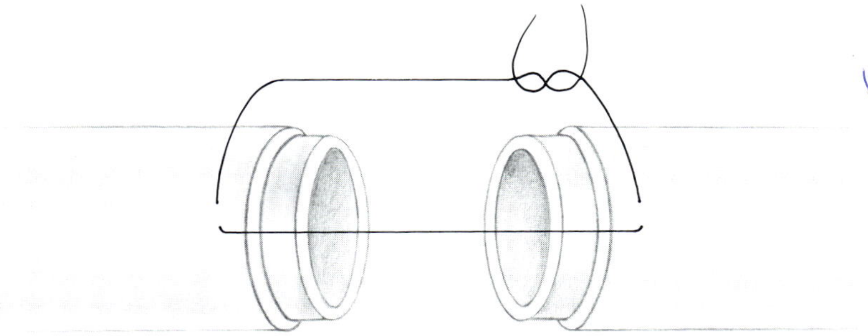

Fig. B–18a

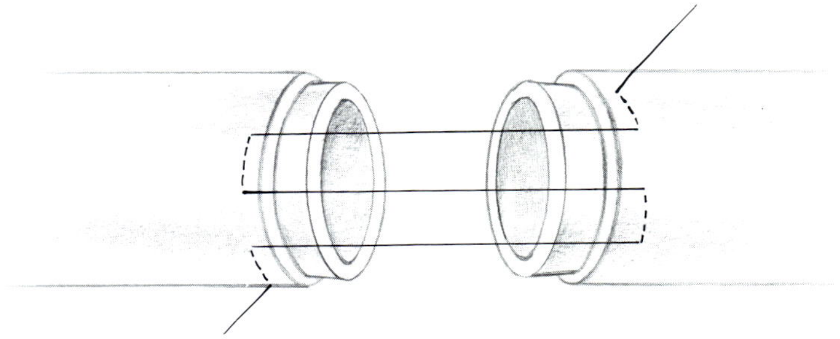

Fig. B–18b

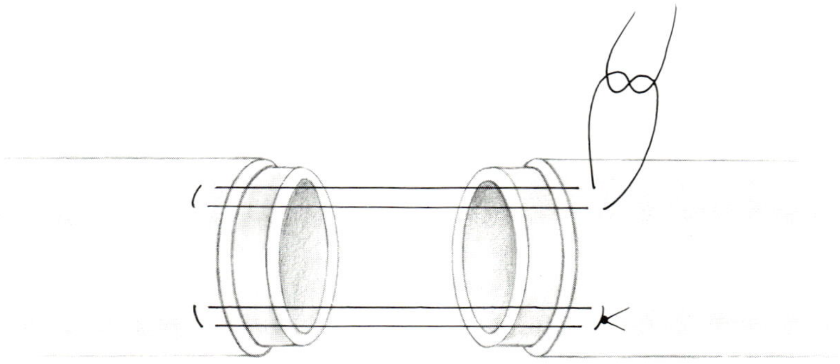

Fig. B–19

difference between the Connell (see Fig. B–21) and a continuous Cushing suture is that the former penetrates into the lumen of the bowel while the latter passes only to the depth of the submucosal layer. The continuous Cushing suture is also much easier and more efficient to accomplish than the Connell.

Halsted Stitch

The Halsted stitch (**Fig. B–19**) also provides excellent seromuscular approximation in a bowel anastomosis. It shares with the Cushing stitch the danger that when tied with excessive tension, it will cause strangulation of a larger bite of tissue than will the Lembert suture.

Continuous Locked Stitch

Fig. B–20 illustrates the approximation of the posterior mucosal layer of a bowel anastomosis with a continuous locked stitch. This stitch assures hemostasis as well as approximation. When hemostasis is not a problem, some surgeons prefer to close this layer with a simple over-and-over continuous stitch (Fig. B–11).

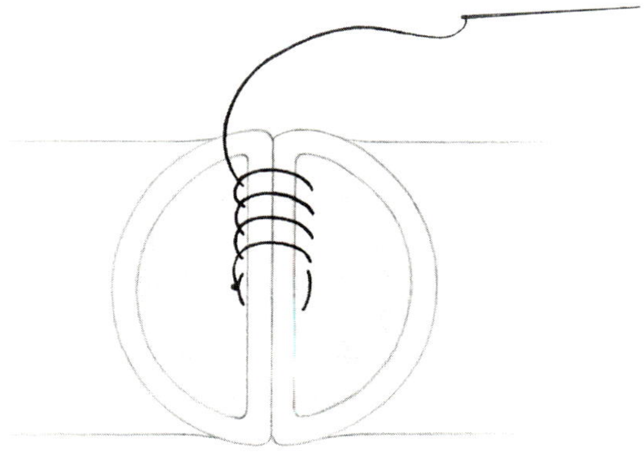

Fig. B–20

Connell Stitch

In 1892 Connell reported that he had devised a way to perform a *one-layer* end-to-end anastomosis of the bowel. For many decades his stitch has been used as the method of inverting the anterior mucosal layer of a *two-layer* bowel anastomosis. The stitch goes from the serosa through all the layers of intestine into the lumen. (**Fig. B–21**), comes out through all the layers on the same side, and passes over to the opposite segment of the bowel, where the same sequence takes place.

Because it forms a loop on the mucosa, the Connell stitch is moderately hemostatic. One should not depend entirely on it for hemostasis, however. As the bowel is inverted, intralumenal bleeding does not remain visible to the surgeon, and may go undetected. Rather than rely on the Connell stitch, it is preferable to ligate the bleeding points on the anterior surface of the bowel with fine catgut, or else to occlude the bleeding points with accurate electrocoagulation. If hemostasis has been achieved in this manner, the Connell technique is not the optimal method of inverting the anterior layer of mucosa in performing bowel anastomosis, as it is more cumbersome tan either the seromucosal suture (Fig. B–16) or a continuous Cushing stitch (Fig. B–18b).

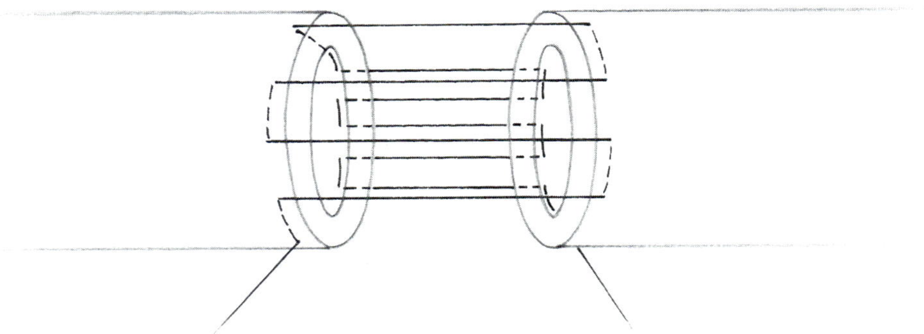

Fig. B–21

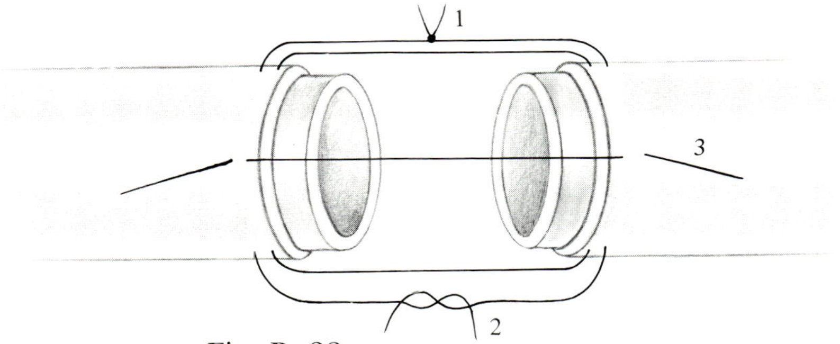

Fig. B–22

Technique of Successive Bisection

The technique that we have named "successive bisection" assures consistently accurate intestinal anastomoses, especially when the diameters of the two segments are not identical. As illustrated in **Fig. B–22**, the first stitch is inserted at the antimesenteric border and the second stitch at the mesenteric border. The third is then inserted at a point that exactly bisects the entire layer. The fourth stitch bisects the distance between the first and third stitches. This pattern is repeated until the anastomotic layer is complete (**Fig. B–23**).

Types of Intestinal Anastomoses

One Layer or Two Layers?

Although there is abundent data confirming that an intestinal anastomosis can be performed safely with either one layer or two layers of sutures, there is, to our knowledge, no consistent body of randomized data conclusively demonstrating the superiority of one or

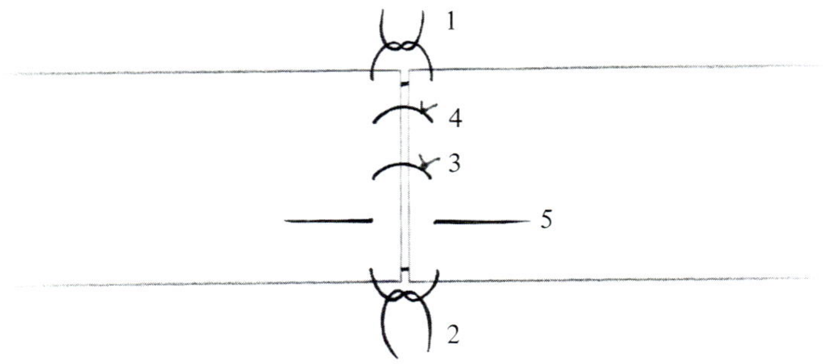

Fig. B–23

the other in humans. It is obvious that the one-layer anastomosis does not turn in as much intestine and, consequently, has a larger lumen than the two-layer. However, in the absence of postoperative leakage, obstruction at the anastomotic site is rare except, perhaps, when the esophagus is involved. It does seem reasonable, though, to assume that if the seromuscular layer sutured by the surgeon suffers from some minor imperfection, then the mucosal sutures may compensate for the imperfection and prevent leakage. While we have experienced good results with one-layer techniques, we recommend in teaching residents, that every surgeon master the standard two-layer technique before considering the other.

End-to-End or End-to-Side?

In most situations, the end-to-end technique is quite satisfactory for joining two segments of bowel. If there is some disparity in diameter, a *Cheatle slit* should be performed on the antimesenteric border of the narrower segment of intestine to enable the two diameters to match each other (**Figs. B–24 and B–25**). In case there is a large disparity in the two diameters, more than 1.5–2 cm, the end-to-side anastomosis has advantages, provided that the anastomosis is not constructed in a manner that permits a blind loop to develop. If the end-to-side anastomosis is placed within 1 cm of the closed end of the intestine, the blind-loop syndrome will not occur. Closing the end of the segment of bowel by suturing requires extra time, but a stapled closure of the bowel end can be accomplished in a matter of seconds and in our experience appears to be just as safe as suturing.

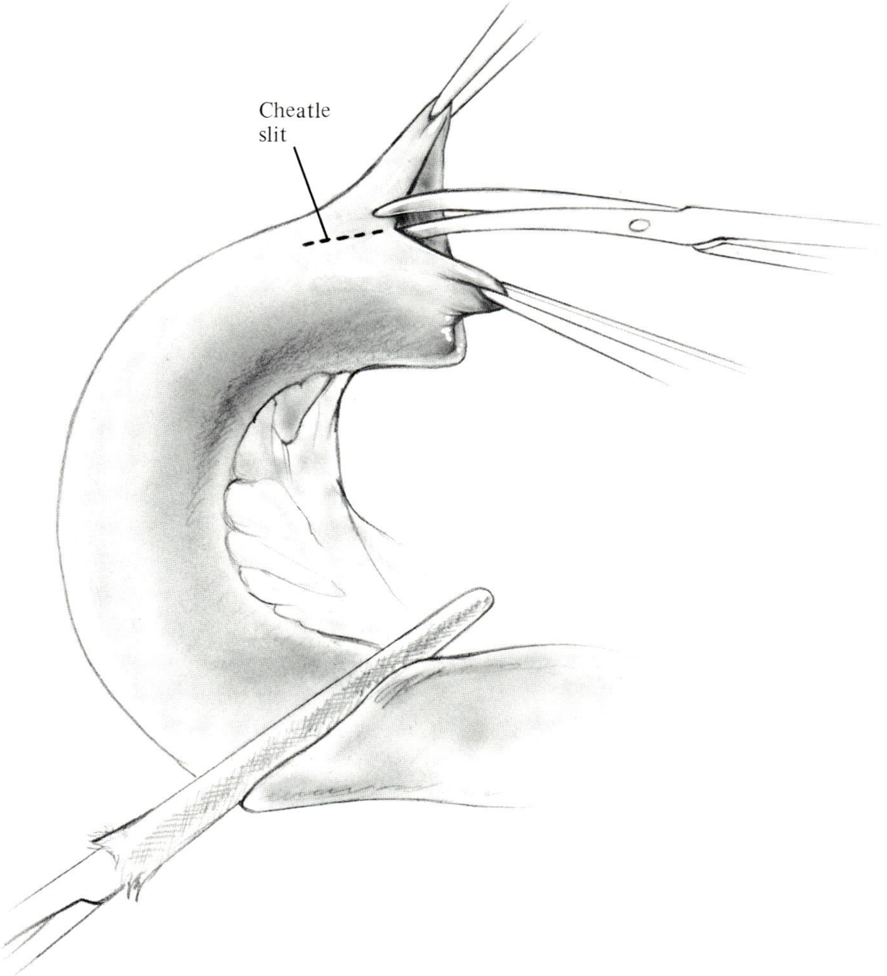

Fig. B–24

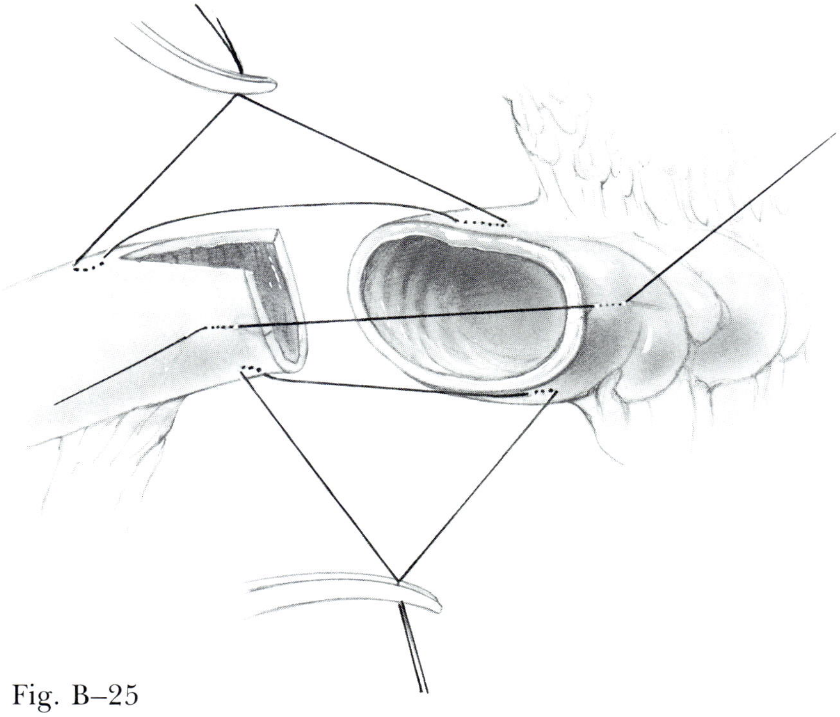

Fig. B–25

There are two instances in which the end-to-side anastomosis is clearly superior to the end-to-end. One is in an esophagogastric anastomosis following esophagogastrectomy. We have reported that in this procedure the incidence of leakage, postoperative stenosis, and mortality are distinctly less with the end-to-side technique. This is probably true also for an esophagojejunal anastomosis. The second instance is in the low colorectal anastomosis. In this procedure the ampulla of the rectum is often much larger in diameter than is the descending colon. Zollinger and Sheppard have reported that the use of the side-to-end Baker technique has virtually eliminated the incidence of postoperative stenosis and leakage. This is confirmed by our experience.

Sutured or Stapled Anastomosis?

A review of 472 stapled suture lines performed at the Booth Memorial Medical Center over a 4-year period, and reported by Chassin et al., demonstrated that the incidence of anastomosis-related complications following stapling was identical to that following sutured anastomoses done over the same period of time by the same surgical staff (see Chap. 4). It was noted, however, that the stapled group contained a much higher incidence of emergency operations, sepsis, bowel gangrene, intestinal obstruction, and carcinomatosis than did the sutured group. When done by surgeons whose techniques are sophisticated, stapling and suturing can achieve equally good results.

Types of Suture Material

Absorbable

Plain Catgut
Plain catgut is not commonly used in modern surgery. Although its rapidity of absorption might seem to be an advantage, this rapidity is the result of an intense inflammatory reaction that produces enzymes for the digestion of the organic material. Plain catgut is acceptable for ligating bleeding points in the subcutaneous tissues and not for very much else.

Chromic Catgut
Chromic catgut has the advantage of a smooth surface, which permits it to be drawn through delicate tissues with minimal friction. It may be depended upon to last for about a week and is suitable only when such rapid absorption is desirable. It is completely contraindicated in the vicinity of the pancreas, where proteolytic enzymes produce premature absorption, and in the closure of abdominal incisions and hernia repair, where it does not hold the tissues long enough for adequate healing to occur. Chromic catgut is useful for the approximation of the mucosal layer in a two-layer anastomosis of the bowel. For this purpose, size 4–0 is suitable. Bear in mind that wound infection will increase the rapidity of catgut digestion.

Polyglycolic Synthetics
Polyglycolic synthetic sutures (PG), such as Dexon or Vicryl, are far superior to catgut because the rate at which they are absorbed is much slower. Even after 15 days, about 20% of the tensile strength remains. Digestion of the polyglycolic sutures is by hydrolysis. Consequently, the proteolytic enzymes in an area of infection have no effect on the rate of absorption of the polyglycolics. Also, the inflammatory reaction they incite is mild as compared with catgut. Their chief drawback is that their surface is somewhat rougher than catgut, which may traumatize tissues slightly when the PG suture material is drawn through the wall of the intestine. This characteristic also *makes the tying of secure knots more difficult* than with catgut. However, these appear to be minor disadvantages, and these products have for many purposes made catgut an obsolete suture material.

Nonabsorbable

Natural Nonabsorbables
Natural nonabsorbable sutures, such as silk, cotton, and linen, have enjoyed a long period of popularity among surgeons the world over. They have the advantage of easy handling and secure knot tying. Once the knots are set, slippage is rare. On the other hand, they produce more inflammatory reaction in tissue than do the monofilament materials (stainless steel, Prolene) or even the braided synthetics. Silk and cotton, although classified as nonabsorbable, do indeed disintegrate in the tissues over a long period of time, whereas the synthetic materials appear to be truly nonabsorbable. In spite of these disadvantages, silk and cotton have maintained worldwide popularity mainly because of their ease of handling and surgeons' long familiarity with them. Because there is no clear-cut data at this time demonstrating that anastomoses performed with synthetic suture material have fewer complications than those performed with silk or cotton, it is not yet necessary for the surgeon to abandon the natural nonabsorbables if he or she can handle them with greater skill. With the exception of the monofilaments, a major disadvantage of nonabsorbable sutures is the formation of chronic draining sinuses and suture granulomas. This is especially marked when material larger than size 3–0 is used in the anterior abdominal fascia or in the subcutaneous tissue.

Synthetic Nonabsorbable Braids
Synthetic braided sutures include those made of Dacron polyester, such as Mersilene, Ticron (Dacron coated with silicone), Tevdek (Dacron coated with Teflon), and Ethibond (Dacron with butilated coating). Braided nylon (Surgilon or Nurolon) is popular in the United Kingdom. All these braided synthetic materials require four or five knots for secure closure, compared to the three required of silk and cotton.

Synthetic Nonabsorbable Monofilaments
Monofilament synthetics like nylon and Prolene are so slippery that as many as 6–7 knots may be required. They and monofilament

stainless steel are the least reactive of all the products available. For this reason, 2–0 or 0 Prolene has been used by some surgeons for the Smead-Jones abdominal closure in the hope of eliminating suture sinuses. Because of the large number of knots, this hope has not been realized, but the sinuses have turned out to be fewer than when nonabsorbable braided materials are used. Prolene size 4–0 on atraumatic needles has been used for the seromuscular layer of intestinal anastomoses. Both Prolene and various braided polyester sutures have achieved great popularity in vascular surgery.

Monofilament Stainless Steel Wire

Monofilament stainless steel wire has many characteristics of the ideal suture material; however, it is difficult to tie. Also, when it has been used for closure of the abdominal wall, patients occasionally have complained of pain at the site of a knot or of a broken suture. True suture sinuses and suture granulomas have been extremely rare when monofilament stainless steel has been used—no more than 1 in 300 cases. (The use of wire in abdominal closure is discussed in Chap. 5.) Size 5–0 monofilament wire has been used by Belsey and Skinner for one-layer esophagogastric anastomoses and by Trimpi for colon anastomoses. Three square throws are adequate for a secure knot in tying this material. If steel wire in the form of a *braid* is used, the incidence of suture sinuses is not less than experienced with braided silk.

Knot-Tying Technique

The "three-point technique" of tying knots is very important in ligating blood vessels. This means that the surgeon's left hand grasping one end of the ligature, the vessel being ligated, and the surgeon's right hand grasping the opposite end of the ligature are positioned in a straight line, as illustrated in **Figs. B–26a and B–26b**. If this is not the case, as the surgeon's hands draw apart in tightening the knot they exert traction against the vessel. In tying deep bleeding points, this traction tears the vessel at the point of ligature and

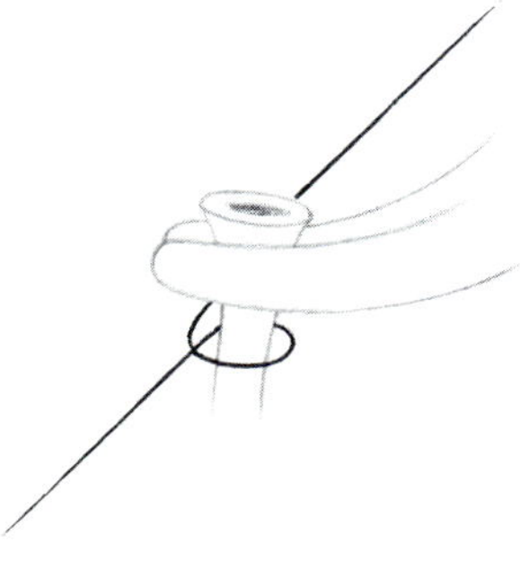

Fig. B–26a

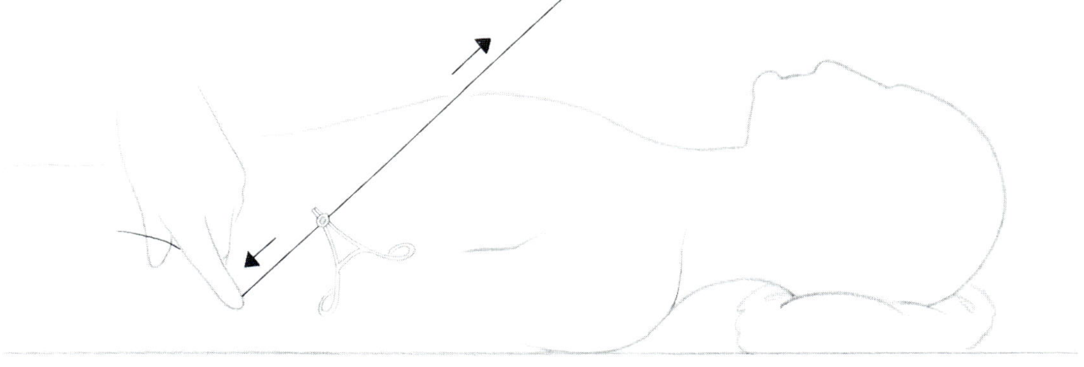

Fig. B–26b

exacerbates bleeding. In tying a deep structure, such as the cystic artery, the surgeon's left index finger should draw the deep end of the ligature deep to the artery so that the left index finger, the cystic artery and the surgeon's right hand always form a straight line.

When using silk or cotton, three square throws provide adequate security. With PG, four throws are necessary. With the various coated polyester sutures, four or five knots must be tied. In using the synthetic materials, many prefer the "surgeon's knot" (**Fig. B–27**) as a first throw.

For heavy monofilament suture material like 0 or 1 Prolene we have used a modification of a fisherman's 3-1-2 knot. First, make a triple throw "surgeon's knot" (**Fig. B–28a**). Then square it with a single throw (**Fig. B–28b**). Complete the knot with the usual double throw "surgeon's knot" (**Fig. B–28c**). This seems to hold without slipping.

When tying a knot in a deep or poorly accessible location, it is vital that the two-hand technique of tying be used. For superficial bleeding points in the skin and subcutaneous tissues, either one- or two-hand knots are efficacious.

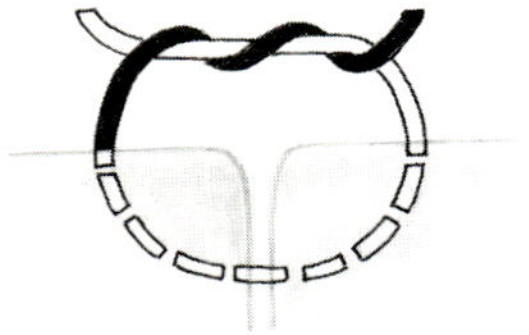

Fig. B–27

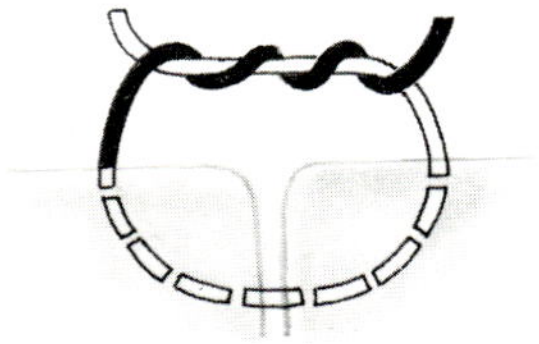

Fig. B–28a

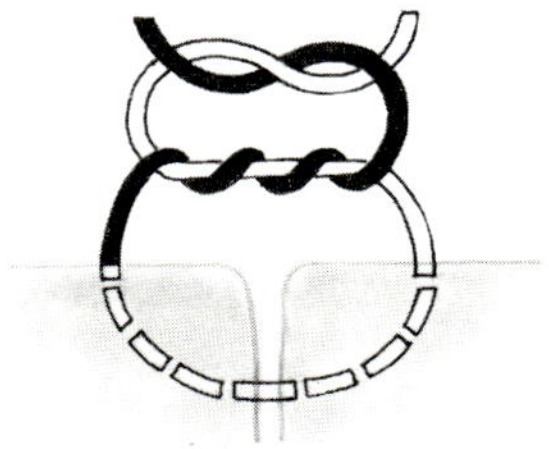

Fig. B–28b

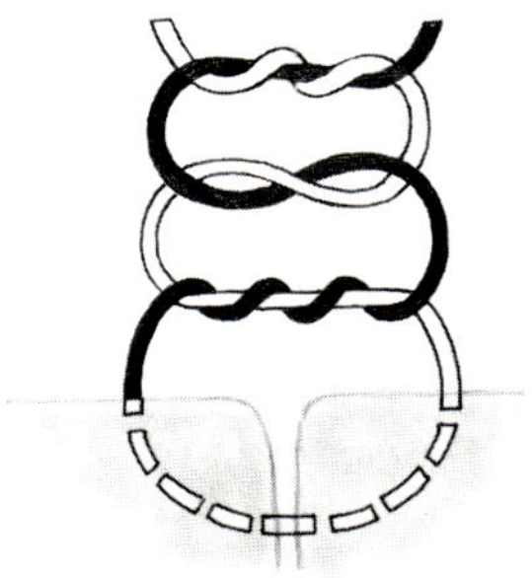

Fig. B–28c

References

Chassin JL (1978) Esophagogastrectomy: data favoring end-to-side anastomosis. Ann Surg 188:22

Connell ME (1892) An experimental contribution looking to an improved technique in enterorrhaphy whereby the number of knots is reduced to two or even one. Med Record 42:335

Zollinger RM, Sheppard MH (1971) Carcinoma of the rectum and the rectosigmoid. Arch Surg 102:335

C Control of Bleeding

Techniques of Achieving Hemostasis

Hemostat and Ligature

A hemostat of the proper length and design is a suitable instrument for occluding most bleeding vessels. This is followed by a ligature of a size compatible with the diameter of the vessel. As demanded by the situation, hemostats the size of a Halsted, Crile, Adson, Kelly, or Mixter may be indicated (see Glossary).

As for the ligature material, surgeons trained in the Halsted tradition have long preferred fine silk because it is less reactive than catgut and eliminates the danger of premature absorption. The advantage of silk and cotton has diminished with the advent of the polyglycollic synthetic absorbable ligatures. The disadvantage of nonabsorbable ligatures is that they may incite the formation of a suture granuloma or suture sinus. It is possible for a sinus to occur after the use of silk deep in the abdomen, although this is rare. Granulomatous nodules have occasionally been palpated on rectal examination following the use of cotton in deep pelvic surgery. Since the polyglycolic materials have low reactivity and slow absorption, they are ideal materials for routine ligatures, if the surgeon has learned to tie secure knots using this material.

The need to ligate a large artery in the presence of an abscess or pancreatitis creates a unique situation. A ligature of braided nonabsorbable material is a foreign body that can readily harbor bacteria in its interstices. When it does, often it erodes into the artery at the site of the ligature and produces hemorrhage. The risk of this type of hemorrhage can be reduced by using heavy polyglycolic absorbable or monofilament (Prolene) ligature material.

In summary, PG ties should be used for most routine ligatures. Cotton or silk provides greater security in tying major vessels such as the left gastric or inferior mesenteric artery. When the mesentery of the sigmoid colon is being divided in the treatment of perforated diverticulitis, use 2–0 PG to ligate the vessels. If the splenic artery is being divided and ligated during the resection of a pseudocyst of the pancreas, use a 2–0 suture-ligature of Prolene.

Ligature-passer

In ligating large vessels such as the inferior mesenteric, the ileocolic, or left gastric, it is convenient to pass a blunt-tip right-angle Mixter clamp behind the vessel. The blunt tip of the clamp separates the adventia of the artery from the surrounding tissue. Preferably, at least 1.5 cm of vessel should be dissected free. When this has been done, use a ligature-passer, which consists of a long hemostat holding the 2–0 cotton ligature, to feed the cotton thread into the jaws of the open Mixter clamp. Then draw the ligature behind the vessel and tie it. Pass the Mixter clamp behind the vessel again, feed a second ligature into its jaws, and ligate the distal portion of the vessel. Divide the vessel, leaving a 1 cm stump distal to the proximal tie and about 0.5 cm on the specimen side. Leaving a long stump of vessel distal to a single tie of 2–0 cotton prevents the ligature from slipping off, even when it is subjected to the continuous pounding of arterial pulse waves. One advantage of a cotton ligature in this situation is its high coefficient of friction, which discourages the ligature or the knot from slipping.

Suture-ligature

Two simple ligatures of 2–0 cotton placed about 3 mm apart, with a free 1 cm stump distal to the ligature, assure hemostasis when ligating the large arteries encountered in gastrointestinal surgery. If there is not a sufficient length of artery to meet these conditions, a 2–0 cotton ligature supplemented by the insertion of a transfixion suture-ligature that pierces the center of the artery 3 mm distal to the simple ligature is almost as good as a free 1 cm stump of artery.

Another type of suture-ligature is used in tissue into which a vessel has retracted. This may occur on the surface of the pancreas, where attempts at grasping a retracted vessel with hemostats can be much more traumatic than a small figure-of-eight suture of atraumatic 4–0 cotton or silk. The same figure-of-eight suture-ligature technique is valuable when a vessel has retracted into a mesentery thickened by obesity or Crohn's disease.

Hemoclip

Metallic clips offer a secure and expedient method of obtaining hemostasis, provided proper application of this technique is accomplished. Hemoclips are applicable *only* when the *entire circumference* of a vessel is visible, preferably *before* the vessel has been lacerated. Applying a clip inaccurately often results in incomplete occlusion of the vessel and continued bleeding, following which the presence of the metal clip obstructs the use of a hemostat or a suture-ligature in the same area. Attempts to remove the clip from a thin-walled vein may increase the rate of bleeding.

When Hemoclips are applied in an area where subsequent steps in the operation require blunt dissection or vigorous retraction—such as in performing a Kocher maneuver—the subsequent surgical maneuvers often dislodge the clips and lacerate the vessels, producing annoying hemorrhage.

Another maneuver that should never be performed is the application of clips in the general area from which blood is oozing, in the hope this will somehow catch the bleeder. Again it must be emphasized that unless a bleeding vessel can be clearly visualized, applying a Hemoclip is counterproductive.

In the absence of these contraindications, the use of Hemoclips is a desirable technique, as for instance in the mediastinum during esophageal dissection, or in the retroperitoneal area during colon resection. The large-size Hemoclip is especially suitable during the presacral mobilization of the rectum for an anterior resection.

Coagulation by Electrocautery

Electrocoagulation is a valuable and rapid means of achieving hemostasis, provided that certain contraindications are observed. Vessels that have an external diameter larger than 2–3 mm should not be electrocoagulated. Just as with Hemoclips, any tissue that will be subjected to blunt dissection or retraction is not suitable for electrocautery, as the friction often wipes away the coagulum, causing bleeding to resume.

In the presence of fat, such as in the subcutis or in the breast, bleeding points should not be electrocoagulated unless a discrete blood vessel has been grasped by a forceps or a hemostat. Otherwise, electrocoagulation in the general area of a bleeder surrounded by fat boils the fat and causes more extensive tissue insult than is necessary. This happens because fat is a poorer conductor of electricity than is muscle or vascular tissue.

When many subcutaneous bleeding points are subjected to electrocoagulation, the extensive tissue insult contributes to wound infection. Although there does not appear to be any randomized, controlled study of the effects of electrocoagulation on human wounds, Cruse noticed a doubled incidence of wound infection in operations done with the electrocautery as compared with those accomplished with a cold knife and hemostats. Very likely this was the result of excessive tissue trauma the electrocautery causes in the fatty layer.

Extensive use of electrocoagulation in muscle tissue, as in opening large incisions in the thoracic cavity, appears to have no deleterious effects. In doing radical mastectomies we have used electrocoagulation to control all the perforating branches of the internal mammary artery. This is an area devoid of fat and also an area where the vessels may be discretely identified and grasped in hemostats before the electrocautery is applied. There has been no instance of postoperative bleeding in a large series of mastectomies. Of course, if a large bulk of tissue is included in the hemostat, the effectiveness of electrocoagulation will be compromised.

In summary, with the exception of fatty tissue and tissues subject to blunt dissection and strong retraction, electrocoagulation of discretely identified vessels is both rapid and effective.

The careful and accurate application of electrocoagulation permits the achievement of complete hemostasis in areas such as the gallbladder bed, the chest wall, and the retroperitoneal tissues, where many tiny veins may continue to ooze even after a period of gauze compression. Individual ligation of each of these innumerable small bleeding points would be rather time consuming.

Physicochemical Methods

Gauze Pack

The physical application of a large, moist gauze pad has been employed for many decades to control diffuse venous oozing. It enhances the clotting mechanism because pressure slows down the loss of blood while the interstices of the gauze help form a framework for the deposition of fibrin. Unfortunately, after the gauze pack is removed, bleeding sometimes resumes.

Oxidized Cellulose

Oxidized regenerated cellulose in the form of gauze (Surgicel) or cottonoid (Oxycel) offer the same advantages as a gauze pack. They may be applied in a thin layer to an oozing surface such as a liver or spleen from which the capsule has been avulsed. Pressure on the cellulose should be applied by an overlying gauze pack. After 10–15 minutes, the gauze pack should be removed and the oxidized cellulose left behind. Used in a thin layer over viable surfaces, the cellulose should undergo uncomplicated absorption. If a wad of cellulose is stuffed into a crack in the liver, however, failure of total absorption and abscess formation may result. Oxidized cellulose is more suitable for surface bleeding than for the control of hemorrhage in a deep crevice.

Avitene

Avitene (microfibrillar collagen) is claimed to be even more effective than oxidized cellulose. It comes in powdered form to be sprinkled on a bleeding surface. Any moisture on instruments or gloves that come into contact with Avitene causes the Avitene to stick to the moist instrument rather than the bleeding surface. If blood oozes through the layer of Avitene, another layer should be applied and pressure exerted over it. When flat surfaces of a denuded spleen or gallbladder bed are oozing, oxidized cellulose seems equally effective as Avitene, and at one-twentieth the cost. Avitene is better for irregular surfaces because it is a powder.

Microfibrillar collagen and oxidized cellulose are extremely valuable when some portion of the splenic capsule has been avulsed during a vagotomy or splenic flexure mobilization. In most cases a splenectomy can be avoided by the use of these substances, occasionally supplemented by the use of sutures.

Control of Hemorrhage, Temporary

In the course of operating, the equanimity of the surgeon is jarred occasionally by a sudden hemorrhage caused by the inadvertent laceration of a large blood vessel. One should have clearly in mind a sequence of steps to execute in such an event, aimed first at temporary control of the bleeding in preparation for definitive steps later. The sequence should go something like this:

1) Finger pressure. The simplest step, especially useful in controlling bleeding from an artery, is the simple application of a fingertip to the bleeding point. In the case of a large vein, such as the axillary or vena cava, pinching the laceration between thumb and index finger is sometimes effective.

2) Elevation of the structure by placing the hand behind it. If step (1) is not applicable, sometimes the left hand may be placed behind a structure such as the hepatoduodenal ligament to control bleeding from the cystic artery or the pancreas or portal vein for bleeding in that area. This may bring temporary control.

3) Compression by hand pressure or gauze-pad pressure. Large lacerations of the liver may be temporarily controlled by compressing this organ between two hands while the patient is being resuscitated. Massive venous bleeding from the presacral space can be controlled by the application of a large gauze pad.

4) Satinsky clamp. When direct pressure is not effective, a partially occluding Satinsky-type vascular clamp may be used to control the laceration of a large vessel.

5) Proximal and distal control. Sometimes, even temporary control of hemorrhage is impossible without proximal and distal occlusion of the vessel. This may involve the aorta or vena cava in some cases. Preferably, vascular clamps should be used, but in their absence umbilical tape is a satisfactory temporary substitute. The aorta may even be clamped in a suprarenal position for 15–20 minutes if no other means of hemostasis is effective. This safe period may be lengthened if iced sterile saline is poured over the kidneys to reduce their metabolic requirements.

Control of Hemorrhage, Definitive

Once temporary control of hemorrhage has been obtained, the surgeon should reassess the strategic situation. The field should be cleared of all instruments and hemostats not relevant to the major problem at hand. If additional exposure is needed, plans should be outlined immediately to accomplish this by extending the incision or by repositioning gauze pads or retractors. Optimal light and suction lines should be obtained. Arrangements should be made with the blood bank for adequate support of the patient. Additional personnel should be recruited as necessary. Dr. Frank C. Spencer, chairman of the department of surgery at New York University, has emphasized that one competent individual must be assigned to "bookkeeping." This individual's only duty should be to keep track of the volume of blood lost as well as the rate of at which it is replaced, and to report this to the operating surgeon at frequent intervals. Otherwise, the surgeon may become so involved with the task at hand that he or she may make inadequate provision for resuscitating the patient.

After all these steps have been completed and the patient's condition has been stabilized, the surgeon can then convert the measures for temporary control of hemorrhage into maneuvers to assure permanent control. This generally involves the application of a partially occluding Satinsky-type clamp to the vessel or the achievement of proximal and distal control with vascular clamps, so that the laceration can be sutured in a definitive fashion with a continuous suture of atraumatic Tevdek or Prolene. No surgeon should undertake to perform major surgery unless he or she has had training and experience in the suturing of large arteries and veins.

D Glossary

Atraumatic suture. Suture material permanently swaged into the end of a disposable needle so as to eliminate the usual double thickness of thread encountered when suture material is threaded through the eye of a needle (see Fig. D–15).

Avitene (microfibrillar collagen hemostat). An absorbable powdery substance that attracts platelets to its fibrils, triggering thrombus formation.

Avicon
P.O. Box 1959
Fort Worth, Texas 76134

Baker tube, Bardic. A plastic tube, 108 cm in length, with an inflatable balloon near its tip which can be manipulated down the small bowel for suction decompression (see Chap. 23).

C. R. Bard
111 Spring Street
Murray Hill, New Jersey 07974

Catheter, Foley. A double-lumen indwelling bladder catheter. The narrower of the two lumens leads to an inflatable balloon at the catheter tip.

Catheter, Swan-Ganz. A balloon-tipped transvenous catheter used to measure pulmonary artery wedge pressure.

Cheatle slit. An incision on the antimesenteric side of the open end of the intestine, designed to increase the circumference of the lumen so that an end-to-end anastomosis can be constructed between it and intestine of a larger diameter (see Figs. B–24 and B–25).

Drain, closed-suction. A fenestrated plastic tube attached to a sterile plastic container which exerts suction after the container is manually compressed. The system is closed to assure sterility (see Fig. D–9).

1. Hemovac-Snyder drain
   Zimmer
   727 North Detroit Street
   Warsaw, Indiana 46580
2. Jackson-Pratt drain
   V. Mueller
   6600 W. Tuohy Avenue
   Chicago, Illinois 60648

Drain, sump. A fenestrated plastic or rubber tube attached to continuous suction. A second channel admits air into the tip of the catheter to prevent tissue being drawn up against the suction vents and occluding them.

1. Shirley sump
   H. W. Andersen Products
   45 E. Main Street
   Oyster Bay, New York 11771
2. Saratoga sump
   Sherwood Medical Industries
   1831 Olive Street
   St. Louis, Missouri 63103

Gomco Thermotic drainage pump. A device which provides intermittent suction at low pressure (either 90 mm or 120 mm of mercury) suitable for sump drains or nasogastric tubes.

Gomco
828 E. Ferry Street
Buffalo, New York 14211

Hartmann operation. See Chap. 41.

Hemoclip. A V-shaped metal clip whose jaws are forced together around a blood vessel for hemostasis.

Edw. Weck
Box 12600
Research Triangle Park, North Carolina 27709

This clip is also manufactured by Ethicon under the name Ligaclip and by U. S. Surgical Corporation under the name Surgiclip.

Hypaque (diatrizoate sodium). An iodinated aqueous contrast medium used instead of barium when performing radiographic contrast enemas or esophagrams in the early postoperative period.

Intestinal bag, Vi-Drape. A sterile 45 × 45 cm plastic bag to contain the small intestine during surgery on the colon.

Med/Surg, Parke-Davis
Park Plaza, P.O. Box 1506
Greenwood, South Carolina 29646

Leg rests, Lloyd-Davies. Used to support the legs and thighs in abduction and in mild flexion for low anterior resection by EEA stapling and abdominal-perineal proctosigmoidectomy (see Fig. D–12).

Downs Surgical
2500 Park Central Boulevard
Decatur, Georgia 30035

Maloney bougies. Mercury-weighted bougies with tapered tips useful in dilating esophageal strictures.

Narco Pilling
Delaware Drive
Fort Washington, Pennsylvania 19034

Marlex mesh. A loosely knitted mesh made of polypropylene filaments, useful to replace defects in the abdominal wall when repairing a large hernia.

Davol
P.O. Box 8500
Cranston, Rhode Island 02920

Mucous fistula. When bowel has been resected but an anastomosis is contraindicated, the proximal segment of intestine is brought out as an enterostomy and the distal cut end of intestine is exteriorized through a stab wound and is called a "mucous fistula" (see Chap. 41).

Oxycel. An oxidized cellulose hemostatic agent which comes in pledget (cotton-type) form and in pads and strips (gauze-type).

Parke-Davis
Park Plaza, P.O. Box 1506
Greenwood, South Carolina 29646

Perioperative antibiotics. Antibiotics administered prior to operation so that adequate blood and tissue concentrations will be achieved to combat intraoperative bacterial contamination. Additional doses are given during or after operation to maintain therapeutic levels for a period of 24 h (see Chap. 2).

Pleur-evac. Disposable sterile plastic device that provides constant negative pressure to catheter inserted into thoracic cavity following thoracotomy.

Krale Division of Deknatel
110 Jericho Turnpike
Floral Park, New York 11001

Retractor, "chain." This device utilizes a sterile chain attached to a lithotomy stirrup to elevate and retract either the left or right costal margin or the sternum (see Fig. D–23).

Retractor, Upper Hand. This retractor is attached to the operating table by a steel bridge. It elevates and draws the sternum or costal margin in a cephalad direction (see Fig. D–22).

Hepco Inc.
Box 5200
Kansas City, Missouri 64112

Silastic. A silicone material useful for drainage tubes because it has low tissue reactivity.

Dow Corning
P.O. Box 1M
Midland, Michigan 48640

Stomahesive peristomal covering. A thin wafer that lies between the peristomal skin and the face-plate of an ileostomy or colostomy applicance and is designed to protect the peristomal skin from digestive juices.

E. R. Squibb
P.O. Box 2013
New Brunswick, New Jersey 08903

Staplers. See Chap. 4 and Figs. D–26 through D–33.

Auto Suture
U. S. Surgical Corporation
2051 W. Main Street
Stamford, Connecticut 06902

A skin stapling device, Proximate, is also manufactured by Ethicon.

Stiches

Lembert	(see Fig. B–17)
Cushing	(see Fig. B–18)
Halsted	(see Fig. B–19)
Seromucosal	(see Fig. B–16)
Smead-Jones	(see Fig. B–13)
Connell	(see Fig. B–21)

Successive bisection. A term used to describe a sequence of inserting anastomotic sutures that will compensate for a minor disparity in the diameters of the two segments of intestine (see Figs. B–22 and B–23).

Surgicel (absorbable hemostat). A "cloth" composed of oxidized regenerated cellulose used adjunctively to assist in control of capillary and venous bleeding; absorbable if used in one or two thicknesses over flat surfaces.

Surgikos (Johnson & Johnson)
2500 Arbrook Boulevard
Arlington, Massachusetts 76010

Suture material

Dermalon—monofilament nylon (Davis and Geck, American Cyanamid, 1 Casper Street, Danbury, Connecticut)
Ethibond—braided Dacron polyester with butilated coating (Ethicon, P.O. Box 151, Somerville, New Jersey 08876
Ethilon—monofilament nylon (Ethicon)
Mersilene—braided Dacron polyester (Ethicon)
Nurolon—braided nylon (Ethicon)
PG—polyglycolic acid, Dexon (Davis and Geck)
—polyglactin, Vicryl (Ethicon)
Prolene—monofilament polypropylene (Ethicon)
Surgilene—monofilament polypropylene (Davis and Geck)
Surgilon—braided nylon coated with silicone (Davis and Geck)
Tevdek—braided Dacron polyester coated with Teflon polytetrafluoroethylene (Deknatel, 110 Jericho Turnpike, Floral Park, New York 11001)
Ticron—braided Dacron polyester coated with silicon (Davis and Geck)

Umbilical tape. Narrow woven cotton tape that comes in widths of from 3 to 10 mm. Useful in ligating the umbilical cord of the newborn infant and in occluding the lumen of the small or large intestine.

Vesseloop. A narrow ribbon (0.9 × 1.5 mm cross section) of siliconized rubber useful in tagging structures like the ureter for later identification in pelvic surgery.

Medgeneral
10800 Lyndale Avenue South
Minneapolis, Minnesota 55420

Water Pik. A device that produces a pulsating jet of water for cleansing.

Teledyne Water Pik
1730 East Prospect Street
Fort Collins, Colorado 80525

Wound protector, Vi-Drape. A sterile plastic drape designed to protect the subcutaneous fat from contamination by intestinal content during abdominal surgery (see Figs. 2–1 and 2–2).

Med/Surg, Parke-Davis
Park Plaza, P.O. Box 1506
Greenwood, South Carolina 29646

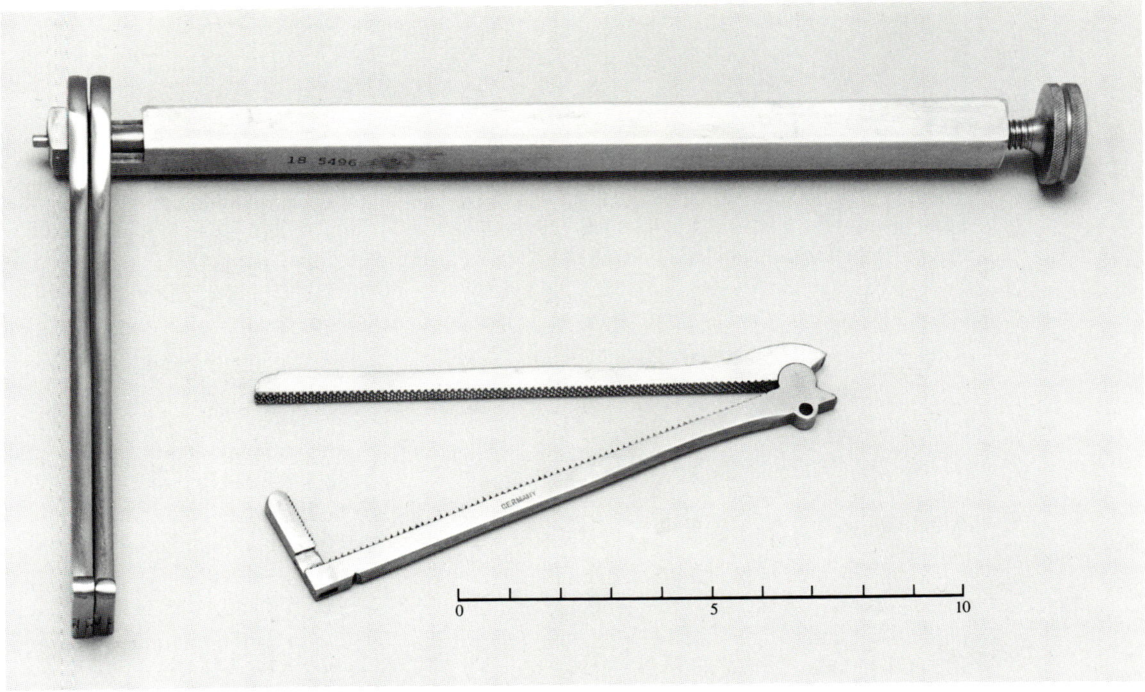

Fig. D–1 Clamp—DeMartel.

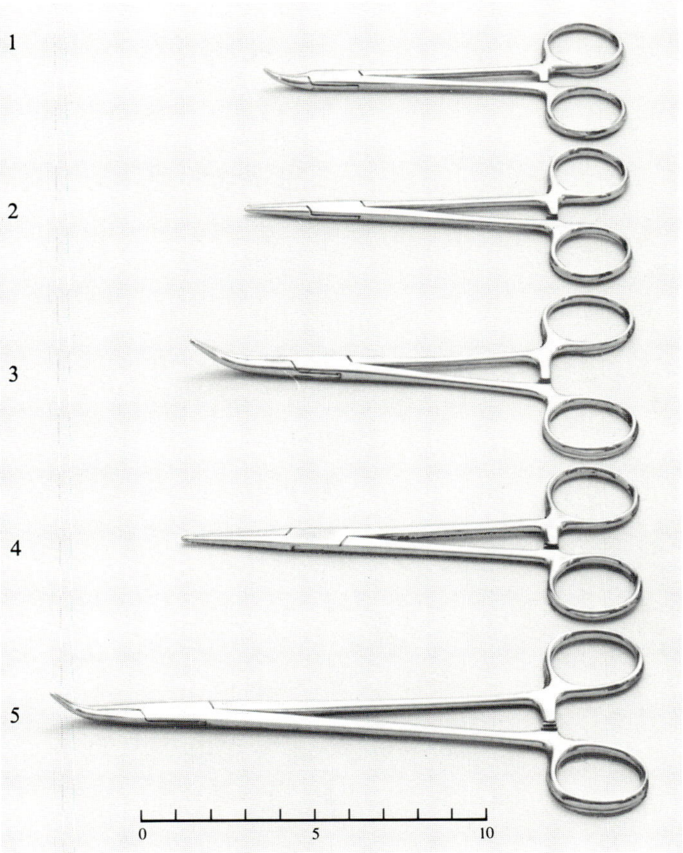

Fig. D–2 Clamps, hemostatic—Halsted (1 and 2), Crile (3 and 4), and Adson (Tonsil) (5).

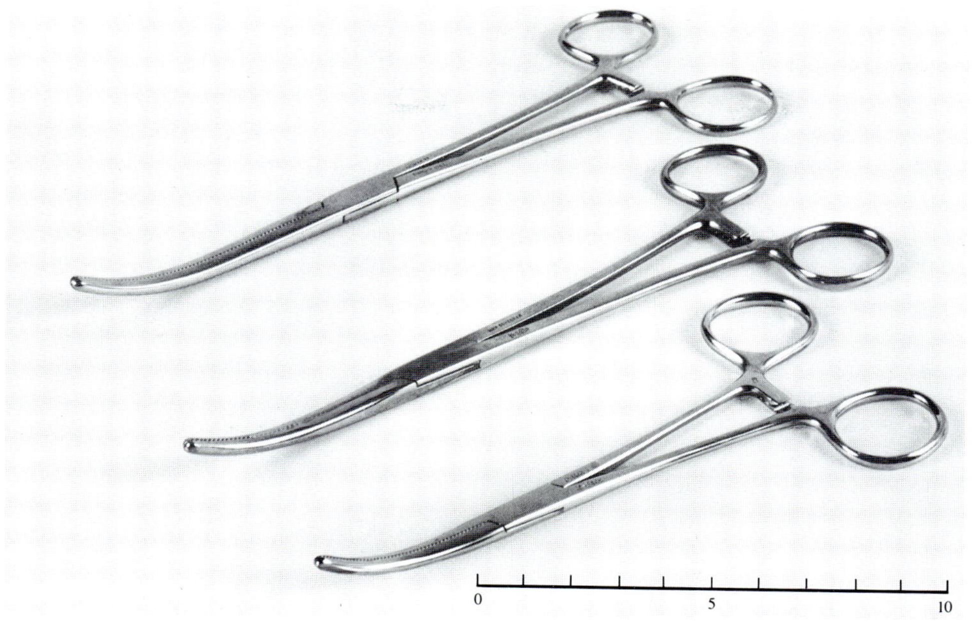

Fig. D–3 Clamps, hemostatic—Kelly.

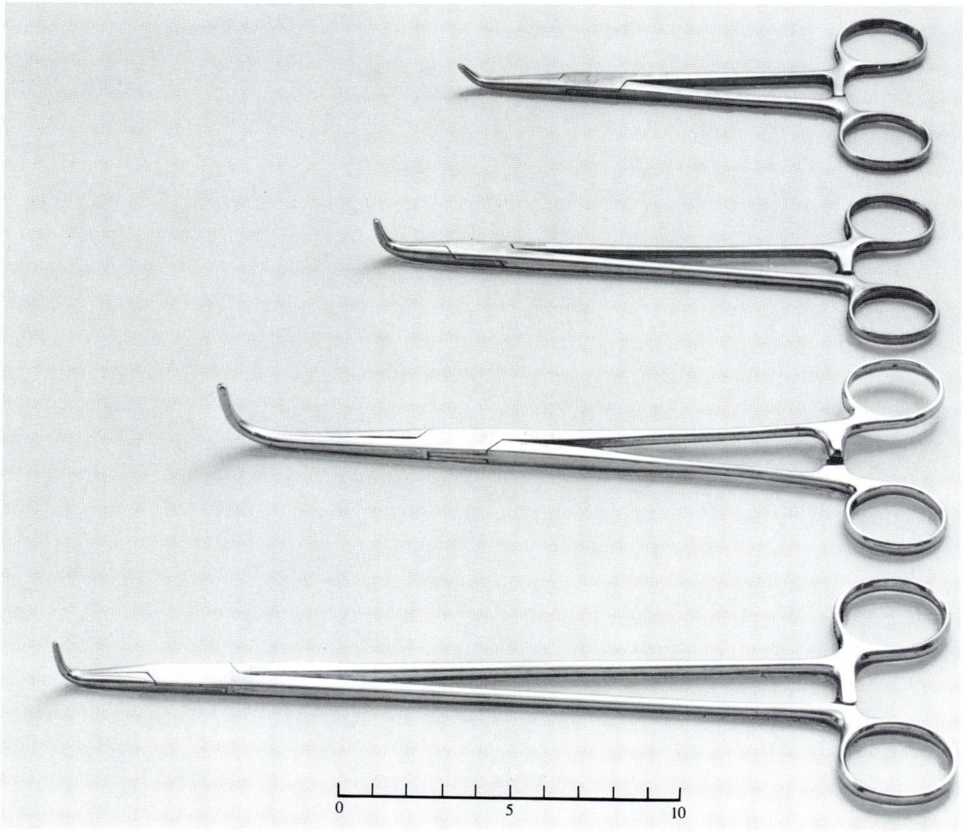

Fig. D–4 Clamps, hemostatic—Mixter Right Angle.

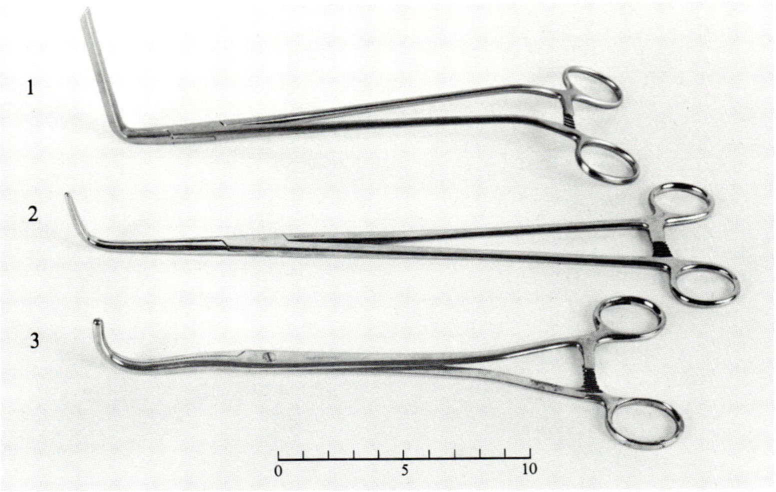

Fig. D–5 Clamps—Kidney Right Angle (1), Bronchus (2), and Moynihan (3).

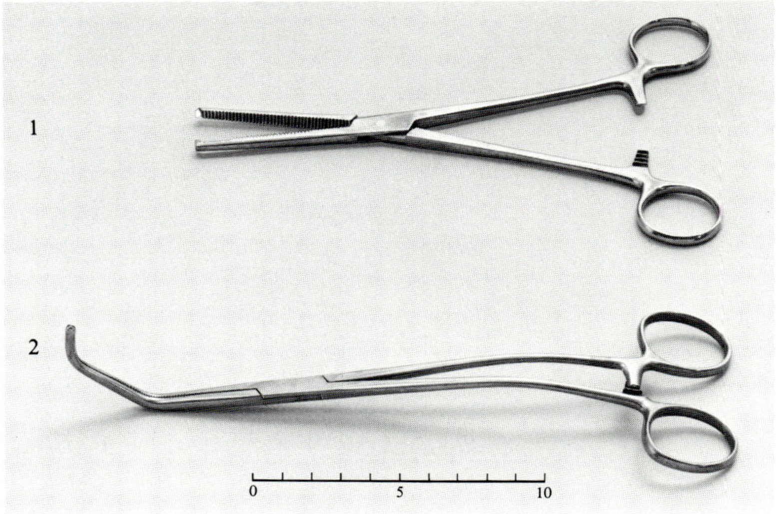

Fig. D–6 Clamps—Kocher (1) and Satinsky (2).

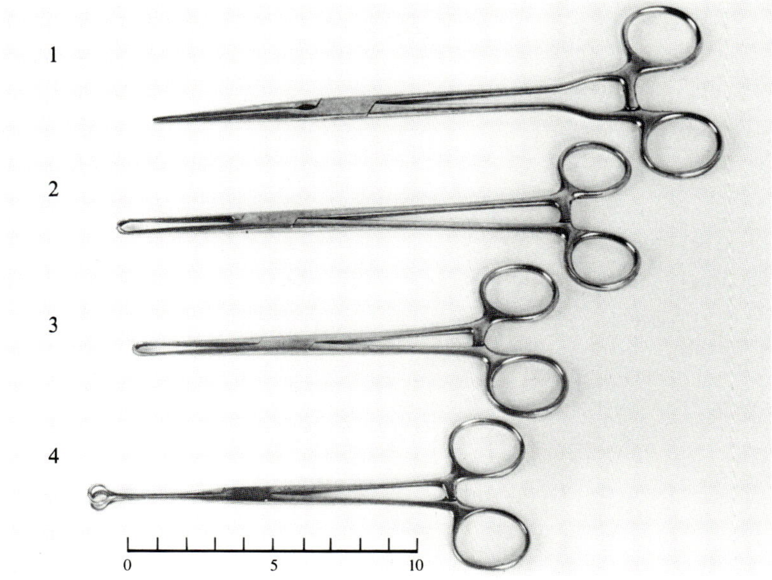

Fig. D–7 Clamps—Allen (1), Allis (2 and 3), and Babcock (4).

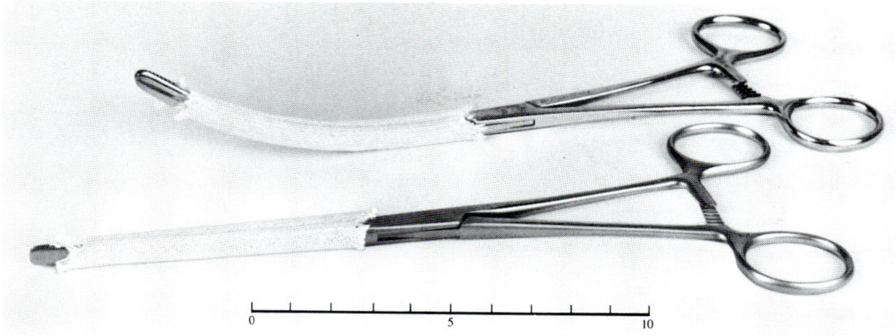

Fig. D–8 Clamps—Doyen Non-Crushing Intestinal, linen-shod.

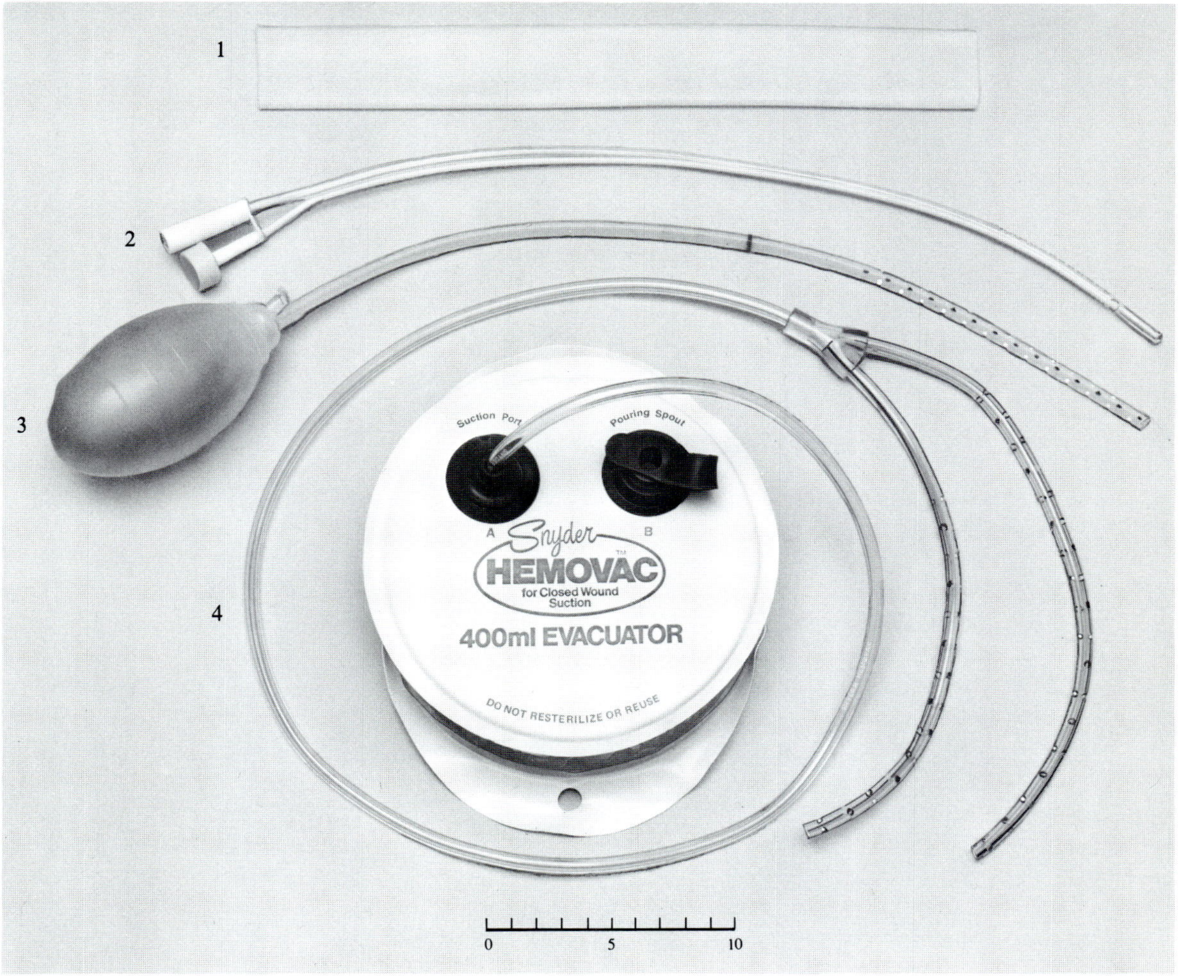

Fig. D–9 Drains—Latex (1), sump, Shirley (2), closed-suction, Jackson-Pratt (3), and Hemovac (4).

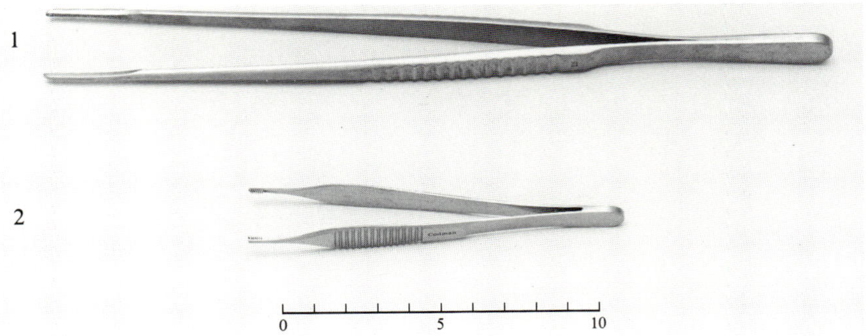

Fig. D–10 Forceps—Debakey (1) and Brown-Adson (2).

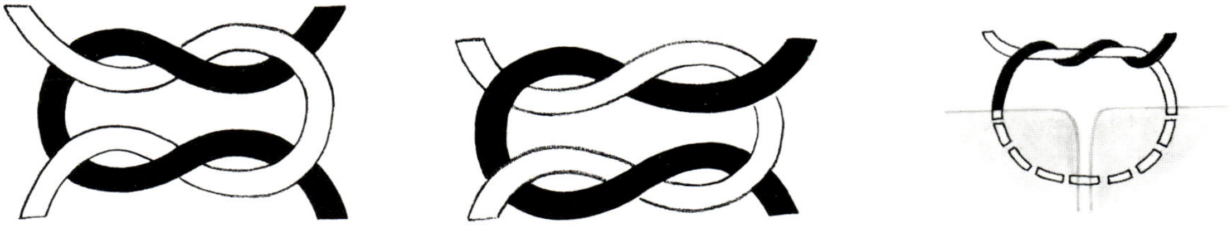

Fig. D–11 Knots—square (1), Grannee (2), and surgeon's (3).

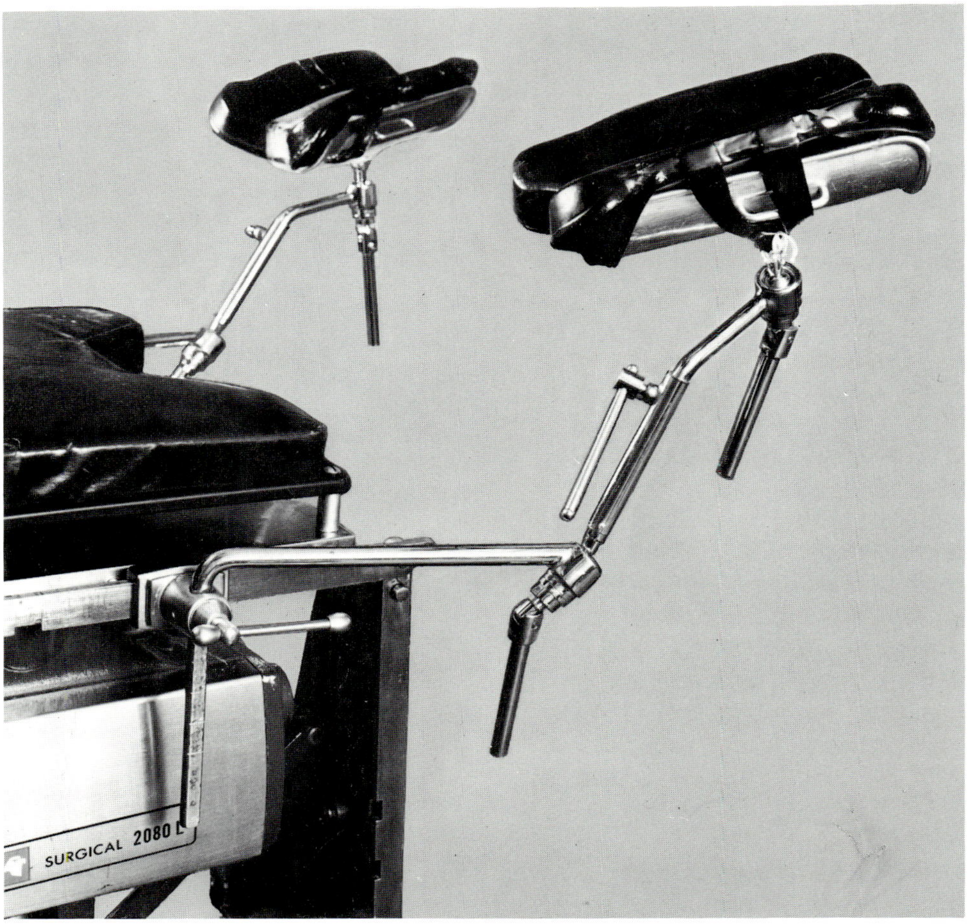

Fig. D–12 Lloyd-Davies leg rests.

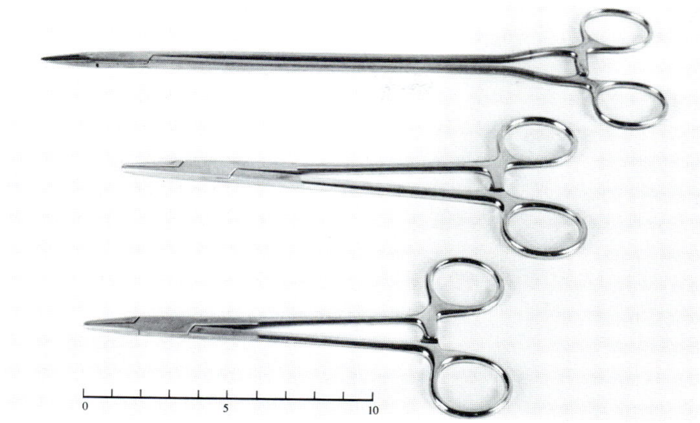

Fig. D–13 Needle-holders, straight.

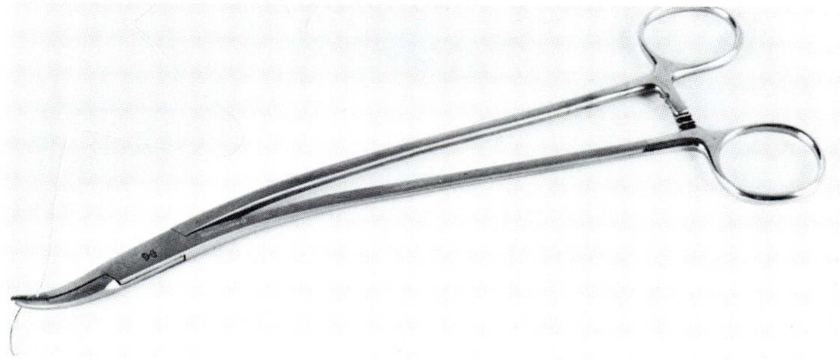

Fig. D–14 Needle-holder, Stratte.

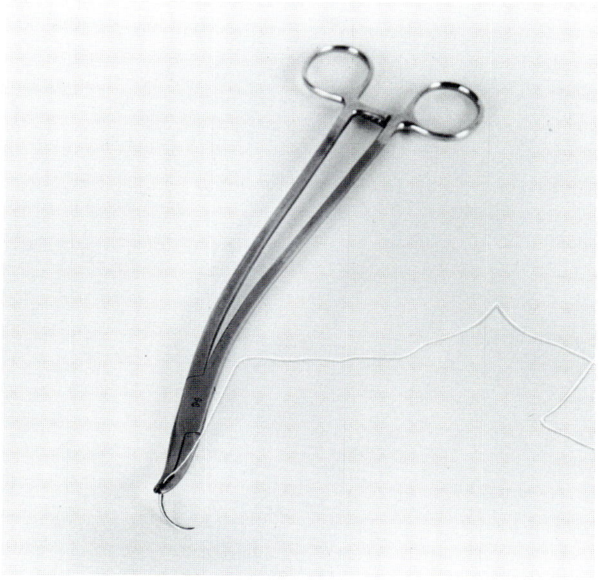

Fig. D–15 Needle-holder, Stratte, grasping an atraumatic suture.

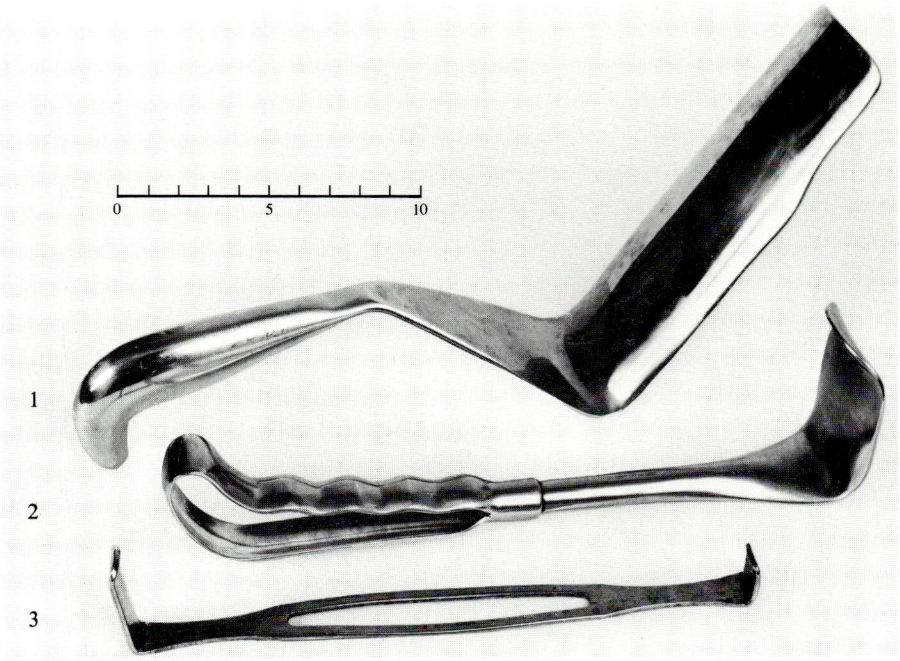

Fig. D–16 Retractors—Lloyd-Davies (1), Richardson (2), and Army-Navy (3).

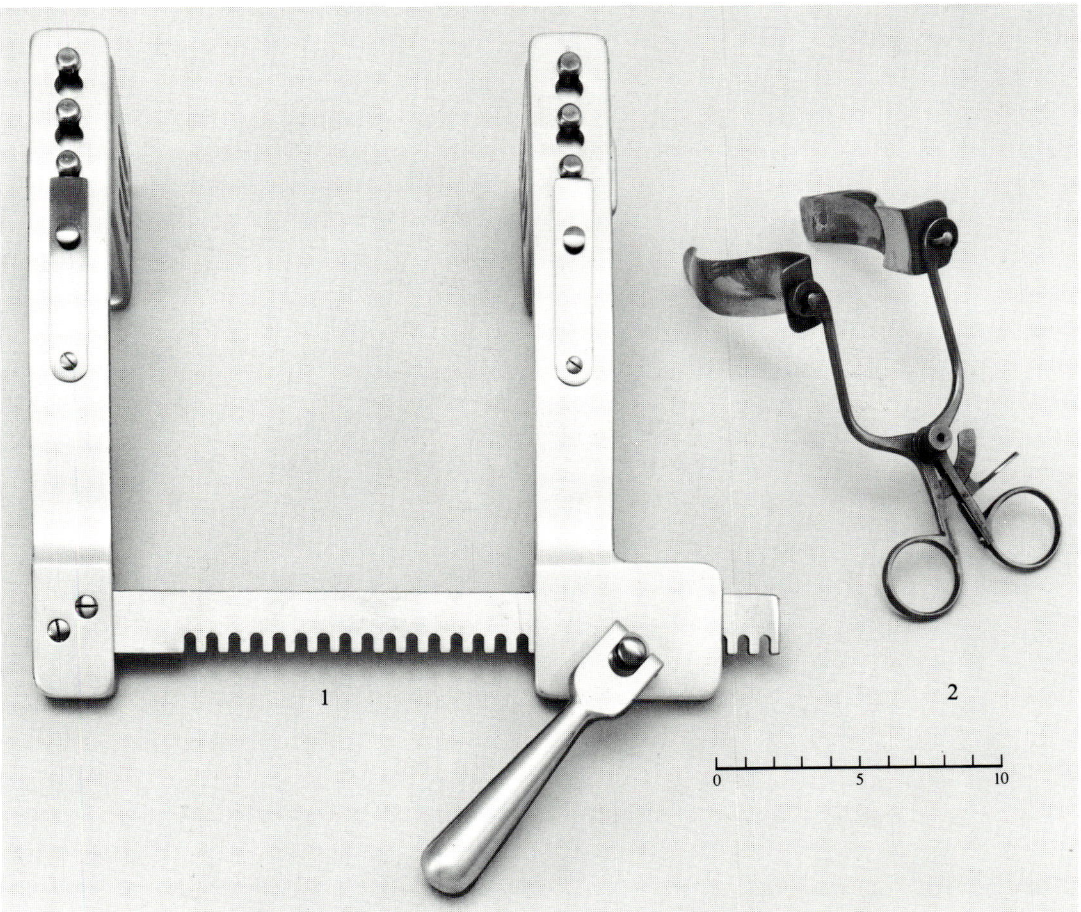

Fig. D–17 Retractors—Finochietto thoracic (1) and Parks rectal (2).

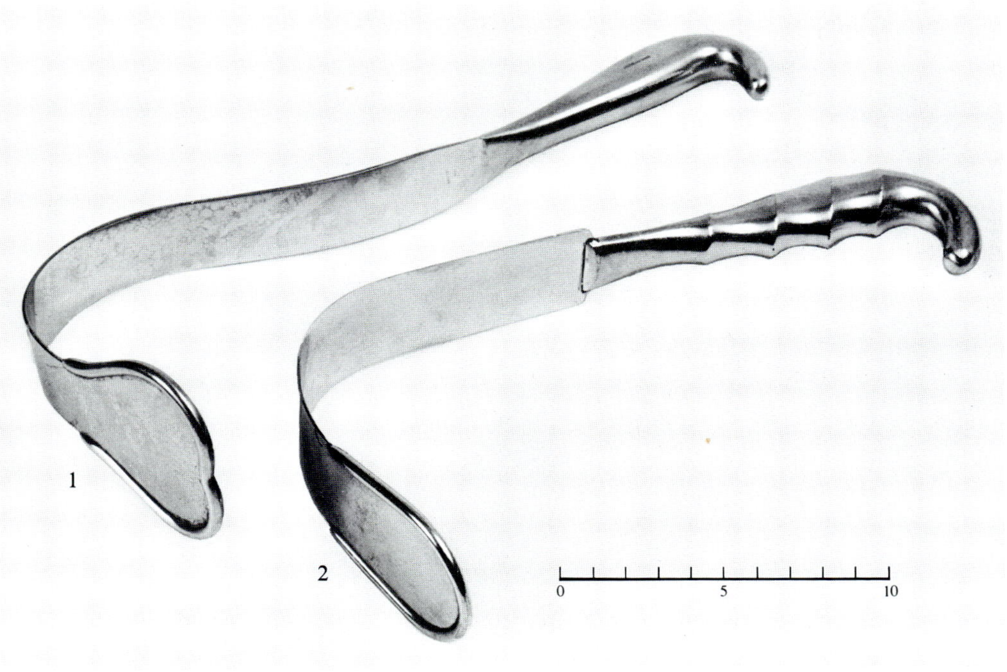

Fig. D–18 Retractors—Harrington (1) and Foss (2).

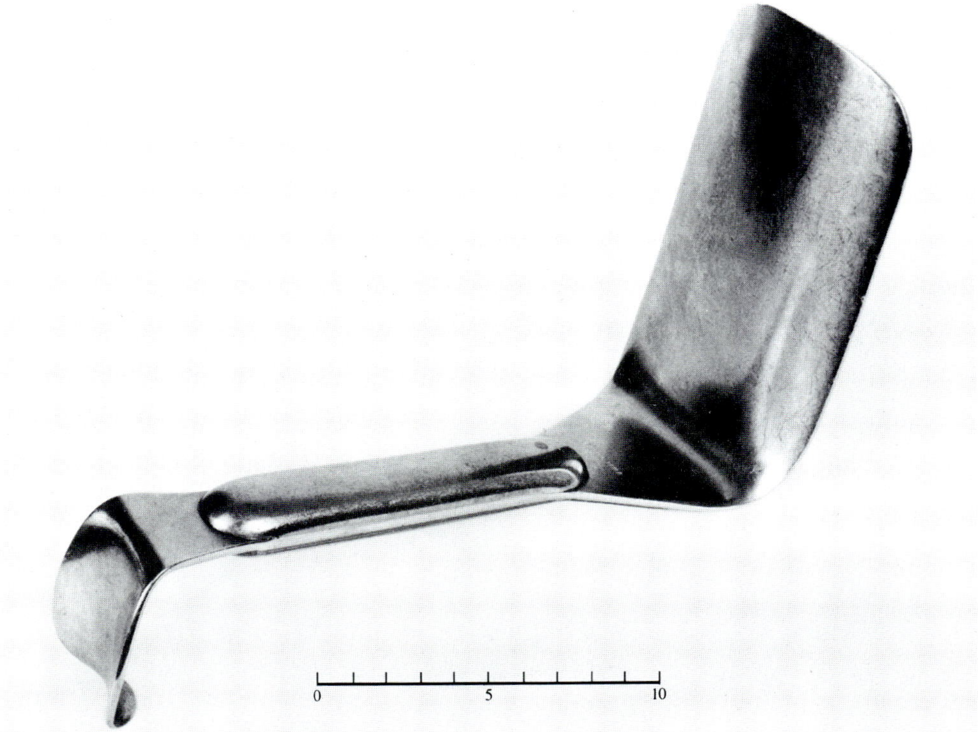

Fig. D–19 Retractor—Weinberg.

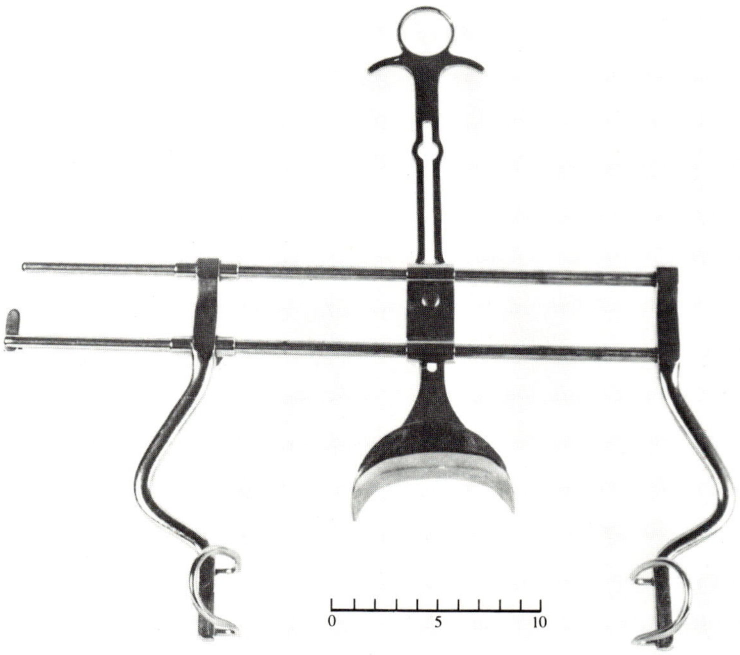

Fig. D–20 Retractor, self-retaining—Balfour.

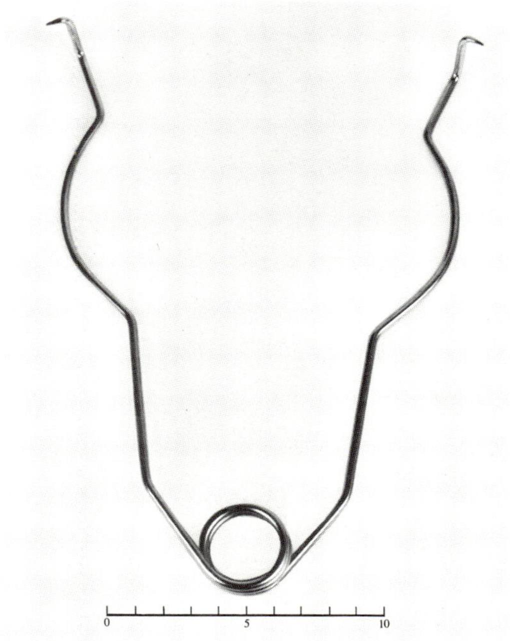

Fig. D–21 Retractor, self-retaining—Farr.

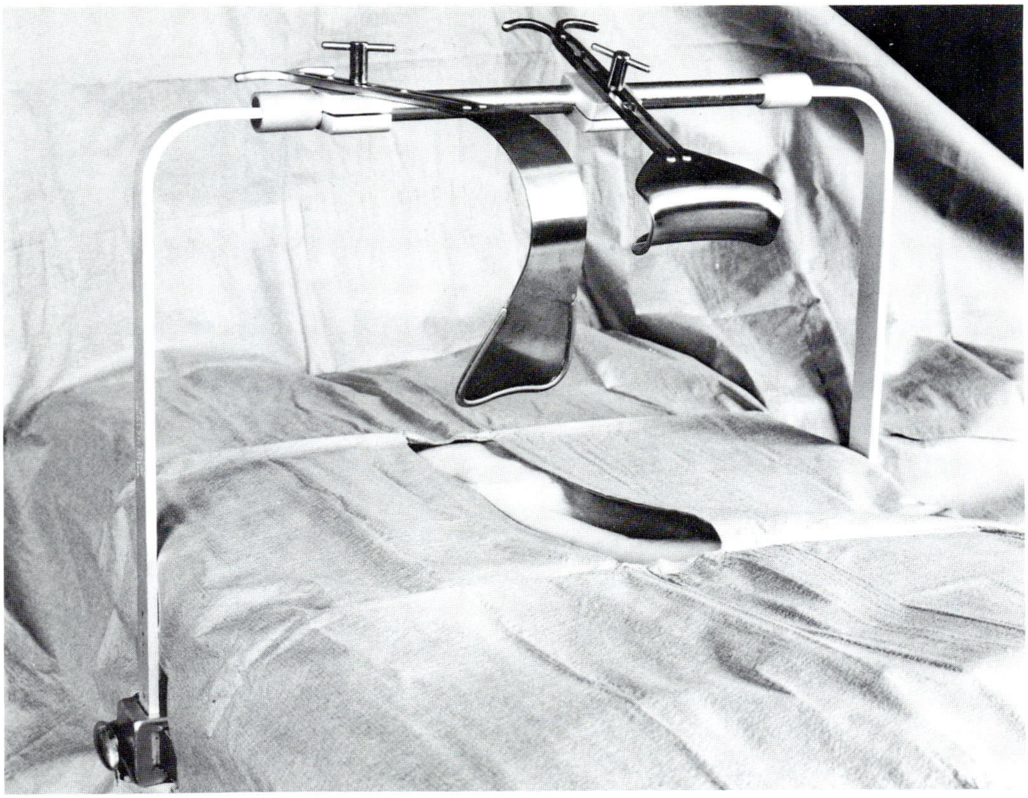

Fig. D–22 Retractor—Upper Hand.

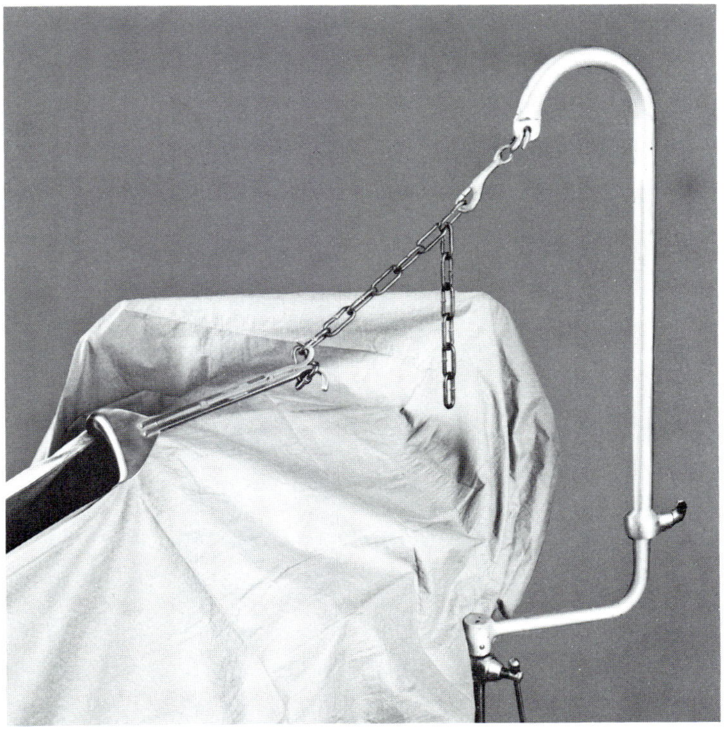

Fig. D–23 Retractor—"chain."

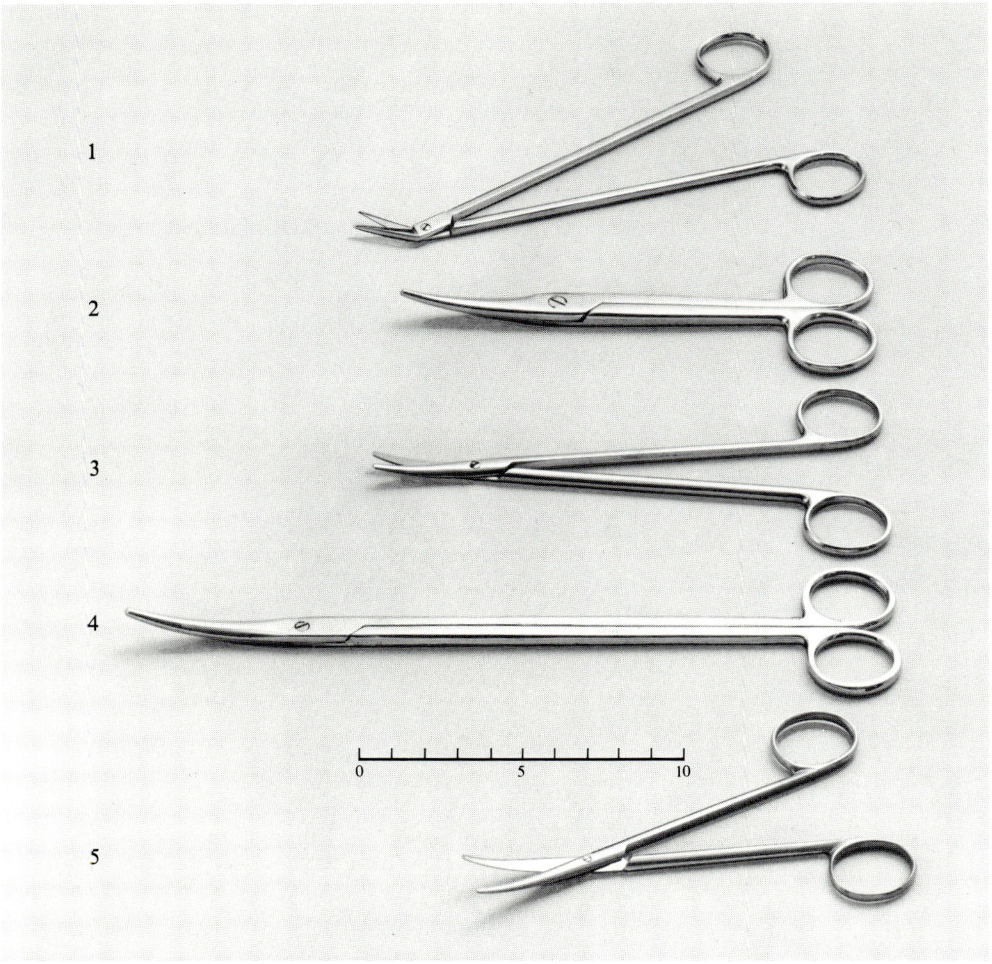

Fig. D–24 Scissors—Potts (1), Mayo (2), and Metzenbaum (3, 4, and 5).

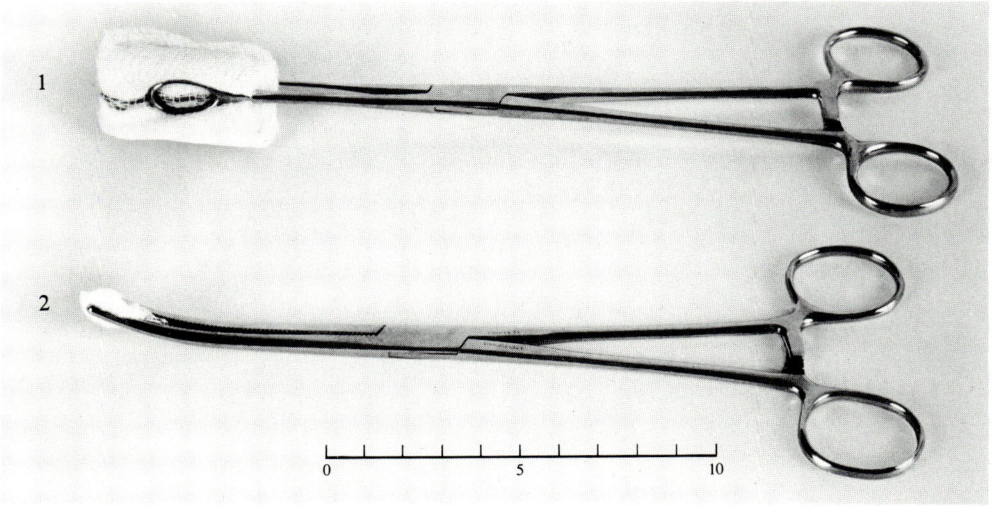

Fig. D–25 Sponge-holder with 10 × 10 cm gauze square (1); peanut-sponge (Kuttner) dissector (2).

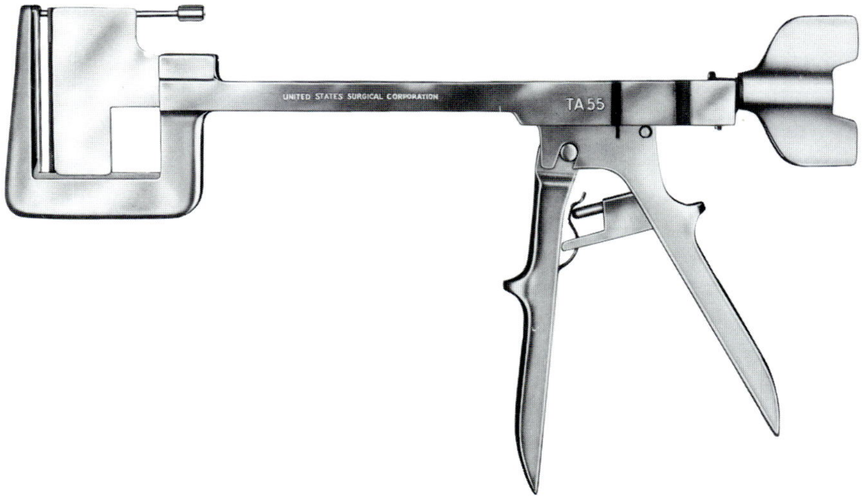

Fig. D–26 Stapler, Auto Suture, TA-55.

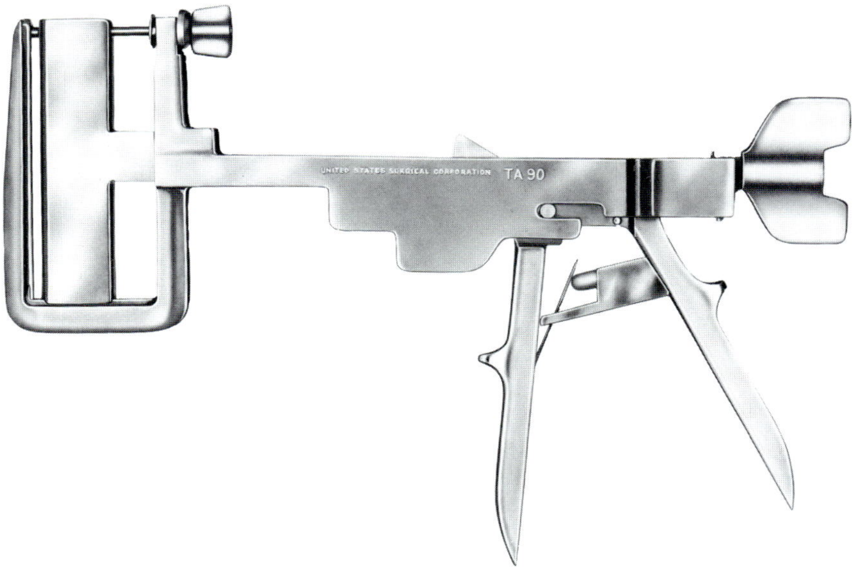

Fig. D–27 Stapler, Auto Suture, TA-90.

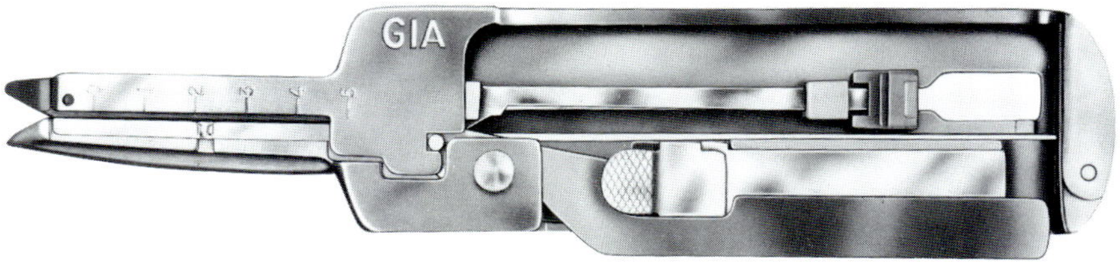

Fig. D–28 Stapler, Auto Suture, GIA.

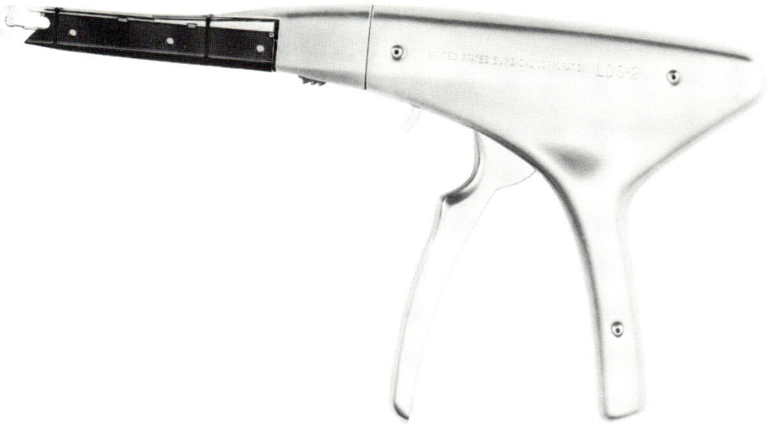

Fig. D–29 Stapler, Auto Suture, LDS.

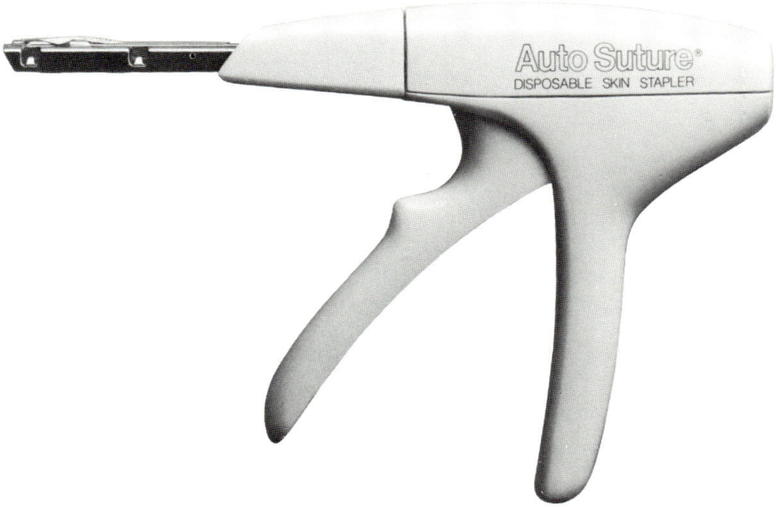

Fig. D–30 Stapler, Auto Suture, skin stapler.

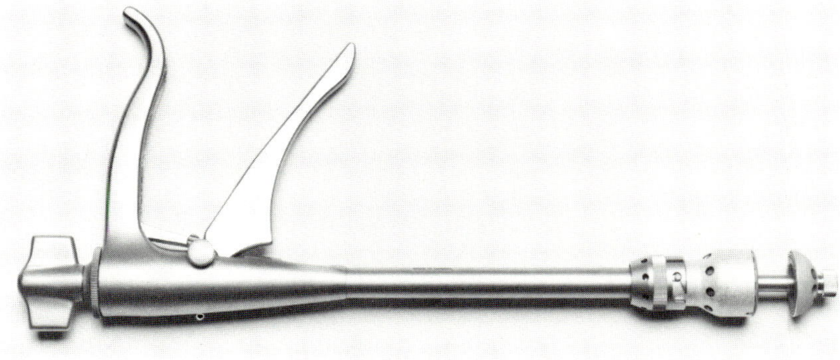

Fig. D–31 Stapler, Auto Suture, EEA.

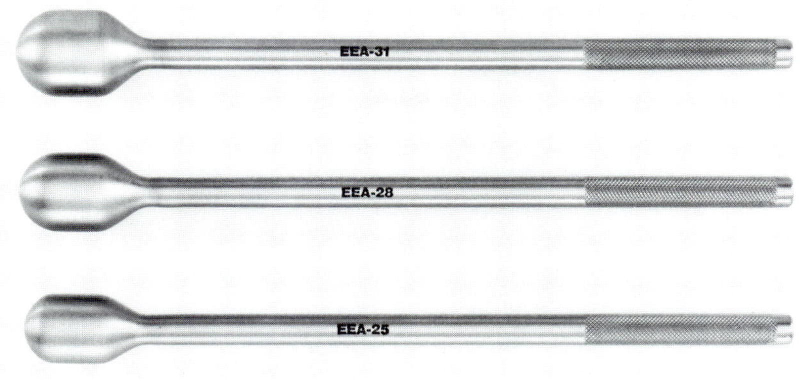

Fig. D–32 Stapler, Auto Suture, EEA sizers.

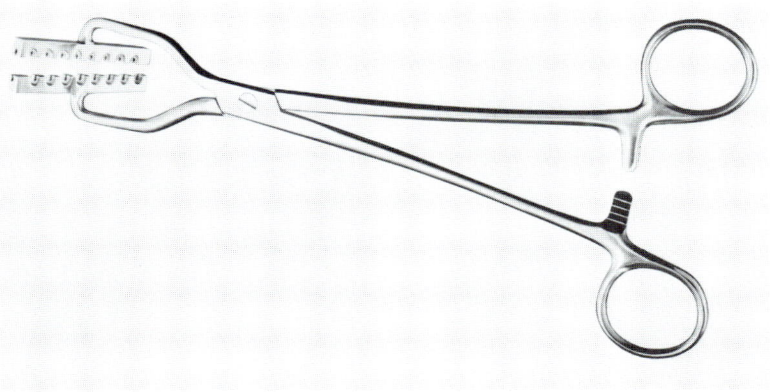

Fig. D–33 Stapler, Auto Suture, purse-string instrument.

Index

D

E

F

G

J

T